10·19·77

The National Directory
for the Performing Arts / Educational

Third Edition

The National Directory for the Performing Arts / Educational

Third Edition

BEATRICE HANDEL, *Editor*

Handel & Sons, Inc.

Janet W. Spencer, *Associate Editor*

Senior Editors

Bette Griffin

H. Michael Stewart

Editorial Assistants

Florence Aptaker
Cynthia R. English
Betty P. Kalmbach
Lorraine M. Noble

A Wiley-Interscience Publication

JOHN WILEY & SONS, New York · Chichester · Brisbane · Toronto

The first edition of this work appeared as part of the
*National Directory for the Performing Arts and Civic
Centers.*

ISBN 0-471-03304-9

Printed in the United States of America

The Honorary Advisory Board for the NATIONAL DIRECTORY FOR THE PER-FORMING ARTS/EDUCATIONAL has been selected for its great contribution to education in the performing arts.

PREFACE

The third edition of this directory provides basic information on all major schools and institutions that offer training in the performing arts.

Entries, arranged alphabetically by state and then by school, give the address, telephone number, and type of support (private, state, etc.). Other information includes areas in which training is offered, performing series sponsored by the institution, performance facilities, number of students, degrees and courses offered, workshops, and financial assistance. New data in this edition identify the names of artists in residence, complete indexing by category, and an alphabetical index, which facilitates use of the directory.

The editors wish to express their appreciation for the prompt and thoughtful response to their questionnaires and will be grateful for notification of any omissions, corrections, or suggestions for additional information.

BEATRICE HANDEL

GUIDE TO USING THE NATIONAL DIRECTORY FOR THE PERFORMING ARTS/EDUCATIONAL

As you use this directory you will find considerable diversity in content on each listing. Just as each artist is an individual, so are the areas of education; for example, you will find all the categories—DANCE, MUSIC, and THEATER—in some of the school listings, but only one or two are listed in other schools. In some instances a wealth of information is given about each arts area of involvement; in others considerably less.

The information about each category varies in relation to the amount of educational activity in that specific arts area. Some schools have listed an activity only if they offer a major and a degree in that subject. Others have included classes for which they have no major or even a department, such as dance classes offered by the physical education department or drama and speech classes in the English department.

As you will notice, there has been notation made for each school in regard to the training offered in visual art, television, and film arts. However, we have not included detailed information about these areas in this edition of *The National Directory for the Performing Arts/Educational.*

The sponsorship or principal support of the school is shown as private, state, county (district), or city. The school's classification as a two-year (junior or community college), four-year (schools with full degree plans, including five-year graduate courses and those offering only junior and senior years to complete a degree), or special (defined by the content of the listing) is given, as is the dean of the division or school supervising the arts activities, when available.

THE DIRECTORY INDICATES

Arts Areas — Dance, instrumental music, vocal music, theater, film arts, television, visual art, and others available at the school are enumerated.

Performing Series — Concerts, lectures, opera, touring plays, poetry readings, and the like, which are sponsored by the school and/or by a faculty or student association, are cited.

Facilities — The name of auditorium, hall, theater, or performance complex is mentioned. Additional information about many of the facilities is available in the companion volume, *The National Directory for the Performing Arts and Civic Centers,* 3rd edition.

Categories — (Dance, Music, Theater) — The schools vary on nomenclature, such as theater or drama. The directory has grouped together under theater such activities as drama and mime. Dance includes creative movement and martial arts.

Faculty — The number given, although frequently approximate, usually includes all those on staff, both full and part time. The chairman or department head is given if possible. In some cases no information was available.

Students — These numbers are also often approximate. Some schools list only major, minor, and graduate students; others include the total number of students serviced by the department, and in a few instances no information was available.

Degrees Offered — Concentrations are included when possible.

Abbreviations used:

A.A.	Associate of Arts	D.M.A.	Doctor of Music
A.S.	Associate of Science	M.A.	Master of Arts
B.A.	Bachelor of Arts	M.F.A.	Master of Fine Arts
B.F.A.	Bachelor of Fine Arts	M.Mus.	Master of Music
B.Mus.	Bachelor of Music	M.Mus.Ed.	Master of Music Education
B.Mus.Ed.	Bachelor of Music Education	M.S.	Master of Science
B.S.	Bachelor of Science	Ph.D.	Doctor of Philosophy

Courses Offered — The range of studies offered is shown.

Special Technical Training — Emphasis areas such as choreography, conducting, electronic music, opera, and acting, are given.

Teaching Certification — If the school's education department for the state in which the school is located offers such courses, it is mentioned.

Financial Assistance — In most instances this refers to general aid by the school, not just the department.

Performing Groups — The listings include the types of performing groups within the departments. It should be noted that participation in these activities is usually not restricted to declared majors or minors.

Workshops/Festivals — Events sponsored or cosponsored by the department or division, including workshops for high school students, educators, and professional artists, are grouped here. Frequently the public is invited to attend the workshops and festivals mentioned.

There are many special schools in the directory that do not contain exactly the same types of information. In these instances the objective has been to give the information segments relative to the activities of that specific school.

Indexes — There are two indexes to assist in the use of the information. The first index is categorical; it gives the school and page number for its full listing for each of the arts areas in which that school offers training. This index is followed by the alphabetical listing of all the schools in the directory.

CONTENTS

UNIVERSITY OF ALABAMA, BIRMINGHAM
University Station, Birmingham   Alabama 35294
205 934-3236

State and 4 Year
Arts Areas: Dance, Instrumental Music, Vocal Music, Theatre, Film Arts, Television and Visual Arts
Performing Series: Commedia; Town & Gown Theater; Ballet UAB; Jazz Ensemble; Chorus
Performance Facilities: Clarks Memorial Theater; Bell Auditorium; Birmingham - Jefferson Civic Center

DANCE

Stevan Grebel, Director, Ballet UAB   *Number Of Faculty:* 3
Number Of Students: 150
Degrees Offered: BA in Dance (through individually designed major program)
Courses Offered: Dance; Modern Dance; Ballet; Jazz Dance; Dance History; Folk Dance; Dance Teaching; Choreography; Theory; Production
Financial Assistance: Scholarships, Work-Study Grants and UAB Financial Aid Programs
Performing Groups: Ballet UAB   *Workshops/Festivals:* Summer Dance Workshop

MUSIC

Dr Sherrill Martin, Head   *Number Of Faculty:* 3
Courses Offered: Fundamentals; Appreciation; Class Voice; Theory; History
Financial Assistance: UAB Financial Aid Programs
Performing Groups: Chorus; Jazz Ensemble

THEATRE

Dr Ward Haarbauer, Chairman, Performing Arts   *Number Of Faculty:* 4
Number Of Students: 30   *Degrees Offered:* BA
Courses Offered: Theater; Acting; Stage Lighting; Costuming; Stage Makeup

DANIEL PAYNE COLLEGE
6415 Washington Blvd, Birmingham   Alabama 35212
205 592-7791

Private and 4 Year   *Arts Areas:* Instrumental Music and Vocal Music

MUSIC

Earlie Bilups, Director   *Degrees Offered:* BMusEd   *Technical Training:* AA
Financial Assistance: Scholarships and Work-Study Grants

GADSDEN STATE JUNIOR COLLEGE
George Wallace Dr, Gadsden   Alabama 35901
205 546-0484 Ext 247

State and 2 Year
Arts Areas: Dance, Instrumental Music, Vocal Music, Theatre, Television and Visual Arts
Performing Series: Performing Artists Series
Performance Facilities: Gadsden State Jr College Theatre

DANCE

Sherry Keeling, Chairman   *Number Of Faculty:* 1   *Number Of Students:* 24
Courses Offered: Ballet; Jazz; Tap   *Financial Assistance:* Work-Study Grants
Performing Groups: Concert Band; Stage Band; Concert Choir; Organ; Piano; Woodwind Ensemble; Brass Ensemble

MUSIC

Edsel Hand, Chairman   *Number Of Faculty:* 4   *Number Of Students:* 74
Financial Assistance: Scholarships and Work-Study Grants

(continued on next page)

Performing Groups: Concert Band, Concert Choir; Organ & Piano; Soloists
Workshops/Festivals: Dist 4 Band Festival; Dist 4 Choir Festival; AMTA Piano Workshop; Brass, Woodwind & Percussion Workshops; Choral Directors Workshop

THEATRE

Mitch DuPont, Chairman   *Number Of Faculty:* 1   *Number Of Students:* 32
Performing Groups: Drama Guys & Gals

JEFFERSON STATE JUNIOR COLLEGE
2601 Carson Rd, Birmingham   Alabama 35215
205 853-1200 Ext 202
State and 2 Year
Arts Areas: Instrumental Music, Vocal Music, Theatre, Television and Visual Arts

MUSIC

Coy E Huggins, Chairman   *Number Of Students:* 600   *Degrees Offered:* AA
Financial Assistance: Assistantships, Scholarships and Work-Study Grants
Performing Groups: Choir; Band

JUDSON COLLEGE
Marion   Alabama 36756, 205 683-2011 Ext 44
Private and 4 Year
Arts Areas: Dance, Instrumental Music, Vocal Music, Theatre and Visual Arts
Performing Series: Concert - Lecture Series
Performance Facilities: Alumnae Auditorium

DANCE

Mrs Beverly Fitts, Chairman   *Number Of Faculty:* 1   *Number Of Students:* 30
Courses Offered: Folk Rhythm; Advanced Rhythms
Financial Assistance: Scholarships and Work-Study Grants
Performing Groups: Terpsichorea
Workshops/Festivals: Annual Recital; J Day Pageant

MUSIC

Dr L Bracey Campbell, Chairman   *Number Of Faculty:* 5
Number Of Students: 90   *Degrees Offered:* BA; BS, Music Education Major
Courses Offered: Organ; Piano; Voice; Music Education
Teaching Certification Available
Financial Assistance: Scholarships and Work-Study Grants
Performing Groups: Judson Ensemble; Judson Singers; Judson - Marion Institute Band
Workshops/Festivals: Christmas Vespers; Faculty & Student Recitals

THEATRE

Miss Linda Hamil, Instructor in Dramatic Art & Speech   *Number Of Faculty:* 1
Number Of Students: 42
Degrees Offered: BA or BS with major in Dramatic Art & Speech
Courses Offered: Speech; Play Production; Color & Design; Oral Interpretation; Stagecraft; Acting; Shakespeare; Modern Drama; Directing; History of Theatre; History of Costume; Special Studies in Drama & Speech; Independent Study
Teaching Certification Available
Performing Groups: Judson Players; Judson Theatre
Workshops/Festivals: Two productions a year; J Day Pageant

LURLEEN B WALLACE STATE JUNIOR COLLEGE
PO Box 1418, Andalusia   Alabama 36420
205 222-6591 Ext 240
State and 2 Year
Arts Areas: Instrumental Music, Vocal Music, Theatre and Visual Arts

(continued on next page)

Performing Series: Cultural Series
Performance Facilities: Jeff Bishop Student Center/LBW Gym

MUSIC

Jerry Padgett, Chairman, Fine Arts Division **Number Of Faculty:** 2
Number Of Students: 35 **Degrees Offered:** AA
Courses Offered: Music Appreciation; Chorus; Music Theory; Community Chorus; Applied Piano; Collegiate Chorale; Applied Voice; Stage Band (Performing Ensemble); Applied Woodwinds; Music Theatre Lab; Applied Brass
Financial Assistance: Scholarships and Work-Study Grants
Performing Groups: LBW Chorus

THEATRE

Sara McAnaulty, Chairman, Language Arts Division

OAKWOOD COLLEGE
Rural Station Alabama 35806, 205 837-1630
Private and 4 Year **Arts Areas:** Instrumental Music and Vocal Music
Degrees Offered: BMus; BMusEd; Vocal Applied
Teaching Certification Available **Financial Assistance:** Scholarships
Performing Groups: Vocal & Instrumental Ensembles

SAMFORD UNIVERSITY
800 Lakeshore, Birmingham Alabama 35209
205 870-2771
Private and 4 Year
Arts Areas: Instrumental Music, Vocal Music, Theatre, Television and Visual Arts
Performing Series: Student Government Concert & Lecture Series

MUSIC

Claude H Rheat, Dean **Number Of Students:** 18
Degrees Offered: BMus, Organ, Voice, Instrumental, Church Music; MMusEd; MA
Teaching Certification Available
Financial Assistance: Scholarships and Work-Study Grants
Performing Groups: A Cappella Choir; University Chorale; Marching Band; Orchestra; Chamber Music
Workshops/Festivals: Opera Workshop

THEATRE

Billy L Harris, Department Head **Number Of Faculty:** 4
Degrees Offered: BA; MA **Teaching Certification Available**
Performing Groups: Samford Masquers

SNEAD STATE JUNIOR COLLEGE
Walnut St, Boaz Alabama 35957
205 593-6521
State and 2 Year
Arts Areas: Dance, Instrumental Music, Vocal Music and Theatre
Performance Facilities: Fielder Auditorium

DANCE

Elaine Brown, Chairman **Number Of Faculty:** 1 **Number Of Students:** 20
Degrees Offered: AA **Performing Groups:** Dance Group
Workshops/Festivals: Ballet Workshop

MUSIC

Glen Mayes, Chairman **Number Of Faculty:** 4 **Degrees Offered:** AA
Financial Assistance: Scholarships
Performing Groups: Choir; Ensemble; Concert Band

(continued on next page)

THEATRE

Nancy Jo Hardy, Chairman **Number Of Faculty:** 1 **Degrees Offered:** AA
Performing Groups: Masquers Drama Club

UNIVERSITY OF SOUTH ALABAMA
307 University Blvd, Mobile Alabama 36688
205 460-6211
  State and 4 Year
  Arts Areas: Dance, Instrumental Music, Vocal Music, Theatre, Film Arts, Television and Visual Arts
  Performance Facilities: The Bethel; The University Theatre for Performing Arts
  Number Of Faculty: 1 **Number Of Students:** 40 **Degrees Offered:** BFA
  Courses Offered: Introductory; Intermediate and Advanced
  Financial Assistance: Scholarships, Work-Study Grants and BEOG
  Performing Groups: Dance Ensemble

MUSIC

Dr Robert F Wermuch, Chairman **Number Of Faculty:** 10
Number Of Students: 100 **Degrees Offered:** BA; BM; BSE
Courses Offered: Applied Music; Woodwinds; Brass; Percussion; Keyboard; Voice; Strings; Literature;
Theory; Education; History
Teaching Certification Available
Financial Assistance: Scholarships, Work-Study Grants and Music Grants
Performing Groups: University Chorale; University Opera Theatre; University Symphonic Band; University
Stage Band; Concert Choir; Summer Chorus & Ensembles; Woodwind; Percussion; String; Piano, Guitar;
Flute; Ancient Instruments
Workshops/Festivals: Piano Workshop

THEATRE

Dr Victor R Cook, Chairman **Number Of Faculty:** 4 **Number Of Students:** 30
Degrees Offered: BA; BFA **Courses Offered:** Playwriting & Direction; Acting
Technical Training: Design, including Theatre Workshop, Technical Theatre & Television
Teaching Certification Available **Performing Groups:** Theatre USA

SOUTHEASTERN BIBLE COLLEGE
1401 S 29th St, Birmingham Alabama 35205
205 251-2311
  Private and 4 Year **Arts Areas:** Instrumental Music and Vocal Music

MUSIC

James Wolfe, Chairman **Number Of Faculty:** 3 **Number Of Students:** 30
Degrees Offered: BA Religious MusEd **Financial Assistance:** Scholarships
Performing Groups: Choir; Instrumental & Vocal Ensembles

SOUTHERN BENEDICTINE COLLEGE
Saint Bernard Alabama 35138, 205 734-4110
  Private and 4 Year
  Arts Areas: Dance, Instrumental Music, Vocal Music, Theatre and Film Arts
  Performing Series: Cultural Activities Series
  Performance Facilities: College Auditorium

DANCE

Mary Ann Trimble, Chairman
The college does not have a Dance Department
Number Of Faculty: 1 **Number Of Students:** 10 **Courses Offered:** Basic Ballet
Technical Training: Basic Ballet **Financial Assistance:** Work-Study Grants

(continued on next page)

MUSIC

Sister Magdalena Craig, OSB, Chairman
Number Of Faculty: 1 Part-time   **Number Of Students:** 25
Degrees Offered: Bachelor & Associate
Technical Training: Piano & Organ   **Financial Assistance:** Work-Study Grants
Performing Groups: Cultural Activities Series

SPRING HILL COLLEGE
Mobile   Alabama 36608, 205 460-2371
Private and 4 Year
Arts Areas: Instrumental Music, Film Arts, Television and Visual Arts
Performance Facilities: Chamber Music Hall; College Theatre; College Inn

MUSIC

Rev Daniel A Creagan, SJ, Chairman, Fine Arts Department
Number Of Faculty: 2   **Number Of Students:** 20
Technical Training: Piano; Classic Guitar; Theory
Performing Groups: Chorus; Collegium Musicum
Workshops/Festivals: Class Guitar Master Class conducted by Manuel Lopez Ramos
Artists-In-Residence/Guest Artists: Maneul Lopez Ramos, Classic Guitarist

---

STILLMAN COLLEGE
Tuscaloosa   Alabama 35402, 205 752-2548
Private and 4 Year
Arts Areas: Instrumental Music, Vocal Music, Theatre and Visual Arts
Performing Series: SC Cultural Series
Performance Facilities: Birthright Auditorium

MUSIC

Number Of Faculty: 4
Degrees Offered: BMusEd; BA, Mus   **Teaching Certification Available**
Financial Assistance: Scholarships   **Performing Groups:** Choir; Band

THEATRE

Janet Dill, Department Head   **Number Of Faculty:** 1
Courses Offered: Play Production; Voice; Diction
Teaching Certification Available   **Financial Assistance:** Scholarships

---

TALLADEGA COLLEGE
627 W Battle St, Talladega   Alabama 35160
205 362-2752
Private and 4 Year   **Arts Areas:** Instrumental Music and Vocal Music
Performing Series: Annual Choir Concerts; Christmas, Easter, Arts Festivals
Performance Facilities: DeForest Chapel; Callanan Gymnasium

MUSIC

Mr Horace Carney, Chairman   **Number Of Faculty:** 4   **Number Of Students:** 20
Degrees Offered: BA
Courses Offered: Concentration in Piano/Organ or Voice; Theory; Music History & Education
Teaching Certification Available
Financial Assistance: Scholarships and Work-Study Grants
Performing Groups: The Talladega College Concert Choir

TROY STATE UNIVERSITY
Troy   Alabama 36081, 205 566-3000
   State and 4 Year
   Arts Areas: Instrumental Music, Vocal Music, Theatre and Visual Arts
   Performing Series: Lyceum Series
   Performance Facilities: Smith Hall Auditorium

MUSIC

Dr John M Long, Chairman   *Number Of Faculty:* 14   *Number Of Students:* 256
Degrees Offered: BME; BS; MME   *Courses Offered:* Full Music Course
Teaching Certification Available
Financial Assistance: Scholarships and Work-Study Grants
Performing Groups: College & Stage Bands; Opera Orchestra; Collegiate & Madrigal Singers; Choir;
Opera Workshop
Workshops/Festivals: Southeast Concert Band Clinic; Southern Invitational Concert Band Festival;
Southern Choral Festival

TUSKEGEE INSTITUTE
Tuskegee   Alabama 35088, 205 727-8011
   Private and 4 Year
   Arts Areas: Instrumental Music, Vocal Music, Theatre and Visual Arts

MUSIC

R E Hicks, Chairman   *Number Of Faculty:* 6
Courses Offered: Fundamentals of Music; Vocal & Instrumental Ensemble; Theory; Choral Conducting;
Public School Music; African & Afro-American Music
Teaching Certification Available   *Performing Groups:* Band; Orchestra; Choir
Performing Groups: Little Theatre
The Little Theatre, an organization which operates under the auspices of the Division of Humanities,
provides opportunities for dramatic expression and personality development through interaction and personal
associations experienced in a variety of productions presented by the Theatre

UNIVERSITY OF MONTEVALLO
Montevallo   Alabama 35115, 205 665-2521 Ext 278
   State and 4 Year
   Arts Areas: Instrumental Music, Vocal Music, Theatre, Television and Visual Arts
   Performing Series: Concert & Lecture Series; Guest Artist Series (Music)

MUSIC

John W Stewart, Chairman   *Number Of Faculty:* 21   *Number Of Students:* 180
Degrees Offered: BM; BME; BA; BS; MM; MME
Courses Offered: Music Education; Performance; Church Music
Teaching Certification Available
Financial Assistance: Assistantships, Scholarships and Work-Study Grants
Performing Groups: Mixed Choir; Chamber Choir; Women's Choir; Concert Band; Brass Ensemble;
Woodwind Ensemble
Workshops/Festivals: Vocal - Choral Festival; Fine Arts Festival

THEATRE

Charles Harbour, Chairman   *Number Of Faculty:* 10   *Number Of Students:* 150
Degrees Offered: BA; BS; BFA; MA
Courses Offered: Speech; Communications Education; Theatre; Dance
Technical Training: Mass Communications; Technical Theatre
Teaching Certification Available
Financial Assistance: Assistantships, Scholarships and Work-Study Grants
Performing Groups: University Theatre; UM Mime Company; Studio Theatre; Dance
Workshops/Festivals: Alabama Drama Institute; UM Invitational Forensic; Trumbauer High School
Drama Forensic Tournament

UNIVERSITY OF ALASKA
COLLEGE OF ARTS & LETTERS
Fairbanks   Alaska 99701, 907 479-7211
State and 4 Year
Arts Areas: Instrumental Music, Vocal Music, Theatre, Television, Visual Arts and Radio
Performance Facilities: Fine Arts Concert Hall

MUSIC

Charles W Davis, Head   *Number Of Faculty:* 10   *Number Of Students:* 55
Degrees Offered: BA; BMus; MA   *Courses Offered:* Music Education; Performance
Teaching Certification Available
Financial Assistance: Scholarships and Work-Study Grants
Performing Groups: Choir of the North; University Chorus; Concert & Jazz Bands; Arctic Chamber Ensemble; University - Fairbanks Symphony; Woodwind & Brass Ensembles; Madrigal Singers; Opera Workshop
Workshops/Festivals: Summer Music Camp; Alaska High School Music Festival

THEATRE

Walter G Ensign, Jr, Head   *Number Of Faculty:* 10   *Degrees Offered:* BA
Teaching Certification Available
Financial Assistance: Scholarships and Work-Study Grants

UNIVERSITY OF ALASKA, ANCHORAGE
2533 Providence Dr, Anchorage   Alaska 99504
907 279-6622 Ext 317
State and 4 Year
Arts Areas: Dance, Instrumental Music, Vocal Music, Theatre and Visual Arts
Performing Series: Performing Arts Series
Performance Facilities: Performing Arts Center Mainstage; Amphitheater, Dance Studio, Classrooms

DANCE

Dewey Ehling, Chairman   *Number Of Faculty:* 6   *Number Of Students:* 350
Courses Offered: Ballet; Modern I, II; Jazz I, II; Belly Dancing; Exercise for Dance
Financial Assistance: Work-Study Grants
Performing Groups: 5 by 2 Dance Company

MUSIC

Jean - Paul Billaud, Chairman   *Number Of Faculty:* 20
Number Of Students: 400   *Degrees Offered:* BA Mus; AA; BMus; BMusEd
Financial Assistance: Internships, Assistantships, Scholarships and Work-Study Grants
Performing Groups: University Singers; Opera Workshop; Stage Band; Anchorage Community Chorus; Chamber Orchestra
Workshops/Festivals: Alaska Festival of Music, Basically Bach Music Festival

THEATRE

Everett Kent, Chairman   *Number Of Faculty:* 6   *Number Of Students:* 25
Degrees Offered: BA Theater
Courses Offered: Theater Practicum; Theater & Management; Acting I, II, III, IV; Stagecraft I, II; Scenery & Lighting Design; Costume Construction & Design I, II; Representative Plays
Technical Training: Scenery & Lighting Design; Basic Stagecraft; Costume Construction; Scene Design

ARIZONA STATE UNIVERSITY
Tempe   Arizona 85281, 602 965-6536 Ext 6536
State and 4 Year
Arts Areas: Dance, Instrumental Music, Vocal Music, Theatre, Film Arts, Television and Visual Arts
Performing Series: Fine Arts; Celebrity; Dance; Great Orchestra; Documentary Film
Performance Facilities: Gammage Center for the Performing Arts

DANCE

Margaret Gisolo, Chairman   *Number Of Faculty:* 4   *Number Of Students:* 100
Degrees Offered: BFA; BAEd; Major in Dance Education
Technical Training: Ballet; Modern Dance; Ethnic Dance
Teaching Certification Available
Financial Assistance: Scholarships and Work-Study Grants
Performing Groups: University Dance Theatre

MUSIC

Dr Andrew Broekema, Chairman   *Number Of Faculty:* 80
Number Of Students: 600
Degrees Offered: BA; BMus; EdD Mus Ed; PhD Mus Ed; MMus Ed
Teaching Certification Available
Financial Assistance: Assistantships, Scholarships and Work-Study Grants
Performing Groups: Concert Bands; Marching Band; Symphony Orchestra; Opera Orchestra; Lyric Opera Theatre; Choral Groups; Jazz Ensembles
Workshops/Festivals: Workshops

THEATRE

Dr William Arnold, Chairman   *Number Of Faculty:* 10
Number Of Students: 200
Degrees Offered: BA Theatre; BFA Theatre with Specialization in Child Drama & Directing; MA Theatre; MA Ed Theatre
Technical Training: Acting; Technical Theatre; Costume Design and Construction; Set Design
Teaching Certification Available
Financial Assistance: Assistantships, Scholarships and Work-Study Grants
Performing Groups: University Theatre; Student Experimental Theatre

UNIVERSITY OF ARIZONA
Tucson   Arizona 85721, 602 884-1301
State and 4 Year
Arts Areas: Dance, Instrumental Music, Vocal Music, Theatre, Film Arts, Television, Visual Arts and Speech
Performing Series: University Artist Series; School of Music Series; University Theater Series
Performance Facilities: University Auditorium; University Theater; Crowder Hall, School of Music

DANCE

Prof Sandra Hamilton, Coordinator   *Number Of Faculty:* 5
Number Of Students: 83   *Degrees Offered:* BFA in Dance
Financial Assistance: Scholarships and Work-Study Grants
Workshops/Festivals: Arts/'77

MUSIC

Dr Robert Werner, Director   *Number Of Faculty:* 43
Number Of Students: 475   *Degrees Offered:* AB; BM; DMA; PhD
Teaching Certification Available
Financial Assistance: Assistantships, Scholarships and Work-Study Grants

(continued on next page)

Performing Groups: Bands; Orchestras; Choirs; Opera Theater; Collegium Musicum; Stage Bands; Ensembles
Workshops/Festivals: Arts/'77; Southern Arizona Regional Festival; Ten Different Workshops

THEATRE

Peter R Marroney, Head   *Number Of Faculty:* 11   *Number Of Students:* 195
Degrees Offered: AB; BFA; MA; MFA
Financial Assistance: Scholarships and Work-Study Grants
Workshops/Festivals: Desert Invitational Drama Festival; Arts/'77

CENTRAL ARIZONA COLLEGE
Signal Peak, Coolidge   Arizona 85228
602 723-4141 Ext 347
County and 2 Year
Arts Areas: Instrumental Music, Vocal Music, Theatre, Visual Arts and Radio, Speech

MUSIC

Dr Charles Hall, Chairman, Creative Arts Department   *Number Of Faculty:* 3
Number Of Students: 75   *Degrees Offered:* AA
Courses Offered: Music Appreciation; Theory Music; Voice; College Choir; Piano; Instrumental; Mariachi Band; Piano, Orchestra/Musical & Barber Shop Ensembles; Guitar; Jazz & Soul Choirs; Community Chorus; Music History; Music Theatre Workshop
Financial Assistance: Scholarships, Work-Study Grants and Fee Waivers
Performing Groups: Jazz; Mariachi Band

THEATRE

Dr Charles Hall, Chairman, Creative Arts Department   *Number Of Faculty:* 1
Number Of Students: 50   *Degrees Offered:* AA
Courses Offered: Acting; Stagecraft; Film Art; Theatre Production Workshop
Technical Training: Stagecraft; Technical Theatre
Financial Assistance: Scholarships and Work-Study Grants
Performing Groups: CAC Players; Community Group

GLENDALE COMMUNITY COLLEGE
6000 W Olive, Glendale   Arizona 85302
602 734-2211
State and 2 Year
Arts Areas: Instrumental Music, Vocal Music, Theatre and Film Arts
Performing Series: Artists Series   *Performance Facilities:* Theatre

MUSIC

Dr Paul Harpen, Chairman   *Number Of Faculty:* 5   *Number Of Students:* 75
Degrees Offered: AA
Financial Assistance: Assistantships and Work-Study Grants
Performing Groups: Choir; Band; Orchestra; Opera Workshop

THEATRE

Dr August Lovenzini, Chairman   *Number Of Faculty:* 4
Number Of Students: 45   *Degrees Offered:* AA
Financial Assistance: Assistantships and Work-Study Grants
Performing Groups: National Collegiate Players

GRAND CANYON COLLEGE
3300 W Camelback Rd, Phoenix   Arizona 85017
602 249-3300
Private and 4 Year
Arts Areas: Instrumental Music, Vocal Music and Theatre
Performance Facilities: Ethington Theater

(*continued on next page*)

MUSIC

Dr Macon Delavan, Chairman   **Number Of Faculty:** 5   **Degrees Offered:** BA
Teaching Certification Available
Financial Assistance: Scholarships, Work-Study Grants and BEOG; SEOG; BIAG
Performing Groups: Oratorio Society; Choralaires; Jubilation; Wind Ensemble; Orchestra; Stage Band
Workshops/Festivals: Arizona Brass Workshop

THEATRE

Roger Miller, Assistant Professor, Speech & Drama   **Number Of Faculty:** 1
Degrees Offered: BA   **Teaching Certification Available**

MESA COMMUNITY COLLEGE
1833 W Southern Ave, Mesa   Arizona 85202
602 833-1261 Ext 241
County and 2 Year
Arts Areas: Dance, Instrumental Music, Vocal Music and Theatre
Performance Facilities: Performing Arts Theatre; Gymnasium; Navajo Room

DANCE

Ms Shirley Luhtala, Chairman, Physical Education Division
Number Of Faculty: 2   **Number Of Students:** 300   **Degrees Offered:** AA
Courses Offered: Choreography; Dance Production I, II; Contemporary Dance; Music for Dance;
Beginning & Intermediate Ballet; Beginning & Intermediate Modern Jazz; Tap Dance Performance
Technical Training: Jazz; Tap; Ballet; Choreography
Financial Assistance: Scholarships and Fee Waivers
Performing Groups: Mesa College Dance Theatre (two concerts per year - also traveling performances)
Workshops/Festivals: 5 x 2 Company (Modern Dance); Bill Evans Dance Co (Modern Dance)

MUSIC

James Hendricks, Chairman   **Number Of Faculty:** 6   **Number Of Students:** 500
Degrees Offered: AA
Courses Offered: Fund of Music; Concert Music; Aural Perception; Integated Elementary Theory;
Perspectives in Jazz & Pop Music; Appreciation & Literature of Music; Electronic Music; Integ Advanced
Theory; Music History & Literature; Music Performance
Technical Training: Music Performance; Elements of Conducting
Financial Assistance: Scholarships, Work-Study Grants and Fee Waivers
Performing Groups: A Cappella Choir; Opera Workshop; Men's Choir; Women's Chorus; Orchestra; Band;
Stage & Jazz Bands; Chamber Singers; Percussion, Brass, Piano & Woodwind Ensembles
Workshops/Festivals: Jazz Workshop; Opera Workshop

THEATRE

Charles Evans, Chairman, Communication & Theatre Art   **Number Of Faculty:** 5
Number Of Students: 50   **Degrees Offered:** AA
Courses Offered: Into Theatre; Beginning Acting; Theatre Make-up; Play Study; Stage Acting; Television
Tech; Theatre Production; Creative Drama; Intermediate Acting; Technical Theatre; Classic Theatre;
Children's & Readers' Theatre
Financial Assistance: Scholarships, Work-Study Grants and Fee Waivers
Performing Groups: Four drama productions per year; One Stagedoor Players Production per year;
Chamber Opera Theatre (Technical); Dance Concert (Technical)
Workshops/Festivals: American College Theatre Festival in December

---

NORTHERN ARIZONA UNIVERSITY
COLLEGE OF CREATIVE ARTS
Box 5755, Flagstaff   Arizona 86001
602 523-3011
State and 4 Year
Arts Areas: Dance, Instrumental Music, Vocal Music, Theatre, Film Arts, Television and Visual Arts
Performing Series: NAU Student Series
Performance Facilities: Creative Arts Symphony House

(continued on next page)

DANCE

Ms J Limpert, Chairman   **Number Of Faculty:** 1   **Number Of Students:** 20
Performing Groups: Dance Clusters
Workshops/Festivals: Spring Dance Festival & Concert

MUSIC

Dr Pat B Curry, Chairman   **Number Of Faculty:** 24   **Number Of Students:** 130
Degrees Offered: BMus Applied; BMusEd; MMusEd
Teaching Certification Available
Financial Assistance: Assistantships, Scholarships and Work-Study Grants
Performing Groups: University Orchestra; Band; String Quartet; Opera; Chamber Ensembles; Chorus
Workshops/Festivals: Summer Music Camp; Summer Music Festival

THEATRE

Dr Robert Stevens, Chairman   **Number Of Faculty:** 15
Number Of Students: 140
Courses Offered: BS Public Address, Radio/TV, Speech Pathology & Audiology, Theatre; BA Public Address, Radio/TV, Theatre; BSEd
Technical Training: Lighting; Makeup; Costuming; Set Designing
Teaching Certification Available
Financial Assistance: Assistantships, Scholarships and Work-Study Grants

---

NORTHLAND PIONEER COLLEGE
PO Box Y, Shaw Low   Arizona 85901
602 537-2976 Ext 32

County and 2 Year   **Arts Areas:** Theatre and Visual Arts
Performing Series: Drama Series; Northland Symphony Orchestra Series
Performance Facilities: Shaw Low Auditorium; Winslow Auditorium; Snowflake Auditorium

THEATRE

Penny Albright, Director   **Number Of Faculty:** 1   **Number Of Students:** 43
Degrees Offered: AA
Courses Offered: Beginning & Intermediate Acting; Play Producting; Children's Theater; Oral Interpretation
Technical Training: Play Productions; Scene Design
Performing Groups: Northland Repertory Theater
Workshops/Festivals: Summer Theater Workshop for High School & College Students

ARKANSAS COLLEGE
PO Box 2317, Batesville   Arkansas 72501
501 793-9813
>   Private and 4 Year
>   *Arts Areas:* Instrumental Music, Vocal Music, Theatre and Television
>   *Performance Facilities:* Brown Chapel Fine Arts Building

MUSIC

>   Mr Herman N Hess, Jr, Chairman   *Number Of Faculty:* 2   *Degrees Offered:* BA
>   *Teaching Certification Available*
>   *Financial Assistance:* Scholarships and Work-Study Grants
>   *Performing Groups:* Arkansas College Lassies and Lads; Arkansas College Choir

THEATRE

>   Dr L J Summers, Jr, Chairman   *Number Of Faculty:* 1   *Degrees Offered:* BA
>   *Teaching Certification Available*
>   *Financial Assistance:* Scholarships and Work-Study Grants
>   *Performing Groups:* Harlequin Theatre

ARKANSAS STATE UNIVERSITY
State University   Arkansas 72467, 501 972-2100
>   State and 4 Year
>   *Arts Areas:* Instrumental Music, Vocal Music, Theatre and Art
>   *Performance Facilities:* Fine Arts Center

MUSIC

>   Don Minx, Division Chairman   *Number Of Faculty:* 22
>   *Number Of Students:* 180   *Degrees Offered:* BMusEd; MMusEd; BMus
>   *Teaching Certification Available*
>   *Financial Assistance:* Assistantships, Scholarships and Work-Study Grants
>   *Performing Groups:* Band; Choir; Ensembles

THEATRE

>   Dr Lyn Bayless, Division Chairman   *Number Of Faculty:* 9
>   *Number Of Students:* 90   *Degrees Offered:* BS Ed; BFA; BA
>   *Teaching Certification Available*

ARKANSAS TECH UNIVERSITY
Russellville   Arkansas 72801, 501 968-0274
>   State and 5 Year
>   *Arts Areas:* Instrumental Music, Vocal Music, Theatre and Visual Arts
>   *Performing Series:* Community Concerts; Folk Music Concerts; Choir Concerts
>   *Performance Facilities:* Witherspoon Arts and Humanities Bldg

MUSIC

>   Gene Witherspoon, Chairman   *Number Of Faculty:* 10
>   *Number Of Students:* 130   *Degrees Offered:* BMusEd; BMus
>   *Teaching Certification Available*
>   *Financial Assistance:* Assistantships, Scholarships and Work-Study Grants
>   *Performing Groups:* Choirs; Bands; Brass; Voice; Piano and Organ Recitals; Woodwind, Brass, String,
>   Percussion Ensembles
>   *Workshops/Festivals:* Band Camps; High School Groups

THEATRE

>   Robert Bolen, Chairman   *Number Of Faculty:* 3   *Number Of Students:* 60

(continued on next page)

Degrees Offered: BA Speech, Theatre   **Teaching Certification Available**
Financial Assistance: Assistantships, Scholarships and Work-Study Grants
Performing Groups: Theatre; Drama

UNIVERSITY OF ARKANSAS, PINE BLUFF
Cedar St, Pine Bluff   Arkansas 71601
501 535-6700 Ext 440
State and 4 Year
Arts Areas: Instrumental Music, Vocal Music, Theatre and Visual Arts
Performing Series: Lyceum Series
Performance Facilities: Isaac Hathaway Fine Arts Center

MUSIC

Dr Grace Wiley, Chairperson   **Number Of Faculty:** 8   **Number Of Students:** 80
Degrees Offered: BA Music; BS MusEd
Teaching Certification Available
Financial Assistance: Scholarships and Work-Study Grants
Performing Groups: Marching & Concert Bands; Jazz Ensemble; Vesper & University Choirs
Workshops/Festivals: Jazz Workshop; State High School Music Festival; State Choral Festival; Opera Workshop

THEATRE

Dr V J Coleman, Chairperson, Department of English, Speech & Drama
Number Of Faculty: 3   **Number Of Students:** 17
Degrees Offered: BA Speech & Drama; BS Speech & Drama Education
Courses Offered: Oral Reading; Dramatic Interpretation & Criticism; History of Costume; Play Production; Survey of the Theatre; Play Directing; Playwriting, Contemporary American Drama; Speech
Teaching Certification Available
Financial Assistance: Scholarships and Work-Study Grants
Performing Groups: Spotlighters Dramatic Society

UNIVERSITY OF ARKANSAS, MONTICELLO
University Ave, Monticello   Arkansas 71655
501 367-6811 Ext 60
State and 4 Year
Arts Areas: Dance, Instrumental Music, Vocal Music, Film Arts and Visual Arts
Performing Series: University of Arkansas at Monticello Concert Association
Performance Facilities: Fine Arts Center; Music Building Recital Hall; Ballroom

DANCE

Number Of Faculty: 1   **Number Of Students:** 20
Courses Offered: Modern Dance; Square & Social Dancing
Performing Groups: Modern Dance

MUSIC

Number Of Faculty: 6
Number Of Students: 100   **Degrees Offered:** BA
Courses Offered: Music Ed Curriculum   **Teaching Certification Available**
Financial Assistance: Scholarships and Work-Study Grants
Performing Groups: Opera Workshop; A Cappela Choir; Grand Chorus; Marching & Concert Band; Stage Band
Workshops/Festivals: Regional Choral Festivals; Regional Band Festivals; Solo & Ensemble Contests

THEATRE

Dr David Lanphier, Head, Speech & Dramatic Arts   **Number Of Faculty:** 3
Number Of Students: 20   **Degrees Offered:** BA
Courses Offered: Minor Theatre Training   **Teaching Certification Available**

(continued on next page)

Financial Assistance: Scholarships and Work-Study Grants
Performing Groups: Bord Treders
Workshops/Festivals: Southeast Arkansas Drama Festival

UNIVERSITY OF ARKANSAS, LITTLE ROCK
33rd & University, Little Rock   Arkansas 72204
501 569-3296
State and 4 Year
Arts Areas: Dance, Instrumental Music, Vocal Music, Theatre and Visual Arts
Performing Series: University Choir; University Chorus; Madrigal Singers; University Band
Performance Facilities: Theater Auditorium; Fine Arts Recital Hall

MUSIC

Dr William Perryman, Acting Chairperson   *Number Of Faculty:* 33
Number Of Students: 125   *Degrees Offered:* BA; BMusEd; BMus
Courses Offered: Music Theory; Music History & Literature; Applied Music - Ensembles; Applied Music - Class; Private Instruction
Teaching Certification Available
Financial Assistance: Scholarships and Work-Study Grants
Performing Groups: Band; Orchestra; Opera Theater; Madrigal Choir; Chorus; Brass Ensemble; Woodwind Ensemble; Recorder Ensemble; Handbell Ensemble
Workshops/Festivals: Opera Workshop

THEATRE

Dr David Ritchey, Chairperson   *Number Of Faculty:* 12
Number Of Students: 65   *Degrees Offered:* BA
Courses Offered: Drama Theory; Drama Performance; Technical Theater; Drama Education
Teaching Certification Available
Artists-In-Residence/Guest Artists: Marjorie Lawrence

UNIVERSITY OF CENTRAL ARKANSAS
Conway   Arkansas 72032, 501 329-2931 Ext 221
State and 4 Year
Arts Areas: Instrumental Music, Vocal Music and Theatre
Performing Series: Public Appearance Series
Performance Facilities: Snow Fine Arts Center Recital Hall & Little Theatre; Waldren Auditorium

MUSIC

Carl Forsberg, Chairman   *Number Of Faculty:* 16   *Number Of Students:* 107
Degrees Offered: BA; BMusEd; MMusEd   *Teaching Certification Available*
Financial Assistance: Assistantships, Scholarships and Work-Study Grants
Performing Groups: Choirs; Orchestra; Bands; Ensembles

THEATRE

C Robert Hawley, Director of Theatre   *Number Of Faculty:* 2
Number Of Students: 47   *Degrees Offered:* BS; BA; BSE
Courses Offered: Intro to Theatre; Acting; Stagecraft & Lighting; Directing; Theatre History; Theatre Workshop; Scene Design; Voice & Phonetics; Theatre Activities; Oral Interpretation
Teaching Certification Available
Financial Assistance: Assistantships, Scholarships and Work-Study Grants
Performing Groups: UCA Players
Workshops/Festivals: Fall High School Speech and Theatre Workshop; Cadron Valley Tournament
Artists-In-Residence/Guest Artists: Kansas City Philharmonic; National Opera Company; Robert Gauralnik

HARDING COLLEGE
Searcy Arkansas 72143, 501 268-6161
> Private and 4 Year
> **Arts Areas:** Instrumental Music, Vocal Music, Theatre, Television and Visual Arts

MUSIC

Dr Erle T Moore, Chairman **Number Of Faculty:** 10 **Number Of Students:** 106
Degrees Offered: BA in Music, Music Ed, Piano, Viola, Violin, Voice
Courses Offered: Music; Music Ed; Piano; Viola; Violin; Voice
Technical Training: Voice; Piano; Wind & String Instruments
Teaching Certification Available **Financial Assistance:** Scholarships
Performing Groups: A Cappella Chorus, Chorale; Concert Band; Marching Band; Orchestra; Belles & Beaux; Pep Band; Stage Band; Woodwind Quintet; String Quartet
Workshops/Festivals: Annual Tahkodah Music Camp

THEATRE

Evan Ulrey, Chairman **Number Of Faculty:** 2 **Degrees Offered:** BA
Courses Offered: Acting; Directing; History; Costume; Makeup; Technical
Teaching Certification Available **Financial Assistance:** Scholarships

HENDRIX COLLEGE
Conway Arkansas 72032, 501 329-6811
> Private and 4 Year
> **Arts Areas:** Instrumental Music, Vocal Music and Theatre
> **Performance Facilities:** Staples Auditorium; Reves Recital Hall; Cabe Theatre Arts Center

MUSIC

Dr George Mulacek, Chairman **Number Of Faculty:** 5 **Number Of Students:** 38
Degrees Offered: BA
Courses Offered: Introduction to Music; Theory; Music Appreciation; Basic Literature and Form; 18th Century Counterpoint; Pedagogy; Introduction to Opera; Chamber & Symphonic Literature; Music in the Elementary School; School Music Methods; Instrumental Music and Technique; Choral Literature & Technique; Orchestration; History of Church Music; Music in Christian Education; Service Playing; Applied Piano, Organ, Voice, Violin, and Wind Instruments; Music History & Literature
Teaching Certification Available
Financial Assistance: Scholarships and Work-Study Grants
Performing Groups: Hendrix College Choir; Madrigal Singers; Chorus; Brass Choir; Wind Ensemble

THEATRE

Dr Rosemary Henenberg, Chairman **Number Of Faculty:** 2
Number Of Students: 25 **Degrees Offered:** BA
Courses Offered: Introduction to Theatre; Contemporary Speaking; Voice & Diction; Oral Interpretation; Advanced Oral Interpretation; Acting; Theatre Practicum; Theatre Production; Integration of Style; Motion Pictures; Stage Directing; Classical & Medieval Theatre; The Drama: 1500 to 1850; Creative Dramatics
Teaching Certification Available
Financial Assistance: Scholarships and Work-Study Grants
Performing Groups: Hendrix Players

PHILLIPS COUNTY COMMUNITY COLLEGE
PO Box 785, Helena Arkansas 72342
501 338-6496 Ext 43
> County and 2 Year
> **Arts Areas:** Instrumental Music, Vocal Music, Theatre and Visual Arts
> **Performance Facilities:** Lily Peter Auditorium

(continued on next page)

MUSIC

William Stiles, Coordinator   **Number Of Faculty:** 3   **Number Of Students:** 60
Degrees Offered: AA
Financial Assistance: Scholarships and Work-Study Grants
Performing Groups: The Collegians (Band); Phillips College Singers
Workshops/Festivals: Marching Band Festival

THEATRE

Eloise Kalb, Coordinator   **Number Of Faculty:** 3   **Number Of Students:** 100
Degrees Offered: AA
Financial Assistance: Scholarships and Work-Study Grants
Performing Groups: Phillips College Players
Workshops/Festivals: Young People's Workshop in the Arts; New Directors' Workshop
Artists-In-Residence/Guest Artists: Larry Spares

SOUTHERN ARKANSAS UNIVERSITY
Magnolia   Arkansas 71753, 501 234-5120
State and 4 Year
Arts Areas: Instrumental Music, Vocal Music, Theatre, Film Arts, Television and Visual Arts
Performing Series: CAB Fine Arts Series
Performance Facilities: Harton Theatre; Dolph Camp Fine Arts Recital Hall

MUSIC

Dr Robert G Campbell, Chairman of Fine Arts   **Number Of Faculty:** 8
Number Of Students: 45   **Degrees Offered:** BA; BMusEd
Courses Offered: Basic courses leading to the Bachelor Degree
Teaching Certification Available
Financial Assistance: Scholarships and Work-Study Grants
Performing Groups: Choral Society; Concert Choir; Madrigal Singers; Marching Band; Symphonic Band; Stage Band
Workshops/Festivals: Orff-Schulwerk; Summer Band Camps

THEATRE

Dr Jerry Cortez, Director of Theatre   **Number Of Faculty:** 3
Number Of Students: 40   **Degrees Offered:** BA; BS Ed with Theatre emphasis
Courses Offered: Basic courses leading to BA - both Production and Theory
Technical Training: Fully equipped theatre & scene shop facilities
Teaching Certification Available
Financial Assistance: Scholarships and Work-Study Grants
Performing Groups: Harton Players; SAU Theatre; Alpha Psi Omega
Workshops/Festivals: Summer Theatre Workshop

ALLAN HANCOCK COLLEGE
800 S College Dr, Santa Maria   California 93454
805 922-6966 Ext 280

Private and 2 Year
Arts Areas: Dance, Instrumental Music, Vocal Music, Theatre, Film Arts and Visual Arts
Performance Facilities: Performing Arts Center Theatre; Sports Pavilion

DANCE

Agnes Grogan, Chairman   *Number Of Faculty:* 4   *Number Of Students:* 300
Degrees Offered: AA Fine Arts
Courses Offered: Beginning Ballet, Jazz, Modern; Intermediate Ballet, Jazz, Modern; Composition;
Performance Lab; Creative Movement for Children; Ethnic Cultural Dance
Financial Assistance: Work-Study Grants
Performing Groups: A H C Dance Department
Workshops/Festivals: Annual Spring Dance Concert; Christmas Concert; Workshops in Tap, Creative
Movement; Performances for Community Groups; Ethnic Cultural Dance Festival

MUSIC

Christopher Kuzell, Chairman   *Number Of Faculty:* 3
Number Of Students: 150   *Degrees Offered:* AA
Courses Offered: Theory; Keyboard; Vocal; Band & Orchestra; History; Appreciation
Performing Groups: Symphony Orchestra; Symphony Band; Choir; Vocal & Instrumental Ensembles;
Studio (Jazz) Band
Workshops/Festivals: District Band & Orchestra Festival; Junior High School Honor Band

THEATRE

Donovan Marley, Director   *Number Of Students:* 130
Degrees Offered: AA; Vocational Certificate in Acting & Theatre Technology
Courses Offered: Pre - professional Acting Training; Pre - professional Technical Theatre Training
Workshops/Festivals: The Solvang Theaterfest; PCPA Theatre Festival

---

AMBASSADOR COLLEGE
300 W Green St, Pasadena   California 91123
213 577-5000

Private and 4 Year
Arts Areas: Dance, Instrumental Music, Vocal Music and Theatre
Performing Series: Ambassador International Cultural Foundation
Performance Facilities: Ambassador Auditorium; Fine Arts Recital Hall

DANCE

R Gerry Long, Chairman   *Number Of Faculty:* 6
Courses Offered: Pointe; Ballet; Jazz; Pas de Deux; Dance Theatre
Financial Assistance: Work-Study Grants
Performing Groups: Ambassador College Dance Theatre

MUSIC

R Gerry Long, Chairman   *Number Of Faculty:* 20   *Number Of Students:* 300
Degrees Offered: BA
Courses Offered: Theory; Literature & History; Orchestration; Composition; Counterpoint; Conducting;
Private Piano; Voice Woodwinds; Strings; Percussion; Guitar; Performing Ensembles
Financial Assistance: Work-Study Grants
Performing Groups: Ambassador Chorale; Ambassador Band; Jazz Ensemble; Ambassador Chamber
Orchestra

BAKERSFIELD COLLEGE
1801 Panorama Dr, Bakersfield   California 93305
805 395-4011
>   County and 2 Year
>   *Arts Areas:* Dance, Instrumental Music, Vocal Music, Theatre, Film Arts and Television

DANCE

Joyce Prewitt, Instructor   *Number Of Faculty:* 1   *Number Of Students:* 55
Degrees Offered: AA   *Courses Offered:* Modern Dance
Financial Assistance: Work-Study Grants
Performing Groups: BC Modern Dance Company
Workshops/Festivals: Summer Musical Dance Workshop; Bi-Annual Dance Workshop

MUSIC

James Mason, Chairman   *Number Of Faculty:* 5   *Number Of Students:* 814
Degrees Offered: AA   *Financial Assistance:* Work-Study Grants
Performing Groups: Chamber Singers; Choir; College Band; Orchestra; Jazz Ensemble; String Ensemble; Symphonic Wind Ensemble
Workshops/Festivals: Vocal Ensemble Festival

THEATRE

Robert Chapman, Chairman   *Number Of Faculty:* 4   *Number Of Students:* 736
Degrees Offered: AA
Technical Training: Community College Acting Workshop/Stagecraft Workshop
Performing Groups: BC Children's Theatre; Renegade Theatre
Workshops/Festivals: Starlight of Kern - Summer Musical

BETHANY BIBLE COLLEGE
800 Bethany Dr, Santa Cruz   California 95060
408 438-3800
>   Private and 4 Year   *Arts Areas:* Instrumental Music and Vocal Music
>   *Performance Facilities:* Redwood Auditorium; Redwood Bowl; Craig Chapel; Twin Lakes Baptist Church

MUSIC

Rev James R Fortunato, Head   *Number Of Faculty:* 4   *Number Of Students:* 39
Degrees Offered: BSMus
Courses Offered: Musicianship; Theory; Harmony; Literature; Piano; Organ; Voice; Accordion; Brass; Woodwind; Strings; Percussion; Song Leading; Conducting; Counterpoint; Choral Arranging; Orchestration; Form & Analysis; Composition; History; Hymnology; Ambassador Choir; Concert Chorale; Band; Ensembles; Church Music Administration; Practicum
Teaching Certification Available
Financial Assistance: Scholarships and Work-Study Grants
Performing Groups: Ambassador Choir; Ambassador Band; Concert Chorale; Bethany Dayspring; Bethanaires; Instrumental Ensembles; Vocal Ensembles
Workshops/Festivals: Sounds of Christmas; Spring Concert; Various small engagements

BUTTE COLLEGE
Route 1, Box 183A, Oroville   California 95965
916 895-2581
>   County and 2 Year
>   *Arts Areas:* Instrumental Music, Vocal Music, Theatre, Film Arts, Television, Visual Arts and Speech Arts
>   *Performance Facilities:* Interim Theatre; Campus Center; BCT Theatre; Theatre in the Glen; Performing Arts Center

MUSIC

Joseph A Rich, Chairman   *Number Of Faculty:* 2   *Degrees Offered:* AA
Courses Offered: Vocal; Instrumental

(continued on next page)

Financial Assistance: Scholarships and Work-Study Grants
Performing Groups: Jazz Bands; Concert Band; Stage Band; Schola Cantorum; Bell Ringers; Choir; A Cappella
Workshops/Festivals: Christmas, Easter & Spring Programs

THEATRE

Joseph A Rich, Chairman   **Number Of Faculty:** 1   **Degrees Offered:** AA
Financial Assistance: Scholarships and Work-Study Grants
Performing Groups: BLT Group; Children's Workshop
Workshops/Festivals: Christmas Theatre

SOUTHERN CALIFORNIA COLLEGE
55 Fair Dr, Costa Mesa   California 92626
714 556-3610
Private and 4 Year
Arts Areas: Instrumental Music, Vocal Music and Theatre
Performing Series: Guest Artist Series
Performance Facilities: College Auditorium

MUSIC

Noel Wilson, Chairman   **Number Of Faculty:** 5   **Number Of Students:** 60
Degrees Offered: BA
Courses Offered: Introduction to Music; Music Theory; Counterpoint; Hymnology; Music History & Literature; Elementary Music Methods; Form & Analysis; Orchestration; Composing & Arranging
Technical Training: Woodwind Techniques; Brass Techniques; Conducting; Advanced Conducting; String Techniques; Percussion Techniques; Piano
Financial Assistance: Scholarships and Work-Study Grants
Performing Groups: College Choir; Vanguards; College Band; Contemporary Instrumental Ensemble

THEATRE

H Keith Ewing, Chairman, Division of Humanities & Fine Arts
Number Of Faculty: 2   **Number Of Students:** 40
Courses Offered: Dramatics; Drama Production; Street Theatre
Financial Assistance: Scholarships and Work-Study Grants
Performing Groups: Street Theatre; Major Production each semester
Artists-In-Residence/Guest Artists: Mary Kinder-Morton; Doug Lawrence

---

THE CALIFORNIA INSTITUTE OF THE ARTS
24700 McBean Pkwy, Valencia   California 91355
805 255-1050
Private and 4 Year
Arts Areas: Dance, Instrumental Music, Vocal Music, Theatre, Film Arts, Television and Visual Arts
Performing Series: Performing Arts Series
Performance Facilities: Modular, Dance, Screening, and Ensemble Theatres

DANCE

Gus Solomons Jr, Artistic Director   **Number Of Faculty:** 5
Number Of Students: 50   **Degrees Offered:** BFA; MFA; Certificate
Courses Offered: Technique; Composition; Technical Theatre; Kinesiology; History; Choreography
Technical Training: Theatre support program in production - related skills
Financial Assistance: Assistantships, Scholarships and Work-Study Grants
Performing Groups: Solomons Company/Dance
Workshops/Festivals: Master Classes in Jazz, Contact Improvisation

MUSIC

Nicholas England, Dean, School of Music   **Number Of Faculty:** 37
Number Of Students: 220   **Degrees Offered:** BFA; MFA; Certificate
Courses Offered: Performance; Composition; General Music Programs

(continued on next page)

Financial Assistance: Assistantships, Scholarships, Work-Study Grants and Special Grants
Performing Groups: Sequoia Quartet; Chamber Orchestra; Chamber Soloists
Workshops/Festivals: Annual Spring Fair; Instrumental Master Classes and Workshops with Guest Artists (Brass, Strings, Woodwinds)

THEATRE

Robert Benedetti, Dean   **Number Of Faculty:** 16   **Number Of Students:** 90
Degrees Offered: BFA; MFA; Certificate
Courses Offered: Acting; Directing; Performance Production Studies
Technical Training: Technical Theatre Program
Financial Assistance: Assistantships, Scholarships and Work-Study Grants
Workshops/Festivals: Annual Spring Fair

CALIFORNIA INSTITUTE OF TECHNOLOGY
Pasadena   California 91125, 213 795-6811
Private and 4 Year
Arts Areas: Instrumental Music, Vocal Music and Theatre
Performing Series: Caltech Presents; Spectrum Productions
Performance Facilities: Dabney Hall of the Humanities; Beckman Auditorium; Ramo Auditorium
Number Of Faculty: 3   **Courses Offered:** Music History; Music Theory
Performing Groups: Band; Choral Groups; Glee Club; Chamber Music Ensemble

CALIFORNIA LUTHERAN COLLEGE
60 W Olson Rd, Thousand Oaks   California 91360
803 492-2411
Private and 4 Year
Arts Areas: Instrumental Music, Vocal Music, Theatre, Film Arts and Television
Performing Series: Artist Series
Performance Facilities: Little Theatre; Gym - Auditorium

MUSIC

C Robert Zimmerman, Chairman   **Number Of Faculty:** 6 Full-time, 17 Part-time
Number Of Students: 300 - 350   **Degrees Offered:** BA
Teaching Certification Available
Financial Assistance: Assistantships, Scholarships, Work-Study Grants and Special Awards
Performing Groups: Concert Choir; Concert Orchestra; All College Choir; Concert Band; Chamber Singers; C L C Conejo Symphony; Kingsmen Quartet; Stage Band; String Ensemble

THEATRE

Richard G Adams, PhD, Chairman
Degrees Offered: BA Drama; BA Communication Arts
Courses Offered: Theatre Arts; Dramatic Literature; Film, Radio, TV
Technical Training: Stagecraft; Lighting; Design; Acting
Teaching Certification Available
Financial Assistance: Assistantships, Scholarships, Work-Study Grants and Special Awards
Performing Groups: Children's Theatre

CALIFORNIA STATE COLLEGE, BAKERSFIELD
9001 Stockdale Highway, Bakersfield   California 93309
805 833-3093
State and 4 Year
Arts Areas: Instrumental Music, Vocal Music and Visual Arts

MUSIC

Dr Vincent Ponko, Jr, Acting Chairman of Fine Arts
Number Of Faculty: 7 Full-time, 7 Part-time   **Number Of Students:** 45
Degrees Offered: BA in Fine Arts with a Concentration in Music
Courses Offered: Music Theory; Music History; Music Education; Applied Music; Performing Organizations

(continued on next page)

Financial Assistance: Assistantships, Scholarships and Work-Study Grants
Performing Groups: Cal State Choir; Madrigals; Wind Ensemble; Chamber Orchestra; Jazz Ensemble; Early Music Ensemble

---

CALIFORNIA STATE COLLEGE, SAN BERNARDINO
5500 State College Pkwy, San Bernardino   California 92407
714 887-6311 Ext 443
State and 4 Year   **Performance Facilities:** Creative Arts Building

MUSIC

Dr Arthur A Moorefield, Chairman   **Number Of Faculty:** 5
Number Of Students: 923   **Degrees Offered:** BA
Teaching Certification Available
Financial Assistance: Internships, Assistantships, Scholarships and Work-Study Grants
Performing Groups: Chamber Orchestra; Band; Jazz Ensemble; Concert Choir; Chamber Singers; Collegium Musicum; South Indian Singing
Workshops/Festivals: High School Choral Festival; Renaissance Festival; Band Festivals

THEATRE

Dr Ronald E Barnes, Chairman   **Number Of Faculty:** 4
Number Of Students: 745   **Degrees Offered:** BA; MA
Teaching Certification Available
Financial Assistance: Assistantships, Scholarships and Work-Study Grants
Performing Groups: Players of the Pear Garden
Workshops/Festivals: High School Theatre Workshop

CALIFORNIA STATE COLLEGE, STANISLAUS
800 Monte Vista, Turlock   California 95380
209 633-2201
State and 4 Year
Arts Areas: Instrumental Music, Vocal Music, Theatre and Visual Arts
Performing Series: Lecture - Concert Series
Performance Facilities: Mainstage Theatre; Studio Theatre

MUSIC

Joseph Bruggman, Chairman   **Number Of Faculty:** 8   **Number Of Students:** 80
Degrees Offered: BA
Courses Offered: Applied Music; History/Literature; Theory/Composition
Technical Training: Elizabethan; Harpsichord; Vocal Chamber Music
Teaching Certification Available
Financial Assistance: Assistantships, Scholarships and Work-Study Grants
Performing Groups: Chorale; Chamber Singers; College Choir; Symphonic Wind Ensemble; Jazz Ensemble; Vocal Ensemble; Brass/Woodwind; Chamber Ensemble
Workshops/Festivals: Renaissance Music Workshops; Public School Teachers Workshops; Solo/Ensemble Festivals; Conducting Workshops; Marching Band Workshops

THEATRE

Jere D Wade, Chairman   **Number Of Faculty:** 4   **Number Of Students:** 40
Degrees Offered: BA
Courses Offered: Acting; Directing; Design; History of Theatre; Theatre Management
Technical Training: The month of January is a separate academic term during which students operate as a resident theatre company
Financial Assistance: Scholarships and Work-Study Grants
Performing Groups: The Theatre Society
Workshops/Festivals: High School Drama Festival

CALIFORNIA STATE UNIVERSITY - DOMINGUEZ HILLS
1000 E Victoria St, Carson   California 90747
213 515-3543
State and 4 Year
Arts Areas: Instrumental Music, Vocal Music, Theatre, Film Arts, Television and Visual Arts
Performing Series: Performing Arts Series
Performance Facilities: University Theatre; Playbox Theatre

MUSIC

Marshall Bialosky, Chairperson   *Number Of Faculty:* 5 Full-time, 8 Part-time
Number Of Students: 350   *Degrees Offered:* BA
Courses Offered: Electronic Music; Instrumental; Vocal; Theory & History; Business of Music Courses
Teaching Certification Available
Financial Assistance: Work-Study Grants and Student Assistants
Performing Groups: Dominguez Chorale; Dominguez Hills Chamber Orchestra; Dominguez Hills College Band; Early Instruments Consort; Victoria Street Ragtime Band
Workshops/Festivals: Southwest Youth Music Festival; American Music Festival

THEATRE

Jack A Vaughn, Professor of Theatre Arts
Number Of Faculty: 3 Full-time, 2 Part-time   *Number Of Students:* 50
Degrees Offered: BA   *Teaching Certification Available*
Financial Assistance: Work-Study Grants and Student Assistants
Performing Groups: Dominguez Theatre Guild
Workshops/Festivals: American College Theatre Festival, Region II; Dominguez Hills School Drama Festival; Southern California Children's Theatre Festival
Artists-In-Residence/Guest Artists: Jack Eddleman; Bella Lewitzky Dance Co; East - West Players

CALIFORNIA STATE UNIVERSITY, CHICO
Chico   California 95929, 916 985-5351
State and 4 Year
Arts Areas: Dance, Instrumental Music, Vocal Music, Theatre, Film Arts, Television and Visual Arts
Performing Series: Faculty Artists Series; Community Concerts
Performance Facilities: Laxson Auditorium; Adams Theatre; Recital Hall; Arena Theatre

DANCE

Charles D Scott, Department of PE   *Number Of Faculty:* 5
Number Of Students: 600
Degrees Offered: BA in Physical Education with emphasis in Dance
Courses Offered: Folk Dance; American Ballet; Dance Performance; Choreography; Square Dance; Ballroom Dance; Modern Dance; Dance Production
Teaching Certification Available
Financial Assistance: Assistantships and Work-Study Grants
Performing Groups: Folk Dance Group and Club; Square Dance Club; Cercle Danse
Workshops/Festivals: Fall - Major Dance Concert; Spring - Student Dance Production

MUSIC

Alfred Loeffler, Chairman   *Number Of Faculty:* 17
Number Of Students: 1628   *Degrees Offered:* BA; MA
Courses Offered: Instrumental; Keyboard; Vocal; Music History; Care & Repair of Instruments; Theory-Composition; Single Subject Credential in Music with Elementary Classroom; Instrumental; Vocal Emphases
Teaching Certification Available
Financial Assistance: Assistantships, Scholarships and Work-Study Grants
Performing Groups: Honor Band; Music Education Conference; Faculty Artist Series
Workshops/Festivals: Fine Arts Festival; Chamber Music Workshop

(continued on next page)

THEATRE

Dr Lloyd S Jones, Chairman, Department of Speech & Drama
Number Of Faculty: 12   **Number Of Students:** 100
Degrees Offered: BA Speech & Drama
Courses Offered: Rhetoric; Public Address; Oral Interpretation; Drama; Speech Pathology
Teaching Certification Available
Workshops/Festivals: One-Act Play Festival; Shakespeare Festival
Artists-In-Residence/Guest Artists: "Women in the Arts"

CALIFORNIA STATE UNIVERSITY, FRESNO
Cedar & Shaw, Fresno   California 93740
209 487-9011
State and 4 Year
Arts Areas: Dance, Instrumental Music, Vocal Music, Theatre, Film Arts and Television
Performance Facilities: John Wright Theatre; Arena Theatre; Amphitheatre; Recital Hall

DANCE

Patricia Thomson, Coordinator, Women's Physical Education Department
Number Of Faculty: 3   **Number Of Students:** 30   **Degrees Offered:** BA; MA
Financial Assistance: Work-Study Grants
Performing Groups: Portable Dance Group
Workshops/Festivals: Annual Dance Concert; Workshops through extension

MUSIC

Ralph C Rea, Acting Chairman   **Number Of Faculty:** 25
Number Of Students: 275   **Degrees Offered:** BA; MA
Courses Offered: Musical Education; Performance; Composition/Theory; History
Teaching Certification Available
Financial Assistance: Scholarships and Work-Study Grants
Performing Groups: Choir; Band; Jazz & Marching Bands; Chamber Singers; Instrumental Chamber Group; Collegium Musicum; Symphony Orchestra
Workshops/Festivals: Festivals and Workshops with MEMC Groups; Annual Special Week with Guest Artists

THEATRE

Ronald D Johnson, Chairman   **Number Of Faculty:** 11
Number Of Students: 140   **Degrees Offered:** BA; MA
Teaching Certification Available
Financial Assistance: Scholarships and Work-Study Grants
Performing Groups: Child Drama Center

CALIFORNIA STATE UNIVERSITY, FULLERTON
Fullerton   California 92634, 718 870-3256
State and 4 Year
Arts Areas: Dance, Instrumental Music, Vocal Music, Theatre, Film Arts, Television and Visual Arts
Performing Series: Performing Artists in Residence
Performance Facilities: Little Theatre; Arena Theatre; Recital Hall

MUSIC

Bentol L Minor, Chairman   **Number Of Faculty:** 58   **Number Of Students:** 600
Degrees Offered: BA; BMus; MA; MM Teaching Certificate
Courses Offered: Theory/Comp; Vocal/Opera; Instrumental; History/Literature; Keyboard; Music Education
Teaching Certification Available
Financial Assistance: Assistantships, Scholarships and Work-Study Grants
Performing Groups: Band; Choir; Orchestra; Jazz Band; Various Ensembles
Workshops/Festivals: Music Teachers' Association; Southern California School Band & Orchestra Association; Western States Music Clinic

(continued on next page)

THEATRE

Dr Alvin J Keller, Chairman   **Number Of Faculty:** 32
Number Of Students: 432
Degrees Offered: BA, MA, MFA (Technical Theatre); Teaching Certificate; BA, MFA in Technical
Production and Design
Courses Offered: Theatre History & Theory; Playwriting; Oral Interpretation; Acting; Directing;
Radio/Television/Film Directing; Technical Production/Design
Technical Training: Dance, Theatre for Children; Secondary Teaching
Teaching Certification Available
Financial Assistance: Internships, Assistantships, Scholarships and Work-Study Grants
Performing Groups: Experimental Theatre; Main Stage Productions; Children's Theatre; Playwrights
Workshop; Advanced Directing Productions; Adjunct Professional Theatre; Cabaret Theatre Company
Workshops/Festivals: High School Theatre Festival; Summer Theatre Workshop
Artists-In-Residence/Guest Artists: James Cunningham and the Acme Dance Company; The LA 4; The
Stanze Peterson Dance Theatre; The LA Mime Company; Tashi - Peter Serkin, Ida Kavafian; Fred Sherry;
Richard Stoltzman

CALIFORNIA STATE UNIVERSITY, LONG BEACH
1250 Bellflower Blvd, Long Beach   California 90840
213 498-4364
State and Five Year
Arts Areas: Dance, Instrumental Music, Vocal Music, Theatre and Visual Arts
Performance Facilities: Studio Theatre; University Theatre

DANCE

Pat Finot, Chairman   **Number Of Faculty:** 4   **Number Of Students:** 120
Degrees Offered: BA in Dance
Courses Offered: Modern Dance Tech; Ballet; Jazz; Tap; Improvisation; Intro Dance Theatre; Dance
Production - Tech; Choreographing; History of Dance; Repertory; Composition; Music for Dance
Technical Training: Teaching; Dance Specialist; Choreographer
Teaching Certification Available
Financial Assistance: Scholarships and Work-Study Grants
Workshops/Festivals: Repertory Workshop; Annual Long Beach Summer School of Dance

MUSIC

Gerald Daniel, Chairman   **Number Of Faculty:** 30   **Number Of Students:** 600
Degrees Offered: BMus; BA; MA
Technical Training: Music Therapy; Commercial Music
Teaching Certification Available
Financial Assistance: Scholarships and Work-Study Grants
Performing Groups: Marching Band; A Cappella Choir; Symphony Orchestra; New Music Ensemble;
Symphonic Band; Chamber Orchestra; University & Chamber Choirs; Men's Chorus; Women's Chorus;
Concert Band; Studio Ensemble

THEATRE

Jerry R Bailor, Acting Chairman   **Number Of Faculty:** 18
Number Of Students: 200   **Degrees Offered:** BA; MA
Courses Offered: Acting; Stage Diction; History; Theory and Criticism; Directing; Puppetry; Mime;
Playwriting
Technical Training: Stagecraft; Makeup; Scene Design; Costume Crafts; Graphics for Theatre; Stage
Lighting
Workshops/Festivals: High School Drama Workshop; High School Drama Festival
Artists-In-Residence/Guest Artists: Bella Lewitzky Dance Company; Los Angeles Chamber Orchestra;
Groupe Vocal de France

CALIFORNIA STATE UNIVERSITY, LOS ANGELES
5151 State University Dr, Los Angeles   California 90032
213 224-3587
State and 4 Year
Arts Areas: Dance, Instrumental Music, Vocal Music, Theatre, Film Arts, Television and Visual Arts
Performance Facilities: State Playhouse Main Theatre; State Playhouse Music Hall

DANCE

Janice Day, Coordinator   *Number Of Faculty:* 2 Full-time, 3 Part-time
Number Of Students: 50
Degrees Offered: BA Physical Ed (Dance option); MA Physical Ed (Concentration in Dance)
Technical Training: Dance Technique classes
Teaching Certification Available   *Performing Groups:* Orchesis
Workshops/Festivals: Master Classes; Dance Workshops

MUSIC

Charles Hubbard, Chairman   *Number Of Faculty:* 24   *Number Of Students:* 500
Degrees Offered: BA; BM; MA
Courses Offered: Music Ed; Performance; Musicology; Composition Options
Technical Training: Teacher Training   *Teaching Certification Available*
Financial Assistance: Scholarships and Work-Study Grants
Performing Groups: Symphony Orchestra; Symphonic Band; Jazz, Woodwind, Brass, String & Percussion
Ensembles; A Cappella Choir; Chamber Singers; University Chorus; Opera Group
Workshops/Festivals: First Choir Band; Various Music Education Workshops

THEATRE

Maris U Ubans, Chairman   *Number Of Faculty:* 9   *Number Of Students:* 285
Degrees Offered: BA; MA
Technical Training: Scenery; Lighting; Costume; Makeup
Teaching Certification Available
Financial Assistance: Assistantships, Scholarships and Work-Study Grants
Performing Groups: Student Experimental Theatre (7-11)
Workshops/Festivals: ACTF; Annual Regional Irene Ryan Acting Awards Performance; Southern
California Children's Theatre Festival; Regional ACTF Festival

CALIFORNIA STATE UNIVERSITY, NORTHRIDGE
18111 Nordhoff St, Northridge   California 91330
213 885-2129
State and 4 Year
Arts Areas: Instrumental Music, Vocal Music, Theatre and Visual Arts

MUSIC

Clarence Wiggins, Chairman   *Number Of Faculty:* 36 Full-Time
Degrees Offered: BA; BM; MA   *Teaching Certification Available*
Financial Assistance: Internships, Assistantships, Scholarships, Work-Study Grants and Music Achievement
Awards
Performing Groups: University, Concert & Matador Field Bands; Symphony Orchestra; Jazz, Chamber
Music & New Music Ensembles; Oratorio, University & Opera Choruses; Opera Theatre; Collegium
Musicum (ancient music)
Workshops/Festivals: Chamber Music Festival

THEATRE

Dr William Schlosser, Chairman   *Number Of Faculty:* 15
Number Of Students: 300   *Degrees Offered:* BA; MA
Technical Training: Productions: Sets, Costumes, Lighting, Makeup
Teaching Certification Available
Financial Assistance: Internships, Assistantships, Scholarships and Work-Study Grants
Performing Groups: Regular Season Productions; Laboratory Theatre
Workshops/Festivals: Shakespeare Workshop; Teenage Drama Workshop

CALIFORNIA STATE UNIVERSITY, SACRAMENTO
6000 J St, Sacramento   California 95819
916 454-6011
State and 4 Year
Arts Areas: Dance, Instrumental Music, Vocal Music and Theatre
Courses Offered: Folk; Square; Modern Social

MUSIC

Norman Lamb, Chairman   *Number Of Faculty:* 26   *Number Of Students:* 241
Degrees Offered: BA; BM; MA   *Teaching Certification Available*
Financial Assistance: Scholarships
Performing Groups: Orchestra; University Chorus; Concert Choir; Symphonic Band; Marching Band;
String Orchestra; Stage Band; University Madrigal Singers; String Ensemble; Woodwind Ensembles; Show
Choir; Percussion, Recorder, Saxophone & Guitar Ensembles
Workshops/Festivals: Opera Workshop; Stan Kenton Clinic; Golden Empire Music Festivals; Festival of
Marching Bands; Workshops for Music Education and Teacher Education in Music

THEATRE

Charles V Hume, Chairman   *Number Of Faculty:* 13   *Number Of Students:* 175
Degrees Offered: BA; MA
Technical Training: Lighting; Makeup; Costuming; Stage Practice
Teaching Certification Available   *Financial Assistance:* Scholarships
Performing Groups: University Theatre; Studio Theatre; Chicano Theatre Group; Sons and Ancestors Black
Theatre; National Collegiate Players; Readers Theatre; Dance Ensemble; One-Acts
Workshops/Festivals: Summer Repertory Theatre; Touring Company

UNIVERSITY OF CALIFORNIA, DAVIS
Davis   California 95616
State and 2 Year
Arts Areas: Dance, Instrumental Music, Vocal Music and Theatre
Performance Facilities: Main Theatre; Wyatt Pavilion Theatre; Freeborn Hall; Lab A; Arena Theatre; Silo

DANCE

E D Berhauer, Professor
Dance program under auspices of Physical Education Department
Number Of Faculty: 2   *Number Of Students:* 30 - 50   *Degrees Offered:* AB; MA
Courses Offered: Composition; History   *Technical Training:* Ballet; Modern
Teaching Certification Available
Financial Assistance: Assistantships and Work-Study Grants
Performing Groups: University Dance Group

MUSIC

Sydney R Charles, Professor   *Number Of Faculty:* 10
Number Of Students: 55   *Degrees Offered:* BA; MA; MAT
Courses Offered: Theory & Composition; History & Literature; Graduate; Performance; Professional
Teaching Certification Available
Financial Assistance: Assistantships, Scholarships and Work-Study Grants
Performing Groups: University Symphony; University Concert Band; University Chorus; Early Music
Ensemble; Chamber Music Ensembles
Workshops/Festivals: Periodic Festivals of Contemporary Music

THEATRE

Robert Fahrner, Professor   *Number Of Faculty:* 15   *Number Of Students:* 108
Degrees Offered: BA; MA; MFA; PhD   *Teaching Certification Available*
Financial Assistance: Assistantships, Scholarships and Work-Study Grants
Performing Groups: University Theatre Season; Studio Season; Premier Season
Workshops/Festivals: Occassional Workshops
Artists-In-Residence/Guest Artists: Rudolf Kolisch

UNIVERSITY OF CALIFORNIA, IRVINE
Irvine California 92717, 714 833-5011

State and 4 Year
Arts Areas: Dance, Instrumental Music, Vocal Music, Theatre, Film Arts and Television
Performance Facilities: Art Gallery; Village Theatre; Little Theatre; Studio Theatre; Concert Hall

DANCE

Mr Eugene Loring, Chairman   *Number Of Faculty:* 13
Number Of Students: 155
Technical Training: Free Style; Jazz; Ballet; Ethnic; Dance; History; Notation; Theory; Music for Dancers; Performance; Choreography
Workshops/Festivals: Dance Workshop; Faculty Dance Concert

MUSIC

Dr Colin Slim, Chairman   *Number Of Faculty:* 10   *Number Of Students:* 60
Degrees Offered: BA; MFA
Performance Oriented Music Majors are auditioned
Courses Offered: Opera, History of Music; Theory; Counterpoint; Conducting; History of Opera, Form & Analysis
Teaching Certification Available
Financial Assistance: Internships, Assistantships, Scholarships and Work-Study Grants
Performing Groups: Pep Band; UCI Orchestra; Wind Ensemble; Chorus; Chamber Ensemble; Brass Ensemble; Stage Band

THEATRE

Dr Robert Cohen, Chairman   *Number Of Faculty:* 10   *Number Of Students:* 160
Degrees Offered: BA Drama; MFA Drama, Technical Major, Lighting, Scene Design, Costume Design
Technical Training: Acting; Directing; Filmmaking; TV Production; Play Writing; Film Writing
Teaching Certification Available
Workshops/Festivals: Drama Workshop; University Theatre

UNIVERSITY OF CALIFORNIA, LOS ANGELES
405 Hilgard Ave, Los Angeles California 90024
213 825-4321

State and 4 Year   *Arts Areas:* Instrumental Music

DANCE

Allegra Fuller Snyder, Chairwoman   *Number Of Faculty:* 29
Number Of Students: 120   *Degrees Offered:* BA; MA; MFA
Courses Offered: Modern; Ballet; Ethnic; Choreography; Notation; Movement; Therapy; Education; History; Music for Dance
Technical Training: Lighting; Costume & Scene Design for Dance Theater
Performing Groups: UCLA Dance Company; Various Specialized Dance Ensembles
Workshops/Festivals: Far Eastern & International Dance Series; Folk & Jazz Dance Series

MUSIC

Marie Louise Gollner, Chairman   *Number Of Faculty:* 80
Number Of Students: 320
Degrees Offered: BA, MA, MFA in Performance Practices; PhD
Courses Offered: History & Literature; Music Education; Systematic Musicology; Instrumental & Vocal; Opera; Ethnomusicology; Composition & Theory
Performing Groups: Symphony Orchestra; Symphonic, Marching & Varsity Bands; UCLA Performing Artists; Baroque Ensemble; Jazz Ensemble; Collegium Musicum; A Cappella Choir; University Chorus; Madrigal Singers; Men's & Women's Glee Clubs; Opera Workshop

THEATRE

John Young, Chairman   *Number Of Faculty:* 48   *Number Of Students:* 550
Degrees Offered: BA; MA; MFA; PhD

(continued on next page)

Courses Offered: All aspects of Theater; Motion Pictures; Television including Acting, Production, Direction, Writing
Technical Training: Scenery, Lighting, Costume, Sound

UNIVERSITY OF CALIFORNIA, SAN DIEGO
La Jolla   California 92093, 714 452-3120
State and 4 Year
Arts Areas: Dance, Instrumental Music, Vocal Music, Theatre, Film Arts, Television and Visual Arts
Performing Series: UCSD Theatre Season
Performance Facilities: Mandeville Center for the Arts; UCSD Theatre; UCSD Studio Theatre

DANCE

Dance program under auspices of Drama Department   *Number Of Faculty:* 3
Financial Assistance: Assistantships, Scholarships and Work-Study Grants
Workshops/Festivals: Summer Session Dance Program

THEATRE

Michael Addison, Professor   *Number Of Faculty:* 13
Number Of Students: 125   *Degrees Offered:* BA in Drama; MFA in Theatre
Courses Offered: Acting/Directing; Voice; Movement; Dance; Dramatic Literature; Design
Technical Training: Broad base of Design & Technical Theatre Courses
Teaching Certification Available
Financial Assistance: Assistantships, Scholarships and Work-Study Grants
Performing Groups: UCSD Theatre; Ensemble Theatre; Teatro Chicano
Workshops/Festivals: Dance Workshop (Summer Session); Theatre Arts Festival (Summer Session)

UNIVERSITY OF CALIFORNIA, SANTA CRUZ
Santa Cruz   California 95064, 408 429-2292
State and 4 Year
Arts Areas: Dance, Instrumental Music, Vocal Music, Theatre, Film Arts, Visual Arts and Electronic, World & Early Music
Performing Series: Senior & Faculty Recitals
Performance Facilities: Concert Hall; Outdoor Quarry Theatre; Theatre; Barn Theatre

MUSIC

Gordon Mumma, Chairman   *Number Of Faculty:* 15   *Number Of Students:* 150
Degrees Offered: BA Music   *Financial Assistance:* Work-Study Grants
Performing Groups: Gamelan; Chorus; Chamber Ensembles; Orchestra; Electronic Arts Ensemble

THEATRE

Audrey Stanley, Chairperson   *Number Of Faculty:* 15
Number Of Students: 200   *Degrees Offered:* BA Theatre Arts

CANADA COLLEGE
4200 Farm Hill Blvd, Redwood City   California 94061
415 364-1212
County and 2 Year
Arts Areas: Dance, Instrumental Music, Vocal Music, Theatre and Visual Arts
Performance Facilities: Main Theater; Flexible Theater

MUSIC

Carl Sitton, Chairman   *Number Of Faculty:* 15   *Number Of Students:* 250
Degrees Offered: AA
Courses Offered: Performance; Literature; Theory; Lower Division Music Major Program
Performing Groups: Peninsula Master Chorale; Canada College Choir; Canada College Singers; San Mateo County Symphony Orchestra; Canada Concert Band; Canada College Orchestra

CERRO COSO COMMUNITY COLLEGE
College Heights Blvd, Ridgecrest   California 93555
714 375-5001
> County and 2 Year
> **Arts Areas:** Instrumental Music, Vocal Music and Theatre
> **Performing Series:** Community Service Program
> **Performance Facilities:** Lecture Center - Auditorium

MUSIC

> Gordon Trousdale, Chairman   **Number Of Faculty:** 6   **Number Of Students:** 411
> **Degrees Offered:** AA
> **Courses Offered:** Music Theory; Music Reading; Intermediate Music Theory; Class Piano A, B, C, D;
> Elementary Voice; Folk Guitar; Orchestra; College Choir; Introduction to Conducting
> **Financial Assistance:** Scholarships and Work-Study Grants
> **Performing Groups:** Cerro Coso/Desert Community Orchestra; Cerro Coso Choir

THEATRE

> Mrs Florence Green, Chairperson   **Number Of Faculty:** 1
> **Number Of Students:** 42   **Degrees Offered:** AA
> **Courses Offered:** Fundamentals of Acting; Introduction to Dramatic Literature; Theatre Laboratory
> **Financial Assistance:** Scholarships and Work-Study Grants
> **Performing Groups:** Theatre 27

CLAREMONT GRADUATE SCHOOL
10th & College, Claremont   California 91711
714 626-8511 Ext 3694
> Private and Graduate Only
> **Arts Areas:** Instrumental Music and Vocal Music
> **Performing Series:** Jazz Series; Artist Course; International Festival
> Garrison Showtime Series; Ballet Film Festival; Theatre Series; Special Events
> **Performance Facilities:** Garrison Theater; Bridges Auditorium

MUSIC

> Frank Traficante, Chairman   **Number Of Faculty:** 16   **Number Of Students:** 22
> **Degrees Offered:** MA
> **Courses Offered:** Music History; Music Composition; Music Performance; Music Education
> **Technical Training:** Instrumental and Vocal Music
> **Teaching Certification Available**
> **Financial Assistance:** Assistantships, Scholarships, Work-Study Grants and Graduate Fellowships
> **Performing Groups:** Collegium Musicum
> **Workshops/Festivals:** Summer Organ Institute; Suzuki Teachers Workshop

COLLEGE OF THE CANYONS
26455 N Rockwell Canyon Rd, Valencia   California 91355
805 259-7800
> County and 2 Year
> **Arts Areas:** Instrumental Music, Vocal Music, Theatre and Visual Arts
> **Performance Facilities:** Student Center Performance Area; Bonelli Amphitheatre
> **Number Of Faculty:** 6   **Number Of Students:** 200   **Degrees Offered:** AA
> **Courses Offered:** Theory; History & Literature; Performance
> **Financial Assistance:** Scholarships and Work-Study Grants
> **Performing Groups:** Choral Groups; Wind Ensembles; Jazz Groups; Vocal & Instrumental Ensembles
> **Workshops/Festivals:** Early Childhood Music Workshop; High School Music Day; Invitational Jazz Festival
> **Number Of Faculty:** 1   **Number Of Students:** 50   **Degrees Offered:** AA
> **Courses Offered:** Introduction to Theatre; Creative Dramatics; Technical Theatre I, II; Acting; Production
> **Financial Assistance:** Scholarships and Work-Study Grants

COLLEGE OF MARIN
Kentfield   California 94904, 415 457-8811

County and 2 Year
Arts Areas: Instrumental Music, Vocal Music, Theatre, Film Arts, Television and Visual Arts
Performing Series: Community Services Series
Performance Facilities: Fine Arts Theatre; Olney Hall; Studio Theatre; Two Choral Halls

MUSIC

Stanley Kraczek, Chairperson   *Number Of Faculty:* 6 Full-time, 6 Part-time
Degrees Offered: AA; Two Year Certificate Program in Commerical Music
Courses Offered: Theory; Ear Training; Music Fundamentals; Applied Music; Analysis and Composition; Technique
Technical Training: Commercial Music Program
Financial Assistance: Scholarships and Work-Study Grants
Performing Groups: Orchestra; Two Bands; Instrumental Ensembles; Collegiate Chorale; College Chorus; Community Chorus; Chamber Singers; Opera Workshop; Jazz Ensemble
Workshops/Festivals: Opera Workshop; Dramatic Musicals; Summer Band Concerts; Full schedule of Student/Community performances

THEATRE

Harvey Susser, Chairman   *Number Of Faculty:* 4 Full-time, 2 Part-time
Number Of Students: 500   *Degrees Offered:* AA
Courses Offered: Introduction to the Theatre; Theory & Practice in Acting; Advanced Acting Techniques; Dramatic Literature & Theatre History; Techniques of Staging; Stage Costume; Rehearsal & Performance; Theatre Practicum; History & Appreciation of Film; Film: The Director's Art; Theatrical Lighting; Stage Design & Technical Organization; Stage Direction; Theatre Management; Stage Makeup: Theory & Practice
Financial Assistance: Scholarships and Work-Study Grants

COLLEGE OF NOTRE DAME
Belmont   California 94002

Private and 4 Year
Arts Areas: Dance, Instrumental Music, Vocal Music and Theatre
Performing Series: Ralston Concert Series
Performance Facilities: Notre Dame Auditorium; Ralston Ballroom; Carriage House Theatre

MUSIC

Birgitte Moyer, Chairman   *Number Of Faculty:* 3 Full-time, 8 Part-time
Number Of Students: 68   *Degrees Offered:* BA; BM; MM; MAT
Teaching Certification Available
Performing Groups: Chamber Orchestra; Chorus; Chamber Singers; Brass Ensemble; Contemporary Ensemble; String Quartet
Workshops/Festivals: California Music Center (Summer Chamber Music Workshop)

THEATRE

Robert Titlow, Chairman   *Number Of Faculty:* 4   *Number Of Students:* 70
Degrees Offered: AB   *Courses Offered:* Performance; Technical; Academic
Technical Training: Acting; Directing; Design
Teaching Certification Available
Financial Assistance: Assistantships, Scholarships and Work-Study Grants
Performing Groups: College of Notre Dame Players

COLLEGE OF SAN MATEO
1700 W Hillsdale Blvd, San Mateo   California 94402
415 574-6288

County and 2 Year
Arts Areas: Dance, Instrumental Music, Vocal Music, Theatre, Film Arts, Television and Visual Arts
Performance Facilities: CSM Little Theatre

(continued on next page)

DANCE

Angela Hudson, Chairman   **Number Of Faculty:** 2   **Number Of Students:** 125
Courses Offered: Folk; Square; Jazz; Modern; Ballet; Movement
Performing Groups: Ballet Theatre; Dance Production Company
Number Of Faculty: 7   **Number Of Students:** 200   **Degrees Offered:** AA
Financial Assistance: Scholarships
Performing Groups: Orchestra; County Symphony; Symphonic Band; Jazz Band; Choir; Chorale; Masterworks Chorale
Number Of Faculty: 4   **Number Of Students:** 150   **Degrees Offered:** AA
Financial Assistance: Scholarships
Performing Groups: Hillbarn Theatre; Children's Theatre; CSM Drama Company

COLLEGE OF THE SEQUOIAS
Mooney Blvd, Visalia   California 93277
209 732-4711 Ext 300
State and 2 Year
Arts Areas: Dance, Instrumental Music, Vocal Music, Theatre, Film Arts and Visual Arts

DANCE

Jean Shewey, Chairman   **Number Of Faculty:** 1   **Number Of Students:** 60
Degrees Offered: AA   **Courses Offered:** Modern; Social; Ballet; Folk & Square
Workshops/Festivals: Jazz Workshop; Modern Dance Workshop

MUSIC

George C Pappas, Dean of Fine Arts   **Number Of Faculty:** 3
Number Of Students: 250   **Degrees Offered:** AA
Courses Offered: Band; Chorus; Chamber Singers; Piano; Theory; Music History; Music Appreciation; Jazz Band
Financial Assistance: Scholarships
Performing Groups: COS Marching Band; Concert Choir; Chamber Singers; Jazz Band

THEATRE

George C Pappas, Chairman   **Number Of Faculty:** 3   **Number Of Students:** 50
Degrees Offered: AA
Courses Offered: Stagecraft; Lighting; Costume; Makeup; Acting; Oral Interpretation; History of the Theatre
Financial Assistance: Scholarships
Performing Groups: Sequoia Players; Music Theatre

COLLEGE OF THE SISKIYOUS
800 College Ave, Weed   California 96094
916 938-4463
County and 2 Year
Arts Areas: Dance, Instrumental Music, Vocal Music and Theatre
Performing Series: Performing Series   **Performance Facilities:** College Theatre
Number Of Faculty: 1 Part-time   **Number Of Students:** 20
Courses Offered: Dance Theatre   **Number Of Faculty:** 2
Number Of Students: 50   **Degrees Offered:** AA
Courses Offered: Theory; Fundamentals, Music Appreciation; Improvisation; Arranging; Various Instrumental & Vocal Courses plus Performance Courses
Financial Assistance: Scholarships and Work-Study Grants
Performing Groups: Vocal/Jazz Ensemble; Concert Choir; Chamber Choir; Jazz Combo; Community Choir; Community Stage Band
Workshops/Festivals: Vocal/Jazz Festival; Area High School and Elementary School Choral and Band Festivals
Number Of Faculty: 2   **Number Of Students:** 40   **Degrees Offered:** AA
Courses Offered: Theatre History; Stagecraft; Acting; Oral Interpretation; Makeup; Puppetry; Radio Workshop; Script Writing

(continued on next page)

Technical Training: Advanced Stagecraft
Financial Assistance: Scholarships and Work-Study Grants
Performing Groups: Summer Repertory Theatre

COMMUNITY MUSIC CENTER
544 Capp St, San Francisco   California 94110
415 647-6015
Private and Community
Arts Areas: Dance, Instrumental Music and Vocal Music
Performance Facilities: Small Recital Hall

DANCE

Grace Johnson, Chairman   **Number Of Faculty:** 2   **Number Of Students:** 77
Courses Offered: Modern Dance; Spanish & Latin-American Dance
Financial Assistance: Scholarships

MUSIC

Landon Young, Chairman   **Number Of Faculty:** 52   **Number Of Students:** 1,046
Courses Offered: Instrumental & Vocal Lessons; Theory & Sightsinging Classes
Financial Assistance: Scholarships
Performing Groups: SF Community Chorus; SF Community Orchestra; SF Children's Chorus; Coro Hispano
Workshops/Festivals: Chinese Music Workshop; Opera Workshop

COMPTON COMMUNITY COLLEGE
1111 E Artesia Blvd, Compton   California 90221
213 635-8081 Ext 303
2 Year and District
Arts Areas: Dance, Instrumental Music, Vocal Music, Theatre, Film Arts, Television, Visual Arts and Full Academic & Vocational Curriculum
Performing Series: Civic Symphony; Jazz Concerts; Children's Programs;
Lecture Series; Film Series; Theatre Arts; Dance Programs
Performance Facilities: Choral Room/Little Theatre; Gymnasium; "The Star" (Outdoor Performances)

DANCE

C Taul, Associate Professor of Physical Ed   **Number Of Faculty:** 2
Number Of Students: 25   **Degrees Offered:** AA
Courses Offered: Modern Dance Techniques; Dramatic Movement; Basic Ballet Techniques
Financial Assistance: Internships, Scholarships and Work-Study Grants
Performing Groups: Corps De Ballet

MUSIC

Manuel Leonardo, PhD, Professor   **Number Of Faculty:** 7
Number Of Students: 536   **Degrees Offered:** AA
Courses Offered: Music Appreciation; History of Music; Fundamentals of Music; Elementary & Intermediate Piano; Wind Instrument Training; Band; Elementary Voice; Choir; Musicianship; Afro-American Music; Beginning Folk & Classical Guitar; Jazz Ensemble; Popular/Jazz Piano; Electric Bass Instrument Training
Financial Assistance: Internships, Scholarships and Work-Study Grants
Performing Groups: CCC Marching Band; CCC Jazz Ensemble; Miz Jones' Group (Vocal)

THEATRE

Pieter J Van Niel, PhD, Associate Professor   **Number Of Faculty:** 2
Number Of Students: 42   **Degrees Offered:** AA
Courses Offered: Acting; Advanced Acting; Modern Drama; Rehearsal & Performance; Introduction to Drama; Project; Beginning Stagecraft; Intermediate & Advanced Stagecraft
Financial Assistance: Internships, Scholarships and Work-Study Grants
Performing Groups: The CCC Drama Group

(continued on next page)

Workshops/Festivals: Regular schedule of Minor and Major Productions, some of which travel to local schools within our District
Artists-In-Residence/Guest Artists: Dr Frances Steiner (Cellist & Symphony Director); R'Wanda Lewis (Dancer); Joyce Carol Thomas (Poet/Playwright)

CYPRESS COLLEGE
9200 Valley View, Cypress   California 90630
714 826-2220 Ext 293
County and 2 Year
Arts Areas: Instrumental Music, Vocal Music, Theatre and Visual Arts
Performance Facilities: Theater Arts Building; Fine Arts Building

MUSIC

Ronald Broadwell, Chairman   **Number Of Faculty:** 9   **Degrees Offered:** AA
Financial Assistance: Scholarships and Work-Study Grants
Performing Groups: Vocal & Instrumental

THEATRE

Mrs Kaleta Brown, Chairman   **Number Of Faculty:** 4   **Degrees Offered:** AA

DE ANZA COLLEGE
21250 Stevens Creek Blvd, Cupertino   California 95014
408 996-4567
2 Year and Community
Arts Areas: Dance, Instrumental Music, Vocal Music, Theatre, Film Arts, Television and Visual Arts
Performing Series: Performing Arts Series; Montage Series; Dance Series; Popular Guitar Series
Performance Facilities: Flint Center for the Performing Arts

DANCE

W Grant Gray, PhD, Chairman   **Number Of Faculty:** 2 Full-time, 7 Part-time
Number Of Students: 450   **Degrees Offered:** AA
Courses Offered: Ballet, Modern; Jazz; Fad; Improvisation; Music & Movement; Children's Dance; Theater Dance; Dance Repertory; Tap
Technical Training: Technical Dance Production
Financial Assistance: Assistantships, Scholarships, Work-Study Grants and Tutor-Departmental Student Work
Performing Groups: De Anza Dancers; The Assortment
Workshops/Festivals: Master Classes by Guest Artists; "Festivity" Scholarship benefit; Professional performing troupes; Film Festival; Field Trips; Technique Classes in Artist Studios

MUSIC

William Cleveland, Division Administrator Fine Arts
Number Of Faculty: 7 Full-time, 8 Part-time   **Number Of Students:** 200
Degrees Offered: AA
Courses Offered: Lower Division Theory, Music Literature, Performance Groups, Jazz Studies, Electronic Music
Financial Assistance: Scholarships and Work-Study Grants
Performing Groups: De Anza College Chorale & Concert Band; Vintage Singers; Jazz Ensembles; String Orchestra
Workshops/Festivals: Instrumental Workshops for Local Musicians and School Student Groups; Choral Festivals (high school and college)

THEATRE

William Cleveland, Division Administrator Fine Arts
Number Of Faculty: 5 Full-time, 3 Part-time   **Number Of Students:** 250
Degrees Offered: AA
Courses Offered: Introduction to Theater Arts; Dramatic Literature; Principles of Acting; Actors Ensemble; Readers' Theater; Directing; Play Production; Painting & Props; Stage Lighting & Sound; Theater

(continued on next page)

Graphics & Scenic Design; Costume History & Fabrics; Theatrical Makeup; Playwriting; Dramatics; Children's Theater; Puppetry; Chicano Dramatic Lit; Stage Diction; Workshop in Chicano Teatro; Rehearsal & Performance
Financial Assistance: Scholarships and Work-Study Grants
Artists-In-Residence/Guest Artists: Ella Fitzgerald; John Carradine; Celeste Holm

---

FOOTHILL COLLEGE
El Monte Rd, Los Altos Hills   California 94022
415 948-8590 Ext 262
County and 2 Year
Arts Areas: Dance, Instrumental Music, Vocal Music, Theatre, Film Arts, Television and Visual Arts
Performing Series: Summer Repertory Theatre Series
Performance Facilities: Foothill College Theatre; Appreciation Hall; Campus Center

DANCE

Marlene Poletti, Chief Instructor   *Number Of Faculty:* 2
Number Of Students: 175   *Degrees Offered:* AA
Technical Training: Modern Jazz; Modern Ballet; Modern Dance; Tap; Mexican Folk; Folk; Social Dancing
Workshops/Festivals: Annual Dance Festival

MUSIC

John Mortarotti, Chairman, Fine Arts Division   *Number Of Faculty:* 7
Number Of Students: 300   *Degrees Offered:* AA
Courses Offered: Music Comprehension; Music History; Musicianship & Harmony; Contemporary Music Styles; Afro - American Music; Music Fundamentals; Jazz Ensemble
Technical Training: Commercial Music Program; Piano Tuning & Repair Program
Financial Assistance: Scholarships
Performing Groups: Chorale; Concert Choir; Jazz Vocal Ensemble; String Orchestra; Orchestra; Woodwind Ensemble; Nora Vista Symphony; Jazz Ensemble; Band; Chamber Ensemble
Workshops/Festivals: Jazz Festival; Workshops featuring top Professional Instrumentalists; Young Conductors' Workshop

THEATRE

John Mortarotti, Chairman, Fine Arts Division   *Number Of Faculty:* 3
Number Of Students: 250   *Degrees Offered:* AA
Courses Offered: Theatre Appreciation; Dramatic Lit; Principles of Acting; Black Theatre; Play Production; Makeup; Stagecraft; Lighting; Design; Voice & Diction; Classic Theatre
Financial Assistance: Scholarships
Performing Groups: Summer Repertory Theatre; Annual Summer Music Theatre; Quarterly Productions

---

FRESNO CITY COLLEGE
1101 E University Ave, Fresno   California 93741
209 442-4600
County and 2 Year
Arts Areas: Dance, Instrumental Music, Vocal Music, Theatre, Film Arts and Visual Arts
Performing Series: Drama, Music, Film Series; Combination Midwinter Festival of the Arts
Performance Facilities: Theatre; Recital Hall; Forum Hall "A"; Forum Hall "B"; Main Hall of Cafeteria

DANCE

Janice Janses, Instructor   *Number Of Faculty:* 2   *Number Of Students:* 100
Courses Offered: Fundamentals of Dance, Tap, Jazz, Ballet
Technical Training: Students work on major dance productions each year
Financial Assistance: Scholarships and Work-Study Grants
Performing Groups: Fresno City College Dance Company; Mexican Folk Dance Troupe; Afro - American Creativity Workshop
Workshops/Festivals: Mini - Concerts and Performances

(continued on next page)

MUSIC

Vincent Moats, Department Head
Number Of Faculty: 5 Full-time, 10 Part-time   **Number Of Students:** 150
Degrees Offered: AA in Instrumental, Vocal, Piano & Guitar
Courses Offered: Instrumental, Vocal, Piano including Performance Lab Activities
Technical Training: Work for credit in or on Summer Musical Theatre Production
Financial Assistance: Scholarships and Work-Study Grants
Performing Groups: College-Community Orchestra; Jazz Ensemble (vocal); Jazz Band; Marching & Studio Bands; Choir; Vocal Ensembles

THEATRE

Tom Wright, Department Head   **Number Of Faculty:** 4
Number Of Students: 200   **Degrees Offered:** AA in Theatre Arts
Courses Offered: Techniques of Acting; Intro to Theatre; Stage Costume & Makeup; Lab; Theatre Literature
Financial Assistance: Scholarships and Work-Study Grants
Performing Groups: Major Productions; Student - directed One - Acts; Reader's Theatre
Workshops/Festivals: Summer Musical Theatre
Artists-In-Residence/Guest Artists: Dance Theatre of Seattle; Eric Hawkins Dance Company

---

FRESNO PACIFIC COLLEGE
1717 S Chestnut, Fresno   California 93702
207 251-7194 Ext 68

2049824

Private and 4 Year
Arts Areas: Instrumental Music, Vocal Music, Theatre and Visual Arts
Performance Facilities: Alumni Hall; College Amphitheater

MUSIC

Curtis Funk, Chairman   **Number Of Faculty:** 11   **Number Of Students:** 40
Degrees Offered: BA Mus   **Courses Offered:** Vocal & Instrumental
Technical Training: Private Instruction in most instruments & voice
Teaching Certification Available
Financial Assistance: Scholarships and Work-Study Grants
Performing Groups: Concert Choir; String Quartet; Jazz Band; Chamber Choir; Wind Ensemble
Workshops/Festivals: Central California Choral Conductors Clinic co-sponsored with Fresno School Music Department

THEATRE

James Becker, Chairman   **Number Of Faculty:** 2   **Number Of Students:** 20
Degrees Offered: BA Drama - Communication   **Teaching Certification Available**
Financial Assistance: Scholarships and Work-Study Grants

FULLERTON COLLEGE
321 E Chapman Ave, Fullerton   California 92632
714 871-8000

State and 2 Year
Arts Areas: Dance, Instrumental Music, Vocal Music, Theatre and Visual Arts
Performing Series: Artist - Lecture Series; Performing Arts Series
Performance Facilities: Campus Theatre; Studio Theatre

DANCE

Florance English, Chairman   **Number Of Faculty:** 4
Performing Groups: Modern & Jazz Groups

MUSIC

Darwin Frederickson, Chairman   **Number Of Faculty:** 14
Number Of Students: 250   **Technical Training:** Commercial Music
Workshops/Festivals: Choral Festival; Jazz Festival; Vocal Jazz Festival

(continued on next page)

THEATRE

George Archambeault, Chairman   **Number Of Faculty:** 4
Number Of Students: 90   **Technical Training:** Stage Technique
Performing Groups: Theatre Workshop & Major Productions
Workshops/Festivals: LA Center Theatre- Improviosational Theatre
Artists-In-Residence/Guest Artists: Marnie Nixon, Vocalist

GAVILAN COLLEGE
5055 Santa Teresa Blvd, Gilroy   California 95020
408 847-1400

County and 2 Year
Arts Areas: Instrumental Music, Vocal Music, Theatre, Film Arts and Visual Arts
Performance Facilities: Theatre

MUSIC

Ron Ward, Director   **Number Of Faculty:** 4   **Degrees Offered:** AA
Courses Offered: All Instruments - Instruction; Voice; Stage Band; Concert Choir
Technical Training: Advanced Musicianship
Financial Assistance: Scholarships and Work-Study Grants
Performing Groups: Community Band; Jazz Band
Workshops/Festivals: Easter Choir Festival; Christmas Feast of Lights (Choir Presentation)

THEATRE

Marilyn Abad, Director   **Number Of Faculty:** 1   **Degrees Offered:** AA
Courses Offered: Actor's Workshop; Stage Production; Independent & Field Study
Financial Assistance: Scholarships and Work-Study Grants
Performing Groups: Actor's Workshop
Workshops/Festivals: Three Productions per year; Co-Sponsors Children's stage productions for area schools
Artists-In-Residence/Guest Artists: Tandy Beal Modern Dance Company; Gilbert and Sullivan Opera Society

---

GROSSMONT COLLEGE
8800 Grossmont College Dr, El Cajon   California 92020
714 465-1700 Ext 321

County and 2 Year
Arts Areas: Dance, Instrumental Music, Vocal Music, Theatre, Film Arts, Television and Visual Arts
Performing Series: Drama, Dance & Music
Performance Facilities: Performing Arts Center; Student Center; Fine Arts Recital Hall; Stagehouse Theatre

DANCE

Dr Lolita D Carter, Director   **Number Of Faculty:** 5
Number Of Students: 400   **Degrees Offered:** AA
Courses Offered: Folk Dance; Modern Dance; Jazz Dance; Ballet; Dance Theatre; Aerobic Dance
Financial Assistance: Scholarships and Work-Study Grants
Performing Groups: Grossmont College Dance Group

MUSIC

Carroll M Reed, Chairman   **Number Of Faculty:** 12   **Number Of Students:** 1500
Degrees Offered: AA
Courses Offered: Great Music Listening; Piano; Guitar; Musicianship; History of Jazz & Modern Music; Harmony; Voice; Fundamentals of Electronic Music; Choir; Band - Orchestra
Financial Assistance: Scholarships and Work-Study Grants
Performing Groups: Orchestra; Concert, Varsity & Stage Bands; Choir; Chamber Chorale - String Ensemble; Brass & Guitar Ensembles; Woodwind Ensemble

THEATRE

Clark G Mires, Chairman, Communication Arts Department
Number Of Faculty: 3   **Number Of Students:** 325   **Degrees Offered:** AA

(*continued on next page*)

Courses Offered: Stagecraft; Makeup & Costume Production; Intro to Theatre; History of the Theatre; Stage & TV Acting; Historic Costume for the Theatre; Costume Construction; Techniques of Directing
Financial Assistance: Scholarships and Work-Study Grants
Performing Groups: Griffin Players

HARTNELL COLLEGE
156 Homestead Ave, Salinas   California 93901
408 758-8211
County and 2 Year
Arts Areas: Dance, Instrumental Music, Vocal Music, Theatre, Film Arts, Television and Visual Arts
Performing Series: Theatre Season Series; Hartnell Presents Lecture & Concert Series; Concert Season Series

DANCE

Dance under auspices of Physical Education Department

MUSIC

Robert Lee, Chairman   **Number Of Faculty:** 8   **Number Of Students:** 225
Degrees Offered: AA
Financial Assistance: Scholarships and Work-Study Grants
Performing Groups: Hartnell College Community Chorus; Hartnell College Chamber Singers; Choir; Chamber Orchestra; Band; Jazz Ensemble; Laborarory Band
Workshops/Festivals: Spring Festival of the Arts; Concert Series

THEATRE

Robert Lee/Ron Danko, Chairmen   **Number Of Faculty:** 5
Number Of Students: 150   **Degrees Offered:** AA
Financial Assistance: Scholarships and Work-Study Grants
Performing Groups: Hartnell Theatre Company; Hartnell Children's Theatre Company
Workshops/Festivals: Children's Theatre Festival; Spring Festival of the Arts; Summer Theatre Program

---

HUMBOLDT STATE UNIVERSITY
Arcata   California 95521, 707 826-3011
State and 4 Year
Arts Areas: Dance, Instrumental Music, Vocal Music, Theatre, Film Arts and Visual Arts
Performance Facilities: Music Recital Hall; Gist Hall Experimental Theatre and Theatre
John Van Duzer Theatre; Studio Theatre

DANCE

Dance program under auspices of Physical Education   **Number Of Faculty:** 2
Number Of Students: 65
Courses Offered: Stage Movement & Mime; Creative Movement for Children; Modern Dance; Square Dance; Folk Dance; Folk Dance Workshop; Children's Dance
Financial Assistance: Work-Study Grants
Performing Groups: Modern & Folk Dance
Workshops/Festivals: Elementary School Lecture/Demonstrations; High School Lecture/Demonstrations

MUSIC

David Smith, Chairman   **Number Of Faculty:** 16   **Number Of Students:** 140
Degrees Offered: BA   **Technical Training:** Reed Making; Instrument Repair
Teaching Certification Available
Financial Assistance: Scholarships and Work-Study Grants
Performing Groups: Humboldt Chorale; Concert Choir; Symphony Orchestra; Symphonic Band; Intermediate Wind Ensemble; Piano Ensemble; Chamber Ensemble; Chamber Singers
Workshops/Festivals: Opera Workshop; General Chamber Music Workshop; Brass Chamber Music Workshop; Sequoia Chamber Music Workshop; Elementary Education Summer Workshop

(continued on next page)

THEATRE

Charles Myers, Chairman, Theatre Arts Department   **Number Of Faculty:** 15
Number Of Students: 155   **Degrees Offered:** BA; MA; MFA
Technical Training: Theatrical Design; Film Production; Costume Pattern Drafting
Teaching Certification Available
Financial Assistance: Scholarships and Work-Study Grants
Performing Groups: University Theatre; Puppetry Group; Improvisational Theatre; Mime Troupe
Workshops/Festivals: Annual International Student Film Festival

---

IMPERIAL VALLEY COLLEGE
Imperial   California 92251, 714 352-8320
State and 2 Year
Arts Areas: Dance, Instrumental Music, Vocal Music, Theatre and Film Arts
Performance Facilities: Multipurpose Building

DANCE

Gary Hulst, Chairman, Physical Education Department   **Number Of Faculty:** 1
Number Of Students: 40   **Degrees Offered:** AA

MUSIC

Rollie Wisbrock, Chairman   **Number Of Faculty:** 23   **Number Of Students:** 75
Degrees Offered: AA
Financial Assistance: Scholarships and Work-Study Grants
Number Of Faculty: 1 Part-time   **Number Of Students:** 30   **Degrees Offered:** AA
Financial Assistance: Scholarships and Work-Study Grants

INTERNATIONAL COLLEGE
1019 Gayley Ave, Los Angeles   California 90024
213 477-6761
Private and 4 Year
Arts Areas: Dance, Instrumental Music, Theatre, Film Arts and Visual Arts

DANCE

Number Of Faculty: 2   **Degrees Offered:** BA; MA; PhD   **Courses Offered:** African; Contemporary

MUSIC

Number Of Faculty: 12   **Degrees Offered:** BA; MA; PhD
Courses Offered: Musical Theater; Computer Graphic/Music; Ethnomusicology; Orchestra Conducting &
Management; Music Criticism; History & Theory; Performance & Theory
Financial Assistance: Loans   **Number Of Faculty:** 5
Degrees Offered: BA; MA; PhD

THEATRE

Financial Assistance: Loans

LANEY COLLEGE
900 Fallon St, Oakland   California 94607
415 834-5740 Ext 325
State and 2 Year
Arts Areas: Dance, Instrumental Music, Vocal Music, Theatre and Television
Performing Series: University Community Service Program
Performance Facilities: Laney College Theatre

DANCE

Elendar Barnes, Instructor   **Number Of Faculty:** 1   **Number Of Students:** 655
Degrees Offered: AA
Financial Assistance: Work-Study Grants

(*continued on next page*)

MUSIC

Elvo D'Amante, Chairman   **Number Of Faculty:** 5   **Number Of Students:** 2,733
Degrees Offered: AA
Courses Offered: Music Fundamentals; Basic Musicianship; Harmony; Introduction to Musical Literature;
Voice; String Ensemble; Opera Workshop; Opera Chorus; College Choir; Elementary & Intermediate
Piano; Vocal Ensemble; College Band; Jazz Workshop; College Orchestra; Instrumental Ensemble; Music
Appreciation; Jazz, Blues and Popular Music in the American Culture; Classic Guitar; Chinese Orchestra
Financial Assistance: Work-Study Grants

THEATRE

Lew Levinson, Chairman   **Number Of Faculty:** 2   **Number Of Students:** 648
Degrees Offered: AA
Courses Offered: Introduction to the Theatre Arts; Principles & Theory of Acting; Theatre; Black
American Theatre History; Rehearsal & Production; Stagecraft; Makeup; Advanced Body Movement &
Mime; Acting Techniques & the History of Street Theatre; Stage Lighting; Introduction to Dramatic
Literature
Financial Assistance: Work-Study Grants

LOMA LINDA UNIVERSITY
Riverside   California 92515, 714 785-2036
Private and 4 Year
Arts Areas: Instrumental Music, Vocal Music and Visual Arts
Performing Series: "Our Own Concert Series"
Performance Facilities: Hole Memorial Auditorium; La Sierra Alumni Pavilion

MUSIC

H Allen Craw, PhD, Chairman, Professor of Music   **Number Of Faculty:** 7
Number Of Students: 30
Degrees Offered: BA (Music Major); B Mus; MA in teaching
Teaching Certification Available
Financial Assistance: Scholarships and Work-Study Grants
Performing Groups: Consort Woodstock Brass Group; University Band; Collegiate Choir; University
Singers; University Chamber Orchestra
Workshops/Festivals: Institute of Orchestral Conducting & Symphonic Performance with Herbert
Blomstedt; Master Workshop in Choral Rehearsal & Performance Techniques with Sir David Willcocks

---

LONE MOUNTAIN COLLEGE, SAN FRANCISCO
2800 Turk Blvd, San Francisco   California 94118
415 752-7000 Ext 243
Private, 4 Year and Graduate Program
Arts Areas: Dance, Instrumental Music, Vocal Music, Theatre, Visual Arts and Video
Performing Series: Music Faculty Concert Series; Dance Faculty Concert Series

MUSIC

Dr Mack Crooks, Chairman   **Number Of Faculty:** 20   **Number Of Students:** 35
Degrees Offered: BA; MA; BM; MM
Courses Offered: Music History; Music Theory; Composition; Ensembles: Vocal & Jazz, Applied Music
Financial Assistance: Scholarships and Work-Study Grants
Performing Groups: Vocal & Jazz Ensembles; Chamber & Early Music Ensemble
Workshops/Festivals: Numerous Workshops by faculty and students throughout the academic year.

THEATRE

Mr Sean McKenna, Chairman   **Number Of Faculty:** 12   **Number Of Students:** 35
Degrees Offered: BA; MA
Courses Offered: Acting; Voice; Movement; Technical Theatre; Playwriting; Directing; Management;
Dramatic Lit; Design; Production
Financial Assistance: Scholarships and Work-Study Grants

LOS ANGELES BAPTIST COLLEGE
PO Box 878, Newhall   California 91322
805 259-3540
   Private and 4 Year   *Arts Areas:* Instrumental Music and Vocal Music

MUSIC

Ken De Jong, Chairman   *Number Of Faculty:* 4   *Number Of Students:* 50
Degrees Offered: BA   *Teaching Certification Available*
Financial Assistance: Scholarships and Work-Study Grants
Performing Groups: Choir; Mixed Ensembles; Instrumental Ensembles

LOS ANGELES HARBOR COLLEGE
1111 Figueroa Pl, Wilmington   California 90744
213 518-1000
   City and 2 Year
   Arts Areas: Dance, Instrumental Music, Vocal Music and Theatre
   Performance Facilities: Mainstage Theater; Arena Theater; Recital Hall

DANCE

Sachiye Nakano, Associate Professor   *Number Of Faculty:* 1
Number Of Students: 100
Courses Offered: Music Analysis & Modern Dance; Modern Dance; Dance Composition; Modern Dance
Production; Ballet
Performing Groups: LA Harbor College Dance Company
Workshops/Festivals: LA Harbor College Dance Company Concert

MUSIC

Robert H Billings, Chairman   *Number Of Faculty:* 9
Number Of Students: 1,200   *Degrees Offered:* AA transfer; AA Commercial Music
Courses Offered: Theory; History; Performance; Commercial
Technical Training: Recording & Commercial Music
Performing Groups: Choir; Chorale; Concert Band; Stage Band; Brass Ensemble; Chamber Ensemble
Workshops/Festivals: Spring Chorale Festival; Annual Summer Musical

THEATRE

Number Of Faculty: 3   *Number Of Students:* 400   *Degrees Offered:* AA
Performing Groups: Annual Summer Musical

LOS ANGELES SOUTHWEST COLLEGE
1600 W Imperial Hwy, Los Angeles   California 90047
213 757-9251
   2 Year and Community
   Arts Areas: Dance, Instrumental Music, Vocal Music, Theatre, Film Arts, Television and Visual Arts

DANCE

Jan Riggs, Instructor
Dance program under auspices of Physical Education Department
Number Of Faculty: 1   *Number Of Students:* 25   *Degrees Offered:* AA
Courses Offered: Modern; Tap
Financial Assistance: Scholarships and Work-Study Grants
Performing Groups: Dance Club

MUSIC

Roland Jackson, Department Head   *Number Of Faculty:* 3
Number Of Students: 100   *Degrees Offered:* AA
Financial Assistance: Scholarships and Work-Study Grants
Performing Groups: Studio Jazz Band; College Choir

(continued on next page)

THEATRE

Dr Merrilee Stafford, Department Head   *Number Of Faculty:* 2
Number Of Students: 50   *Courses Offered:* AA
Financial Assistance: Scholarships and Work-Study Grants
Workshops/Festivals: One Play per Semester

LOS ANGELES VALLEY COLLEGE
5800 Fulton Ave, Van Nuys   California 91401
213 781-1200
County and 2 Year
Arts Areas: Dance, Instrumental Music, Vocal Music, Theatre, Film Arts, Television and Visual Arts

DANCE

Dance program under auspices of Physical Education Department

MUSIC

Richard Carlson, Professor   *Number Of Faculty:* 13
Number Of Students: 600   *Degrees Offered:* AA
Financial Assistance: Scholarships
Performing Groups: Rock Marching Band; Studio Jazz Band; Symphony Orchestra; Two Choral Groups
Workshops/Festivals: Opera Workshop; High School Jazz Band Ensemble

THEATRE

E Peter Mauk, Professor   *Number Of Faculty:* 6   *Number Of Students:* 300
Degrees Offered: AA   *Financial Assistance:* Scholarships
Performing Groups: Valley Collegiate Playerss
Workshops/Festivals: High School One-Act Play Festival

MIRA COSTA COMMUNITY COLLEGE
1 Bernard Dr, Oceanside   California 92054
714 757-2121
County and 2 Year
Keith L Broman Dean of Continuing Education
Arts Areas: Dance, Instrumental Music, Vocal Music, Theatre and Visual Arts
Performing Series: College Community Orchestra Series; Drama Series; Chamber Music Series; Concert Association Series
Performance Facilities: Little Theatre; Gymnasium

DANCE

Keith Broman, Dean   *Number Of Faculty:* 3 Part-time
Number Of Students: 150   *Degrees Offered:* AA; AS
Courses Offered: Ballet 1,2,3,4; Modern & Theatrical Dance
Financial Assistance: Work-Study Grants
Performing Groups: Students perform, if qualified, with the North County Ballet Company
Workshops/Festivals: North County Ballet; Bab Banas Modern Dance Workshop; Hartford Ballet

MUSIC

Howard Ganz, Chairman   *Number Of Faculty:* 4   *Number Of Students:* 400
Degrees Offered: AA; AS
Courses Offered: Harmony; Counterpoint; History; Performance; Jazz; Band; Orchestra; Chorus & Smaller Ensembles
Technical Training: Electronic Music
Financial Assistance: Scholarships and Work-Study Grants
Performing Groups: Spartan Singers; MCC Jazz Band; College Orchestra; College Chorus; Various Small Ensembles
Workshops/Festivals: North County Jazz Festival; Orchestra Talent Competition; Church Choir Festival

(continued on next page)

THEATRE

Mary Lou Gombar, Chairman   **Number Of Faculty:** 3   **Number Of Students:** 150
Degrees Offered: AA; AS
Courses Offered: Theater Appreciation; Oral Interpretation; Dramatic Literature; Children's Theater; Creative Dramatics; Voice & Diction; Playwriting; Acting; Mime; Makeup; Costume Design & Construction; Stage Craft; Scene Design & Puppetry
Financial Assistance: Scholarships and Work-Study Grants
Performing Groups: Mime Troupe; MCC Drama Company; Community - College Theater; Reader's Theater
Workshops/Festivals: Puppetry Workshop with Bruce Chesse ; Mime with Miko

---

MODESTO JUNIOR COLLEGE
College Ave, Modesto   California 95350
209 526-2000 Ext 270
County and 2 Year
Arts Areas: Dance, Instrumental Music, Vocal Music, Theatre, Film Arts, Television and Visual Arts
Performing Series: MJC Presents! Series; Special Events Sponsored by Community Services Office
Performance Facilities: Auditorium; Recital Hall; Gymnasium; Cabaret - West

DANCE

Douglas Hodge, Chairman
Dance program under auspices of Physical Education Department
Number Of Faculty: 2 Part-time   **Degrees Offered:** AA
Financial Assistance: Scholarships and Work-Study Grants

MUSIC

Dr Robert W Larson, Chairman   **Number Of Faculty:** 7   **Degrees Offered:** AA
Financial Assistance: Scholarships and Work-Study Grants
Performing Groups: Orchestra; Wind Symphony; Opera Theater; Vocal Jazz Ensemble; Masterworks Chorus; Symphonic Choir
Workshops/Festivals: Festival of Winds; Vocal Jazz Festival

THEATRE

Curtis A Ennen, Chairman   **Number Of Faculty:** 3   **Degrees Offered:** AA
Financial Assistance: Scholarships and Work-Study Grants
Workshops/Festivals: Annual Performing Arts Workshop; MJC Summer Theater

---

MOUNT SAINT MARY'S COLLEGE
12001 Chalon Rd, Los Angeles   California 90049
213 476-2237
Private and 4 Year
Arts Areas: Instrumental Music, Vocal Music and Visual Arts
Performance Facilities: Mount Saint Mary's College Theater; Jose Drudis Biada Hall - Art Gallery

MUSIC

Sister Teresita Espinosa, Chairman   **Number Of Faculty:** 10
Number Of Students: 40   **Degrees Offered:** BA; BMus
Courses Offered: Performance; Theory & Composition
Technical Training: Music History; Music Education; Church Music
Teaching Certification Available
Financial Assistance: Scholarships and Work-Study Grants
Performing Groups: Mount - Community Orchestra; Mount Chorus; Women's Chamber Ensemble; Chamber Music Group
Workshops/Festivals: Spring Choral Festival; Chamber Music Seminar

MOUNT SAN ANTONIO COLLEGE

1100 N Grand Ave, Walnut   California 91789
714 598-2811

2 Year and Public, Community
Arts Areas: Dance, Instrumental Music, Vocal Music, Theatre, Film Arts, Television and Visual Arts
Performing Series: Lively Arts Concert Series - Fall, Spring, Summer; Lively Arts Children's Series
Performance Facilities: Little Theatre; Gymnasium; Auditorium

DANCE

Beth Spicer, Instructor
Dance program under auspices of Physical Education Department
Number Of Faculty: 5   **Number Of Students:** 200   **Degrees Offered:** AA
Financial Assistance: Scholarships, Work-Study Grants and BEOG; NDSL

MUSIC

Lewis Forney, Chairperson   **Number Of Faculty:** 9 Day, 7 Evening
Number Of Students: 350   **Degrees Offered:** AA; AS
Financial Assistance: Scholarships, Work-Study Grants and BEOG, NDSL
Performing Groups: College Choir; Men's & Women's Glee Clubs; Stage, Concert & Jazz Band; Concert Singers
Workshops/Festivals: Annual Paul Weston Scholarship Concert; Christmas Concert; Spring Music Festival Concert; Annual Music at Noon Concerts; Artists-in-Residence Series

THEATRE

Carter Doran, Instructor   **Number Of Faculty:** 9 Day, 9 Evening
Number Of Students: 450   **Degrees Offered:** AA; AS
Financial Assistance: Scholarships, Work-Study Grants and BEOG, NDSL
Performing Groups: MSAC Players; Tarradiddle Travellers; Reader's Theatre; Forensics

MOUNT SAN JACINTO COLLEGE

21400 Hwy 79, San Jacinto   California 92383
741 654-7321 Ext 235

State and 2 Year
Arts Areas: Dance, Instrumental Music, Vocal Music, Theatre and Film Arts
Performing Series: Major Dramatic Plays; Opera; Musical Concerts
Performance Facilities: Little Theatre; Music Room; Arena Theatre

DANCE

Louis Canter, Dean of Academic Instruction   **Number Of Faculty:** 1
Number Of Students: 60   **Degrees Offered:** AA; AS
Courses Offered: Modern Dance
Financial Assistance: Scholarships and Work-Study Grants

MUSIC

Louis Canter, Dean of Academic Instruction   **Number Of Faculty:** 4
Number Of Students: 175   **Degrees Offered:** AA; AS
Courses Offered: Guitar I; Music Fundamentals; Music Theory; Beginning Piano; Intermediate Piano; Jazz Improvisation; Concert Band; Wind & Percussion Instruments; College Singers; Opera Workshop; History & Appreciation of Music
Financial Assistance: Scholarships and Work-Study Grants
Performing Groups: Performing Arts Guild; Orchestra; Band; Chorus; Opera
Workshops/Festivals: Summer Music Camp

THEATRE

Louis Canter, Dean of Academic Instruction   **Number Of Faculty:** 1
Number Of Students: 85   **Degrees Offered:** AA; AS
Courses Offered: Stage Diction; Fundamentals of Acting; Advanced Acting Techniques; Drama Workshop;

(continued on next page)

Technical Theatre; Introduction & History of Theatre Arts
Financial Assistance: Scholarships and Work-Study Grants
Performing Groups: Theatre Guild

MUSIC & ARTS INSTITUTE OF SAN FRANCISCO
2622 Jackson St, San Francisco   California 94115
415 567-1445

Private and 4 Year   *Arts Areas:* Instrumental Music and Vocal Music
Performing Series: Special Events Series
Performance Facilities: Recital Hall

MUSIC

Ross McKee, Director   *Number Of Faculty:* 23   *Number Of Students:* 89
Degrees Offered: BM; Post-Graduate Studies
Courses Offered: Applied Music: Voice, Piano, Musical Instruments; Accompanying/Coaching; Piano Pedagogy; Music Theory; Composition
Financial Assistance: Assistantships, Scholarships, Work-Study Grants and Extended Payment Plan
Performing Groups: Soloists; Duo-Piano Consortium; Guitar Ensemble; Instrumental Ensemble
Workshops/Festivals: Master Classes; Special Events

THEATRE

Walter Teschan, Chairman
Artists-In-Residence/Guest Artists: Rey De La Torre; Hermann Reutter

NAPA COLLEGE
2277 Napa Valley Hwy, Napa   California 94558
707 255-2100 Ext 274

County and 2 Year
Arts Areas: Dance, Instrumental Music, Vocal Music, Theatre, Film Arts, Television and Visual Arts
Performing Series: Napa College Concert Series; Music Department Concert Series; NC Film Series
Performance Facilities: Little Theatre

DANCE

Olga Schneider, Instructor   *Number Of Faculty:* 1   *Number Of Students:* 25

MUSIC

Michael R Tausig, Chairman   *Number Of Faculty:* 6   *Number Of Students:* 300
Degrees Offered: AA   *Courses Offered:* Theory; Vocal; History; Instrumental
Financial Assistance: Scholarships and Work-Study Grants
Performing Groups: Concert Choir; Swing Chorale; Jazz Ensemble; Chamber Singers; Treble Chorus; Wind Ensemble; Concert Band; Orchestra

THEATRE

Jan Molen, Director   *Number Of Faculty:* 3   *Number Of Students:* 30
Degrees Offered: AA
Financial Assistance: Scholarships and Work-Study Grants
Performing Groups: NAPA Drama Department Presents

OHLONE COLLEGE
PO Box 909, Fremont   California 94538
415 657-2100

2 Year and Community College District
Arts Areas: Dance, Instrumental Music, Vocal Music, Theatre and Television
Performing Series: Summer Performing Arts Festival; Recital Series; String Orchestra Concert Series; Repertory Theatre

(continued on next page)

MUSIC

Dr G S Smith, Chairperson   *Number Of Faculty:* 11   *Number Of Students:* 580
Degrees Offered: AA
Financial Assistance: Work-Study Grants
Performing Groups: State Bands; Chamber Ensemble; College Chorus; Cantorum Chorus; Chamber Chorus; String Orchestra; Band
Workshops/Festivals: Choral, Chamber & Instrumental Workshops; Spring Festival of Contemporary Choral Literature

THEATRE

G Craig Jackson, Chairperson   *Number Of Faculty:* 2
Number Of Students: 86   *Degrees Offered:* AA
Technical Training: Technical Theatre; Lighting & Sound Set Design
Financial Assistance: Scholarships and Student Help Work Assignments
Performing Groups: Rehearsal & Performance Classes; Repertory Theatre
Workshops/Festivals: Summer Performing Arts Festival

ORANGE COAST COLLEGE
2701 Fairview Rd, Costa Mesa   California 92626
714 556-5725
State and 2 Year
Arts Areas: Dance, Instrumental Music, Vocal Music, Theatre, Film Arts, Television and Visual Arts
Performance Facilities: Auditorium; Fine Arts Halls; Drama Lab Theater

DANCE

Dorothy Duddridge, Chairman   *Number Of Faculty:* 5
Financial Assistance: Scholarships

MUSIC

Paul Cox, Chairman   *Number Of Faculty:* 12   *Degrees Offered:* AA
Financial Assistance: Scholarships
Performing Groups: College Choir; Chorale; Chamber Singers; Symphonic Chorale; Symphony Orchestra; Concert Band; Jazz Ensemble
Workshops/Festivals: OCC Jazz Festival; Stan Kenton Clinic; Orange County Honor Band; High School Invitational Choir Festival

THEATRE

Number Of Faculty: 4   *Financial Assistance:* Scholarships
Performing Groups: Environmental Theatre Group; Mime; Performance & Rehearsal Classes
Workshops/Festivals: High School Invitational Theatre Festival

---

PACIFIC UNION COLLEGE
Angwin   California 94508, 707 965-6211
Private and 4 Year
Arts Areas: Instrumental Music, Vocal Music and Visual Arts
Performing Series: Concert Series; Candlelight Series
Performance Facilities: Pacific Auditorium; Irwin Hall; Paulin Hall

MUSIC

James Kempstel, Chairman   *Number Of Faculty:* AA
Degrees Offered: BMus; MMus; BMusEd
Courses Offered: Music Education; Performance; Piano Pedagogy; History; Literature
Teaching Certification Available
Financial Assistance: Scholarships and Work-Study Grants
Performing Groups: Pro Musica; Collegeiate Choral; PUC Orchestra; Brass Ensemble
Workshops/Festivals: Kato Havas String Workshop; Choral Workshop; Invitational Band Workshop

UNIVERSITY OF THE PACIFIC
3601 Pacific Ave, Stockton   California 95211
209 946-2311

Private and 4 Year
Arts Areas: Instrumental Music, Vocal Music and Theatre
Performance Facilities: The Long Theatre; Little Theatre; Fallon House Summer Theatre
University Center Theatre; Rotunda Theatre; Conservatory of Music Auditorium

DANCE

Dr Sy M Kahn, Chairman, Drama Department
Dance program under auspices of Drama Department
Number Of Faculty: 1   **Degrees Offered:** Drama BA with emphasis in Dance
Financial Assistance: Scholarships and Work-Study Grants

MUSIC

Ira Lehn, Dean, Conservatory of Music   **Number Of Faculty:** 35
Number Of Students: 200   **Degrees Offered:** BMusEd; MMusEd; DMusEd
Courses Offered: Performance; Music Education; Music Therapy; Music History; Music
Theory-Composition
Teaching Certification Available
Financial Assistance: Scholarships, Work-Study Grants and Talent Awards
Performing Groups: Ensembles in Residence: The Pacific Arts Woodwind Quintet, The Sierra String
Quartet
Workshops/Festivals: Five week-long Summer Music Camps for Junior & Senior Students

THEATRE

Sy Kahn, Chairman   **Number Of Faculty:** 7   **Number Of Students:** 60
Degrees Offered: BA   **Teaching Certification Available**
Performing Groups: The Columbia Company
Workshops/Festivals: Summer Resident theatre group at Fallon House in Columbia State Park, Columbia,
CA (eight weeks)

PALOMAR COLLEGE
1140 W Mission, San Marcos   California 92069
714 744-1150 Ext 447

State and 2 Year
Arts Areas: Dance, Instrumental Music, Vocal Music, Theatre, Film Arts, Television and Visual Arts
Performance Facilities: Drama Laboratory; Dance Studio; Multi - purpose Dome

DANCE

Billie Hutchings, Instructor   **Number Of Faculty:** 1   **Degrees Offered:** AA
Courses Offered: Modern; Folk; Ballet; Creative; Choreography; Notation
Technical Training: Choreography; Staging; Lighting; Publicity
Financial Assistance: Scholarships and Work-Study Grants
Performing Groups: Dance Ensemble
Workshops/Festivals: Spring Concert; Christmas

MUSIC

Robert Gilson, Chairperson   **Number Of Faculty:** 7   **Degrees Offered:** AA
Courses Offered: Harmony; Counterpoint; Piano; Organ; Strings; Jazz Theory & Arranging; Voice; Brass;
Woodwinds; Percussion; Electronics; Guitar; Ensemble; Choir; Band
Financial Assistance: Scholarships and Work-Study Grants
Performing Groups: Concert Choir; Chamber Singers; Chorale; Jazz-Rock Vocal Ensemble; Stage Band;
Concert Band; Orchestra; Brass & Strings Ensembles
Workshops/Festivals: Contemporary Music Festival; Annual Jazz Concert

(continued on next page)

THEATRE

Ray Dahlin, Chairperson **Number Of Faculty:** 2 **Degrees Offered:** AA
Courses Offered: Light & Sound; Costume & Makeup; Reader's Theatre - Verse Choir; Costume History; Children's Theatre; Black Theatre; Acting; Pantomime; Playwriting; Direction; Oral Interpretation
Financial Assistance: Scholarships and Work-Study Grants
Performing Groups: Forensics Square; Summer Theater Workshop
Workshops/Festivals: Summer Workshop

PASADENA CITY COLLEGE
1570 E Colorado Blvd, Pasadena California 91106
213 578-7216
County and 2 Year
William B Shanks, Chairman, Communication Department
Arts Areas: Instrumental Music, Vocal Music, Theatre, Television, Visual Arts and Radio
Performance Facilities: Main Stage; Little Theatre; Harbeson Hall

DANCE

Suzanne Macauley, Chairman, Women's Physical Education
Number Of Faculty: 4 **Number Of Students:** 500 **Degrees Offered:** AA
Courses Offered: Modern Dance; Production; Theory; Modern Dance & Ballet Techniques; Jazz; Afro - American Jazz; Ethnic; Mexican Folkloric; Tap; Dance Staging; Choreography; Makeup; Lighting
Financial Assistance: Scholarships
Performing Groups: Modern Dance Production Group
Workshops/Festivals: Works in Progress; Spring Concert; Special demonstrations for community by Mexican Ballet Folkloric

MUSIC

Robert M Fleury, Director **Degrees Offered:** AA **Technical Training:** Opera
Financial Assistance: Scholarships

THEATRE

William B Shanks, Chairman, Communication Department **Number Of Faculty:** 5
Number Of Students: 200 **Degrees Offered:** AA
Courses Offered: Acting; Directing; Makeup; Stage Technology; Mime
Technical Training: Stage Technology; Makeup
Performing Groups: Four plays in Little Theatre each year; Major musical with music department every two years

---

PEPPERDINE UNIVERSITY, SEAVER COLLEGE
24255 Pacific Coast Hwy, Malibu California 90265
213 456-4000
Private and 4 Year
Arts Areas: Instrumental Music, Vocal Music, Theatre, Television, Visual Arts and Radio
Performance Facilities: Elkins Auditorium; Chapel; Fine Arts Theatre; Concert Hall; Opera House

MUSIC

Dr James Smythe, Humanities & Fine Arts Division
Number Of Faculty: 5 Full-time, 10 Adjunct **Number Of Students:** 60
Degrees Offered: BA MusEd; BA in Theory; BA in Performance; BA in Literature
Courses Offered: Theory & Musicianship; History; Music Education Courses; Counterpoint; Conduction; Analytical Techniques; Orchestration
Technical Training: All applied music training in performance
Teaching Certification Available
Financial Assistance: Assistantships, Scholarships and Special Achievement Awards
Performing Groups: Orchestra; Wind & Jazz Ensembles; Pep Band; Brass Quintet; Woodwind & String Quartet; A Cappella Chorus; Madrigal Singers; University Chorus; Faculty Performances - Soloists & Ensembles
Workshops/Festivals: String Workshops; Brass & Woodwind Workshops; Piano Workshops

(continued on next page)

THEATRE

Dr Stewart M Hudson, Chairman, Communication   **Number Of Faculty:** 3
Number Of Students: 30   **Degrees Offered:** BA
Courses Offered: Intro to Theatre; Scenes; American Musical Theatre; Developing the Actor; Voice & Movement; Advanced Acting; Stagecraft; Play Production; Theatre History
Technical Training: Play Production; Directing; Set Construction
Teaching Certification Available   Financial Assistance: Scholarships
Performing Groups: Pepperdine Players   **Workshops/Festivals:** Summer Theatre
Artists-In-Residence/Guest Artists: Pavel Farkas - Violinist; Penta Brass

POINT LOMA COLLEGE
3900 Lomaland Dr, San Diego   California 92106
714 222-6474 Ext 344
    Private and 4 Year
    Arts Areas: Instrumental Music, Vocal Music and Visual Arts
    Performance Facilities: Salomon Hall

MUSIC

Dr Reuben Rodeheaver, Chairman, Division of Fine Arts
Number Of Faculty: 17   **Number Of Students:** 700   **Degrees Offered:** BA
Courses Offered: Applied Music; Ensembles; Theory/Composition; Music Education
Teaching Certification Available   Financial Assistance: Grants for Lessons
Performing Groups: College Orchestra; Crusader Band; Choral Union; Crusader Chorale; Treble Choir; Concert Choir; Point Loma Singers; Instrummental Ensemble; Brass Choir
Workshops/Festivals: Church Music Conference
Artists-In-Residence/Guest Artists: Miss Esther Saxon; Dr David Uerkvitz; Christopher Lindbloom

RIO HONDO COLLEGE
3600 Workman Mill Rd, Whittier   California 90608
213 692-0921 Ext 361
    State and 2 Year
    Arts Areas: Dance, Instrumental Music, Vocal Music, Theatre, Film Arts, Television and Visual Arts
    Performing Series: CAPES
    Performance Facilities: Rio Hondo College Wray Theatre

DANCE

John R Jacobs, Chairman   **Number Of Faculty:** 2   **Number Of Students:** 80
Courses Offered: Folklorico; Modern; Folk; Foreign
Financial Assistance: Scholarships
Performing Groups: Modern; Folklorico; Folk; Foreign
Workshops/Festivals: Dance & Ballet Folklorico Workshops

MUSIC

John R Jacobs, Chairman   **Number Of Faculty:** 12   **Number Of Students:** 600
Degrees Offered: AA   **Technical Training:** Commercial Music
Teaching Certification Available
Performing Groups: Choir; Concert Band; Orchestra; Chamber Singers; All Ensembles; Jazz Band; Varsity Band
Workshops/Festivals: Music Festivals & Workshops

THEATRE

John R Jacobs, Chairman   **Number Of Faculty:** 6   **Number Of Students:** 250
Degrees Offered: AA   **Technical Training:** Acting
Financial Assistance: Scholarships
Performing Groups: Acting & Musical Theatre Productions; Mime; Children's Theatre
Workshops/Festivals: Acting & Theatre Workshops

RIVERSIDE CITY COLLEGE
4800 Magnolia Ave, Riverside   California 92506
714 684-3240

City and 2 Year
Arts Areas: Dance, Instrumental Music, Vocal Music, Theatre and Visual Arts
Performing Series: Noon Concert Series; Performances of Student Groups
Performance Facilities: Landis Auditorium; Backstage Theater

DANCE

Mrs Kathy Farris, Chairman   **Degrees Offered:** AA
Courses Offered: Folk Dance; Jazz; Modern
Workshops/Festivals: Annual Professional Dance (modern) Concert; Folk Dance Workshop

MUSIC

Richard Stover, Chairman, Division of Fine & Applied Arts
Number Of Faculty: 5   **Degrees Offered:** AA
Courses Offered: Harmony; Counterpoint; Conducting; Music History & Literature; Chorus; Chamber Singers; Instrumental; Guitar; Piano; Organ
Workshops/Festivals: Voice Workshop; Chamber Singers Festival; Jazz Workshop

THEATRE

Gary Schultz, Chairman   **Number Of Faculty:** 3   **Degrees Offered:** AA
Courses Offered: Rehearsals & Performance; Theater for Deaf; Children's Theater for Teachers; Introduction to Theater; Oral Interpretation; History; Acting; Stagecraft; Readers' Theater
Workshops/Festivals: One-act Play Tournament for High Schools

SAN DIEGO CITY COLLEGE
1313 Twelfth Ave, San Diego   California 92101
714 238-1181

City, 2 Year and Public, Coeducational Community College
Arts Areas: Instrumental Music, Vocal Music, Theatre, Film Arts, Television, Visual Arts and Radio Broadcasting
Performing Series: Film Series; Performing Arts Series

DANCE

Betty Hock, Assistant Athletic Director   **Number Of Faculty:** 2
Financial Assistance: Scholarships

MUSIC

Douglas Dailard, Chairman, Creative Arts Department   **Number Of Faculty:** 2
Degrees Offered: AA   **Financial Assistance:** Scholarships
Performing Groups: Stage Band; Chamber Singers; Jazz Ensemble; Concert Choir

THEATRE

Douglas Dailard, Chairman, Creative Arts Department   **Number Of Faculty:** 2
Degrees Offered: AA

SAN FRANCISCO CONSERVATORY OF MUSIC
1201 Ortega St, San Francisco   California 94122
415 564-8086

Private and 4 Year   **Arts Areas:** Instrumental Music and Vocal Music
Performance Facilities: Ruth & Marco Hellman Hall

MUSIC

Richard Howe, Dean   **Number Of Faculty:** 62   **Number Of Students:** 180
Degrees Offered: BM; MM; Music Diploma
Courses Offered: All Instruments; Voice; Orchestra; Chamber Music; New Music; Early Music;

(continued on next page)

Conducting; Composition; Opera Workshop; Theory
Financial Assistance: Assistantships, Scholarships and Work-Study Grants
Performing Groups: The Francesco Trio; The New Music Ensemble; Early Music Ensemble; Opera Workshop; Conservatory Orchestra; Chamber Music Players
Workshops/Festivals: Chamber Music/West Festival (summer chamber music festival); Master Classes by Rampal, Dempster, Schwartz, Fleisher, Leonhardt, Nelsova, Lorimer, Bellson
Artists-In-Residence/Guest Artists: The Francesco Trio; Jean Pierre Rampal; Stuart Demptster; Gustav Leonhardt; Leon Fleisher; Michael Lorimer; Louis Bellson; Zara Nelsova

SAN FRANCISCO STATE UNIVERSITY
1600 Holloway, San Francisco   California 94132
415 469-2075

State and 4 Year
Arts Areas: Dance, Instrumental Music, Vocal Music, Theatre, Film Arts, Television, Visual Arts and Radio
Performing Series: Artists Series
Performance Facilities: McKenna Theatre; Arena Theatre; Little Theatre; Brown Bag Theatre; Knuth Concert Hall

DANCE

Dance program under auspices of Physical Education Department
Courses Offered: Modern Dance; Jazz; Afro-Haitian; Ballet; Ethnic; Folk; Ballroom; Square Dance
Financial Assistance: Assistantships, Scholarships and Work-Study Grants
Performing Groups: EMBAJE (Dance Club)
Workshops/Festivals: Technique Workshops; Production Workshops; Master Classes

MUSIC

Warren Rasmussin, Chairperson   *Number Of Faculty:* 44
Degrees Offered: BMus; BA; BMusEd; MA; Teaching Certificate
Financial Assistance: Assistantships, Scholarships and Work-Study Grants
Performing Groups: Orchestra; Band; A Cappella Choir; Women's Choir; Men's Glee Club; Instrumental Ensemble; Chamber Music; Choral Union; String Orchestra; Chamber Choir; Piano Ensemble; Jazz Ensemble; Collegium Musicum
Workshops/Festivals: Opera Workshop; Recitals; Composition Workshop

THEATRE

Jack Byers, Chairperson   *Number Of Faculty:* 25
Degrees Offered: BA; MA in Drama
Technical Training: Costuming; Makeup; Lighting; Directing; Scene Design; Acting
Teaching Certification Available
Performing Groups: Brown Bag Theatre Company; Players' Club
Workshops/Festivals: Acting Workshop; Mime Theatre Workshop; Arena Theatre Staging Workshop; Musical Theatre Workshop

UNIVERSITY OF SAN FRANCISCO
2130 Fulton St, San Francisco   California 94117
415 666-6133

Private and 4 Year
Arts Areas: Dance, Instrumental Music, Vocal Music, Theatre, Film Arts and Visual Arts
Music, Film Arts & Visual Arts are offered through a cooperative program with Lone Mountain and Academy of Art Colleges
Performance Facilities: McLaren Center; USF Memorial Gym; Loyola Gym; Gill Theatre

DANCE

Kathileen A Gallagher, Director
Program offered through Physical Education Department
Number Of Faculty: 3   *Number Of Students:* 150 - 200
Courses Offered: Jazz: Ballet; Modern; Folk

(continued on next page)

THEATRE

James J Dempsey, SJ, Director of USF College Players   **Number Of Faculty:** 4
Number Of Students: 60   **Degrees Offered:** BA in Communication Arts
Performing Groups: USF College Players

SAN JOAQUIN DELTA COLLEGE
5151 Pacific Ave, Stockton   California 95207
209 478-2011
County and 2 Year
Arts Areas: Dance, Instrumental Music, Vocal Music, Theatre, Film Arts, Television, Visual Arts and Radio
Performing Series: Drama (including Ethnic Theatre); Music; Dance
Performance Facilities: Drama Theatre; Auidtorium; Recital Hall

MUSIC

Number Of Faculty: 16   **Number Of Faculty:** 5   **Number Of Students:** 200
Degrees Offered: AA
Performing Groups: Band; A Cappella Choir; Chorale; Piano Ensemble

THEATRE

Number Of Faculty: 4   **Number Of Students:** 180   **Degrees Offered:** AA
Performing Groups: Applied Drama Class

SANTA BARBARA CITY COLLEGE
CONTINUING EDUCATION DIVISION
914 Santa Barbara St, Santa Barbara   California 93101
805 962-8144
City and 2 Year
Arts Areas: Instrumental Music, Vocal Music, Theatre, Television and Visual Arts
Performance Facilities: Alhecama Theatre; SBCC West Campus Theatre; Abravanel Hall; Music Academy
of the West

DANCE

Mrs Dorothy Eberle, Program Planning Assistant, Discovery in Movement
Number Of Faculty: 3   **Number Of Students:** 50

MUSIC

Dr Joseph A Bagnall, Assistant Dean   **Number Of Faculty:** 17
Number Of Students: 1,600
Workshops/Festivals: Who's Afraid of Opera; Jazz Showcase with Kenton Alumni

THEATRE

Mrs Dorothy Eberle, Program Planning Assistant
Number Of Faculty: 14 Part-time   **Number Of Students:** 300
Artists-In-Residence/Guest Artists: Dr Jan Popper; Ann Richards; Buddy Childers; Ladd McIntosh;
Mundell Lowe; Shelley Mann; David Ligare; BArton Emmet; Dr Maurice Faulkner; Natalie Limonick; Dr
Carl Zytowski

SANTA MONICA COLLEGE
1900 Pico Blvd, Santa Monica   California 90405
213 450-5150
2 Year and Community College District
Arts Areas: Dance, Instrumental Music, Vocal Music, Theatre, Film Arts, Television and Visual Arts

DANCE

Linda Gold, Chairman   **Number Of Faculty:** 2   **Number Of Students:** 43
Degrees Offered: AA

(continued on next page)

Courses Offered: Modern Dance; Ballet; Folk Dance; Jazz; Tap
Financial Assistance: Work-Study Grants
Workshops/Festivals: Musical Comedy Workshop

MUSIC

Rule Beasley, Chairman **Number Of Faculty:** 6 **Number Of Students:** 130
Degrees Offered: AA
Performing Groups: Concert Chorale; Chamber Choir; Concert Choir; Chamber Orchestra; Jazz Ensemble; Concert Band; Marching Band
Workshops/Festivals: Musical Theatre Workshop

THEATRE

Joe Brown, Chairman **Number Of Faculty:** 4 **Number Of Students:** 140
Degrees Offered: AA *Workshops/Festivals:* Musical Comedy Workshop

SANTA ROSA JUNIOR COLLEGE
1501 Mendocino Ave, Santa Rosa California 95401
707 527-4011
State and 2 Year
Arts Areas: Instrumental Music, Vocal Music, Theatre and Visual Arts

MUSIC

Dr Curtis Sprenger, Chairperson **Number Of Faculty:** 6
Degrees Offered: AA
Financial Assistance: Scholarships and Work-Study Grants

THEATRE

Dr Homer T Bower, Chairperson **Number Of Faculty:** 5 *Degrees Offered:* AA

SCRIPPS COLLEGE
Claremont California 91711, 714 626-8511 Ext 3045
Private and 4 Year
Arts Areas: Dance, Instrumental Music, Vocal Music, Theatre, Film Arts and Visual Arts
Performing Series: Bessie Bartlett Frankel Chamber Music Series
Performance Facilities: Garrison Theatre; Strut & Fret Theatre; Balch Auditorium
Humanities Auditorium; Pattison Recital Hall; Beatrice Richardson Dance Studio; Bowling Green Lawn

DANCE

Linda L Levy, Assistant Professor **Number Of Faculty:** 3
Number Of Students: 166 *Degrees Offered:* BA
Courses Offered: Technique; Composition; Accompaniment; Production; Improvisation; Ballet; Repertory; Kinesiology; Pedagogy; Notation; History
Financial Assistance: Scholarships, Work-Study Grants and College & Federal Loans
Performing Groups: Scripps College Dance Theatre
Workshops/Festivals: Master's Classes

SIERRA COLLEGE
5000 Rocklin Rd, Rocklin California 95677
916 624-3333
2 Year and Community
Arts Areas: Instrumental Music, Vocal Music, Theatre, Film Arts and Visual Arts
Performance Facilities: Auditorium/Theatre; Choral Room; Band Room

MUSIC

Donald Whitehead, Instructor **Number Of Faculty:** 3 *Degrees Offered:* AA
Courses Offered: Voice; Brass Ensemble; Woodwind; Harmony; Music; Music Appreciation
Financial Assistance: Scholarships and Work-Study Grants

(continued on next page)

THEATRE

Mike Hunter/Charlotte Starbird, Instructors   **Number Of Faculty:** 2
Degrees Offered: AA
Courses Offered: Acting; Stagecraft; Makeup; Theatre; Puppetry

---

SKYLINE COLLEGE
3300 College Dr, San Bruno   California 94066
415 355-7000 Ext 123
County and 2 Year
Arts Areas: Dance, Instrumental Music, Vocal Music, Theatre and Visual Arts
Performance Facilities: Main Theatre; Studio Theatre

DANCE

Ruth Welles, Instructor, Physical Education   **Number Of Faculty:** 1
Degrees Offered: AA
Financial Assistance: Work-Study Grants

MUSIC

Number Of Faculty: 5   **Number Of Students:** 30 - 40   **Degrees Offered:** AA
Financial Assistance: Scholarships and Work-Study Grants
Performing Groups: College Choir; Symphonic Band; Jazz Band; Bay Bones; Music Theatre

THEATRE

Number Of Faculty: 3   **Number Of Students:** 10 - 15   **Degrees Offered:** AA
Technical Training: Lighting; Stagecraft
Financial Assistance: Scholarships and Work-Study Grants
Performing Groups: Children's Theatre

SONOMA STATE COLLEGE
1801 E Cotati Ave, Rohnert Park   California 94928
707 664-2416
State and 4 Year
Arts Areas: Dance, Instrumental Music, Vocal Music and Theatre
Performing Series: Performing Arts Series
Performance Facilities: Ives Hall; Warren Auditorium & Room 119; Studio Theatre; Dance Studio;
Gymnasium

DANCE

Dance program under auspices of Theatre Arts
Degrees Offered: BA in Theatre Arts with emphasis in Dance
Performing Groups: Dance Ensemble   **Workshops/Festivals:** Summer Dance Festival

MUSIC

Dr E Gardner Rust, Chairman   **Number Of Faculty:** 29
Number Of Students: 191   **Degrees Offered:** BA
Technical Training: Private instructions on all instruments
Teaching Certification Available
Financial Assistance: Scholarships and Work-Study Grants
Performing Groups: Chamber Orchestra; Chamber Music Workshop; Concert Jazz Ensemble; Jazz
Workshop; Opera Workshop; African Music & Dance Ensemble; Wind Ensemble; Chorus; Madrigals; Brass
Choir
Workshops/Festivals: Redwood Empire Jazz Festival; Summer Chamber Music for Strings; Redwood
Empire Choral Festival

THEATRE

Robin Jackson, Chairman   **Number Of Faculty:** 10   **Number Of Students:** 121
Degrees Offered: BA   **Courses Offered:** Drama; Dance; Design

(continued on next page)

Financial Assistance: Scholarships and Work-Study Grants
Performing Groups: Theatre Ensemble
Artists-In-Residence/Guest Artists: National Ballet Company of Illinois

---

UNIVERSITY OF SOUTHERN CALIFORNIA
3518 University Ave, Los Angeles California 90007
213 741-2311
Private and 4 Year
Arts Areas: Dance, Instrumental Music, Vocal Music, Theatre, Film Arts, Television and Visual Arts
Performing Series: Chamber Series; Performing Artist Series
Performance Facilities: Bovard Auditorium; Bing Theater; Eileen Norris Cinema Theatre; Stop Gap
Theatre

DANCE

Jeanne Flood, Supervisor   *Number Of Faculty:* 6   *Number Of Students:* 500
Degrees Offered: BA, MA Physical Education major with Dance Specialization
Courses Offered: Modern; Ballroom; Folk; Ballet; Jazz; Tap; Dance History; Choreography; Dance
Production & Performance; Creative Movement for Children
Technical Training: Choreography; Modern; Ballroom; Folk; Ballet; Jazz; Tap
Teaching Certification Available
Financial Assistance: Assistantships, Scholarships and Work-Study Grants
Performing Groups: Ballroom Dance Team; Hallmark Dancers; Dance Theatre Group
Workshops/Festivals: Visiting Artist Series Workshop; Jazz Workshop; Ethnic Dance Workshop

MUSIC

Howard Rarig, Director   *Number Of Faculty:* 118   *Number Of Students:* 850
Degrees Offered: BMus; BA; MMus; MMusEd; MA; DMA; PhD
Technical Training: Study in Tunis, Vienna, and other foreign countries; Opera; Church Music
Teaching Certification Available
Financial Assistance: Assistantships, Scholarships and Work-Study Grants
Performing Groups: Symphony Orchestra; Vocal & Instrumental Ensembles; Trojan Marching Band;
Trojan Concert Band; University Orchestra; Chamber Orchestra; University Chamber Singers; Opera
Chorus; University Chorus; Opera Theatre
Workshops/Festivals: Autumn Arts Festival; Recording Arts Workshop; Choral Conductors Workshop;
Advanced Workshop in Orff - Schulwerk; Gregor Piatigorsky Seminar

THEATRE

Richard Toscan, Interim Chairman   *Number Of Faculty:* 18
Number Of Students: 200   *Degrees Offered:* BA; BFA; MA; MFA; PhD
Courses Offered: Acting; Design; Directing; Playwriting; Voice
Technical Training: Professionally oriented study; Study abroad
Financial Assistance: Assistantships, Scholarships and Work-Study Grants
Performing Groups: Experimentation in Theatre; Masters Company; BFA Company (Advanced Theatre
Workshop); Main Stage; Lunchtime Theatre
Workshops/Festivals: Acting & Directing Workshops; Edinborough Theatre Festival
Artists-In-Residence/Guest Artists: William Kraft; Jan Degaetani; Pepe Romero

---

SOUTHWESTERN COLLEGE
900 Otay Lakes Rd, Chula Vista California 92010
714 421-6700 Ext 289
County and 2 Year
Arts Areas: Dance, Instrumental Music, Vocal Music, Theatre and Film Arts
Performing Series: Southwestern Presents
Performance Facilities: Mayan Hall Theatre; Arena Theatre

DANCE

Johanna Weikel, Director   *Number Of Faculty:* 3 Full-time, 4 Part-time
Number Of Students: 700   *Degrees Offered:* AA

(continued on next page)

Courses Offered: Folk & Round; Ethnic Dance; African; Ballroom Dance; Ballet, Modern Dance; Adv Modern; Modern Jazz Dance; Tap; Square
Financial Assistance: Scholarships and Work-Study Grants
Performing Groups: Round; Ballet; Folk; Jazz: Modern
Workshops/Festivals: Folk Dance Festival; Annual Spring Concert; Mini Concerts; College Hour Dance Workshops

MUSIC

James C Merrill, Director   **Number Of Faculty:** 13   **Number Of Students:** 700
Degrees Offered: AA
Financial Assistance: Scholarships and Work-Study Grants
Performing Groups: Concert Band; Jazz Ensemble; Rock Ensemble; Choir; Chamber Singers; Small Chamber Groups
Workshops/Festivals: Clinics; Solo & Ensemble Festival; Band & Orchestra Festival; Jazz Festival

THEATRE

William Virchia, Director   **Number Of Faculty:** 7   **Number Of Students:** 300
Degrees Offered: AA Drama
Financial Assistance: Scholarships and Work-Study Grants
Performing Groups: Opera Workshop; Musical Workshop; Classical Drama; Delta Psi Omega; Children's Touring Company; Mime Company; Acting Lab
Workshops/Festivals: Mime Festival; One Act Play Festival; Craig Noel Classical Audition Festival in conjunction with Old Globe Theatre

---

STANFORD UNIVERSITY
Stanford   California 94305, 415 497-2300
Private and 4 Year
Arts Areas: Dance, Instrumental Music and Vocal Music
Performance Facilities: Memorial Auditorium; Dinkelspiel Auditorium; Annenberg Auditorium; Kresge Auditorium

DANCE

Inge Weiss, Chairman
Dance program under auspices of Physical Education Department
Number Of Faculty: 11
Courses Offered: Rhythm & Movement; Modern Dance; Ballet for Contemporary Dance; Improvisation; Folk Dance; Ethnic Dance
Teaching Certification Available   **Financial Assistance:** Scholarships

MUSIC

Albert Cohen, Professor & Chairman   **Number Of Faculty:** 41
Number Of Students: 180   **Degrees Offered:** BA; MA; PhD; DMA
Courses Offered: Music Theory & Composition; History & Literature of Music; Performance
Teaching Certification Available
Financial Assistance: Assistantships, Scholarships and Work-Study Grants
Performing Groups: Early Music Singers; Renaissance Wind Band; New Music Ensemble ; University Chorus; University Orchestra; Chamber Orchestra; Univ Choir; Stanford Chorale; Glee Club; University Bands; Wind Ensemble; Jazz Band; Percussion Ensemble; Brass Choir; Sports Activity Bands; Chamber Music; Piano Accompanying
Workshops/Festivals: Various Workshops during Summer Session

THEATRE

Charles Lyons, Chairman   **Number Of Faculty:** 19
Degrees Offered: BA Teaching Drama; MA Teaching Drama; MFA; PhD Drama & Humanities
Technical Training: Stage Lighting; Costume Design
Teaching Certification Available   **Financial Assistance:** Scholarships
Workshops/Festivals: Drama Workshop
Artists-In-Residence/Guest Artists: Walter Ducloux; Thomas Binkley; Wendy Hilton

UNITED STATES INTERNATIONAL UNIVERSITY

10455 Pomerado Rd, San Diego   California 92131
714 271-4300 Ext 431

Private and 4 Year
Arts Areas: Dance, Instrumental Music, Vocal Music, Theatre, Visual Arts and Musical Theatre
Performing Series: City Stage Performances
Performance Facilities: City Stage; City College Auditorium

DANCE

John Hart, Chairman   *Number Of Faculty:* 5   *Number Of Students:* 85
Degrees Offered: BFA; MFA
Courses Offered: Ballet; Modern; Jazz; Musical Theatre Dance
Financial Assistance: Scholarships and Work-Study Grants

THEATRE

Gordon Hilker, Director, Professional Training   *Number Of Faculty:* 5
Number Of Students: 60   *Degrees Offered:* BFA
Courses Offered: Acting; Directing; Speech

UNIVERSITY OF CALIFORNIA, RIVERSIDE

PO Box 112, Riverside   California 92521
714 787-3594

State and 4 Year
Arts Areas: Dance, Instrumental Music, Vocal Music and Theatre
Performance Facilities: University Theatre; Studio Theatre; Dance Studio; International Lounge; Watkins House

DANCE

Fred Strickler, Associate Professor   *Number Of Faculty:* 2
Number Of Students: 30   *Degrees Offered:* BA
Courses Offered: Choreography; History; Theory; Performance; Technique
Technical Training: Modern Dance; Ballet; Tap
Financial Assistance: Scholarships and Work-Study Grants
Performing Groups: UCR Modern Dance Group
Workshops/Festivals: California Dance Artists Series

MUSIC

William H Reynolds, Professor   *Number Of Faculty:* 34
Number Of Students: 85 - 90   *Degrees Offered:* BA; MA
Courses Offered: Theory; Composition; History; Performance
Technical Training: Vocal & Instrumental Performance; Carillon Performance
Financial Assistance: Scholarships and Work-Study Grants
Performing Groups: Choral Society; Madrigal Singers; Collegium Musicum; Symphony Orchestra; Varsity Band; Chamber Ensembles
Workshops/Festivals: Contemporary Music Festival

THEATRE

Dr Richard D Risso, Professor   *Number Of Faculty:* 8
Number Of Students: 60 - 70
Degrees Offered: MA; MFA Acting; BA; BA Acting Track; BA Tech/Design Track
Courses Offered: Studio; Non - Studio; Acting
Technical Training: Sound; Light; Set & Costume Construction; Scenic Painting

UNIVERSITY OF REDLANDS
1200 E Colton Ave, Redlands   California 92373
714 793-2121 Ext 326
Private and 4 Year
Arts Areas: Dance, Instrumental Music, Vocal Music, Theatre and Visual Arts
Performing Series: Faculty Recitals; Student Recitals; Ensemble Programs; Theatre Productions
Performance Facilities: Watchorn Hall; Chapel; Wallichs Theatre

MUSIC

Wayne R Bohrnstedt, Director   *Number Of Faculty:* 14
Number Of Students: 125   *Degrees Offered:* BM; BA; MM; MA
Teaching Certification Available
Financial Assistance: Assistantships and Scholarships

THEATRE

Dr Paul Little, Chairman   *Number Of Faculty:* 3   *Number Of Students:* 40
Degrees Offered: BA

UNIVERSITY OF SOUTHERN CALIFORNIA
Los Angeles   California 90007, 213 741-2526
Community   *Arts Areas:* Dance, Instrumental Music, Vocal Music and Theatre
The Community School of Performing Arts is designed to meet the needs of anyone that wants to take
courses in music, dance or drama, other than for university credit.

DANCE

Technical Training: Ballet; Modern; Creative; Tap

MUSIC

Marienne Uszler, Chairman
Technical Training: Suzuki Program in Violin & Piano

THEATRE

Delle & David Colloff, Chairmen   *Financial Assistance:* Scholarships
Workshops/Festivals: Summer Workshop

VICTOR VALLEY COLLEGE
PO Box 00, Victorville   California 92392
714 245-4271 Ext 264
State and 2 Year
Arts Areas: Instrumental Music, Vocal Music, Theatre, Film Arts and Visual Arts
Performing Series: Band; Symphony Orchestra; Vocal Recitals; Three Plays; Annual Musical Comedy
Performance Facilities: Gym

MUSIC

Selmer Spitzer, Chairman   *Number Of Faculty:* 2   *Number Of Students:* 100
Degrees Offered: AA   *Financial Assistance:* Work-Study Grants

THEATRE

Polly Fitch, Chairman, Department of Drama & Speech Communication
Number Of Faculty: 3   *Number Of Students:* 350   *Degrees Offered:* AA
Financial Assistance: Work-Study Grants

WEST HILLS COLLEGE
300 Cherry Lane, Coalinga   California 93210
209 935-0801
State and 2 Year
Arts Areas: Dance, Instrumental Music, Vocal Music, Theatre and Visual Arts
Performance Facilities: West Hills College Little Theatre

DANCE

Dr anie Jones, Chairman   *Number Of Faculty:* 1   *Number Of Students:* 40
Courses Offered: Basic Modern Dance

MUSIC

Dr Bernice Isham, Chairman   *Number Of Faculty:* 2   *Number Of Students:* 150
Degrees Offered: AA; AS
Courses Offered: Piano; Fundamentals of Music; Theory; Voice; Chorus; Music History; Jazz Band; Stage Band; Symphony; Opera Workshop; Beginning Instruments; Guitar; Field Experience; Pop Rock
Financial Assistance: Scholarships and Work-Study Grants
Performing Groups: Chorus; Choir; Madrigal Singers; Community Chorus; Opera Workshop; Stage & Jazz Bands; Theatre; Community Theatre
Workshops/Festivals: High School Band Day; Band Workshop; Madrigal Festival; Christmas Festival

THEATRE

Dr Janie Jones, Chairman   *Number Of Faculty:* 1   *Number Of Students:* 25
Degrees Offered: AA; AS
Courses Offered: Makeup; Theatre History; Theatre Workshop; Acting; Stage Lighting & Sound; Theatre Crafts; Scene Design; Directed Study
Performing Groups: Drama Club; Community Theatre; College Productions

WEST VALLEY COLLEGE
14000 Fruitvale Ave, Saratoga   California 95070
408 867-2200
2 Year and Community
Arts Areas: Instrumental Music, Vocal Music, Theatre and Visual Arts

MUSIC

Ken Jewell, Chairman   *Number Of Faculty:* 4   *Degrees Offered:* AA
Performing Groups: Santa Clara Valley Symphony; West Valley Symphony; Community Chorale; Concert Choir; Chorus; Jazz Bands

THEATRE

Jack Senteney, Chairman   *Number Of Faculty:* 3   *Degrees Offered:* AA
Performing Groups: Standard Performance once or twice a semester; Road Apples Repertory Company

WESTMONT COLLEGE
955 La Paz Rd, Santa Barbara   California 93108
805 969-5051
Private and 4 Year
Arts Areas: Dance, Instrumental Music, Vocal Music and Theatre
Performing Series: Artist Series
Performance Facilities: Recital Hall; Gymnasium; Intermediate Hall

DANCE

Erlyne Whiteman, Instructor   *Number Of Faculty:* 1   *Number Of Students:* 15
Degrees Offered: BA   *Courses Offered:* Dance; Body Movement

MUSIC

Dr Howard Stevenson, Professor   *Number Of Faculty:* 4
Number Of Students: 40   *Degrees Offered:* BA

(continued on next page)

Courses Offered: Theory; Composition; History; Conducting Ensembles; Lessons
Financial Assistance: Scholarships and Work-Study Grants
Performing Groups: Two College Choirs; Madrigal Group; Brass Choir; Ensembles
Workshops/Festivals: Hymn Festival; Christmas Concerts; Spring Festival of Music

THEATRE

Everett Vande Beek, Associate Professor   **Number Of Faculty:** 1 ½
Number Of Students: 20   **Degrees Offered:** BA
Courses Offered: History; Production; Beginning Acting
Workshops/Festivals: Three Productions per Year

ADAMS STATE COLLEGE

Alamosa Colorado 81101, 303 589-7011

State and 4 Year
Arts Areas: Instrumental Music, Vocal Music, Theatre and Visual Arts
Performing Series: Artists & Lecture Series

MUSIC

Gordon B Childs, Coordinator *Degrees Offered:* BMus; BMusEd; MMus; MMusEd
Teaching Certification Available
Workshops/Festivals: Music Theatre Workshop

THEATRE

James V Biundo, Chairman, Humanities *Degrees Offered:* BA; MA
Teaching Certification Available *Performing Groups:* Adams State Players

---

ARAPAHOE COMMUNITY COLLEGE

5900 S Santa Fe Dr, Littleton Colorado 80120
303 794-1550 Ext 320

State and 2 Year
Arts Areas: Vocal Music, Theatre, Television and Visual Arts
Performing Series: ACC Concert Series, Brown Bag Concerts

MUSIC

Kevin Kennedy, Coordinator *Number Of Faculty:* 1 *Number Of Students:* 90
Degrees Offered: AA
Courses Offered: Theory and Analysis, History, Choral Groups, Applied Music
Financial Assistance: Scholarships and Work-Study Grants
Performing Groups: College Choir, Madrigal Singers

THEATRE

Joan Shields, Coordinator *Number Of Faculty:* 1 *Number Of Students:* 35
Degrees Offered: AA *Courses Offered:* Introduction to Theatre, Acting
Financial Assistance: Scholarships and Work-Study Grants
Performing Groups: Drama Club

ASPEN MUSIC SCHOOL

Aspen Colorado 81611, 303 925-3254

Winter Address: 1860 Broadway, New York, NY 10023
Private and 9-Week Summer School
Arts Areas: Instrumental Music, Vocal Music and Opera
Performing Series: Festival Concerts, Chamber Music Series, Student Concerts Series
Performance Facilities: Aspen Amphitheater, Music Hall, Opera Hall, Wheeler Opera House

DANCE

Dance class offered through Opera Workshop

MUSIC

Jorge Mester, Music Director *Number Of Faculty:* 80
Number Of Students: 800
Degrees Offered: College credit through University of Colorado
Courses Offered: Rudiments of Music, Ear Training, Calligraphy, Orchestration, Counterpoint, Survey in Analysis, Keyboard Studies, Music Literature, Music & Ideas, The Baroque, The Renaissance, Ideas for String Players, Video Analysis for Violinists, Chamber Music Master Class, String Quartet Performance Seminar, Harpsichord, Accompanying, Introduction to Jazz Arranging, Improvisation
Technical Training: Voice, Composition, Applied Music, Conducting

(continued on next page)

Financial Assistance: Scholarships and Fellowships
Performing Groups: Aspen Festival Orchestra, Festival Chorus, Aspen Chamber Symphony, Aspen Philharmonia, Repertory Orchestra, Conductors' Workshop Orchestra, String Ensemble, Aspen Jazz-Rock Ensemble, Wind Ensemble
Workshops/Festivals: Opera Workshop, Choral Institute, Electronic Music Workshop, Conference on Contemporary Music

THEATRE

Acting classes offered through Opera Workshop
Artists-In-Residence/Guest Artists: Jan DeGaetani, Claude Frank, Lee Luvisi, Cleveland Quartet, Zara Nelsova, Oscar Ghiglia, American Brass Quintet

COLORADO COLLEGE
Colorado Springs   Colorado 80903, 473-2233 Ext 242
Private and 4 Year
Arts Areas: Dance, Instrumental Music, Vocal Music, Theatre, Film Arts and Visual Arts
Performing Series: Summer Opera Festival, Summer Dance Courses with Hanya Holm
Performance Facilities: Armstrong Theatre

DANCE

Norman Cornick, Chairman   **Number Of Faculty:** 1
Workshops/Festivals: Annual "Nutcracker Suite"

MUSIC

Dr Albert Seay, Chairman   **Number Of Faculty:** 21   **Number Of Students:** 500
Degrees Offered: BA
Technical Training: Electronic Music, Ethnomusicology
Teaching Certification Available   **Financial Assistance:** Work-Study Grants
Performing Groups: Colorado College Choir, Collegium Musicum, New Music Ensemble, String Ensemble

THEATRE

William E McMillen, Chairman   **Number Of Faculty:** 5
Number Of Students: 125   **Degrees Offered:** BA
Financial Assistance: Work-Study Grants
Performing Groups: Colorado College Players
Workshops/Festivals: Rocky Mountain CT Conference; Theatre Workshop

COLORADO MOUNTAIN COLLEGE, EAST CAMPUS
Leadville   Colorado 80461, 303 486-2015
County and 2 Year
Arts Areas: Instrumental Music, Vocal Music, Theatre and Visual Arts
Performing Series: Concert - Lecture Series
Performance Facilities: College Auditorium   **Degrees Offered:** AA

COLORADO MOUNTAIN COLLEGE, WEST CAMPUS
Glenwood Springs   Colorado 81601, 303 945-7481
County and 2 Year
Arts Areas: Dance, Instrumental Music, Vocal Music, Theatre, Film Arts and Visual Arts
Performance Facilities: Crystal Theater, College Auditorium

DANCE

Number Of Faculty: 1   **Number Of Students:** 20
Courses Offered: Ballet, Modern Dance, Jazz Dance

MUSIC

Financial Assistance: Scholarships and Work-Study Grants
Number Of Faculty: 3   **Number Of Students:** 50

(continued on next page)

Courses Offered: Private Lessons, Vocal and Instrumental, Sight Reading & Ear Training, Theory & Harmony, Coaching, Piano Repertory and Chorale
Financial Assistance: Scholarships and Work-Study Grants
Performing Groups: Bach Chorale, College Chorale
Workshops/Festivals: Voice Clinic

THEATRE

Number Of Students: 30   *Number Of Faculty:* 1
Courses Offered: Fundamentals of Theatre, Acting, Production, Stage Movement, Performance Workshop
Financial Assistance: Scholarships and Work-Study Grants

COLORADO STATE UNIVERSITY
Fort Collins   Colorado 80523, 303 491-5116
State and 4 Year
Arts Areas: Dance, Instrumental Music, Vocal Music, Theatre, Film Arts, Television and Visual Arts
Performing Series: Performing Arts Council, Fine Arts Series, Special Events Board
Performance Facilities: Johnson Hall Theatre, Lory Student Center Theatre, Moby Auditorium - Gymnasium

DANCE

Irmel W Fagan, Associate Professor
Dance Division is in Department of Physical Education, College of Professional Studies
Number Of Faculty: 4   *Number Of Students:* 500 - 750
Degrees Offered: BS in PE, Dance concentration
Courses Offered: Ballet, Ballroom Dancing, Modern Dance, Tap Dance, Character Dance, Folk Dance, Square Dance, Dance Techniques, Movement & Rhythm Analysis, Dance Choreography, Dance Production, Theory of Teaching Dance, Dance History, Dance in Religion, Dance Accompaniment, Dance Therapy
Technical Training: Dance Education with Performance emphasis
Teaching Certification Available
Financial Assistance: Assistantships, Scholarships and Work-Study Grants
Performing Groups: Rocky Mountain Dance Theatre, La Petit Chambre Ballet Company
Workshops/Festivals: Workshops in dance for the handicapped, methods of teaching dance in high school and college, teaching dance and rhythm in elementary school, dance therapy, modern dance

MUSIC

Dr R L Garretson, Chairman
Music Division is in College of Arts, Humanities, & Social Studies
Number Of Faculty: 26   *Number Of Students:* 268
Degrees Offered: BA Mus in Performance, MusEd, Mus Therapy; MA in Applied Mus, MusEd, Mus History & Literature, Theory & Composition, Sacred Mus
Courses Offered: Theory; Chorus; Band; Applied Music and Voice; Music History and Literature; Technique; Conducting; Elementary - High School Music
Teaching Certification Available
Financial Assistance: Assistantships and Scholarships
Performing Groups: CSU Bands, Chamber Singers, Musica Nova, Opera Theatre, Theatre Chamber Orchestra, Univeristy Chorus, University Orchestra, University Singers, Wind Ensemble, Women's Chorus
Workshops/Festivals: Organ Workshop, Opera Theatre

THEATRE

Dr Porter Woods, Director, University Theatre
Theatre Division is in Department of Speech & Theatre Arts, College of Arts, Humanities & Social Sciences
Number Of Faculty: 5   *Number Of Students:* 300   *Degrees Offered:* BA, MA
Courses Offered: Introduction to Theatre, Acting, Technical Theatre, Design, History of Theatre, Directing, Repertory Theatre Workshop, Dramatic Theory, Seminar in Classical Theatre, Seminar in Contemporary Theatre
Teaching Certification Available
Financial Assistance: Assistantships and Scholarships
Performing Groups: University Theatre, Small World Players

COLORADO WOMEN'S COLLEGE
Montview & Quebec, Denver   Colorado 80220
303 394-6012

Private and 4 Year
Arts Areas: Dance, Instrumental Music, Vocal Music, Theatre and Visual Arts
Performance Facilities: W Dale & W Ida Houston Fine Arts Center

DANCE

Rita Berger, Chairman   *Number Of Faculty:* 2   *Number Of Students:* 30
Technical Training: Dance Technique   *Performing Groups:* Dance Productions

MUSIC

Thomas MacCluskey, Chairman   *Number Of Faculty:* 3   *Number Of Students:* 30
Degrees Offered: BA Music   *Technical Training:* Music Industry
Teaching Certification Available
Financial Assistance: Scholarships and Work-Study Grants
Performing Groups: Chamber Orchestra; Concert Choir; Madrigals; Balinese Gamelan; Woodwind
Ensemble; String Ensemble
Workshops/Festivals: Mountain Plains Music Festival

THEATRE

Dr Richard Kelly, Chairman   *Number Of Faculty:* 4   *Number Of Students:* 35
Degrees Offered: BA Theatre Arts
Technical Training: Stagecraft; Sound Lighting; Stage Management
Teaching Certification Available
Financial Assistance: Scholarships and Work-Study Grants
Performing Groups: Fun & Games; Children's Theatre; Readers' Theatre
Workshops/Festivals: Children's Theatre Workshop; Departmental Play Festival

UNIVERSITY OF COLORADO, BOULDER
Boulder   Colorado 80302

State and 4 Year
Arts Areas: Dance, Instrumental Music, Vocal Music, Theatre, Film Arts, Television and Visual Arts

DANCE

Martin Cobin, Chairman
Theater and dance programs combined in Theatre - Dance Department
Degrees Offered: BA; BS in Dance

MUSIC

Warner Imig, Dean   *Number Of Faculty:* 50   *Number Of Students:* 500
Degrees Offered: BA; BMus; MM; MMusEd; D Musical Arts; PhD Musicology and MusEd
Teaching Certification Available
Financial Assistance: Assistantships, Scholarships, Work-Study Grants and Fellowships
Performing Groups: Symphony; Chamber Orchestra; Marching Band; Symphonic Band; Concert Band;
Jazz Ensembles; Festival Chorus; University Chorus; Modern Choir; University Singers; Women's Chorus;
Chamber Chorale; Collegium Musicum; Operas, Musicals
Workshops/Festivals: Opera, String, Choral and Band Workshops; All-State Orchestra; Piano Forums

COMMUNITY COLLEGE OF DENVER, NORTH CAMPUS
3645 W 112th Ave, Westminister   Colorado 80030
303 466-8811

State and 2 Year
Arts Areas: Instrumental Music, Vocal Music and Theatre
Performance Facilities: Recital Facility
Degrees Offered: AA   *Financial Assistance:* Work-Study Grants

UNIVERSITY OF DENVER
University Park, Denver   Colorado 80208
303 753-2143

Private and 4 Year
Arts Areas: Dance, Instrumental Music, Vocal Music, Theatre, Film Arts, Television and Visual Arts
Performing Series: University Programs Board Series
Performance Facilities: General Classroom Building Auditorium; Proscenium Stage

MUSIC

Dr Roger Dexter Fee, Director   *Number Of Faculty:* 32
Number Of Students: 200   *Degrees Offered:* BA; BME; BMus; MA
Courses Offered: Performance; Music Theory; Composition; Music History and Literature; Music Education
Teaching Certification Available
Performing Groups: University & Chamber Orchestras; Jazz Bands (2); University Chorale; Chamber Singers; Glee Clubs; Chamber Ensembles; Symphonic Band; Wind Ensemble, Opera Workshop
Workshops/Festivals: Orff Schulwerk; Suzuki Workshop; Paul Christiansen Choral School; In-Residence Studies in Opera at Santa Fe; International Clarinet Clinic, 20th Century Music Conference in Aspen

THEATRE

Lewis Crickard, Acting Chairman   *Number Of Faculty:* 10
Number Of Students: 120   *Degrees Offered:* BA; MA; PhD
Technical Training: Actual Production in Scene Design, Lighting, and Costume
Teaching Certification Available
Financial Assistance: Assistantships, Scholarships and Work-Study Grants
Performing Groups: University Theatre; Children's Theatre
Workshops/Festivals: Summer Theatre Festival
Artists-In-Residence/Guest Artists: Donald H Keats, Composer-in-Residence

---

EL PASO COMMUNITY COLLEGE
2200 Bott Ave, Colorado Springs   Colorado 80904
303 471-7546

State and 2 Year   *Arts Areas:* Theatre and Television
Performance Facilities: Auditorium; Little Theatre

THEATRE

Eugene W Tedd, Instructor   *Number Of Faculty:* 1   *Number Of Students:* 30
Degrees Offered: AA   *Courses Offered:* Intro; Acting; Production
Technical Training: Stagecraft (Set, Lighting, Makeup)
Performing Groups: Saturday Players
Workshops/Festivals: Children's Theatre; Community Theatre; Musical Theatre

---

FORT LEWIS COLLEGE
College Heights, Durango   Colorado 81301
303 247-7010

State and 4 Year
Arts Areas: Instrumental Music, Vocal Music and Theatre
Performing Series: Denver or Utah Symphony
Performance Facilities: Theatre and Fine Arts Auditorium; Field House

MUSIC

Richard Strawn, Chairman   *Number Of Faculty:* 4   *Number Of Students:* 85
Degrees Offered: BA Music with Instrumental Emphasis; BA Music with Vocal Emphasis
Teaching Certification Available
Financial Assistance: Scholarships and Work-Study Grants
Performing Groups: Orchestra; Chorus; Band; Various Vocal and Chamber Ensembles
Workshops/Festivals: Summer Music Camp; Clinics for Various Instruments

(continued on next page)

THEATRE

Kenneth E Bordner, Chairman   **Number Of Faculty:** 3   **Number Of Students:** 70
Degrees Offered: Student Constructed Major in Theatre
Financial Assistance: Assistantships, Scholarships and Work-Study Grants
Workshops/Festivals: Annual High School Workshop

LAMAR COMMUNITY COLLEGE
2400 South Main, Lamar   Colorado 81052
303 336-2248
State and 2 Year
Arts Areas: Dance, Instrumental Music, Vocal Music and Theatre
Performance Facilities: Theatre; Auditorium; Gymnasium

DANCE

Bart Queary, Area Chairman, Communications and Fine Arts
Number Of Faculty: 3   **Number Of Students:** 68   **Degrees Offered:** AA
Courses Offered: Ballroom Dance; Folk & Square Dance; Modern Dance
Financial Assistance: Scholarships and Work-Study Grants

MUSIC

Bart Queary, Area Chairman, Communications and Fine Arts
Number Of Faculty: 3   **Number Of Students:** 68   **Degrees Offered:** AA
Courses Offered: Chorus; Elementary Music; Band; Music History
Technical Training: Applied Music Instruction
Financial Assistance: Scholarships and Work-Study Grants
Performing Groups: College Chorus; College Band; Women's Trio; Men's Quartet
Workshops/Festivals: Travel Group; Chamber Choir; High School Assemblies; Service Club Entertainment

THEATRE

Bart Queary, Area Chairman, Communications and Fine Arts
Number Of Faculty: 3   **Number Of Students:** 68   **Degrees Offered:** AA
Courses Offered: Speech; Drama; Acting; Argument and Debate
Technical Training: Special Studies; Staging; Makeup
Performing Groups: Drama Club; Delta Psi Omega
Workshops/Festivals: Community Service Club Entertainment; College Semester Theatre Production

LORETTO HEIGHTS COLLEGE
Denver   Colorado 80236, 303 936-8441
Private and 4 Year
Arts Areas: Instrumental Music, Vocal Music and Theatre
Courses Offered: Dance Appreciation; Introduction to Ballet Technique; Modern Dance Technique;
Advanced Ballet Technique
Degrees Offered: BA
Performing Groups: College Chorus; Studio Singers; Pacesetters
Degrees Offered: BA   **Performing Groups:** Theatre Productions

MESA COLLEGE
North Ave at 12th St, Grand Junction   Colorado 81501
303 248-1020
State and 4 Year
Arts Areas: Dance, Instrumental Music, Vocal Music, Theatre and Visual Arts
Performance Facilities: Walter Walker Fine Arts Center

DANCE

Ann Sanders, Instructor   **Number Of Faculty:** 1   **Number Of Students:** 200
Courses Offered: Square & Folk, Social, Modern, Modern Jazz; Ballet; Tap; Creative; Repertory;
Independent Study

(continued on next page)

Technical Training: Modern; Ballet; Jazz; Creative Activities; Special Workshops
Financial Assistance: Scholarships and Work-Study Grants
Performing Groups: Mesa Repertory Dance Company
Workshops/Festivals: Summer Dance Workshop; Visiting Dance Companies (for concerts & workshops)

MUSIC

Darrell C Blackburn, Head   **Number Of Faculty:** 5
Number Of Students: 90 - 100   **Degrees Offered:** BA Performing Arts
Courses Offered: Vocal; Instrumental; Ensembles; Theory; History; Conducting; Methods; Independent Study
Technical Training: Music Theatre; Electronic Music; Opera Workshop
Financial Assistance: Scholarships and Work-Study Grants
Performing Groups: Mesa College Community Choir; Mesa College Civic Symphony Orchestra; Mesa College Jazz Ensemble; Mesa College Concert Choir; Mesa College Modern Choir
Workshops/Festivals: Symphony & Choral Concerts; Opera Workshop; Young Artist Competition

THEATRE

Wm S Robinson, Head, Department of Speech & Drama   **Number Of Faculty:** 3
Number Of Students: 100   **Degrees Offered:** BA Performing Arts
Courses Offered: Acting; Costuming; Dance; Theatre Problems; History; Management; Styles; Staging; Lighting; Scene Design; Creative Play (Dance & Drama); Independent Study
Technical Training: Lighting; Sound; Design & Construction; Directing; Special Theatres
Financial Assistance: Scholarships and Work-Study Grants
Performing Groups: Mesa College Theatre; Mesa Summer Players; Children's Theatre; Music Theatre
Workshops/Festivals: Summer Theatre; Traveling Operas & Special Theatre; Folk Festivals

---

METROPOLITAN STATE COLLEGE
1006 11th St, Denver   Colorado 80204
303 629-3215
State and 4 Year
Arts Areas: Dance, Instrumental Music, Vocal Music, Theatre, Film Arts, Television, Visual Arts and Communication Arts
Performance Facilities: Theatre; Theatre Arts Shops; Communication Laboratories; Audio Visual Studios

DANCE

W Thomas Cook, Chairman   **Number Of Faculty:** 8   **Number Of Students:** 85
Degrees Offered: BA   **Technical Training:** Internships
Teaching Certification Available
Financial Assistance: Internships, Scholarships and Work-Study Grants
Performing Groups: Metropolitan State Players; Auraria Production Company
Workshops/Festivals: Play Production Workshop; Makeup Workshop; Stagecraft Workshop; Costuming Workshop; Mayfest; Historic Denver

MUSIC

Dr Hal Tamblyn, Professor   **Number Of Faculty:** 9 Full-time, 26 Part-time
Number Of Students: 700   **Degrees Offered:** BA in MusEd or Performance
Teaching Certification Available
Financial Assistance: Scholarships and Work-Study Grants
Performing Groups: Metropolitan Singers; Concert Choir; Jazz Bands; Wind Ensemble; Concert Band; MSC Symphony & String Orchestras; Community Arts & Jefferson Symponies; Woodwind & Brass Quintets; Brass & Percussion Ensembles; String Quartet; Chamber Ensemble

THEATRE

W Thomas Cook, Chairman   **Number Of Faculty:** 8   **Number Of Students:** 85
Degrees Offered: BA
Technical Training: Costuming; Makeup; Stagecraft; Lighting; Stage Design
Teaching Certification Available
Financial Assistance: Scholarships and Work-Study Grants

(continued on next page)

Performing Groups: Metropolitan State Players Auraria Production Company
Workshops/Festivals: Play Production Workshop; Makeup Workshop; Costuming Workshop; Mayfest; Historic Denver

---

NORTHEASTERN JUNIOR COLLEGE
Sterling   Colorado 80751, 303 522-6600 Ext 671
County and 2 Year   **Arts Areas:** Vocal Music, Theatre and Visual Arts
Performance Facilities: Theatre

MUSIC

Robert Wagner, Vocal; C R Stasenka, Instrumental
Number Of Faculty: 2 Full-time, 1 Part-time   **Number Of Students:** 20
Degrees Offered: AA   **Courses Offered:** Lower-division music courses
Financial Assistance: Scholarships and Work-Study Grants
Performing Groups: Choir; College Singers; Chamber Group; Instrumental Ensembles; Stage Band; Varsity Band; Symphonette
Workshops/Festivals: Sterling Arts Council

THEATRE

Ronald Bailey, Director   **Number Of Faculty:** 1   **Number Of Students:** 15
Degrees Offered: AA   **Courses Offered:** Lower-division theatre courses
Financial Assistance: Scholarships and Work-Study Grants
Performing Groups: College Players

UNIVERSITY OF NORTHERN COLORADO
Greeley   Colorado 80631, 303 351-1890
State and 4 Year
Arts Areas: Instrumental Music, Vocal Music, Theatre and Visual Arts

DANCE

Dance program under auspices of Physical Education Department
Courses Offered: Social Dance; Modern Dance; Folk Dance; American Square & Couple Dance

MUSIC

James E Miller, Dean   **Number Of Faculty:** 40
Degrees Offered: BA; BMus; MA; MMusEd   **Teaching Certification Available**
Performing Groups: Jazz Ensemble; Symphony Orchestra; Chamber Orchestra; Lab Orchestra; Brass Choir; String Ensemble; Brass; Woodwind; Percussion; Piano & Guitar Ensembles; Concert Choir; Chorus; Women's Concert Choir; Varsity Glee Club; Symphonic Wind Band; Concert Band; Marching Band; Varsity Band
Workshops/Festivals: Festival Week of Music; Summer Opera; Opera Workshop; Chorus and Orchestra Workshop

THEATRE

John W Willcoxon, Chairman   **Number Of Faculty:** 7   **Degrees Offered:** BA
Teaching Certification Available
Performing Groups: The Little Theatre of the Rockies; Children's Theatre; Reader's Theatre; Musical Theatre; Dance Theatre; Art & Technical Theatre

---

OTERO JUNIOR COLLEGE
18th & Colorado, La Junta   Colorado 81050
303 384-4446
State and 2 Year
Arts Areas: Instrumental Music, Vocal Music, Theatre and Visual Arts
Performance Facilities: Theatre - Auditorium Complex
Degrees Offered: AA
Financial Assistance: Scholarships and Work-Study Grants

UNIVERSITY OF SOUTHERN COLORADO
2200 Bonforte Blvd, Pueblo   Colorado 81001
303 549-2552

State and 4 Year
Arts Areas: Dance, Instrumental Music, Vocal Music, Theatre, Film Arts, Television and Visual Arts
Performing Series: Artist Series
Performance Facilities: Hoag Music Hall; Arena Theater

DANCE

James Duncan, Director, Center for Creative and Performing Arts
Number Of Faculty: 1   *Number Of Students:* 55
Courses Offered: Ballet; Modern Dance
Technical Training: With Pueblo Civic Ballet
Financial Assistance: Scholarships and Work-Study Grants
Workshops/Festivals: Workshops co-sponsored with Sangre de Cristo Arts Center

MUSIC

Ralph Levy, Chairman   *Number Of Faculty:* 11   *Number Of Students:* 120
Degrees Offered: BS; BA   *Courses Offered:* Music Ed; Performance; Theory
Teaching Certification Available
Financial Assistance: Scholarships and Work-Study Grants
Performing Groups: Estudiantina; Ragtime & Piano Ensembles; Stage Band; Single Reed Choir; Orchestra; Symphonic Jazz Ensemble; Three Bands; Concert Choir; "Together" Vocal Ensemble; Guitar Ensemble
Workshops/Festivals: Summer Music Institute; Piano Ensemble Competition; Opera Workshop

THEATRE

Kenneth Plonkey, Co-ordinator   *Number Of Faculty:* 2
Number Of Students: 20   *Degrees Offered:* BS; BA
Teaching Certification Available
Financial Assistance: Scholarships and Work-Study Grants
Performing Groups: Socolo Players
Workshops/Festivals: Summer Theater; High School Theatre Workshop
Artists-In-Residence/Guest Artists: Markowski & Cedrone, Duo Pianists

TRINIDAD STATE COLLEGE
Trinidad   Colorado 81082, 303 846-5531

State and 2 Year
Arts Areas: Instrumental Music, Vocal Music and Theatre
Performing Series: Cultural Events Series
Performance Facilities: College Auditorium   *Number Of Faculty:* 3
Number Of Students: 60   *Degrees Offered:* AA Music
Financial Assistance: Scholarships and Work-Study Grants
Performing Groups: Vocal and Instrumental Ensembles

THEATRE

Margaret Brennan, Chairman
Performing Groups: College Players; Delta Psi Omega

WESTERN STATE COLLEGE
Gunnison   Colorado 81230, 303 943-2186

State and 4 Year
Arts Areas: Instrumental Music, Vocal Music, Theatre, Film Arts and Visual Arts
Performing Series: Concert - Lecture Series
Performance Facilities: Western State College Auditorium

MUSIC

David Sweetkind, Chairman   *Number Of Faculty:* 9   *Number Of Students:* 200
Degrees Offered: BA; MA   *Teaching Certification Available*

(continued on next page)

(*Western State College — cont'd*)

Financial Assistance: Assistantships, Scholarships and Work-Study Grants
Performing Groups: Band; Orchestra; Chorus; Instrumental Ensembles; Madrigal Singers; Opera Workshop

THEATRE

Jess W Gern, Chairman   **Number Of Faculty:** 6   **Number Of Students:** 200
Degrees Offered: BA; MA   **Teaching Certification Available**
Financial Assistance: Assistantships, Scholarships and Work-Study Grants
Performing Groups: Mountaineer Players

ALBANO BALLET AND PERFORMING ARTS ACADEMY, INC
15 Girard Ave, Hartford   Connecticut 06105
203 232-8898
> Private and Special
> *Arts Areas:* Dance, Instrumental Music, Vocal Music and Theatre
> *Performance Facilities:* Resident Stage & Auditorium

DANCE

> Joseph Albano, Chairman   *Number Of Faculty:* 6   *Number Of Students:* 300
> *Degrees Offered:* Two-year teacher training Dance Diploma program
> *Teaching Certification Available*
> *Financial Assistance:* Internships and Work-Study Grants
> *Performing Groups:* Albano Youth Ballet Company; Albano Ballet Company of America, Inc

MUSIC

> Audrey Anweiler, Chairman   *Number Of Faculty:* 5   *Number Of Students:* 50
> *Degrees Offered:* Two-year Music Diploma; two-year Voice Diploma
> *Financial Assistance:* Internships and Work-Study Grants
> *Performing Groups:* Recitals; Operas; Musicals

THEATRE

> Rolayne Kapelner, Chairperson   *Number Of Faculty:* 3
> *Number Of Students:* 50   *Degrees Offered:* Two-year Drama Diploma
> *Financial Assistance:* Internships and Work-Study Grants
> *Performing Groups:* Albano Drama Ensemble

ALBERTUS MAGNUS COLLEGE
700 Prospect St, New Haven   Connecticut 06511
203 777-6631 Ext 357
> Private and 4 Year
> *Arts Areas:* Instrumental Music, Vocal Music, Theatre and Visual Arts

MUSIC

> Gordon Emerson, Chairman   *Number Of Faculty:* 1   *Degrees Offered:* BA; AA
> *Courses Offered:* Music Classes and Private Instruction
> *Financial Assistance:* Scholarships and Work-Study Grants
> *Performing Groups:* Albertus Magnus Glee Club; Patchwork Can Ensemble

THEATRE

> Maxine Schlingman, Chairman   *Number Of Faculty:* 3
> *Teaching Certification Available*
> *Financial Assistance:* Scholarships and Work-Study Grants
> *Performing Groups:* Campus Theatre Players

ANNHURST COLLEGE
Woodstock   Connecticut 06281, 203 928-7773 Ext 31
> Private and 4 Year   *Arts Areas:* Instrumental Music and Vocal Music
> *Performance Facilities:* Cultural Center Auditorium; Cultural Center Little Theater

MUSIC

> Eva Szacik, Acting Chairman   *Number Of Faculty:* 3   *Degrees Offered:* BA
> *Financial Assistance:* Scholarships and Work-Study Grants
> *Performing Groups:* Glee Club; Sylvans; Band

UNIVERSITY OF BRIDGEPORT
84 Iranistan Ave, Bridgeport   Connecticut 06002
203 576-4397

Private and 4 Year
Arts Areas: Dance, Instrumental Music, Vocal Music, Theatre, Film Arts and Visual Arts
Performance Facilities: Andre & Clara Mertens Theatre; Lecture, Recital Hall

DANCE

Margo Knis, Chairman   *Financial Assistance:* Assistantships and Scholarships

MUSIC

Professor Richard De Baise, Chairman   *Number Of Faculty:* 20
Number Of Students: 200   *Degrees Offered:* BA; BFA; BM; BMusEd; MMusEd
Teaching Certification Available
Financial Assistance: Assistantships, Scholarships and Work-Study Grants
Performing Groups: Jazz Ensemble; Concert Band; Concert Choir; String Quartet

THEATRE

W Ellard Taylor, Chairman   *Number Of Faculty:* 10   *Number Of Students:* 60
Degrees Offered: BA; BFA
Courses Offered: Acting; Directing; Technical Theatre
Financial Assistance: Assistantships, Scholarships and Work-Study Grants
Performing Groups: University Players

CENTRAL CONNECTICUT STATE COLLEGE
1615 Stanley St, New Britain   Connecticut 06050
203 827-7000

State and 4 Year
Arts Areas: Dance, Instrumental Music, Vocal Music and Theatre
Performing Series: CCSC Music Series; CCSC Theatre Series
Performance Facilities: College Theatre; Welte Auditorium

DANCE

Dance program under auspices of Physical Education Department

MUSIC

Henley Denmead, Chairperson   *Number Of Faculty:* 13 Full-time, 7 Part-time
Number Of Students: 80   *Degrees Offered:* BS
Courses Offered: Complete Curriculum in Instrumental and Vocal Music
Teaching Certification Available
Financial Assistance: Assistantships and Work-Study Grants
Performing Groups: Wells String Quartet; CCSC Concert Choir; Women's Chorus; College - Community
Orchestra; Wind Ensemble; Chamber Singers; Marching Band
Workshops/Festivals: Summer Chamber Music Workshop

THEATRE

Dr Clyde Bassett, Chairperson   *Number Of Faculty:* 7
Number Of Students: 60   *Degrees Offered:* BFA
Courses Offered: Complete Curriculum in Acting, Directing, Design and Technical Theater
Technical Training: Complete Technical Theatre Courses
Teaching Certification Available
Financial Assistance: Assistantships, Scholarships and Work-Study Grants
Workshops/Festivals: Summer Theatre Workshop

CONNECTICUT COLLEGE

New London   Connecticut 06320, 203 442-5391

Private and 4 Year

Arts Areas: Dance, Instrumental Music, Vocal Music, Theatre, Film Arts and Visual Arts
Performing Series: Concert & Artist Series
Performance Facilities: Palmer Auditorium; Dana Hall

DANCE

Martha Myers, Chairman   *Number Of Faculty:* 5   *Number Of Students:* 40
Degrees Offered: BA; MFA
Courses Offered: Techniques; Composition; Improvisation; History of Dance; Practice Teaching; History of Human Movement; Performing Styles; Production
Technical Training: Modern; Ballet; Jazz
Financial Assistance: Scholarships and Work-Study Grants
Performing Groups: Advanced Improvisational Lab
Workshops/Festivals: Touring Professional Dance Companies (2 Concerts Annually)

MUSIC

William Dale, Professor of Music   *Number Of Faculty:* 9
Number Of Students: 271   *Degrees Offered:* BA; MA; MAT
Courses Offered: Theory; Music History; Composition; Applied Music
Technical Training: Instrumental Study; Performance/Repertory Class
Financial Assistance: Scholarships and Work-Study Grants
Performing Groups: Connecticut College Chorus; Harkness Chapel Choir; Connecticut College Orchestra; Jazz Ensemble

THEATRE

Linda Herr, Co-Director   *Number Of Faculty:* 3   *Number Of Students:* 35
Degrees Offered: BA; MA in Educational Theater for the Deaf
Courses Offered: Acting; Directing
Technical Training: Costuming; Lighting; Design
Financial Assistance: Scholarships and Work-Study Grants
Performing Groups: Ensemble Workshop
Workshops/Festivals: Department Productions; Theater I Workshops & Productions
Artists-In-Residence/Guest Artists: St Paul Chamber Orcherstra; Philharmonica Hungarian; Cincinnati Orchestra; Les Menestriers; Tokyo String Quartet

UNIVERSITY OF CONNECTICUT

Storrs   Connecticut 06268, 203 486-3016

State and 4 Year

Arts Areas: Dance, Instrumental Music, Vocal Music, Theatre, Film Arts, Television and Visual Arts
Performing Series: Major Concert Series; Chamber Music Series; Dance Series
Performance Facilities: Jorgensen, Mobius, and Studio Theatres; Jorgensen Auditorium; Mehden Recital Hall

DANCE

Dr John H Herr, Chairman
Dance program is intergrated with Theatre program
Financial Assistance: Assistantships

MUSIC

Dr Edward G Evans, Jr, Chairman
Number Of Faculty: 28 Full-time, 37 Part-time   *Number Of Students:* 324
Degrees Offered: B Mus, Applied Music, Music History, Theory & Composition; BS Mus Ed; BFA, Music; MA Applied Music, Theory, Composition, Historical Musicology, Pedagogy, Psychoacoustics, Music Education; PhD Music
Teaching Certification Available
Financial Assistance: Assistantships, Scholarships and Work-Study Grants

(continued on next page)

Performing Groups: Symphonic Wind Ensemble; Concert Band; Marching Band; Chorus; Concert Choir; Chamber Singers; Choral Society; Orchestra; Small Ensembles; Collegium Musicum; Black Voices of Freedom
Workshops/Festivals: Orff Workshop; Kodaly Workshop; Opera Workshop

THEATRE

Dr John H Herr, Chairman   **Number Of Faculty:** 17   **Number Of Students:** 230
Degrees Offered: BFA; MA; MFA
Financial Assistance: Assistantships, Scholarships and Work-Study Grants
Performing Groups: The Ragbaggers (Children's Theatre); The Mobius Ensemble
Workshops/Festivals: ATA Regional Theatre Festival, 1975; The New England Theatre Conference, 1978

EASTERN CONNECTICUT STATE COLLEGE
83 Windham St, Willimantic   Connecticut 06226
203 456-2231
State and 4 Year
Arts Areas: Instrumental Music, Vocal Music, Film Arts, Television and Visual Arts
Performance Facilities: Shafer Auditorium

MUSIC

Robert Lemons, Chairperson   **Number Of Faculty:** 5   **Degrees Offered:** BA
Courses Offered: Introductory and Advances Courses; Theory and Applied
Teaching Certification Available
Financial Assistance: Internships, Scholarships and Work-Study Grants
Performing Groups: Choral Group; Concert Band; Orchestra; Woodwind Ensemble

THEATRE

William Lannon, Director of the Harry Hope Theatre   **Number Of Faculty:** 1

HARTFORD COLLEGE FOR WOMEN
Hartford   Connecticut 06105, 203 236-1215
Private and 2 Year   **Arts Areas:** Theatre

THEATRE

Paul De Sole, Chairman   **Degrees Offered:** AA
Performing Groups: Dramatic Club

THE HARTFORD CONSERVATORY
834-846 Asylum Ave, Hartford   Connecticut 06105
203 246-2588
Private and 2 Year
Arts Areas: Dance, Instrumental Music and Vocal Music
Performance Facilities: Hosmer Auditorium; Welch Music Room

DANCE

Mary Giannone, Coordinator of Dance   **Number Of Faculty:** 8
Number Of Students: 30   **Degrees Offered:** Two Year Diploma in Dance
Courses Offered: Ballet; Modern (Limon, Cunningham); Jazz; Composition; Anatomy for Dancers; History of Dance; Music Theory & Analysis; Dance Pedagogy & Apprentice Teaching
Financial Assistance: Scholarships and Work-Study Grants
Performing Groups: Hartford Conservatory Modern Dance Ensemble

MUSIC

Geraldine Douglass, Director   **Number Of Faculty:** 48
Number Of Students: 750   **Degrees Offered:** Two-Year Diploma in Performance

(continued on next page)

Courses Offered: Curricula in Keyboard Instruments, Voice, Orchestral Instruments in Traditional Study and Jazz and Pop Music
Financial Assistance: Work-Study Grants
Artists-In-Residence/Guest Artists: The Connecticut Ballet Company; Connecticut Dance Theatre

UNIVERSITY OF HARTFORD
West Hartford   Connecticut 06117, 203 206-5411
Private and 4 Year
Arts Areas: Instrumental Music, Vocal Music and Theatre
Performance Facilities: Auerbach Auditorium

MUSIC

Elizabeth Warner, Dean, Hartt School of Music   *Number Of Faculty:* 70
Degrees Offered: BMus; BMusEd; MMus; MMusEd; DMusArts; MMus Composition
Teaching Certification Available
Financial Assistance: Assistantships, Scholarships and Work-Study Grants
Performing Groups: Hartt Collegium Musicum; Hartt Concert Band; Hartt Symphonic Wind Ensemble; Hartt Symphony Orchestra; Hartt Repertory Orchestra; Hartt Chamber Singers; Hartt Chorale

THEATRE

Gerald Forbes, Chairman   *Number Of Faculty:* 11   *Degrees Offered:* BA
Teaching Certification Available
Financial Assistance: Internships, Assistantships, Scholarships and Work-Study Grants
Performing Groups: University Players
Workshops/Festivals: Summer Repertory Theatre

MATTATUK COMMUNITY COLLEGE
650 Chase Pkwy, Waterbury   Connecticut 06795
203 757-9661 Ext 223
State and 2 Year   *Arts Areas:* Vocal Music and Theatre
Performance Facilities: Opera House Facilities   *Number Of Faculty:* 1
Number Of Students: 100   *Degrees Offered:* AA
Financial Assistance: Work-Study Grants
Performing Groups: Mattatuck Chorus; Mattatuck Chamber Singers
Workshops/Festivals: Spring Festival; Music Workshops   *Number Of Faculty:* 2
Number Of Students: 50   *Degrees Offered:* AA
Financial Assistance: Work-Study Grants   *Performing Groups:* Stage Society
Workshops/Festivals: Spring Festival

MITCHELL COLLEGE
Pequot & Montauk Aves, New London   Connecticut 06320
203 443-2811
Private and 2 Year   *Arts Areas:* Theatre and Puppetry
Performance Facilities: Clarke Center

THEATRE

Jennifer O'Donnell, Instructor   *Number Of Faculty:* 1
Number Of Students: 30 - 50   *Courses Offered:* Dramatic Production
Technical Training: On-the-Job Technical Training
Performing Groups: Richard Mansfield Players

NEW HAVEN DANCE CENTER
612 Chapel St, New Haven   Connecticut 06511
203 865-4649
Private and Special   *Arts Areas:* Dance

(continued on next page)

(New Haven Dance Ctr — cont'd)

DANCE

Emy de Pradines, Director   **Number Of Faculty:** 9
Technical Training: Ballet; Modern Ethnic Dance; Modern Dance; Jazz; Character; Mime; Pointe; Adagio
Music Appreciation

UNIVERSITY OF NEW HAVEN
300 Orange Ave, West Haven   Connecticut 06516
203 934-6321
Private and 4 Year
Arts Areas: Instrumental Music, Vocal Music, Theatre and Ethnomusicological Field Training
Performing Series: World Music Concert Series
Performance Facilities: Ensemble Rooms; Practice Rooms

MUSIC

Dr Michael G Kaloyanides, Chairman   **Number Of Faculty:** 5
Number Of Students: 115   **Degrees Offered:** BA in World Music
Courses Offered: History & Literature; Theory; Performance; Research
Technical Training: Techniques & Methodology in Ethnomusicology
Financial Assistance: Scholarships and Work-Study Grants
Performing Groups: Orchestra; Wind Ensemble; Greek Rebetic Ensemble; Chorus; Jazz Ensemble; West
African Drumming Ensemble
Workshops/Festivals: World Music Concert Series
Artists-In-Residence/Guest Artists: George Mgrdichian; Mohammed El Akkad; Namino Torii; Abraham
Adzenyah; Sumarsam; Laxmi G Tewari; T Viswanathan; B Ranganatham; Jean Redpath

---

QUINNIPIAC COLLEGE
Mt Carmel Ave, Hamden   Connecticut 06518
203 288-5251
Private and 4 Year
Arts Areas: Instrumental Music, Vocal Music, Theatre and Radio
Performing Series: Concert - Lecture Series

MUSIC

Richard Burwell, Chairman   **Degrees Offered:** BA
Financial Assistance: Scholarships   **Performing Groups:** Glee Club
Workshops/Festivals: Jazz Workshop; Intercollegiate Jazz Festival
Financial Assistance: Scholarships   **Performing Groups:** Quinnipiac Theatre
Workshops/Festivals: Theatre Workshop

SOUTHERN CONNECTICUT STATE COLLEGE
501 Crescent, New Haven   Connecticut 06515
203 397-2101
State and 4 Year
Arts Areas: Instrumental Music, Vocal Music, Theatre and Visual Arts
Performance Facilities: John Lyman Auditorium; Drama Laboratory
Workshops/Festivals: Dance Workshop   **Number Of Faculty:** 11
Degrees Offered: BA   **Number Of Faculty:** 7   **Number Of Students:** 225
Degrees Offered: BA   **Performing Groups:** The Crescent Players

---

TRINITY COLLEGE
300 Summit St, Hartford   Connecticut 06106
203 527-3151 Ext 431
Private and 4 Year
Arts Areas: Dance, Instrumental Music, Vocal Music, Theatre and Visual Arts
Performance Facilities: Goodwin Theatre

(continued on next page)

DANCE

Judy Dworin, Program Director   **Number Of Faculty:** 1 Full-time, 3 Part-time
Number Of Students: 80 - 100   **Degrees Offered:** BA
Courses Offered: Dance History; Composition; Improvisation; Repertory
Financial Assistance: Assistantships, Scholarships and Work-Study Grants

MUSIC

Gail Rehman, Program Director   **Number Of Faculty:** 3 Full-time, 1 Part-time
Number Of Students: 180 - 225   **Degrees Offered:** BA
Courses Offered: Music History; Music Literature; Theory; Composition
Technical Training: Instrumental; Voice   **Teaching Certification Available**
Financial Assistance: Assistantships, Scholarships and Work-Study Grants
Performing Groups: Band; Choir

THEATRE

George E Nichols, Program Director
Number Of Faculty: 2 Full-time, 1 Part-time   **Number Of Students:** 60 - 80
Degrees Offered: BA
Courses Offered: Theatre History and Literature; Acting; Directing; Playwriting
Technical Training: Production Participation; Oral Interpretation
Financial Assistance: Assistantships, Scholarships and Work-Study Grants
Performing Groups: The Jesters
Workshops/Festivals: Summerstage; Summer Repertory Theatre and Courses; productions throughout the academic year
Artists-In-Residence/Guest Artists: Connie Kreemer; Shulamit Saltzman; Carter McAdams

U S COAST GUARD ACADEMY
Mohegan Ave, New London   Connecticut 06320
203 443-6045
4 Year and Federal Academy
Arts Areas: Dance, Instrumental Music, Vocal Music and Theatre
Performing Series: US Coast Guard Band Concert Series
Performance Facilities: Auditorium; Outdoor Shell; Chapel

DANCE

Jill Holt, FISTD, Instructor   **Number Of Faculty:** 1
Number Of Students: 30   **Courses Offered:** Modern; Tap

MUSIC

D L Janse, Director Cadet Musical Activities   **Number Of Faculty:** 3
Number Of Students: 300   **Courses Offered:** 12 Choral Band performing groups
Technical Training: Voice Class; Group and Individual Training
Performing Groups: Singing Idlers; Glee Club; Chapel Choirs; NL Trio; Barbershoppers; Brigade Band; Cadet Band Windjammers; Nite Caps; Wind Ensemble; Brass Choir; Informal Bands

THEATRE

D L Janse, Chairman   **Number Of Faculty:** 1   **Number Of Students:** 30
Performing Groups: Cadet Musical Activity Musical Production Club; Cadet Musical Activity Drama Production Club

WESLEYAN UNIVERSITY
Middletown   Connecticut 06457, 203 347-9411
Private and 4 Year
Arts Areas: Dance, Instrumental Music, Vocal Music, Theatre, Film Arts and Visual Arts
Performing Series: Crowell Concert Series; World Music Series
Performance Facilities: Crowell Concert Hall; World Music Hall; Center for Arts Theatre; '92 Theatre

(continued on next page)

DANCE

William R Ward, Chairman   **Degrees Offered:** BA
Courses Offered: Improvisation; History and Criticism; Compositon; Music for Dance, Teaching, Choreography Workshop
Financial Assistance: Scholarships and Work-Study Grants
Performing Groups: Sonomama; The Corner Store
Workshops/Festivals: Day of Dance; Winter Dance Concert; Music for Dance and Dance Teaching Workshop

MUSIC

Richard K Winslow, Chairman   **Number Of Faculty:** 11
Degrees Offered: BA; MA; PhD
Courses Offered: Stylistic Analysis (W Europe Art Music); World Music (Afro-American, S Indian, Javanese, Japanese, W African, European Folk, Yiddish, W Asian); Private Instruction; Musicology; Theory and Composition; Group Instruction
Financial Assistance: Scholarships and Work-Study Grants
Performing Groups: Gamelan; Wesleyan Singers; Choir; Orchestra; Big Band (jazz); Woodwind Quintet
Workshops/Festivals: Navaratri Festival; World Music Performances; Performances and Workshops by Visiting Artists

THEATRE

William R Ward, Chairman   **Number Of Faculty:** 11   **Degrees Offered:** BA; MA
Courses Offered: Acting, Production, and Directing Techniques; Criticism; Playwriting; Design; Lighting; Vocal Music for Theater; Costuming Experimental Theater; Black Theater; Improvisation; Stage Movement
Financial Assistance: Scholarships and Work-Study Grants
Performing Groups: Second Stage
Artists-In-Residence/Guest Artists: Music: 27 Artists-in-Residence (World Music) and Visiting Teachers (European Art Music)
Theater: Eileen Blumenthal; Greta Slobin
Dance: Pamela Finney; Laura Pawel

WESTERN CONNECTICUT STATE COLLEGE
181 Whit St, Danbury   Connecticut 06810
203 792-1400
State and City
Arts Areas: Dance, Instrumental Music, Vocal Music, Theatre, Film Arts, Television and Visual Arts

DANCE

Margaret Lipscomb, Instructor   **Number Of Faculty:** 1
Number Of Students: 16   **Performing Groups:** Modern Dance
Workshops/Festivals: Three Yearly Workshops

MUSIC

Richard Moryle, Chairman   **Number Of Faculty:** 13   **Number Of Students:** 150
Degrees Offered: BMus; BS MusEd   **Teaching Certification Available**
Financial Assistance: Scholarships and Work-Study Grants
Performing Groups: Chorus; Band; Orchestra; Choir; Jazz Ensemble; Percussion Ensemble

THEATRE

Richard Reinold, Chairman   **Number Of Faculty:** 10   **Degrees Offered:** BA
Performing Groups: Children's Theatre; Speech and Theatre Groups
Workshops/Festivals: Annual Arts Festival; Several Theatre & Children's Theatre Workshops

---

YALE UNIVERSITY
96 Wall St, New Haven   Connecticut 06520
203 426-4771
State and 4 Year
Arts Areas: Instrumental Music, Vocal Music, Theatre, Television and Visual Arts
Performance Facilities: Yale Repertory Theatre; University Theatre

(continued on next page)

DANCE

Mrs John Barnett, Director   **Number Of Faculty:** 6   **Number Of Students:** 500
Technical Training: Beginning Ballet; Advanced Ballet; Jazz; Tap Dancing; Beginning Modern;
Intermediate Modern; Advanced Modern
Performing Groups: Yale Concert Dancers
Workshops/Festivals: Master Classes with Professionals

MUSIC

Phillip F Nelson, Dean   **Number Of Faculty:** 79   **Number Of Students:** 320
Degrees Offered: BA; MMus; MAEd; PhD; MPh
Technical Training: Conducting Opera; Electronic Music
Teaching Certification Available
Financial Assistance: Internships, Assistantships, Scholarships and Work-Study Grants
Performing Groups: Yale Philharmonic Orchestra; Wind Ensembles; String Ensembles; Choir; Chamber
Music
Workshops/Festivals: Opera Workshop; Body Movement; Summer Festival, Norfolk, Conn

THEATRE

Robert Brustein, Chairman   **Number Of Faculty:** 55   **Number Of Students:** 225
Degrees Offered: BA, Theatre History; MFAA; DFA, Dramatic Literature & Criticism; PhD, Acting
Technical Training: Playwriting; Acting; Directing; Design; Theatre Design & Technology; Theatre
Administration
Teaching Certification Available
Financial Assistance: Internships, Assistantships, Scholarships and Work-Study Grants
Performing Groups: Yale Repertory Theatre, professional company in which third year students perform;
Theatre Ensembles
Workshops/Festivals: Workshop Productions

DELAWARE

BRANDYWINE COLLEGE
Box 7139 Concord Dike, Wilmington   Delaware 19803
203 478-3000
>   Private and 2 Year
>   *Arts Areas:* Instrumental Music, Vocal Music, Theatre and Visual Arts
>   *Performing Series:* Cultural Events Series
>   *Performance Facilities:* College Auditorium
>   AA Liberal Arts, Scholarships and Work - Study Grants; No Arts Majors

---

DELAWARE STATE COLLEGE
Dover   Delaware 19901, 302 678-5155
>   State and 4 Year
>   *Arts Areas:* Instrumental Music, Vocal Music, Theatre and Visual Arts

MUSIC

Number Of Faculty: 5   *Degrees Offered:* BA; BMusEd; MMusEd
Teaching Certification Available
Financial Assistance: Assistantships, Scholarships and Work-Study Grants
Performing Groups: Orchestra; Band; Chorus; Vocal and Instrumental Ensembles

THEATRE

Number Of Faculty: 3   *Degrees Offered:* BA; MA
Teaching Certification Available
Financial Assistance: Assistantships, Scholarships and Work-Study Grants
Performing Groups: College Theatre

UNIVERSITY OF DELAWARE
Newark   Delaware 19711, 302 738-2351
>   Private and 4 Year
>   *Arts Areas:* Dance, Instrumental Music, Vocal Music and Theatre

DANCE

Debra Loewen, Coordinator   *Number Of Faculty:* 1   *Number Of Students:* 60
Degrees Offered: BA in Theatre with Dance Emphasis
Financial Assistance: Work-Study Grants   *Performing Groups:* New Space Company

MUSIC

Henry L Cady, Chairman   *Number Of Faculty:* 19 Full-time, 18 Part-time
Number Of Students: 160
Degrees Offered: BA; BMus in Applied Music, Music Education, Theory and Composition
Teaching Certification Available
Financial Assistance: Assistantships, Scholarships and Work-Study Grants
Performing Groups: Instrumental Groups; Orchestra; Wind, Jazz, and Percussion Ensembles; Symphonic Band; Marching Band; Chamber Trios; Quartets; Quintets; Concert Choir; University Singers; Chorale; Choral Union
Workshops/Festivals: Solo and Ensemble Music Festival, Instrumental and Piano Divisions; Contemporary Music Festival; Master Classes by Visiting Artists; Choral Workshops by Guest Conductors

THEATRE

Brian Hansen, Chairman   *Number Of Faculty:* 11   *Number Of Students:* 75
Degrees Offered: BA
Courses Offered: Performance; Technical Design; Dance; Theatre Education; Black Theatre

(continued on next page)

Technical Training: University Theatre Season
Teaching Certification Available   **Performing Groups:** University Theatre; E52
Workshops/Festivals: Fall Conference for High School Students; Spring One-Act Festival

---

WESLEY COLLEGE
College Square, Dover   Delaware 19901
302 674-4000

Private and 2 Year
Arts Areas: Instrumental Music, Vocal Music and Visual Arts

MUSIC

Robert W Bailey, Chairman   **Number Of Faculty:** 1   **Degrees Offered:** AA
Financial Assistance: Scholarships

THEATRE

James K Young, Chairman   **Number Of Faculty:** 1   **Degrees Offered:** AA
Performing Groups: Wesley Players; Delta Psi Omega

WILMINGTON COLLEGE
320 DuPont Pkwy, Newcastle   Delaware 19720
302 328-9401

Private and 4 Year   **Arts Areas:** Theatre and Visual Arts
Performing Series: Concert - Lecture Series
Performance Facilities: College Auditorium

THEATRE

Degrees Offered: AA; BA   **Financial Assistance:** Scholarships and Work-Study Grants
Performing Groups: Wilmington College Players

WILMINGTON MUSIC SCHOOL
4101 Washington St, Wilmington   Delaware 19802
302 762-1132

Private and Special   **Arts Areas:** Instrumental Music and Vocal Music
Performance Facilities: Wilmington Music School Auditorium

MUSIC

Stephen Gunzenhauser, Executive Director   **Number Of Faculty:** 48
Number Of Students: 640   **Degrees Offered:** Pre-College Diploma
Financial Assistance: Scholarships
Performing Groups: String Club; Stage Band Combo; Chamber Orchestra; Training Orchestra
Workshops/Festivals: Jazz Workshop; Arden Chamber Players Series; Delaware Trio Workshop;
Musicianship Seminar; Composition Seminar

THE AMERICAN UNIVERSITY ACADEMY FOR THE PERFORMING ARTS
Massachusetts Ave & Nebraska Ave, NW, Washington   District of Columbia 20016
202 686-2315
   Private and 4 Year
   Charles Crowder, Chairman, Department of Performing Arts
   Arts Areas: Dance, Instrumental Music, Vocal Music, Theatre, Film Arts, Television, Visual Arts and Arts
   Management
   Performance Facilities: Woods Brown Amphitheatre; Clendenen Theatre; MacDonald Recital Hall

DANCE

Naima Prevots, Director   *Number Of Faculty:* 3 Full-time, 2 Part-time
Number Of Students: 100   *Degrees Offered:* BA; BS; MA
Courses Offered: Three years History & Philosophy of Dance plus full track in Dance Composition;
Anatomy; Effort Shape; Dynamic Alignment; Kineseology
Technical Training: Full track Modern Dance and Classical Ballet
Teaching Certification Available
Financial Assistance: Internships, Assistantships, Scholarships, Work-Study Grants and Cooperative
Education
Performing Groups: Dance Theatre
Workshops/Festivals: Summer Academy of Performing Arts

MUSIC

George Schuetze, Director   *Number Of Faculty:* 8   *Number Of Students:* 85
Degrees Offered: BMus; BA; B MusEd; MA
Courses Offered: Full track in Music History/Musicology and in Music Theory
Technical Training: Full track in all areas of Applied Music
Teaching Certification Available
Financial Assistance: Internships, Assistantships, Work-Study Grants and Cooperative Education
Performing Groups: Ensembles in Brass, Percussion, Woodwinds, Jazz; University Chorale; University
Singers; University Orchestra
Workshops/Festivals: Master Classes by Prominent Visitors; Summer Academy of Performing Arts

THEATRE

Kenneth Baker, Director   *Number Of Faculty:* 5 Full-time, 1 Part-time
Number Of Students: 60   *Degrees Offered:* BA; BS; MA
Courses Offered: Emphasis on Acting/Directing with supportive coursework in History, Creative Theory,
Technical Theatre
Technical Training: Full track in Acting/Directing
Financial Assistance: Internships, Assistantships, Scholarships, Work-Study Grants and Cooperative
Education
Performing Groups: University Players
Workshops/Festivals: Summer Academy of Performing Arts

THE CATHOLIC UNIVERSITY OF AMERICA
Washington   District of Columbia 20064, 202 635-5000
   Private and 4 Year
   Arts Areas: Dance, Instrumental Music, Vocal Music, Theatre and Film Arts
   Performing Series: Guest Artist Series
   Performance Facilities: Ward Recital Hall; Hartke Theatre; McMahon Auditorium; Malony Auditorium

DANCE

Jone Dowd, Coordinator   *Number Of Faculty:* 1   *Number Of Students:* 25
Technical Training: Dance Classes & Gymnastics

(continued on next page)

MUSIC

Dr Thomas Mastroianni, Dean   **Number Of Faculty:** 80
Number Of Students: 556   **Degrees Offered:** BMus; BA; MMus; MA; DMA; PhD
Courses Offered: General Choral; Instrumental; Theory; Composition; Music Therapy; Music Education; Pedagogy
Teaching Certification Available
Financial Assistance: Assistantships, Scholarships and Work-Study Grants
Performing Groups: University Symphony Orchestra; Wind Symphony; A Cappella Choir; Concert Orchestra; Trombone Choir; Collegium Musicum; Contemporary Chamber, Brass, Jazz, Percussion and Guitar Ensembles; Cardinalaires
Workshops/Festivals: Suzuki Workshop; Kodaly & Orff Workshops; Jazz Workshops; Music Therapy Workshops, Music in the Liturgy Workshops

THEATRE

William H Graham, Chairman   **Number Of Faculty:** 17
Number Of Students: 265   **Degrees Offered:** BA; BFA; MA; MFA
Technical Training: Provided by working on actual productions
Performing Groups: National Players Touring Company (the longest-running - 29 years - theatrical repertory touring company in the US); The Gilbert V Hartke, OP Theatre; The Callan Laboratory Theatre
Workshops/Festivals: Communications workshops for professional men & women; High School Institutes; Acting Conservatory

---

DISTRICT OF COLUMBIA TEACHERS COLLEGE
Harvard & 11th Sts NW, Washington   District of Columbia 20009
202 362-1501
Private and 4 Year   **Arts Areas:** Theatre and Visual Arts

THEATRE

T W Brown, Chairman   **Number Of Faculty:** 1   **Number Of Students:** 40
Financial Assistance: Scholarships and Work-Study Grants
Performing Groups: DCTC Players

FEDERAL CITY COLLEGE
916 G St NW, Washington   District of Columbia 20001
292 727-2943
City and 4 Year
Arts Areas: Dance, Instrumental Music, Vocal Music, Theatre, Film Arts, Television and Visual Arts
Performance Facilities: Environmental Theatre

DANCE

Wilmer Johnson, Chairman, Physical Education Department
Number Of Faculty: 1   **Number Of Students:** 50
Dance program under auspices of Physical Education Department
Degrees Offered: BA with Concentration in Dance
Teaching Certification Available   **Financial Assistance:** Work-Study Grants

MUSIC

William E Moore, Chairman   **Number Of Faculty:** 14   **Number Of Students:** 180
Degrees Offered: BMusEd   **Teaching Certification Available**
Financial Assistance: Work-Study Grants
Performing Groups: Federal City College Chorale; The Voices; Jazz Lab Band
Workshops/Festivals: String Competition

THEATRE

Robert E West, Acting Chairman   **Number Of Faculty:** 4
Number Of Students: 80
Degrees Offered: BA with Concentration in Production, Directing
Financial Assistance: Work-Study Grants

GALLAUDET COLLEGE

7th & Florida Ave NE, Washington   District of Columbia 20002
202 447-0605

Private and 4 Year   *Arts Areas:* Theatre
Performance Facilities: Gallaudet Auditorium
The only liberal arts college for the deaf in the world.

THEATRE

Gilbert C Eastman, Chairman   *Number Of Faculty:* 4   *Degrees Offered:* BA
Technical Training: Theatre for the Deaf
Performing Groups: Gallaudet College Theatre

GEORGE WASHINGTON UNIVERSITY

Washington   District of Columbia 20006, 202 676-6000

Private and 4 Year   *Arts Areas:* Dance, Instrumental Music and Theatre
Performance Facilities: Marvin Theatre

DANCE

Dr Sharon Leigh Clark, Dance Program Director   *Number Of Faculty:* 3
Number Of Students: 65   *Degrees Offered:* BA; MA
Teaching Certification Available   *Financial Assistance:* Assistantships
Performing Groups: The Dance Company
Workshops/Festivals: Guest Artist Series

MUSIC

Prof George Steiner, Chairman   *Number Of Faculty:* 38
Degrees Offered: BA; MA   *Teaching Certification Available*
Performing Groups: University Choir; Orchestra

THEATRE

Nathan Garner, Theatre Program Chairman   *Number Of Faculty:* 5
Number Of Students: 60   *Teaching Certification Available*
Financial Assistance: Assistantships and Work-Study Grants
Performing Groups: University Theatre
Workshops/Festivals: Guest Artist Series

GEORGETOWN UNIVERSITY

State One, 3620 P St, NW, Washington   District of Columbia 20057
202 333-1789

Private and 4 Year   *Arts Areas:* Theatre and Visual Arts
Performing Series: University Concerts
Performance Facilities: Trinity Theatre; State One

THEATRE

Donn B Murphy, Chairman   *Number Of Faculty:* 1   *Number Of Students:* 20
Degrees Offered: BA, Theatre minor   *Financial Assistance:* Work-Study Grants
Performing Groups: Mask & Bauble Theatre

HOWARD UNIVERSITY

2400 Sixth St, NW, Washington   District of Columbia 20059
202 636-6100

Private and 4 Year
Arts Areas: Instrumental Music, Vocal Music and Theatre

MUSIC

Dr Doris McGinty, Chairman   *Number Of Faculty:* 37
Number Of Students: 234   *Degrees Offered:* BMus; BMusEd; MMus; MMusEd

(continued on next page)

Courses Offered: Applied Music; Composition; History & Literature; Jazz Studies; Music Therapy; Piano; Voice; Guitar; Violin or Violincello or Orchestral Instruments
Technical Training: Instrument Repair; Piano Tuning and Repair; Legal Protection of Music
Financial Assistance: Assistantships, Scholarships and Work-Study Grants
Performing Groups: Howard University Jazz Ensemble; Collegium Musicum; Brasswinds Ensemble; Concert Band; Woodwind Ensemble
Workshops/Festivals: Choral Workshop

THEATRE

Prof Theodore Cooper, Chairman   **Number Of Faculty:** 13
Number Of Students: 135   **Degrees Offered:** BFA
Courses Offered: Playwriting; Directing; Acting; Technical Production; Theatre Education
Financial Assistance: Assistantships, Scholarships and Work-Study Grants
Performing Groups: Howard Players

IMMACULATA COLLEGE OF WASHINGTON
4300 Nebraska Ave NW, Washington   District of Columbia 20016
202 966-0040
Private and 2 Year
Arts Areas: Instrumental Music, Vocal Music and Theatre

MUSIC

Degrees Offered: AA
Financial Assistance: Scholarships and Work-Study Grants

THEATRE

E Wierdak, Chairman   **Number Of Faculty:** 3   **Degrees Offered:** AA
Financial Assistance: Scholarships and Work-Study Grants
Performing Groups: Players Club

MARJORIE WEBSTER JUNIOR COLLEGE
Kalmia Rd & Sixth NW, Washington   District of Columbia 20012
202 882-4400
Private and 2 Year
Arts Areas: Instrumental Music, Vocal Music and Theatre

MUSIC

Degrees Offered: A Mus
Financial Assistance: Scholarships and Work-Study Grants

MODERN SCHOOL OF MUSIC
Washington   District of Columbia 20010, 202 726-3763
Private and 4 Year   **Arts Areas:** Instrumental Music and Vocal Music
Degrees Offered: BA

MOUNT VERNON COLLEGE
2100 Foxhill Rd, Washington   District of Columbia 20007
202 331-3444
Private and 4 Year
Arts Areas: Dance, Instrumental Music, Vocal Music, Theatre, Film Arts, Television and Visual Arts
Performance Facilities: Florence Hollis Hand Chapel

THEATRE

William Barlow, Chairman   **Number Of Faculty:** 6   **Number Of Students:** 40
Degrees Offered: AA; BA
Financial Assistance: Scholarships and Work-Study Grants
Performing Groups: Curtain Callers

TRINITY COLLEGE
Washington   District of Columbia 20017, 202 269-2270
Private and 4 Year
Arts Areas: Dance, Instrumental Music, Vocal Music, Theatre and Visual Arts
Performing Series: Annual Concert Series
Performance Facilities: O'Connor Auditorium; O'Connor Art Gallery

MUSIC

Dr Sharon Shafer, Assistant Professor   *Number Of Faculty:* 7
Number Of Students: 187   *Degrees Offered:* BA
Courses Offered: Voice; Piano; Violin; Flute; Conducting; Theory, History, Appreciation; Pedagogy
Technical Training: Praciticums with National Symphony, Radio Stations and Choral Groups
Teaching Certification Available
Financial Assistance: Scholarships and Work-Study Grants
Performing Groups: Concert Choir; Chamber Ensemble; Opera Workshop
Workshops/Festivals: Opera Workshop; Performance Choral Seminars; Music Workshops for High School Students
Artists-In-Residence/Guest Artists: Zetta Finkelstein, Piano; Loretta Goldberg, Piano

BARRY COLLEGE
11300 NE 2nd, Miami Shores   Florida 33161
305 758-3392

Private and 4 Year
Arts Areas: Instrumental Music, Vocal Music, Theatre and Visual Arts

MUSIC

Sister Madonna Oliver, Chairman   **Number Of Faculty:** 3
Number Of Students: 69   **Degrees Offered:** BA, Applied, Theory
Technical Training: Liturgical Singing   **Teaching Certification Available**
Financial Assistance: Scholarships and Work-Study Grants
Performing Groups: Glee Club; Recitals; Choir; Chamber Ensembles

THEATRE

Sister Marie Carol Hurley, Chairman   **Number Of Faculty:** 2
Number Of Students: 46   **Degrees Offered:** BA
Teaching Certification Available
Financial Assistance: Scholarships and Work-Study Grants
Performing Groups: Barry College Playhouse

BETHUNE - COOKMAN COLLEGE
640 Second Ave, Daytona Beach   Florida 32014
904 255-1401 Ex 220

Private and 4 Year   **Arts Areas:** Instrumental Music and Vocal Music

MUSIC

Dr David S Collins, Chairman   **Number Of Faculty:** 8
Number Of Students: 62   **Degrees Offered:** BA Mus; BA MusEd
Teaching Certification Available
Financial Assistance: Internships, Scholarships and Work-Study Grants
Performing Groups: College Concert Choir; College Marching Band; Concert Band; Stage Band

BISCAYNE COLLEGE
16400 NW 32nd Ave, Miami   Florida 33054
305 625-1561 Ext 163

Private and 4 Year
Arts Areas: Instrumental Music, Vocal Music and Theatre

MUSIC

Degrees Offered: BA Mus; BMus; MMus; DMA; PhD   **Financial Assistance:** Scholarships
Performing Groups: Choir; Vocal & Instrumental Groups

BROWARD COMMUNITY COLLEGE
225 East Las Olas, Ft Lauderdale   Florida 33312
305 467-6700

State and 2 Year
Arts Areas: Dance, Instrumental Music, Vocal Music, Theatre, Film Arts, Television and Visual Arts
Performing Series: Artist Series; Special Events Series
Performance Facilities: Bailey Concert Hall

DANCE

Jimmy Woodle, Chairman of Humanities Division   **Number Of Faculty:** 1
Number Of Students: 40
Financial Assistance: Scholarships and Work-Study Grants
Performing Groups: Modern Dance Group

(continued on next page)

MUSIC

Jimmy O Woodle, Acting Department Head
Number Of Faculty: 6 Full-time, 21 Part-time   **Number Of Students:** 800
Degrees Offered: AA Instrumental Music
Courses Offered: Voice & Instrumental Lessons; Service Playing Fundamentals of Music; Theory; Music Appreciation; Technique Classes; Music History
Technical Training: Voice & Instrumental Lessons; Service Playing
Financial Assistance: Scholarships and Work-Study Grants
Performing Groups: Concert Choir; College Singers; Opera Workshop; Jazz Ensemble; Symphonic Band; Broward Symphony Orchestra; Chamber Ensemble; Adult Jazz Band
Workshops/Festivals: Festival of the Arts

THEATRE

Mildred Mullikin, Head   **Number Of Faculty:** 4   **Number Of Students:** 200
Degrees Offered: AA
Courses Offered: Theatre Productions; Theatre Western Cult; Stagecraft; Makeup; Pantomime; Voice & Diction; Fencing; Ballet; Acting; Contemporary Drama
Technical Training: Design; Make-up; Acting
Financial Assistance: Scholarships and Work-Study Grants
Performing Groups: Pantomime Players; Children's Theatre
Workshops/Festivals: Broward Theatre Alliance Workshop

CENTRAL FLORIDA COMMUNITY COLLEGE
PO Box 1388, Ocala   Florida 32670
904 237-2111
County and 2 Year
Arts Areas: Instrumental Music, Vocal Music, Theatre and Visual Arts
Performing Series: Concert Series; Theater Series; Film Series
Performance Facilities: Fine Arts Auditorium

MUSIC

Gene A Lawton, Chairman   **Number Of Faculty:** 5   **Number Of Students:** 400
Degrees Offered: AA; AS
Courses Offered: College-transfer in Music, General College, Adult Education
Technical Training: Church Music Course
Financial Assistance: Assistantships and Scholarships
Performing Groups: Chorale; Variations; Civic Chorus; Studio Band; Stage Band One; Musical Theater Workshop
Workshops/Festivals: Church Music

THEATRE

George W Statler, Chairman   **Number Of Faculty:** 1   **Number Of Students:** 44
Degrees Offered: AA
Courses Offered: Introduction to the Theater; Oral Interpretation; Speech; Play Production; Advanced Play Production; Independent Study
Financial Assistance: Assistantships and Scholarships
Workshops/Festivals: Summer Theater Workshop; Spring Mime Workshop

---

CHIPOLA JUNIOR COLLEGE
Marianna   Florida 32446, 904 526-2761
State and 2 Year
Arts Areas: Instrumental Music, Vocal Music, Theatre and Visual Arts
Performing Series: Music & Dance   **Performance Facilities:** Auditorium

MUSIC

Lawrence R Nelson, Chairman   **Number Of Faculty:** 3   **Number Of Students:** 40
Degrees Offered: AA

(continued on next page)

Courses Offered: Theory; Sight Singing; Keyboard Harmony; Music History; Styles and Forms; College Chorus; Chamber Chorus
Technical Training: Applied Music
Financial Assistance: Scholarships and Work-Study Grants
Performing Groups: College Chorus; Chamber Chorus; Instrumental Ensemble
Workshops/Festivals: Festival of The Performing Arts

THEATRE

Virgil D Oswald, Sr, Director   **Number Of Faculty:** 1
Number Of Students: 15   **Degrees Offered:** AA
Courses Offered: Introduction to Theatre; Fundamentals of Acting; Play Production
Financial Assistance: Scholarships and Work-Study Grants
Performing Groups: Village Players

DAYTONA BEACH JUNIOR COLLEGE
Daytona Beach   Florida 32015, 904 255-1476
State and 4 Year
Arts Areas: Instrumental Music, Vocal Music and Theatre
Performance Facilities: College Auditorium
Degrees Offered: AA, Instrumental Music
Financial Assistance: Scholarships and Work-Study Grants

THEATRE

Alan Perrins, Chairman   **Degrees Offered:** AA, Drama
Performing Groups: DBJC Theatre

ECKERD COLLEGE
34 St 7 54 Ave, S, St Petersburg   Florida 33733
813 867-1166 Ext 471
Private and 4 Year
Arts Areas: Dance, Instrumental Music, Vocal Music, Theatre and Visual Arts

DANCE

Number Of Faculty: 1   **Degrees Offered:** BA
Courses Offered: Technique; Choreography; Ethnic
Financial Assistance: Work-Study Grants

MUSIC

Williams Waters, Coordinator   **Number Of Faculty:** 2 Full-time, 10 Part-time
Degrees Offered: BA
Courses Offered: Theory; History; Applied Music; Vocal and Instrumental Ensembles
Teaching Certification Available
Financial Assistance: Scholarships and Work-Study Grants
Performing Groups: Sandpipers; Concert Choir

THEATRE

James Carlson, Coordinator   **Number Of Faculty:** 3   **Degrees Offered:** BA
Courses Offered: Theory; Criticism; Performance; Crafts
Teaching Certification Available   Performing Groups: Eckerd College Theatre
Workshops/Festivals: Residency program with the Pallisades Theatre Company, the Florida Studio Theatre, and guest artists and companies; campus - community workshops

---

EDISON COMMUNITY COLLEGE
College Pkwy, Fort Myers   Florida 33901
813 481-2121
State and 2 Year
Arts Areas: Instrumental Music, Vocal Music, Theatre and Visual Arts
Performing Series: Arts Series

(continued on next page)

Performance Facilities: Doris Corbin Auditorium

MUSIC

Number Of Faculty: 2   *Number Of Students:* 200   *Degrees Offered:* AA
Financial Assistance: Scholarships
Performing Groups: Choir; Band; Jazz Ensemble; Orchestra
Workshops/Festivals: Arts Series

THEATRE

Number Of Faculty: 3   *Number Of Students:* 100   *Degrees Offered:* AA
Performing Groups: Drama Group   *Workshops/Festivals:* Arts Series

---

FLORIDA AGRICULTURAL & MECHANICAL UNIVERSITY
PO Box 235, Tallahassee   Florida 32307
904 599-3831
State and 4 Year
Arts Areas: Instrumental Music, Vocal Music, Theatre and Visual Arts
Performance Facilities: Lee Hall Auditorium; CW Wood Theatre

DANCE

Beverly Barber, Chairman
Dance program under auspices of Physical Education Department
Number Of Faculty: 1   *Number Of Students:* 4
Technical Training: Graham Method   *Financial Assistance:* Work-Study Grants
Performing Groups: Orchesis Club

MUSIC

Dr William P Foster, Chairman   *Number Of Faculty:* 14
Number Of Students: 161
Degrees Offered: BS Choral, Instrumental Music; BA Music
Teaching Certification Available   Financial Assistance: Work-Study Grants
Performing Groups: Choir; Men's Glee Club; Women's Glee Club; Marching Band; Symphonic Band; Jazz
Lab Band; Percussion Ensembles

THEATRE

Ronald O Davis, Chairman   *Number Of Faculty:* 2   *Number Of Students:* 62
Degrees Offered: BA   *Technical Training:* Makeup and Lighting for Blacks
Teaching Certification Available   Financial Assistance: Work-Study Grants
Performing Groups: The Florida A & M University Playmakers Guild

---

FLORIDA ATLANTIC UNIVERSITY
500 NW 20th St, Boca Raton   Florida 33432
305 395-5100
State and 4 Year
Arts Areas: Instrumental Music, Vocal Music and Theatre
Performing Series: Cultural & Entertainment Series

MUSIC

Eugene W Crabb, Chairman   *Degrees Offered:* BA in Music, Music Ed
Teaching Certification Available
Financial Assistance: Scholarships and Work-Study Grants
Performing Groups: Instrumental & Vocal Groups

THEATRE

Joe Conaway, Chairman   *Degrees Offered:* BA in Theatre
Teaching Certification Available
Financial Assistance: Scholarships and Work-Study Grants
Performing Groups: University Theatre

FLORIDA COLLEGE
Temple Terrace   Florida 33617, 813 988-5131
　Private and 2 Year
　Arts Areas: Instrumental Music, Vocal Music and Theatre
　Performing Series: Faculty Concert Series; Guest Artists Concert Series
　Performance Facilities: Hutchinson Memorial Auditorium

MUSIC

James G Walker, Chairman   *Number Of Faculty:* 5   *Number Of Students:* 149
Degrees Offered: AA
Courses Offered: Sight Singing & Ear Training; Music Appreciation; Band; Piano; Musicianship; Chorus; Church Music; Piano Literature; Theory; Freshman & Sophmore Brasses, Percussion, Woodwinds; Private Voice & Piano
Technical Training: Vocal; Instrumental; Piano
Financial Assistance: Scholarships and Work-Study Grants
Performing Groups: Florida College Chorus; Florida College Public Relations Group "Friends"; Florida College Band

THEATRE

Nancy Bingham, Chairman   *Number Of Faculty:* 2   *Number Of Students:* 39
Degrees Offered: AA   *Courses Offered:* Drama Workshop; Basic Issues in Drama
Financial Assistance: Scholarships and Work-Study Grants
Performing Groups: Footlighters

FLORIDA INTERNATIONAL UNIVERSITY
Tamiami Trail   Florida 33199, 305 552-2895
　State and 2 Year
　Arts Areas: Instrumental Music, Vocal Music, Theatre and Visual Arts
　Performing Series: University Theatre

MUSIC

Dr Philip H Fink, Chairman   *Number Of Faculty:* 6 Full-time, 20 Part-time
Number Of Students: 95   *Degrees Offered:* BM, BS; MS Music Education
Teaching Certification Available
Financial Assistance: Scholarships and Work-Study Grants
Performing Groups: FIU Community Chorus; FIU Community Orchestra; FIU Civic Wind Ensemble; Studio Jazz Ensemble
Workshops/Festivals: Think Guitar and Choral Institutes

THEATRE

Philip Giberson, Director   *Number Of Faculty:* 4   *Number Of Students:* 60
Degrees Offered: BFA
Technical Training: Acting/Directing; Design/Tech; Teacher Prep; Film
Teaching Certification Available
Financial Assistance: Internships, Assistantships, Scholarships and Work-Study Grants

FLORIDA JUNIOR COLLEGE
Jacksonville   Florida 32205, 904 389-1321
　State and 2 Year
　Arts Areas: Dance, Instrumental Music, Theatre and Visual Arts
　Performing Series: Concert - Lecture Series
　Performance Facilities: College Auditorium
　Degrees Offered: AA
　Financial Assistance: Scholarships and Work-Study Grants

FLORIDA KEYS COMMUNITY COLLEGE
Key West   Florida 33040, 305 296-9081
   State and 2 Year   *Arts Areas:* Instrumental Music and Visual Arts
   Performance Facilities: College Auditorium

MUSIC

P A Davison, Chairman   *Number Of Faculty:* 2   *Number Of Students:* 75
Degrees Offered: AA
Courses Offered: Music Theory; Music History & Literature; Piano; Voice; Chorus
Financial Assistance: Scholarships, Work-Study Grants and BEOG
Performing Groups: Choral

THEATRE

Jay Drury, Chairman   *Number Of Faculty:* 1
Courses Offered: Introduction to Theatre
Financial Assistance: Scholarships and Work-Study Grants

FLORIDA MEMORIAL COLLEGE
15800 NW 42nd Ave, Miami   Florida 33054
305 625-4141
   Private and 4 Year   *Arts Areas:* Instrumental Music and Vocal Music

MUSIC

Roosevelt Williams, Chairman   *Number Of Faculty:* 2
Number Of Students: 18   *Degrees Offered:* BS MusEd
Courses Offered: Piano; Voice   *Teaching Certification Available*
Financial Assistance: Work-Study Grants
Performing Groups: College Chorale; College Ensemble

FLORIDA SOUTHERN COLLEGE
Lake Hollingsworth Dr, Lakeland   Florida 33802
813 683-5521 Ext 244
   Private and 4 Year
   Arts Areas: Dance, Instrumental Music, Vocal Music, Theatre and Film Arts
   Performing Series: Festival of Fine Arts
   Performance Facilities: Branscomb Memorial Auditorium

DANCE

Janet Santosuosso, Chairman   *Number Of Faculty:* 1   *Number Of Students:* 20
Degrees Offered: BA Mus; MusEd, Sacred Music
Teaching Certification Available
Financial Assistance: Internships, Assistantships, Scholarships and Work-Study Grants
Performing Groups: Concert Band; FSC Chorale; Bell Choir; Chapel Choir; Southern Singers; Dixieland Band; Stage Band
Workshops/Festivals: District State Band; Choral Festivals; Youth Music Workshop

THEATRE

Mel Wooton, Chairman   *Number Of Faculty:* 3   *Number Of Students:* 260
Degrees Offered: BA   *Teaching Certification Available*
Financial Assistance: Assistantships, Scholarships and Work-Study Grants
Performing Groups: Vagabonds
Workshops/Festivals: Show'mester (New York Semester) Summer Theatre

FLORIDA STATE UNIVERSITY
Fine Arts Bldg, Tallahassee   Florida 32306
904 644-2525
State and 4 Year
Arts Areas: Dance, Instrumental Music, Vocal Music, Theatre, Film Arts, Visual Arts and Radio
Performing Series: Leisure Program Artist Series
Performance Facilities: Fine Arts Building, Studio, and Conradi Theatres; Mac Arthur Center

DANCE

Dr Nancy Smith, Chairman   *Number Of Faculty:* 5   *Number Of Students:* 300
Degrees Offered: BFA; MFA
Audition Requirements must be met for admission into the program.
Technical Training: Modern; Ballet; Dance Composition; History & Philosophy of Dance; Music & Choreography
Teaching Certification Available   *Financial Assistance:* Work-Study Grants
Performing Groups: Dance Theatre

MUSIC

Wiley Housewright, Dean   *Number Of Faculty:* 86   *Number Of Students:* 2986
Degrees Offered: BMus in Performance, Composition, Theory, History, Music Therapy, Literature; BMusEd; MMus in Performance, Theory, Composition, History & Literature, Music Therapy; MMusEd; BMusEd; BA Mus; PhD in Performance, Composition & Theory, Music Education; Music Theory & Musicology
Teaching Certification Available
Financial Assistance: Internships, Assistantships, Scholarships and Work-Study Grants
Performing Groups: Symphony; Chamber Orchestra; University Singers; Choral Union; Chamber Choir; Chorus; Madrigals; Pop - Jazz Ensemble; Opera Chorus; Symphonic Band; Marching Chiefs; Woodwind Ensemble - Brass Ensemble; Jazz Groups
Workshops/Festivals: Opera Workshop

THEATRE

Richard G Gallon, Dean   *Number Of Faculty:* 19   *Number Of Students:* 300
Degrees Offered: BA; BFA; MA; BFA; PhD
Financial Assistance: Internships, Assistantships and Work-Study Grants
Performing Groups: Asolo State Theatre; Black Players; Asolo Children's Theatre; Pied Pipers
Workshops/Festivals: Workshop with visiting professionals; Hosting; The American College Theatre Festival

FLORIDA TECHNOLOGICAL UNIVERSITY
PO Box 25000, Orlando   Florida 32816
305 275-9101
State and 4 Year
Arts Areas: Instrumental Music, Vocal Music, Theatre, Film Arts, Television and Visual Arts

MUSIC

J Gary Wolf, Chairman   *Number Of Faculty:* 24   *Number Of Students:* 175
Degrees Offered: BA Mus, MusEd; MA MusEd
Courses Offered: Applied Music; Theory/History; Major & Minor Ensembles; Opera; Music Education
Technical Training: Applied Music; Composition; Opera
Teaching Certification Available
Financial Assistance: Assistantships, Scholarships and Work-Study Grants
Performing Groups: Basically Baroque (Faculty Artist-in-Residence Ensemble); University/Community Orchestra; University Symphonic Band; Jazz Lab Band; University Chorus; Chamber Singers; Opera Ensemble
Workshops/Festivals: Annual Oboe, Clarinet, Bassoon Workshops (summer); Annual Piano Workshop; Matthay Piano Festival; Festival of Contemporary Music (annual) with the Florida Symphony Orchestra

THEATRE

Harry W Smith, Chairman   *Number Of Faculty:* 4   *Number Of Students:* 50
Degrees Offered: BA

(continued on next page)

Courses Offered: Acting/Directing; Design/Tech; History; Criticism; Film
Technical Training: Practicum Classes   **Teaching Certification Available**
Financial Assistance: Assistantships, Scholarships and Work-Study Grants
Performing Groups: Village Players

UNIVERSITY OF FLORIDA
Gainesville   Florida 32611, 904 392-0207
State and 4 Year
Arts Areas: Dance, Instrumental Music, Vocal Music, Theatre and Visual Arts
Performing Series: President's Music Festival; Student Government Productions; Florida Players Productions
Performance Facilities: University Auditorium; Music Building Facilities; Constans Theatre
Number Of Students: 8   **Degrees Offered:** BFA
Performing Groups: Florida Dance Company (under Theatre Department)

MUSIC

Dr Budd Udell, Chairman   **Number Of Faculty:** 27   **Number Of Students:** 250
Degrees Offered: BMusEd; BMus; BA; MMusEd; MAEd; PhD; EdD
Teaching Certification Available
Financial Assistance: Assistantships, Scholarships, Work-Study Grants and Grants
Performing Groups: Choir; Bands (including Marching, Jazz, Symphonic); Orchestras; Small Ensembles
Workshops/Festivals: President's Music Festival; Opera Workshop; Gatorland Music Clinic

THEATRE

Dr James Hooks, Chairman   **Number Of Faculty:** 8   **Number Of Students:** 1,300
Degrees Offered: BA; BFA; BA Ed; MFA; PhD   **Teaching Certification Available**
Financial Assistance: Internships, Assistantships, Scholarships and Work-Study Grants
Performing Groups: Florida Players; Florida Dance Company
Workshops/Festivals: Florida Players Productions (including Summer Repertory Theatre)

GULF COAST COMMUNITY COLLEGE
5230 W Highway 98, Panama City   Florida 32401
904 769-1551
State and 2 Year
Arts Areas: Instrumental Music, Vocal Music and Theatre
Performance Facilities: Fine Arts Auditorium   **Number Of Faculty:** 3
Degrees Offered: AA Music
Courses Offered: Instrument Training; Voice Training; Music Appreciation; Survey of Music Literature
Financial Assistance: Assistantships, Scholarships and Work-Study Grants
Performing Groups: Stage Band; College - Community Orchestra; College Singers

HILLSBOROUGH COMMUNITY COLLEGE, YBOR CAMPUS
PO Box 22127, Tampa   Florida 33622
813 879-7222 Ext 406
State and 2 Year
Arts Areas: Instrumental Music, Vocal Music, Theatre and Visual Arts
Performance Facilities: Fine Arts Building

MUSIC

C Richard Rhoades, Chairman   **Number Of Faculty:** 2 Full-time, 10 Part-time
Number Of Students: 300   **Degrees Offered:** AA
Courses Offered: Fundamentals of Music; History of Music; Vocal & Performance Ensembles; Band; Chorus; Theory
Financial Assistance: Scholarships
Performing Groups: Stage Band; Concert Band; Chorus Jazz Band; Vocal Ensemble
Workshops/Festivals: Ybor City Arts Festival

(continued on next page)

THEATRE

Marvin Kirschman, Chairman   **Number Of Faculty:** 1   **Number Of Students:** 150
Degrees Offered: AA
Courses Offered: Intro to Theatre Arts; Stage Workshop; Acting I & II
Financial Assistance: Scholarships
Workshops/Festivals: Yearly Drama Presentation

INDIAN RIVER JUNIOR COLLEGE
Virginia Ave, Fort Pierce   Florida 33450
305 464-2000
State and 2 Year
Arts Areas: Instrumental Music, Theatre and Visual Arts
Degrees Offered: AA
Financial Assistance: Scholarships and Work-Study Grants
Courses Offered: Introduction; Play Production; Acting; Technical
Financial Assistance: Scholarships and Work-Study Grants
Performing Groups: Indian River Theatre

JACKSONVILLE UNIVERSITY
College of Fine Arts, Jacksonville   Florida 32211
904 744-3950
Private and 4 Year
Arts Areas: Dance, Instrumental Music, Vocal Music, Theatre and Visual Arts

DANCE

Dr Davis Sikes, Chairman   **Number Of Faculty:** 2   **Number Of Students:** 30
Degrees Offered: BA; BFA
Financial Assistance: Internships, Scholarships and Work-Study Grants

MUSIC

Dr James Hoffren, Chairman   **Number Of Faculty:** 32
Number Of Students: 147   **Degrees Offered:** BMus; BFA; BMusEd; BA
Teaching Certification Available
Financial Assistance: Scholarships and Work-Study Grants
Performing Groups: Band; Chorus; Orchestra; Stage Band; String Quartets; Dolphinnaires

THEATRE

Dr Davis Sikes, Chairman   **Number Of Faculty:** 3   **Number Of Students:** 60
Degrees Offered: BA; BFA   **Teaching Certification Available**

LAKE CITY COMMUNITY COLLEGE
Lake City   Florida 32055, 904 752-1822
State and 2 Year
Arts Areas: Instrumental Music, Vocal Music, Theatre and Visual Arts

MUSIC

Larry Elshoff, Chairman, Humanities Department   **Number Of Faculty:** 2
Number Of Students: 100   **Degrees Offered:** AA Music
Financial Assistance: Scholarships and Work-Study Grants
Performing Groups: College Choir; Collegiate Consort; Hand Bell Choir; Stage Band; Concert Band;
Various Quartets, Ensembles
Workshops/Festivals: MAD (Music, Art, Drama) Festival

THEATRE

Larry Elshoff, Chairman, Humanities Department   **Number Of Faculty:** 1
Number Of Students: 40   **Degrees Offered:** AA

(continued on next page)

Financial Assistance: Scholarships and Work-Study Grants
Performing Groups: Emerald City Players (Children's Theatre Troup); LCCC Theatre
Workshops/Festivals: MAD Festival

LAKE SUMTER COMMUNITY COLLEGE
Leesburg   Florida 32748, 904 787-3747
State and 2 Year
Arts Areas: Instrumental Music, Vocal Music, Theatre and Visual Arts
Performance Facilities: College Auditorium   **Degrees Offered:** AA
Financial Assistance: Scholarships and Work-Study Grants
Performing Groups: Choral Ensemble; Instrumental Ensembles

MANATEE JUNIOR COLLEGE
5840 26th St, W, Bradenton   Florida 33507
813 755-1511
State and 2 Year
Arts Areas: Instrumental Music, Vocal Music, Theatre, Film Arts and Visual Arts
Performance Facilities: Neel Auditorium; Studio 84

MUSIC

Dr Charles Johnson, Co-ordinator   **Number Of Faculty:** 6 - 8
Degrees Offered: AA
Courses Offered: Fundamentals of Music; College Band; College Choir; Organ; Guitar; Music Theory;
Piano; Voice; Music History; Ensemble
Financial Assistance: Scholarships and Work-Study Grants
Performing Groups: College Choir; Lancer Sound & Studio Bands; String & Percussion Ensembles;
Madrigal Singers
Workshops/Festivals: Sacred Music Festival

THEATRE

John James, Director   **Number Of Faculty:** 4   **Number Of Students:** 30
Degrees Offered: AA
Courses Offered: Film Workshop; Cinema Arts; History Appreciation of Theater; Stage Makeup;
Stagecraft; Introduction to Theatre
Performing Groups: MJC Players   **Workshops/Festivals:** Four Plays Yearly

MIAMI - DADE COMMUNITY COLLEGE - NEW WORLD CENTER
300 N E Second Ave, Miami   Florida 33132
305 577-6740
County and 2 Year   **Arts Areas:** Dance, Instrumental Music and Theatre
Performance Facilities: Auditorium; Room 1261

DANCE

Number Of Faculty: 1   **Number Of Students:** 30   **Courses Offered:** Dance & Mime
Financial Assistance: Assistantships, Scholarships and Work-Study Grants
Performing Groups: New World Dance Group

MUSIC

Paula Milton, Chairperson, Creative Arts   **Number Of Faculty:** 1
Number Of Students: 30   **Degrees Offered:** AA
Financial Assistance: Assistantships, Scholarships and Work-Study Grants
Workshops/Festivals: Lunchtime Lively Arts Concerts (every Wednesday)

THEATRE

Number Of Faculty: 1   **Number Of Students:** 82   **Degrees Offered:** AA
Financial Assistance: Assistantships, Scholarships and Work-Study Grants
Performing Groups: Promethean Players
Artists-In-Residence/Guest Artists: Dave Gossoff; Teresa Alvarez; Jane Steinsnyder; Ruth Greenfield

MIAMI - DADE COMMUNITY COLLEGE - NORTH CAMPUS
11380 N W 27th Ave, Miami   Florida 33167
305 685-4314
State and 2 Year
Arts Areas: Instrumental Music, Vocal Music and Theatre
Performance Facilities: Pawley Theatre

MUSIC

John Alexander, Chairperson   *Number Of Faculty:* 15 Full-time, 35 Part-time
Number Of Students: 5,607   *Degrees Offered:* AA Mus; AS in Commercial Music
Financial Assistance: Scholarships and Work-Study Grants
Performing Groups: Band; Orchestra; Gospel Ensemble; Brass Ensemble; Jazz Band; String Ensemble; Woodwind Ensemble; Choir; Hi - Lites Vocal Ensemble; Flute & Percussion Ensembles

THEATRE

John Alexander, Chairperson   *Number Of Faculty:* 5
Number Of Students: 506   *Degrees Offered:* AA
Financial Assistance: Scholarships and Work-Study Grants
Performing Groups: Pen Players

MIAMI - DADE COMMUNITY COLLEGE, SOUTH CAMPUS
11011 SW 104th St, Miami   Florida 33176
305 596-1203
State and 2 Year
Arts Areas: Dance, Instrumental Music, Vocal Music, Theatre and Visual Arts

DANCE

Sherry Penn, Chairman   *Number Of Faculty:* 1   *Number Of Students:* 40
Financial Assistance: Assistantships, Scholarships and Work-Study Grants

MUSIC

David Lee Roberts, Chairman   *Number Of Faculty:* 10
Number Of Students: 194
Courses Offered: All standard Freshman/Sophomore music courses
Financial Assistance: Scholarships and Work-Study Grants
Performing Groups: Caravan Singers; College Choir; Concert & Stage Bands; Symphonic Orchestra; Guitar Ensemble; Jazz Singers; Woodwind & Brass Ensembles
Workshops/Festivals: Madrigal Supper

THEATRE

Edward Anderson, Chairman   *Number Of Faculty:* 5   *Number Of Students:* 50
Degrees Offered: AA
Courses Offered: Acting; Stagecraft; Costuming; Makeup; Theatre History; Lighting
Financial Assistance: Scholarships and Work-Study Grants
Performing Groups: Caravan Players
Artists-In-Residence/Guest Artists: Mark Cohen; Chuck Toman; William Williams; June Blum & Audrey Flak; Walter Hopps; Duane Hanson

UNIVERSITY OF MIAMI
Coral Gables   Florida 33124, 305 284-2433
Private and 4 Year
Arts Areas: Dance, Instrumental Music, Vocal Music and Theatre

DANCE

Jerry Ross, Director
Dance program under auspices of Theatre Department
Technical Training: Ballet; Jazz; Tap; Modern

(continued on next page)

MUSIC

William F Lee, Dean   ***Number Of Faculty:*** 65   ***Number Of Students:*** 800
Degrees Offered: BA Mus; BMus; MMus; DMA; PhD
Teaching Certification Available
Financial Assistance: Internships, Assistantships, Scholarships, Work-Study Grants and Endowed Scholarships
Performing Groups: Jazz Guitar Ensemble; Marching Band; Symphonic Band; Concert Band; Jazz Band· Brass Choir; Wind Ensemble; Studio Jazz Orchestra; Percussion Ensemble; Chamber Music; Symphony Orchestra; Collegium Musicum; Tuba Ensemble; Guitar Ensemble; Small Jazz Ensemble; Rock Ensemble; Jazz Performance Seminar; Contemporary Music Ensemble; University - Civic Chorale; Concert Choir; Chamber Singers I & II; Choral Conducting Workshop; Singing Hurricanes; Opera Workshop; Men & Women's Glee Clubs; Jazz Vocal I & II; Graduate Chorale
Workshops/Festivals: Summer Music Study, enrichment courses, and activities through camps and workshops

THEATRE

Herman Diers, Chairman   ***Number Of Faculty:*** 16   ***Number Of Students:*** 170
Degrees Offered: BA; BFA; MA; MFA
Technical Training: For Professional Performance; Musical Comedy
Teaching Certification Available
Financial Assistance: Internships, Assistantships, Scholarships and Work-Study Grants
Performing Groups: Associated with Coconut Grove Playhouse; The Players Repertory
Workshops/Festivals: Summer Dinner Theatre on Campus

NEW COLLEGE OF THE UNIVERSITY OF SOUTH FLORIDA
5700 N Tamiami Trail, Sarasota   Florida 33580
813 355-7671 Ext 258
State and 4 Year
Arts Areas: Instrumental Music, Visual Arts and Musicology
Performance Facilities: Music Room; Hamilton Center; Van Wezel Performing Arts Hall

MUSIC

Dr E David Dykstra, Chairman, Humanities Division   ***Number Of Faculty:*** 4
Degrees Offered: BA
Courses Offered: Harmony; Counterpoint; Fugue; Form & Analysis; Orchestration; Composition
Financial Assistance: Scholarships and Work-Study Grants
Performing Groups: New College String Quartet
Workshops/Festivals: New College Music Festival

NORTH FLORIDA JUNIOR COLLEGE
Madison   Florida 32340, 904 973-2288 Ext 55
State and 2 Year
Arts Areas: Instrumental Music, Vocal Music, Theatre and Visual Arts
Performing Series: Flight Arrow Series of Lectures and Performances
Performance Facilities: Fine Arts Auditorium; Van H Priest Community Center

MUSIC

Number Of Faculty: 2   ***Number Of Students:*** 20   ***Degrees Offered:*** AA
Courses Offered: Theory; Voice and Piano; Peforming Groups
Financial Assistance: Work-Study Grants and Activity Scholarships
Performing Groups: Sentinal Singers; Chorus; Instrumental Ensemble

THEATRE

Number Of Faculty: 1   ***Number Of Students:*** 20   ***Degrees Offered:*** AA
Courses Offered: Acting; Directing; Technical Theater; Introduction to Drama Workshop

(continued on next page)

Technical Training: Lighting; Scene Construction
Financial Assistance: Work-Study Grants
Workshops/Festivals: Summer Drama Workshops in Madison or in the six-county area that the college serves

---

UNIVERSITY OF NORTH FLORIDA
PO Box 17074, Jacksonville   Florida 32216
904 646-2960

State and Two Year Upper Level
Arts Areas: Instrumental Music, Vocal Music and Visual Arts
Performing Series: Concert & Lecture Series
Performance Facilities: Lecture - Performance Hall; Lecture - Performance Auditorium

MUSIC

Number Of Faculty: 4   **Number Of Students:** 100   **Degrees Offered:** BA
Courses Offered: Piano; Organ; Voice; Applied Music; Music History; Counterpoint; Form & Analysis; Conducting
Teaching Certification Available
Financial Assistance: Assistantships, Scholarships and Work-Study Grants
Performing Groups: University Chorus; University Singers; Opera Workshop

THEATRE

Courses Offered: Acting; Performance & Production; Theatre Perspectives
Financial Assistance: Assistantships, Scholarships and Work-Study Grants
Performing Groups: Venture Theatre

OKALOOSA - WALTON JUNIOR COLLEGE
Niceville   Florida 32578, 904 678-5112

State and 2 Year
Arts Areas: Dance, Instrumental Music, Vocal Music, Theatre and Visual Arts
Performing Series: Okaloosa Community Concert Association; Area Music Associations Concerts
Performance Facilities: Auditorium; Library Recital Hall; Music Rehearsal/Recital Hall; Mall Recital Hall

DANCE

Dance program under auspices of Physical Education Department
Number Of Faculty: 1   **Number Of Students:** 60
Financial Assistance: Scholarships and Work-Study Grants
Workshops/Festivals: West Florida Square & Round Dance Workshops in cooperation with Lyceum Programs

MUSIC

Dr J Richard Warren, Chairman, Fine & Performing Arts/Humanities
Number Of Faculty: 5 Full-time, 2 - 4 Part-time   **Number Of Students:** 90
Degrees Offered: AA
Courses Offered: Theory; History/Literature; Applied; Organizations; General Appreciation; Techniques Classes
Technical Training: Applied; Related Professional
Financial Assistance: Assistantships, Scholarships and Work-Study Grants
Performing Groups: Stage Band; Concert Band; Concert Chorus; Chamber Choir; Vocal and Instrumental Ensembles
Workshops/Festivals: Area Music Association Workshops, Festivals, Contests, Concerts; American Arts Festival

THEATRE

Dr J Richard Warren, Chairman, Fine & Performing Arts/Humanities
Number Of Faculty: 1   **Number Of Students:** 50   **Degrees Offered:** AA
Courses Offered: Theatre (appreciation); Acting I - II; Amateur Theatre
Financial Assistance: Assistantships, Scholarships and Work-Study Grants
Performing Groups: Proscenium Playhouse

PALM BEACH ATLANTIC COLLEGE
West Palm Beach   Florida 33401, 305 883-8592

State and 4 Year   **Arts Areas:** Theatre   **Degrees Offered:** AA
Financial Assistance: Scholarships and Work-Study Grants
Performing Groups: PBAC Theatre

PALM BEACH JUNIOR COLLEGE
4200 Congress Ave, Lake Worth   Florida 33461
305 965-8000

State and 2 Year
Arts Areas: Instrumental Music, Vocal Music, Theatre and Visual Arts
Performance Facilities: Palm Beach Junior College Auditorium; PBJC Gym
Workshops/Festivals: Dance Workshops

MUSIC

Letha Madge Royce, Chairperson   **Number Of Faculty:** 14
Number Of Students: 130   **Degrees Offered:** AA; AS
Financial Assistance: Scholarships and Work-Study Grants
Performing Groups: Brass Ensemble; Concert Band; Concert Choir; Community Orchestra; Guitar
Ensemble; Jazz Ensemble; Pacesetters
Workshops/Festivals: Opera Workshop; Jazz Ensemble

THEATRE

Watson B Duncan, III, Chairperson   **Number Of Faculty:** 3
Number Of Students: 37   **Degrees Offered:** AA
Financial Assistance: Work-Study Grants   **Performing Groups:** PBJC Players
Workshops/Festivals: One-Act Play Festival; Oral Interpretation Festival for County High Schools;
Production Workshops

PENSACOLA JUNIOR COLLEGE
1000 College Blvd, Pensacola   Florida 32561
904 476-5410 Ext 294

State and 2 Year
Arts Areas: Dance, Instrumental Music, Vocal Music, Theatre, Television and Visual Arts
Performing Series: Lyceum Series
Performance Facilities: Health Building; Fine Arts Auditorium

DANCE

Heather Shepley, Chairman   **Number Of Faculty:** 1   **Number Of Students:** 40
Financial Assistance: Scholarships

MUSIC

Sidney Kennedy, Head   **Number Of Faculty:** 8   **Number Of Students:** 80
Degrees Offered: AA; AS
Courses Offered: Theory; Literature; All Applied; Conducting
Technical Training: All areas of Applied Music
Financial Assistance: Scholarships
Performing Groups: Concert Choir; Band (Concert); Jazz Ensemble; Oratorio Society; Civic Band;
Woodwind Quintet
Workshops/Festivals: Opera Workshop

(continued on next page)

THEATRE

Sidney Kennedy, Head   **Number Of Faculty:** 2   **Degrees Offered:** AA
Courses Offered: Introduction to Theatre; Acting; Scenery & Design
Financial Assistance: Scholarships

ROLLINS COLLEGE

Winter Park   Florida 32789, 305 646-2000 Ext 2501
Private and 4 Year
Arts Areas: Instrumental Music, Vocal Music and Theatre
Performing Series: Bach Festival; Annie Russell Theatre Productions
Performance Facilities: Russell and Stone Theatres; Crummer and Bush Auditoriums

MUSIC

Ross Rosazza, Head   **Number Of Faculty:** 6   **Number Of Students:** 165
Degrees Offered: BA
Courses Offered: Applied, all fields; Comprehensive Musicianship I, II, III, IV; General courses of musico-historio nature
Teaching Certification Available   Financial Assistance: Scholarships
Performing Groups: Baroque String Ensemble; Brass Ensemble; Woodwind Quintet; Chapel Choir

THEATRE

Robert O Juergens, Head   **Number Of Faculty:** 6   **Number Of Students:** 75
Degrees Offered: BA
Courses Offered: Introduction to Theatre; History of Theatre; Acting I & II; Stage Craft; Set Design; Lighting Design; Costume Design; Senior Practicum; Dramatic Literature; Dramatic Film; Playwriting
Financial Assistance: Scholarships   **Performing Groups:** The Rollins Players
Workshops/Festivals: Thespian State Conference

SAINT JOHNS RIVER JUNIOR COLLEGE
FLORIDA SCHOOL OF THE ARTS

5001 St Johns Ave, Palatka   Florida 32077
904 328-1571
State and 2 Year
Arts Areas: Dance, Instrumental Music, Vocal Music, Theatre and Visual Arts
Performance Facilities: Fine Arts Auditorium

DANCE

Degrees Offered: AA
Financial Assistance: Internships, Assistantships, Scholarships and Work-Study Grants

MUSIC

Degrees Offered: AA
Financial Assistance: Assistantships, Scholarships and Work-Study Grants

THEATRE

Degrees Offered: AA
Financial Assistance: Internships, Assistantships, Scholarships and Work-Study Grants

---

SAINT LEO COLLEGE
Hwy 52, Saint Leo   Florida 33574
904 588-2800 Ext 326
   Private and 4 Year
   Arts Areas: Dance, Instrumental Music, Vocal Music, Theatre and Visual Arts
   Performing Series: College - Community Artist Series
   Performance Facilities: College Theatre; Selby Auditorium; Marion Bowman Activities Center

DANCE

Number Of Faculty: 1   *Number Of Students:* 12   *Degrees Offered:* BA
Performing Groups: Modern Concert Dance Company; Dance Ensemble
Workshops/Festivals: May Performance Tour

MUSIC

Number Of Faculty: 9   *Number Of Students:* 32   *Degrees Offered:* BA
Financial Assistance: Scholarships and Work-Study Grants
Performing Groups: Oratorio Chorus; College Choir; Saint Leo Singers; Wind Ensemble; Stage Band; Percussion Ensemble; Collegium Musicum

THEATRE

Number Of Faculty: 2   *Number Of Students:* 12   *Degrees Offered:* BA
Financial Assistance: Scholarships and Work-Study Grants
Performing Groups: College Theatre; May Performance
Workshops/Festivals: May Performance Tour

SAINT PETERSBURG COLLEGE
Saint Petersburg   Florida 33733, 813 544-2551
   State and 2 Year   *Arts Areas:* Theatre and Visual Arts

THEATRE

Robert E Jones, Chairman   *Number Of Faculty:* 3   *Number Of Students:* 200
Degrees Offered: AA
Financial Assistance: Scholarships and Work-Study Grants
Performing Groups: Playmakers

SOUTH FLORIDA JUNIOR COLLEGE
Avon Park   Florida 33825, 813 453-6661
   State and 2 Year
   Arts Areas: Instrumental Music, Vocal Music and Theatre

MUSIC

Buford G Jasper, Chairman   *Number Of Faculty:* 2   *Number Of Students:* 20
Degrees Offered: AA
Courses Offered: Piano; Voice; Theory; Music Applied; Guitar
Financial Assistance: Scholarships and Work-Study Grants

THEATRE

Lynn McNeil, Chairman   *Number Of Faculty:* 1   *Number Of Students:* 40
Degrees Offered: AA   *Courses Offered:* Theatre History; Drama; Speech

UNIVERSITY OF SOUTH FLORIDA
Tampa   Florida 33620, 813 974-2301
State and 4 Year
Arts Areas: Dance, Instrumental Music, Vocal Music, Theatre, Film Arts and Visual Arts
Performing Series: Artist Series/Dance Residency; Film Art Series; Summer Chamber Music Program
Performance Facilities: University Theatre; Theatre Centre; Fine Arts Auditorium

DANCE

Nancy Cole, Intermin Chairman   **Number Of Faculty:** 6
Number Of Students: 250   **Degrees Offered:** BA
Courses Offered: Modern Dance, Ballet; Dance History; Music for Dance; Introduction to Dance; Pas De Deux; Jazz; Character; Choreography
Technical Training: Modern Dance; Ballet
Financial Assistance: Scholarships and Service Awards
Workshops/Festivals: Student Dance Workshops and Dance Concerts

MUSIC

Vance Jennings, Chairman   **Number Of Faculty:** 32   **Number Of Students:** 300
Degrees Offered: BA; MM
Courses Offered: Applied Music; Ensembles; Music Theory; Music History; Conducting
Financial Assistance: Assistantships and Scholarships
Performing Groups: Chamber Singers; Jazz Laboratory Band; Brass Choir; Brass Quintet; Woodwind Quintet; Piano Ensemble; String Quartet; Horn Quartet; Clarinet Choir; Percussion Ensemble; Marimba Ensemble; Flute Choir; New Music Ensemble; University Orchestra; University Singers; Opera Workshop; Choral Union; Wind Ensemble I & II; University Band; University Community Chorus
Workshops/Festivals: Chorale Associates Workshop; Festival of Winds

THEATRE

Nancy Cole, Chairman   **Number Of Faculty:** 8, with 6 affiliates
Number Of Students: 150   **Degrees Offered:** BA
Courses Offered: Acting; Improvisation; History; Voice; Performance; Puppetry; Playwriting; Costume; Makeup; Lighting; Management
Financial Assistance: Assistantships and Scholarships
Performing Groups: Theatre USF; Student Production Board
Workshops/Festivals: International Thespian Conference

STETSON UNIVERSITY
DeLand   Florida 32720, 904 734-4121
Private and 4 Year
Arts Areas: Instrumental Music, Vocal Music and Theatre
Performing Series: Artists and Lecturers Series
Performance Facilities: Edmunds Center; Elizabeth Hall; Stover Theatre

MUSIC

Paul Langston, Dean   **Number Of Faculty:** 17   **Number Of Students:** 160
Degrees Offered: BA; BMus; BMusEd
Courses Offered: Comprehensive Musicianship; Theory; Music History & Literature; Piano; Violin; Viola; Cello; Church Music, Music Education; Music Ensembles; Opera; Organ
Teaching Certification Available
Financial Assistance: Scholarships and Work-Study Grants
Performing Groups: Symphonic Orchestra; Symphonic Wind Ensemble; Jazz Ensemble; University Chorus; Concert Choir; Opera Workshop; Brass Choir; Woodwind Ensemble
Workshops/Festivals: Summer Orchestral Music Institute; Church Music Workshop

THEATRE

Dr James Wright, Chairman   **Number Of Faculty:** 4
Number Of Students: 75 - 100   **Degrees Offered:** BA
Courses Offered: Speech and Theatre Workshops, Stagecraft; Lighting; Children's Theatre; Makeup and

(continued on next page)

Costume; Play Directing; Theatre History; Acting; Dramatic Criticism; Summer Theatre
Technical Training: Costume; Makeup; Lighting; Set Design & Building
Teaching Certification Available
Financial Assistance: Scholarships and Work-Study Grants
Performing Groups: Stover Theatre University Players; Children's Theatre

UNIVERSITY OF TAMPA
401 W Kennedy, Tampa   Florida 33606
813 253-8861 Ext 217
Private and 4 Year
Arts Areas: Dance, Instrumental Music, Vocal Music, Theatre, Visual Arts and Arts Management
Performing Series: Ballroom Concert Series (chamber music); Gallery Recitals (chamber music)
Performance Facilities: Ballroom; Fletcher Lounge; Scarfone Gallery

DANCE

Anzia Arsenault, Instructor   *Number Of Faculty:* 2   *Number Of Students:* 65
Courses Offered: Beginning, Intermediate and Advanced Modern/Classical Ballet
Financial Assistance: Work-Study Grants
Performing Groups: Tampa Ballet Company
Workshops/Festivals: Tampa Ballet Company Series

MUSIC

Richard W Rodean, Chairman   *Number Of Faculty:* 5   *Number Of Students:* 60
Degrees Offered: BMus
Courses Offered: All courses leading to Theory, Studio, and Education Majors
Technical Training: Education and Studio courses
Teaching Certification Available
Financial Assistance: Scholarships and Work-Study Grants
Performing Groups: Jazz & Chamber Music Ensembles; Bands; Show Chorus; Concert Choir

THEATRE

Gary Luter, Instructor   *Number Of Faculty:* 2
Courses Offered: Introduction Courses to Drama
Financial Assistance: Scholarships and Work-Study Grants
Artists-In-Residence/Guest Artists: Esther Glazer - Violin; Tampa Ballet Company; Spanish Little Theatre
(all Artists-in-Residence)

UNIVERSITY OF WEST FLORIDA
Pensacola   Florida 32504, 904 476-9500 Ext 319
State and 2 Year
Arts Areas: Instrumental Music, Vocal Music, Theatre, Film Arts, Television and Visual Arts
Performing Series: Music Hall Artist Series; West Florida Music Festival; Lyceum Series
(student-sponsored)
Performance Facilities: University Theatre; Music Hall

MUSIC

Grier M Williams, Chairman   *Number Of Faculty:* 5   *Number Of Students:* 40
Degrees Offered: BA   *Courses Offered:* Music, Music Ed
Teaching Certification Available
Financial Assistance: Scholarships and Work-Study Grants
Performing Groups: University Singers; Chamber Singers; Festival Chorus, Intercollegiate Band; Civic
Band; Intercollegiate Jazz Band
Workshops/Festivals: West Florida Music Festival; Various Instrumental, Vocal and Piano Workshops

THEATRE

Grier M Williams, Chairman   *Number Of Faculty:* 3   *Number Of Students:* 30
Degrees Offered: BA

(continued on next page)

Courses Offered: Professional; Educational; Technical Theatre; Children's Theatre
Teaching Certification Available
Financial Assistance: Scholarships and Work-Study Grants
Performing Groups: Actor's Factory
Artists-In-Residence/Guest Artists: New Orleans Symphony; Michel Debost; Bulgarian String Quartet; Consortium Antiquum (Antwerp); Ossian Ellis

ABRAHAM BALDWIN AGRICULTURAL COLLEGE
Tifton   Georgia 31794, 404 386-0666

State and 2 Year
Arts Areas: Instrumental Music, Vocal Music, Theatre and Visual Arts
Performing Series: Mutual Concert Association
Performance Facilities: Main Auditorium

MUSIC

Degrees Offered: AA   *Financial Assistance:* Scholarships and Work-Study Grants

THEATRE

James M Burt, Chairman   *Degrees Offered:* AA
Financial Assistance: Scholarships and Work-Study Grants
Performing Groups: ABAC Players

ACADEMY THEATRE SCHOOL OF PERFORMING ARTS
1374 W Peachtree, Atlanta   Georgia 30309
404 892-0355

Private and Special   *Arts Areas:* Theatre
Performance Facilities: Mainstage Theater; Six large classroom spaces

THEATRE

Frank Wittow, Artistic Director   *Number Of Faculty:* 12   *Number Of Students:* 150
Courses Offered: Acting; Voice; Movement for Actors (Mime, Tumbling)
Technical Training: Scene Design; Lighting Design; Costume Design; Stage Management
Financial Assistance: Work-Study Grants and Apprenticeship Program
Performing Groups: Children's Theatre Company; State Tour Team; Second Space Company

AGNES SCOTT COLLEGE
Decatur   Georgia 30030, 404 373-2571

Private and 4 Year
Arts Areas: Dance, Instrumental Music, Vocal Music, Theatre and Visual Arts
Performance Facilities: Winter Theatre in Dana Fine Arts Building; Presser Hall

DANCE

Marylin B Darling, Assistant Professor of Physical Education
Dance is part of Physical Education and Theatre Departments
Number Of Faculty: 1   *Courses Offered:* Dance History
Technical Training: Beginning & Intermediate Contemporary Dance, Ballet, Jazz, Tap, Folk Dance, Square Dance, Social Dance
Performing Groups: Studio Dance Theatre
Workshops/Festivals: Master Classes by professional dance companies

MUSIC

Dr Ronald L Byrnside; Charles A Dana, Chairmen   *Number Of Faculty:* 9
Degrees Offered: BA
Courses Offered: Music Appreciation; Theory & History; Church Music
Technical Training: Piano; Organ; Harpsichord; Voice; Strings; Woodwinds; Guitar
Financial Assistance: Scholarships
Performing Groups: Glee Club; Madrigal Singers; Opera Workshop; Baroque Ensemble; Recorder Society
Workshops/Festivals: Agnes Scott College Composition Contest; Metropolitan Atlanta Music Teachers Association; Atlanta Flute Club

THEATRE

Dr Jack T Brooking; Annie Louise Harrison Waterman, Chairpersons
Number Of Faculty: 3   *Degrees Offered:* BA

(continued on next page)

Courses Offered: History & Literature; Technical Theatre; Acting & Directing
Technical Training: Acting; Voice & Diction; Backstage & Technical Operations
Financial Assistance: Scholarships
Performing Groups: Blackfriars Student Theatre Group
Workshops/Festivals: Guest actors, directors, costumers speak to theatre classes
Artists-In-Residence/Guest Artists: Atlanta Chamber Players

ALBANY STATE COLLEGE
504 College Dr, Albany   Georgia 31705
912 435-3411
State and 4 Year
Arts Areas: Instrumental Music, Vocal Music, Theatre and Visual Arts
Performing Series: Lyceum Programs

MUSIC

James H Marquis, Chairman   **Number Of Faculty:** 5   **Number Of Students:** 70
Degrees Offered: BMus; BMusEd
Teaching Certification Available
Financial Assistance: Scholarships and Work-Study Grants
Performing Groups: College Marching & Concert Band; College Choir; Jazz Orchestra; Various Ensembles

THEATRE

Donniel A Doster, Chairman   **Degrees Offered:** BA
Teaching Certification Available
Financial Assistance: Scholarships and Work-Study Grants
Performing Groups: Albany State College Players

ANDREW COLLEGE
Cuthbert   Georgia 31740, 912 732-2171
Private and 2 Year   **Arts Areas:** Instrumental Music and Vocal Music
Performance Facilities: College Auditorium; Music Hall

MUSIC

Larry Belt, Chairman   **Number Of Faculty:** 6   **Number Of Students:** 40
Degrees Offered: AA; AS   **Courses Offered:** Music; Voice
Financial Assistance: Scholarships and Work-Study Grants
Performing Groups: Choir; Choraliers; Stage Band

ARMSTRONG STATE COLLEGE
11935 Abercorn St, Savannah   Georgia 31406
912 925-4200
State and 4 Year
Arts Areas: Instrumental Music, Vocal Music, Theatre and Visual Arts
Performing Series: Performing Series
Performance Facilities: Fine Arts Center Auditorium; Jenkins Hall Auditorium; Fine Arts Center Lecture -
Recital Hall

MUSIC

J Harry Persee, Head   **Number Of Faculty:** 5   **Number Of Students:** 40
Degrees Offered: BA; BMusEd
Technical Training: Opera; Applied Keyboard; Voice; Woodwind; Brass and Percussion
Teaching Certification Available
Financial Assistance: Assistantships, Scholarships and Work-Study Grants
Performing Groups: ASC Chorus; Symphonic Wind Ensemble; Jazz Ensemble; Opera Workshop
Workshops/Festivals: Annual District High School Band Festival; Instrumental Clinics in connection with
appearance of Guest Artists

(continued on next page)

THEATRE

John Suchower, Director   **Number Of Faculty:** 2   **Number Of Students:** 60
Degrees Offered: Concentration in Speech & Drama offered through Language & Literature Department, leading to BA in Language & Literature
Courses Offered: Acting; Play Production
Technical Training: Acting; Directing; All Phases of Stage Production
Financial Assistance: Assistantships, Scholarships and Work-Study Grants
Performing Groups: The Masquers
Workshops/Festivals: ASC Summer Theatre; First District High School One-Act Play Festival; Theatre Workshops and Student - Directed Plays

---

BERRY COLLEGE
Mount Berry   Georgia 30149, 404 232-5374
Private and 4 Year
Arts Areas: Dance, Instrumental Music, Vocal Music, Theatre, Film Arts and Visual Arts
Performing Series: Cultural Affairs
Performance Facilities: Ford Auditorium; Trustees Hall Auditorium; Green Hall Auditorium; Krannert Center Ballroom

DANCE

Dance program under auspices of Physical Education Department

MUSIC

Darwin White, Head   **Number Of Faculty:** 8   **Number Of Students:** 100
Degrees Offered: BA; BM Performance; BMMusic Ed
Teaching Certification Available
Financial Assistance: Scholarships and Work-Study Grants
Performing Groups: Concert Choir; Berry Singers; Symphonic Band; Jazz Ensemble; Brass Choir; Brass Quintet; Woodwind Quintet
Workshops/Festivals: May Fine Arts Festival

THEATRE

Dr Leroy Clark, Director   **Number Of Faculty:** 2   **Number Of Students:** 98
Degrees Offered: BA Drama; BA Speech - Drama combination
Teaching Certification Available
Financial Assistance: Scholarships and Work-Study Grants
Performing Groups: Berry Players; Theatre Laboratory

BRENAU COLLEGE
Washington St, Gainesville   Georgia 30501
404 532-4341 Ext 204
Private and 4 Year
Arts Areas: Dance, Instrumental Music, Vocal Music, Theatre and Visual Arts
Performing Series: Community Concert Series; Brenau Centennial Series
Performance Facilities: Pearce Auditorium; Little Theatre; Brenau Amphitheater

DANCE

Diane B Callahan, Director, Gainesville School of Ballet
Number Of Faculty: 3   **Number Of Students:** 200   **Degrees Offered:** BA
Financial Assistance: Scholarships and Work-Study Grants
Performing Groups: Gainesville School of Ballet
Workshops/Festivals: Annual Gainesville School of Ballet Dance Festival

MUSIC

David Lee Johnson, Director   **Number Of Faculty:** 6   **Number Of Students:** 45
Degrees Offered: BMEd; BA
Courses Offered: Music Education; Performing Musicium; Pedagogy
Teaching Certification Available

(*continued on next page*)

Financial Assistance: Scholarships and Work-Study Grants
Performing Groups: Chamber Choir; Women's Concert Choir

THEATRE

Elizabeth Hedrick, Director   *Number Of Faculty:* 2   *Number Of Students:* 10
Degrees Offered: BA   *Courses Offered:* Theatre/Drama
Financial Assistance: Scholarships and Work-Study Grants
Performing Groups: Playmakers
Workshops/Festivals: Highland's Summer Stock Playhouse at Gainesville
Artists-In-Residence/Guest Artists: Richard Collins; Elizabeth Holmes Feldmann

---

COLUMBUS COLLEGE
Algonquin Dr, Columbus   Georgia 31907
404 568-2030
   State, 4 Year and Graduate Program
   Arts Areas: Dance, Instrumental Music, Vocal Music and Theatre
   Performance Facilities: Experimental Theatre; Fine Arts Hall Auditorium

DANCE

Dance program under auspices of Theatre Department   *Number Of Faculty:* 1
Courses Offered: Classic Ballet   *Financial Assistance:* Scholarships

MUSIC

Dr Andrew Galos, Head   *Number Of Faculty:* 22   *Number Of Students:* 160
Degrees Offered: BM & MEd in Art & Music   *Teaching Certification Available*
Financial Assistance: Scholarships
Performing Groups: Faculty Concert Series; College Orchestra; Jazz Band; College Choir; Flute Ensemble;
Woodwinds, Trio and other Chamber Ensembles; Women's Glee Club; Activities Band
Workshops/Festivals: Students Cultural Events Series; Master Classes & Workshops with various Music
Masters; Piano Teachers Workshop; American Music Festival; District III Instrumental Solo & Ensemble
Festival

THEATRE

Dennis Ciesil, Head   *Number Of Faculty:* 3½   *Number Of Students:* 30
Degrees Offered: BA
Courses Offered: Theatre History; Dramatic Literature; Acting; Directing; Design; Playwriting
Technical Training: Lighting; Stagecraft; Scene Painting; Makeup
Financial Assistance: Scholarships
Performing Groups: Studio Theatre; Main - Stage Theatre
Workshops/Festivals: High School Drama Festival; Workshops in Stagecraft, Directing and Acting

---

COVENANT COLLEGE
Lookout Mountain   Georgia 37350, 404 831-6531
   Private and 4 Year   *Arts Areas:* Instrumental Music and Vocal Music
   Performance Facilities: Auditorium; Recital Hall

MUSIC

John Hamm, Chairman   *Number Of Faculty:* 3 Full-time, 5 Part-time
Number Of Students: 25   *Degrees Offered:* BA; BMus
Courses Offered: Liberal Arts; Music Ed; Applied
Teaching Certification Available
Financial Assistance: Scholarships and Work-Study Grants
Performing Groups: Chorus; Wind Ensemble; Brass Choir

DEKALB COMMUNITY COLLEGE
555 N Indian Creek Dr, Clarkston   Georgia 30021
404 292-1520 Ext 255

County and 2 Year
Arts Areas: Instrumental Music, Vocal Music, Theatre and Visual Arts
Performing Series: Music Guest Artist Series
Performance Facilities: Fine Arts Auditorium; Studio Theatre

MUSIC

Dr Thomas J Anderson, Head   *Number Of Faculty:* 9 Full-time, 5 Part-time
Number Of Students: 100   *Degrees Offered:* AA
Courses Offered: History & Literature; Theory & Keyboard Harmony; Applied Music; Performing Organizations
Financial Assistance: Assistantships, Scholarships and Work-Study Grants
Performing Groups: DCC Concert Band; DeKalb Symphony Orchestra; DeKalb Wind Ensemble; DeKalb Jazz Ensemble; DeKalb Opera Theatre; DeKalb College Singers; DCC Percussion Ensemble; DCC Brass Ensemble; DCC Woodwind Ensemble
Workshops/Festivals: Summer Music Workshop for High School Students

THEATRE

Mrs Faye Clark, Head   *Number Of Faculty:* 4   *Number Of Students:* 30
Degrees Offered: AA   *Courses Offered:* Acting; Stagecraft
Artists-In-Residence/Guest Artists: Klaus Hellwig; Trio d'Anches; Cologne; Tartini Trio; Zagreb String Quartet; Atlanta Chamber Players

EMORY UNIVERSITY
Atlanta   Georgia 30322, 404 329-6216

Private and 4 Year
Four-year undergraduate division of Emory University
Arts Areas: Instrumental Music, Vocal Music, Theatre and Visual Arts
Performing Series: Flora Glenn Candler Concert Series
Performance Facilities: Glenn Memorial Auditorium; AMUC Auditorium

MUSIC

Dr William W Lemonds, Chairman   *Number Of Faculty:* 3 Full-time, 2 Part-time
Number Of Students: 150   *Degrees Offered:* BMus
Courses Offered: Music History; Music Theory; Applied Music
Financial Assistance: Assistantships, Scholarships and Work-Study Grants
Performing Groups: Glee Club; Women's Chorale; Chamber Singers; Collegium Musicum; Atlanta - Emory Orchestra; Wind Ensemble; Emory Consort; Emory Baroque Trio; Emory Bach Ensemble
Workshops/Festivals: Flora Glenn Candler Concert Series; Summer Music Festival

THEATRE

Dr Fergus G Currie, Director   *Number Of Faculty:* 2
Technical Training: On the job training leading to technical assistants positions
Financial Assistance: Assistantships, Scholarships and Work-Study Grants
Performing Groups: Emory University Theatre; Emory University Summer Theatre; Emory University Children's Theatre; Ad Hoc Productions; Professional Workshop
Workshops/Festivals: One-Act Play Festival; Guest Artist Series

GAINESVILLE JUNIOR COLLEGE
Gainesville   Georgia 30501, 404 536-5226

State and 2 Year
Arts Areas: Instrumental Music, Vocal Music and Theatre

MUSIC

T J Byrnes, Head   *Number Of Faculty:* 2
Degrees Offered: AA Music; AA Music Ed

(continued on next page)

Financial Assistance: Scholarships and Work-Study Grants
Performing Groups: Choral and Instrumental Groups

THEATRE

Ed Cabell, Director   **Number Of Faculty:** 2   **Degrees Offered:** AA
Financial Assistance: Scholarships and Work-Study Grants

GEORGIA COLLEGE
Milledgeville   Georgia 31061, 912 453-4226
State and 4 Year
Arts Areas: Instrumental Music, Vocal Music, Theatre and Visual Arts
Performing Series: Lyceum Series; Community Concert Association; Music Department sponsored special events
Performance Facilities: Russell Auditorium; Porter Auditorium

MUSIC

Dr Robert F Wolfersteig, Chairman
Number Of Faculty: 9 Full-time, 1 Part-time   **Number Of Students:** 50 - 60
Degrees Offered: BM in Performance; BMusEd; B Mus Therapy
Courses Offered: Applied; Theory; Music History & Literature; Conducting; Literature; Choral Literature; Arranging; Orchestration; Counterpoint; Ensembles
Teaching Certification Available
Financial Assistance: Scholarships and Work-Study Grants
Performing Groups: Georgia College Stage Band; Concert Band; Woodwind Choir; Brass Choir; Women's Chorale; Mixed Chorus; Aeolian Singers
Workshops/Festivals: Jazz Workshop; Instrumental Clinics; Keyboard Clinics
Artists-In-Residence/Guest Artists: Leonard Pennario; John Wells; Jack Trussell; New Christy Minstrels; New York Pro Arte Orchestra

---

GEORGIA SOUTHERN COLLEGE
Statesboro   Georgia 30458, 912 681-5600 Ext 434
State and 4 Year
Arts Areas: Instrumental Music, Vocal Music, Theatre, Television and Broadcasting
Performing Series: Campus Life Enrichment Series; Departmental Concert Series by Music Department
Performance Facilities: Mc Croan Auditorium; Puppet Theatre; Foy Fine Arts Building Recital Hall

MUSIC

Dr Jack W Broucek, Chairman   **Number Of Faculty:** 11
Number Of Students: 105
Degrees Offered: BM Performance, School Music, Theory/Composition, Music History; BA Music; BS Ed; M Ed; MST; Six Year Certificate; EdS Music Education
Technical Training: Performance; Teaching; Electronic Music
Teaching Certification Available
Financial Assistance: Scholarships and Work-Study Grants
Performing Groups: Concert Band; Jazz Ensemble; Orchestra; Opera Theatre; Choral Groups; Faculty Ensembles
Workshops/Festivals: Piano Teachers; Marching Clinic; Summer Music Camp

THEATRE

Dr Clarence Mc Cord, Chairman   **Number Of Faculty:** 7
Number Of Students: 70   **Degrees Offered:** BA; BS
Courses Offered: Drama; Speech; Broadcasting; Public Relations; Puppetry
Technical Training: Lighting; Staging, Scenic Design; Performance; Teaching
Teaching Certification Available
Financial Assistance: Scholarships and Work-Study Grants
Performing Groups: Masquers; Puppetry Guild
Workshops/Festivals: High School Drama Debate Workshops; High School Forensics Meets

GEORGIA SOUTHWESTERN COLLEGE
Americus   Georgia 31709, 912 928-1350
State and 4 Year
Arts Areas: Instrumental Music, Vocal Music, Theatre and Visual Arts
Performing Series: Student Union Board Cultural Activities
Performance Facilities: Jackson Hall

MUSIC

Dr Donald W Forrester, Chairman   *Number Of Faculty:* 4
Number Of Students: 25   *Degrees Offered:* BS Mus Ed
Teaching Certification Available
Financial Assistance: Scholarships and Work-Study Grants
Performing Groups: Chorus; Band; Ensemble   *Workshops/Festivals:* Quarterly Concerts by each group

THEATRE

Byron Nichols, Chairman   *Number Of Faculty:* 3   *Number Of Students:* 13
Degrees Offered: BSEd in Speech & Theater   *Teaching Certification Available*
Financial Assistance: Scholarships and Work-Study Grants
Performing Groups: Quarterly Dramatic Theater Production; Quarterly Dinner Theater Production

GEORGIA STATE UNIVERSITY
University Plaza, Atlanta   Georgia 30303
404 658-2291
State and 4 Year
Arts Areas: Dance, Instrumental Music, Vocal Music, Theatre, Film Arts, Television and Visual Arts
Performing Series: GSU Department of Music Faculty Artists Recital Series
Performance Facilities: Recital Hall; Arts Complex

DANCE

Courses Offered: Master Classes in Ballet, Modern & Jazz; Lecture - Demonstrations by Atlanta
Contemporary Dance Company
Workshops/Festivals: Dance Workshops

MUSIC

Steven D Winick, Interim Chairman   *Number Of Faculty:* 42
Number Of Students: 375   *Degrees Offered:* BMus; MMus
Courses Offered: Voice Performance; Orchestral Instrument; Keyboard Performance; Music Theory; Music
Literature; Music Education; Choral Conducting
Teaching Certification Available
Financial Assistance: Scholarships and Work-Study Grants
Performing Groups: Orchestra; Concert Choir; University Chorus; Symphonic Band; Symphonic Wind
Ensemble; Jazz Ensemble; Chamber Music Ensemble
Workshops/Festivals: Seminars in Music Education Series; Atlanta Choral Workshop; Comprehensive
Summer High School Band & Chorus Workshop

THEATRE

Hilda G Dyches, Chairman   *Number Of Faculty:* 13   *Degrees Offered:* AB
Courses Offered: Theatre History, Creative Dramatics; Reader's Theatre; Theatre Management; Technical
Theatre; Acting; Directing; Mime
Financial Assistance: Assistantships, Scholarships and Work-Study Grants
Workshops/Festivals: Theatre Workshops for high school students
Artists-In-Residence/Guest Artists: Florence Kopleff

UNIVERSITY OF GEORGIA
Athens   Georgia 30601, 404 542-2836
State and 4 Year
Arts Areas: Instrumental Music, Vocal Music and Theatre
Performance Facilities: University Theatre   *Number Of Faculty:* 21
Degrees Offered: BA; BFA; BMus

(continued on next page)

THEATRE

Leighton M Ballew, Director   **Number Of Faculty:** 22
Degrees Offered: BFA; BA   **Performing Groups:** University Theatre

---

LA GRANGE COLLEGE

LaGrange   Georgia 30240, 404 882-2911
Private and 4 Year
Arts Areas: Dance, Vocal Music, Theatre and Visual Arts
Performing Series: Summer Theater; Spring Fine Arts Festival
Performance Facilities: Price Theater

MUSIC

David E Blalock, Choral Director   **Number Of Faculty:** 1
Number Of Students: 14
Financial Assistance: Scholarships and Work-Study Grants
Performing Groups: Something Special

THEATRE

Dr Max C Estes, Chairman   **Number Of Faculty:** 3   **Number Of Students:** 30
Degrees Offered: BA Speech & Drama
Courses Offered: Essentials of Acting; Directing; Playwriting; Drama
Technical Training: Technical Theater; Scene Design; Stage Management; Choreography
Financial Assistance: Scholarships and Work-Study Grants
Performing Groups: Curtain Raisers
Workshops/Festivals: Drama Workshop; Summer Theater

MACON JUNIOR COLLEGE

US 80 & I-475, Macon   Georgia 31206
912 474-2700 Ext 285
State and 2 Year   **Arts Areas:** Vocal Music, Theatre and Visual Arts
Performance Facilities: Auditorium

MUSIC

Dr Jack L Hutcheson, Associate Professor
Number Of Faculty: 1 Full-time, 1 Part-time   **Number Of Students:** 25
Degrees Offered: AA
Courses Offered: Music Theory; Applied Courses in Voice, Piano, Organ & Guitar
Financial Assistance: Scholarships and Work-Study Grants
Performing Groups: Macon Junior College Chorus; Macon Junior College Pop Chorus
Workshops/Festivals: Spring Musical

THEATRE

Dr Charles Pecor, Assistant Professor of Speech   **Number Of Faculty:** 1
Number Of Students: 15   **Degrees Offered:** AA in Speech & Drama
Courses Offered: Introduction to Drama & Theatre; Fundamentals of Speech
Financial Assistance: Scholarships and Work-Study Grants
Performing Groups: Macon Junior College Drama Club

MERCER UNIVERSITY, ATLANTA

3000 Flowers Rd, Atlanta   Georgia 30341
404 451-0331 Ext 54
Private and 4 Year
Arts Areas: Instrumental Music, Vocal Music, Theatre, Visual Arts and Church Music
Performance Facilities: Fine Arts Auditorium   **Number Of Faculty:** 3
Number Of Students: 75   **Degrees Offered:** BA; BMus
Teaching Certification Available
Financial Assistance: Scholarships and Work-Study Grants

(continued on next page)

Performing Groups: Concert Choir; PM Singers; Sound Lab; Piano Ensemble; Guitar Ensemble
Workshops/Festivals: Pace Piano Workshop; GMEA Choral Festival

THEATRE

Linda Langenbruch, Chairman   **Number Of Faculty:** 1   **Number Of Students:** 10
Financial Assistance: Work-Study Grants   **Performing Groups:** Mercer Players

---

MIDDLE GEORGIA COLLEGE
Sara St, Cochran   Georgia 31014
912 934-6221 Ext 285
State and 2 Year
Arts Areas: Dance, Instrumental Music, Vocal Music and Theatre
Performing Series: Cultural Performing Arts & Concert Series
Performance Facilities: College Auditorium; Russell Hall Performing Arts Theatre

DANCE

Ms Nancy Weber, Instructor   **Number Of Faculty:** 1   **Number Of Students:** 20
Degrees Offered: AA Physical Education
Courses Offered: Folk & Square Dance; Beginning & Intermediate Modern Dance, Ballet, Ballroom, Tap Jazz

MUSIC

Nat Frazier, Professor   **Number Of Faculty:** 2   **Number Of Students:** 30
Degrees Offered: AA Music; Two-Year Career Program: Sacred Choral Music
Financial Assistance: Scholarships and Work-Study Grants
Performing Groups: Vocal & Instrumental Ensembles

THEATRE

Nelson Carpenter, Associate Professor   **Number Of Faculty:** 2
Number Of Students: 15   **Degrees Offered:** AA Speech & Drama
Courses Offered: Play Production; Acting; Survey of Theatre History; Stagecraft; Forensic Events
Financial Assistance: Scholarships and Work-Study Grants
Performing Groups: Middle Georgia Players

MOREHOUSE COLLEGE
Atlanta   Georgia 30314, 404 681-2800
Private and 4 Year
Arts Areas: Instrumental Music, Vocal Music and Theatre

MUSIC

Number Of Faculty: 2   **Number Of Students:** 28   **Degrees Offered:** BMus
Teaching Certification Available
Financial Assistance: Scholarships and Work-Study Grants
Performing Groups: Various Ensembles; Concerts   **Degrees Offered:** BMus

THEATRE

Teaching Certification Available
Financial Assistance: Scholarships and Work-Study Grants
Performing Groups: Drama Club

MORRIS BROWN COLLEGE
643 Hunter St, NW, Atlanta   Georgia 30314
404 525-7831
Private and 4 Year
Arts Areas: Instrumental Music, Vocal Music and Visual Arts
Number Of Faculty: 4   **Number Of Students:** 60   **Degrees Offered:** BMus
Teaching Certification Available
Financial Assistance: Scholarships and Work-Study Grants

NORTH GEORGIA COLLEGE
Dahlonega   Georgia 30533, 404 864-3391 Ext 317
State and 4 Year
Arts Areas: Instrumental Music, Vocal Music, Visual Arts and Arts & Music Ed; Craft Marketing
Performance Facilities: Student Union Auditorium; Sanford Hall Auditorium

MUSIC

Mike O'Neal, Coordinator   *Number Of Faculty:* 3   *Number Of Students:* 18
Degrees Offered: BS Music Ed   *Teaching Certification Available*
Financial Assistance: Scholarships and Work-Study Grants
Performing Groups: North Georgia College Chorale
Workshops/Festivals: Arts to the People

THEATRE

Joe Morgan, Coordinator   *Number Of Faculty:* 1   *Number Of Students:* 10
Financial Assistance: Scholarships and Work-Study Grants
Performing Groups: North Georgia College Play Makers
Workshops/Festivals: Arts to the People

PIEDMONT COLLEGE
Demorest   Georgia 30535, 404 723-3911
Private and 4 Year
Arts Areas: Instrumental Music, Vocal Music, Theatre and Visual Arts

MUSIC

Number Of Faculty: 1   *Number Of Students:* 20
Degrees Offered: BMus
Financial Assistance: Scholarships and Work-Study Grants

THEATRE

Number Of Faculty: 1   *Number Of Students:* 23
Degrees Offered: BA
Financial Assistance: Scholarships and Work-Study Grants

SAVANNAH STATE COLLEGE
Savannah   Georgia 31404
State and 4 Year   *Arts Areas:* Instrumental Music and Vocal Music
Performing Series: Concert & Lecture Series   *Degrees Offered:* BMusEd
Performing Groups: Choir; Marching Band; Brasss Concert Band

SHORTER COLLEGE
Shorter Hill, Rome   Georgia 30161
404 232-2463
Private and 4 Year
Arts Areas: Instrumental Music, Vocal Music, Theatre and Television
Performing Series: Faculty, Guest, Alumni & Student Recital Series
Performance Facilities: Little Theatre; Brookes Chapel

MUSIC

John Ramsaur, Head   *Number Of Faculty:* 15   *Number Of Students:* 138
Degrees Offered: BMus; BMusEd; B Church Mus; BA with major in Music
Technical Training: Voice; Organ; Piano   *Teaching Certification Available*
Financial Assistance: Scholarships, Work-Study Grants and Extensive Loan Program

(continued on next page)

Performing Groups: Chorale; Pop Ensemble; Madrigal Singers
Workshops/Festivals: Opera Workshop

THEATRE

Pauline Noble, PhD, Head, Department of Language, Literature & Speech
Number Of Faculty: 3   *Number Of Students:* 27   *Degrees Offered:* BA
Technical Training: Speech Therapy; Drama
Financial Assistance: Scholarships, Work-Study Grants and Extensive Loan Program
Performing Groups: Reader's Theatre; Shorter Players
Workshops/Festivals: Jr & Sr Speech Recitals; Speech Festival; Several Workshops

---

SOUTH GEORGIA COLLEGE
Douglas   Georgia 31533, 912 384-1100 Ext 296
State and 2 Year
Arts Areas: Instrumental Music, Vocal Music, Theatre and Visual Arts
Performance Facilities: Large Auditorium; Two Small Auditoriums; Ballroom

DANCE

Number Of Faculty: 3   *Degrees Offered:* AA
Financial Assistance: Scholarships and Work-Study Grants

MUSIC

Number Of Faculty: 1   *Degrees Offered:* AA
Financial Assistance: Scholarships and Work-Study Grants
Performing Groups: College - Community Choir
Workshops/Festivals: Annual Musical Play

THEATRE

Number Of Faculty: 1 *Degrees Offered:* AA
Financial Assistance: Scholarships and Work-Study Grants
Performing Groups: College Theatre
Workshops/Festivals: Four full scale productions each year

SPELMAN COLLEGE
350 Spelman Lane, S W, Atlanta   Georgia 30314
404 681-3643
Private and 4 Year
Arts Areas: Dance, Instrumental Music, Vocal Music and Theatre
Performance Facilities: Sisters Chapel; Fine Arts Auditorium/Theatre; Fine Arts Choral Rehearsal Room; Read Hall

DANCE

Mozel Spriggs, Coordinator   *Number Of Faculty:* 2
Courses Offered: History & Philosophy of Dance; Rhythmic Analysis; Methods & Ballet; Modern; Folk; Modern Jazz
Financial Assistance: Work-Study Grants
Performing Groups: The Atlanta University Dance Theater; Dance Heritage Repertory Workshop
Workshops/Festivals: Intercultural Dance Enrichment Seminars; International Dance Festival; International Dance Workshops

MUSIC

Roland L Allison, Chairman   *Number Of Faculty:* 8   *Number Of Students:* 38
Degrees Offered: BA
Courses Offered: Music History; Music Theory; Class Piano; Class Voice; Choral Conducting; Music Education; Applied Music; Ensembles

(continued on next page)

Financial Assistance: Scholarships, Work-Study Grants and NDSL; Private Awards
Performing Groups: Spelman College Glee Club; Spelman College Wind Ensemble; Atlanta University Center Chamber Orchestra

THEATRE

Dr Frederick D Hall, Jr, Chairman   *Number Of Faculty:* 4
Number Of Students: 17   *Degrees Offered:* BA
Courses Offered: Principles of Acting; Oral Interpretation; Survey of European Drama; Introduction to Theater; Stagecraft; Play Analysis; Styles of Acting; Theory of Drama; Technical Production; Modern Drama
Technical Training: Technical Production
Financial Assistance: Scholarships, Work-Study Grants and NDSL; Private Awards
Performing Groups: Morehouse - Spellman Players
Workshops/Festivals: Summer Theater Workshop; Host to District High School Drama Festival
Artists-In-Residence/Guest Artists: Heinz Trutzschler

TIFT COLLEGE
Forsyth   Georgia 31029, 912 994-6689
Private and 4 Year
Arts Areas: Instrumental Music, Vocal Music and Theatre

MUSIC

R Lee Collins, Acting Head   *Number Of Faculty:* 4   *Number Of Students:* 25
Degrees Offered: BA
Courses Offered: Voice; Piano; Organ; Music Ed; Church Music
Teaching Certification Available
Financial Assistance: Scholarships and Work-Study Grants
Performing Groups: College Choir; Wind Ensemble

THEATRE

Betty Stacey, Head, Fine Arts   *Number Of Faculty:* 2
Number Of Students: 10 - 15   *Degrees Offered:* BA   *Courses Offered:* Speech
Teaching Certification Available   *Performing Groups:* Studio Players

---

VALDOSTA STATE COLLEGE
Division of Fine Arts, Valdosta   Georgia 31601
912 244-6340 Ext 245
State and 4 Year
Arts Areas: Instrumental Music, Vocal Music, Theatre, Television and Visual Arts
Performing Series: Valdosta Entertainment Assn; College Union Board Concerts; College Concert & Lecture Series
Performance Facilities: Whitehead Auditorium; Sawyer Theatre

MUSIC

Dr William F Bunch, Chairman   *Number Of Faculty:* 10
Number Of Students: 90   *Degrees Offered:* BMus; BA; BFA
Teaching Certification Available
Financial Assistance: Assistantships, Scholarships and Work-Study Grants
Performing Groups: Stage Band; Concert Band; Community Orchestra; Concert Choir; Serenaders
Workshops/Festivals: Band Clinic

THEATRE

Dr W Ren Christie, Chairman   *Number Of Faculty:* 8   *Number Of Students:* 75
Degrees Offered: BFA   *Teaching Certification Available*
Financial Assistance: Assistantships and Work-Study Grants
Workshops/Festivals: One - Act Play Festival; Summer Theatre Workshop

(continued on next page)

WESLEYAN COLLEGE
4760 Forsyth Rd, Macon   Georgia 31201
912 477-1110 Ext 311
    Private and 4 Year
    Arts Areas: Instrumental Music, Theatre and Visual Arts
    Performance Facilities: Porter Auditorium

MUSIC

Dr Sylvia Ross, Chairman   *Number Of Faculty:* 8   *Number Of Students:* 70
Degrees Offered: BMus; BMusEd; BA   *Teaching Certification Available*
Financial Assistance: Scholarships and Work-Study Grants
Performing Groups: Glee Club; Wesleyannes; Recorder Ensemble

THEATRE

George McKinney, Chairman   *Number Of Faculty:* 2   *Number Of Students:* 5
Degrees Offered: BA
Financial Assistance: Scholarships and Work-Study Grants

WEST GEORGIA COLLEGE
Carrollton   Georgia 30117, 404 834-4411 Ext 466
    County and 4 Year
    Arts Areas: Instrumental Music, Vocal Music, Theatre and Visual Arts
    Performing Series: Faculty Series; Chamber Series; Student Series; Visiting Artist Series
    Performance Facilities: Cashen Hall; College Auditorium; Studio Theater

MUSIC

Number Of Faculty: 12   *Number Of Students:* 65   *Degrees Offered:* BMus
Teaching Certification Available
Financial Assistance: Scholarships and Work-Study Grants
Performing Groups: Concert Choir Band; Chamber Singers; Men's Chorus; Women's Chorus; Woodwind
Ensemble; Brass Ensemble; String Ensemble
Workshops/Festivals: Fine Arts Festival

THEATRE

Number Of Faculty: 5
Number Of Students: 30   *Degrees Offered:* BA
Teaching Certification Available
Financial Assistance: Scholarships and Work-Study Grants
Performing Groups: WGC Theatre; Readers Theatre; Experimental Theatre

YOUNG HARRIS COLLEGE
Young Harris   Georgia 30582, 404 379-2161
    Private and 2 Year
    Arts Areas: Instrumental Music, Vocal Music, Theatre and Visual Arts
    Performing Series: Cultural Events Series
    Performance Facilities: College Auditorium

MUSIC

Degrees Offered: AA Music
Technical Training: Opera   *Performing Groups:* Vocal and Instrumental Ensemble

THEATRE

Jean English, Chairman   *Degrees Offered:* AA
Performing Groups: Delta Gamma Drama Society

BRIGHAM YOUNG UNIVERSITY - HAWAII CAMPUS
55 - 220 Kaluni St, Laie   Hawaii 96762
808 293-9211

Private and 4 Year   **Arts Areas:** Vocal Music, Theatre and Visual Arts
Performing Series: Lyceum Series   **Performance Facilities:** BYU - HC Auditorium

MUSIC

Number Of Faculty: 3   **Degrees Offered:** BA
Courses Offered: Vocal; Instrumental   **Teaching Certification Available**
Financial Assistance: Scholarships and Talent Awards
Performing Groups: A Capella Choir; University Chorale; Chamber Choir; Jazz Ensemble; Symphonic Band; Windward Symphony
Workshops/Festivals: Fine Arts Festival

THEATRE

Number Of Faculty: 1   **Degrees Offered:** AA   **Financial Assistance:** Scholarships
Performing Groups: Repetory Theatre   **Workshops/Festivals:** Fine Arts Festival

CHAMINADE UNIVERSITY OF HONOLULU
3140 Waialae Ave, Honolulu   Hawaii 96816
808 732-1471

Private, 4 Year and MBA Program Available
Arts Areas: Instrumental Music, Vocal Music, Theatre and Visual Arts
Performance Facilities: Eihen Multipurpose Facility

MUSIC

Number Of Faculty: 3   **Degrees Offered:** BA; BFA   **Teaching Certification Available**
Financial Assistance: Work-Study Grants
Performing Groups: Chaminade Singers; Chaminade University Jazz Ensemble

THEATRE

Number Of Faculty: 2   **Degrees Offered:** BA; BGS
Courses Offered: Drama; Theatre Practice
Financial Assistance: Work-Study Grants
Performing Groups: Chaminade Theatre Group
Workshops/Festivals: Statewide Shakespeare Festival

HAWAII LOA COLLEGE
PO Box 764, Kancohe   Hawaii 96744
808 235-3641 Ext 111

Private and 4 Year   **Arts Areas:** Theatre and Visual Arts

THEATRE

William Mayhew, Assistant Professor   **Number Of Faculty:** 1
Number Of Students: 15   **Degrees Offered:** BA
Courses Offered: Theatre Theory & Practice

UNIVERSITY OF HAWAII
2444 Dole St, Honolulu   Hawaii 96822
808 948-7677

State and 4 Year
Arts Areas: Dance, Instrumental Music, Vocal Music and Theatre
Performance Facilities: John F Kennedy Theatre; Experimental Theatre

(continued on next page)

DANCE

Carl Wolz, Director of the Dance Program
Number Of Faculty: 4 Full-time, 10 Part-time   *Number Of Students:* 450
Degrees Offered: BA; MFA
Financial Assistance: Assistantships and Scholarships
Performing Groups: University Dance Theatre; Hawaii Dance Theatre; Performing Ensembles in Hawaiian, Javanese, & Phillippine Dance
Workshops/Festivals: Festival of Ethnic Music & Dance; Inter Arts; Workshops in many dance genres with visiting dance artists from all over the world

MUSIC

Ricardo Trimillos, Chairman   *Number Of Faculty:* 23 Full-time, 35 Lecturers
Number Of Students: 325   *Degrees Offered:* BA; BMus; BEd; MA; MMus
Technical Training: In cooperation with East West Center Culture Learning
Teaching Certification Available
Financial Assistance: Assistantships, Scholarships, Work-Study Grants and East West Center Grants
Performing Groups: Javanese Gamelan; Javanese Dance; Philippine Music; Philippine Dance; Japanese Gagaku; Japanese Sankyoku; Hawaiian Ancient Hula & Chant; Korean Dance; Oceanic Dance; University Band; Symphony Orchestra; Collegium Musicum; Opera Workshop; Choir; Chamber Singers
Workshops/Festivals: Festival of Ethnic Music & Dance (biannual); Inter Arts; Summer Workshops for Educators in Ethnic Music & Dance; Workshops in Various Ethnic Traditions; Workshops in Particular Instruments; Workshop with Dr H Reutter (Stuttgart) in Vocal Performance

THEATRE

Edward A Langhans, Chairman   *Number Of Faculty:* 11
Number Of Students: 125   *Degrees Offered:* BA; MA; MFA; PhD
Technical Training: Stagecraft; Stage Lighting; Technical Theatre Workshop; Costume Design; Theatre Management
Financial Assistance: Assistantships, Scholarships and Work-Study Grants
Performing Groups: University of Hawaii Theatre; Kumu Kahua (original plays); Director's Company

---

UNIVERSITY OF HAWAII AT HILO - HILO COLLEGE
PO Box 1357, Hilo   Hawaii 96720
808 961-9311
State and 4 Year
Arts Areas: Instrumental Music, Vocal Music and Theatre
Performance Facilities: University of Hawaii Theater

MUSIC

Kenneth W Staton, Assistant Professor   *Number Of Faculty:* 3
Number Of Students: 50   *Degrees Offered:* BA
Courses Offered: Instrumental; Choral; Voice; Theory; History; Music Education
Teaching Certification Available
Financial Assistance: Scholarships and Work-Study Grants
Performing Groups: Repertory Singers; Hilo College Choir; Wind Ensemble Brass Ensemble; Stage Band
Workshops/Festivals: East Hawaii Music Workshop

THEATRE

Robert Spanabel, Assistant Professor   *Number Of Faculty:* 1
Number Of Students: 10   *Degrees Offered:* BA
Courses Offered: Theater Practicum; Beginning Acting
Performing Groups: The Theater Company

BOISE STATE UNIVERSITY
1910 University, Boise Idaho 83725
208 385-3957

State and 4 Year
Arts Areas: Dance, Instrumental Music, Vocal Music, Theatre, Film Arts, Television and Visual Arts
Performance Facilities: Special Events Center; Subal Theatre; Music Auditorium

DANCE

Dance program under auspices of Physical Education Department
Number Of Faculty: 1   *Number Of Students:* 30
Courses Offered: Modern Dance; Stage Movement

MUSIC

Wilbur Elliott, Chairman   *Number Of Faculty:* 18   *Number Of Students:* 140
Degrees Offered: BA; BA Secondary Ed; BMus; MA Secondary Ed
Technical Training: Composition; Synthesis   *Teaching Certification Available*
Financial Assistance: Internships, Scholarships and Work-Study Grants
Performing Groups: Orchestra; Marching Bands; Concert Band; Opera Theatre; Choir; Meistersingers; Musical Theatre
Workshops/Festivals: Marching Band Workshops; M E N C Annual Conference; I M T F Annual Festival

THEATRE

Robert Ericson, Chairman   *Number Of Faculty:* 6   *Number Of Students:* 65
Degrees Offered: BA; BA Secondary Ed
Courses Offered: Acting; Directing; Designing; Theatre History; Dramatic Literature
Technical Training: Light Design; Costuming
Teaching Certification Available
Financial Assistance: Internships, Scholarships and Work-Study Grants
Performing Groups: Theatre Repertory; Children's Theatre
Workshops/Festivals: Idaho Invitational Theatre Arts Festival

IDAHO STATE UNIVERSITY
Pocatello Idaho 83209, 208 236-2431

State and 4 Year
Arts Areas: Instrumental Music, Vocal Music, Theatre, Film Arts, Television and Visual Arts
Performance Facilities: Frazier Auditorium; Powell Little Theatre

MUSIC

Dr Alan E Stanek, Chairman   *Number Of Faculty:* 8
Degrees Offered: BA; BS; BMus
Courses Offered: Elements of Music; Theory of Music; Music in General Culture; Class Piano; Class Voice; Musical Pagentry; Diction; Class Instrument Instruction; History & Literature of Music; Form & Analysis; Conducting; Elementary School Music Curriculum; Vocal School Music Methods; Instrumental School Music Methods; Orchestration; Eighteen & Nineteenth Century Music; Recent & Contemporary Music; Counterpoint; Choral Literature; Major Performance Pedagogy & Literature; Material for Teaching Music Appreciation; Composition
Teaching Certification Available
Financial Assistance: Scholarships and Work-Study Grants
Performing Groups: Symphony Orchestra; Marching Band; Concert Band; Concert Choir; Opera Workshop; Jazz Lab Band; Jazz Vocal Ensemble; Percussion Ensemble
Workshops/Festivals: Summer Workshops for Teachers

THEATRE

Dr Allen P Blomquist, Director   *Number Of Faculty:* 8
Degrees Offered: BA; BS; BFA; MA

(continued on next page)

Courses Offered: Appreciation of Dramatic Arts; Theatre Graphics; Stagecraft; Theatre Production; Stage Lighting; Makeup; Stage Costume Construction; Acting; Theatre Management; The Art of the Film; Puppetry; Theatre Backgrounds; Stage Costume History & Design; Materials & Methods for High School Speech Arts; Problems in Acting; Stage Direction; Creative Dramatics; Modern European Theatre; American Theatre; Basic Pattern Drafting for Stage Costuming; Acting Styles; Scene Design; Playwriting; Advanced Contemporary Theatre

Teaching Certification Available

Financial Assistance: Scholarships and Work-Study Grants

Performing Groups: Theatre ISU; Alpha Psi Omega

THE COLLEGE OF IDAHO
Caldwell   Idaho 83605, 208 459-5011

Private and 4 Year

Arts Areas: Instrumental Music, Vocal Music, Theatre and Visual Arts

Performing Series: Caldwell Fine Arts Series

Performance Facilities: Jewett Auditorium; Blatchley Little Theatre

DANCE

Folk Dance under auspices of Physical Education Department

MUSIC

Dr Richard D Skyrm, Chairman   *Number Of Faculty:* 11

Number Of Students: 200   *Degrees Offered:* BA

Courses Offered: Applied Music; Theory; Music History; Music Education

Teaching Certification Available

Financial Assistance: Scholarships and Work-Study Grants

Performing Groups: Concert Choir; Chamber Singers; Opera Workshop; College - Community Symphony; Jazz Ensemble

Workshops/Festivals: Annual Artist in Residence; Opera Workshop; Caldwell Fine Arts Series

THEATRE

Dr D Jerry White, Professor   *Number Of Faculty:* 1   *Number Of Students:* 30

Degrees Offered: Minor in theater   *Courses Offered:* Drama; Literature; Stage

Teaching Certification Available

Financial Assistance: Scholarships and Work-Study Grants

Performing Groups: Scarlet Masque

UNIVERSITY OF IDAHO
Moscow   Idaho 83843, 208 885-6465

State and 4 Year

Arts Areas: Dance, Instrumental Music, Vocal Music, Theatre, Film Arts and Television

Performing Series: Theatre Artist Series

Performance Facilities: Performing Arts Center, Phase 1

DANCE

Diane Walker, Chairman   *Number Of Faculty:* 5   *Number Of Students:* 10

Courses Offered: Ballet; Folk   *Teaching Certification Available*

Financial Assistance: Scholarships and Work-Study Grants

Performing Groups: University Dance Theatre

Workshops/Festivals: Northwest Dance Symposium

MUSIC

Floyd Peterson, Chairman   *Number Of Faculty:* 21   *Number Of Students:* 180

Degrees Offered: BA; BMus; MMus; MA; MAEd   *Teaching Certification Available*

Financial Assistance: Assistantships, Scholarships and Work-Study Grants

Performing Groups: University Symphony Orchestra; Concert Choir; University Concert Band; Idaho Chamber Orchestra; University Wind Ensemble; University Singers; Vandal Marching Band; University Jazz Ensemble; Brass Choir; Chamber Music; Collegium Musicum; Percussion Ensemble

(continued on next page)

Workshops/Festivals: Inland Empire Music Festival; Various Workshops; High School Camp; Opera Workshop

THEATRE

Edmund M Chavez, Chairman   **Number Of Faculty:** 3   **Number Of Students:** 40
Degrees Offered: BA; BS; MA   **Teaching Certification Available**
Financial Assistance: Assistantships, Scholarships and Work-Study Grants

---

NORTH IDAHO COLLEGE
1000 W Garden Ave, Coeur D'Alene   Idaho 83814
208 667-7422
Private and 2 Year
Arts Areas: Instrumental Music, Vocal Music, Theatre and Television
Performance Facilities: College Auditorium

MUSIC

Number Of Faculty: 4   **Number Of Students:** 120   **Degrees Offered:** AA
Financial Assistance: Scholarships and Work-Study Grants
Performing Groups: Vocal and Instrumental Ensembles

THEATRE

Number Of Faculty: 2   **Number Of Students:** 50   **Degrees Offered:** AA
Performing Groups: Drama Group

NORTHWEST NAZARENE COLLEGE
Nampa   Idaho 83651, 208 467-8406
Private and 4 Year   **Arts Areas:** Instrumental Music and Vocal Music
Performing Series: Nampa Concert Series Co-Sponsor
Performance Facilities: Lecture - Demonstration Hall

MUSIC

Dr D E Hill, Chairman   **Number Of Faculty:** 8   **Number Of Students:** 1100
Degrees Offered: BA
Courses Offered: Theory; History of Music; Composition; Related Theory Courses
Teaching Certification Available
Financial Assistance: Scholarships and Work-Study Grants
Performing Groups: Concert Choir; Crusader Choir; Northwesterners; Concert Band; Brass Ensemble; Lab Band; String Ensemble; Collegium
Workshops/Festivals: Suzuki Workshop

RICKS COLLEGE
Rexburg   Idaho 83440, 208 356-2011
Private and 2 Year
Arts Areas: Dance, Instrumental Music, Vocal Music, Theatre, Film Arts, Television and Visual Arts
Performing Series: Entertainment Series

MUSIC

Dr C LaMar Barrus, Chairman   **Number Of Faculty:** 20
Number Of Students: 125   **Degrees Offered:** AA
Financial Assistance: Assistantships and Scholarships
Performing Groups: Symphony Orchestra; Symphonic Band; Concert Band; Jazz Ensemble; Vikaliers Choir; A Cappella Choir; College Choir; Women's Choir; Chamber Music Group; Ensemble Groups
Workshops/Festivals: Opera Workshop

THEATRE

Robert W Nelson, Chairman   **Number Of Faculty:** 5   **Number Of Students:** 72
Degrees Offered: AA   **Technical Training:** Stage Lighting; Scenic Design
Financial Assistance: Assistantships and Scholarships
Performing Groups: Act I (The Drama Club)
Workshops/Festivals: Summer Workshop for high school students

---

COLLEGE OF SOUTHERN IDAHO
Box 1238, Twin Falls   Idaho 83301
208 733-9554
2 Year and District
Arts Areas: Instrumental Music, Vocal Music, Theatre and Visual Arts

MUSIC

Lawrence M Curtis, Associate Professor   **Number Of Faculty:** 3
Degrees Offered: AA
Courses Offered: Theory of Music; Fundamentals of Music; Music Appreciation; Music History; Applied Music
Financial Assistance: Scholarships and Work-Study Grants
Performing Groups: Concert Band; College and Community Symphony Orchestra; Instrumental Ensemble; Concert Choir; Vocal Ensemble

THEATRE

Fran A Tanner, Professor of Speech & Drama   **Number Of Faculty:** 2
Degrees Offered: AA
Courses Offered: Theatre Appreciation; Fundamentals of Acting; Intermediate Acting; Oral Interpretation; Reader's Theatre; Stagecraft; Stage Lighting; Play Production; Reader's Theatre Practicum; Stage Makeup
Financial Assistance: Scholarships and Work-Study Grants
Performing Groups: Reader's Theatre

AMERICAN CONSERVATORY OF MUSIC
116 S Michigan Ave, Chicago   Illinois 60603
312 263-4161 Ext 215

Private and 4 Year   *Arts Areas:* Instrumental Music and Vocal Music
Performance Facilities: Recital Hall

MUSIC

Number Of Faculty: 160   *Number Of Students:* 2,000   *Degrees Offered:* BMus; MMus; DMA
Courses Offered: Piano; Voice; Theory; Instrument
Teaching Certification Available   *Financial Assistance:* Scholarships

AUGUSTANA COLLEGE
639 38th St, Rock Island   Illinois 61201
309 794-7000

Private and 4 Year
Arts Areas: Instrumental Music, Vocal Music, Theatre and Television
Performing Series: Cultural Activities Series; Faculty Recital Series; Faculty Exchange Series; Augustana Players
Performance Facilities: Centennial Hall; Larson Hall; Potter Hall

MUSIC

Alan B Hersch, Chairman   *Number Of Faculty:* 11   *Number Of Students:* 81
Degrees Offered: BMus; BMusEd
Courses Offered: Music History & Literature; Music Ed, Applied Music
Financial Assistance: Scholarships and Work-Study Grants
Workshops/Festivals: Augustana Band Festival; Augustana Jazz Band Festival; Various Workshops

THEATRE

Dan E Spaugh, Director   *Number Of Faculty:* 2   *Number Of Students:* 50
Degrees Offered: BA in Speech
Technical Training: Basic technical courses including Lighting, Design
Financial Assistance: Scholarships and Work-Study Grants
Performing Groups: Augustana Players; Alpha Psi Omega

AURORA COLLEGE
347 Gladstone, Aurora   Illinois 60507
312 892-6431

Private and 4 Year   *Arts Areas:* Vocal Music, Theatre and Piano
Performance Facilities: Stanley H Perry Theatre; Lowry Chapel; Studio Theatre

MUSIC

Charlotte Peichl, Chairman   *Number Of Faculty:* 5   *Number Of Students:* 50
Courses Offered: Voice I-IV; Piano I-IV; Organ I-IV; Music Appreciation; Opera Appreciation
Financial Assistance: Scholarships
Performing Groups: Vocal Ensemble; New Life Singers
Workshops/Festivals: Fine Arts Festival; Music Festival; Council of West Suburban Colleges

THEATRE

Susan Pellowe, Director   *Number Of Faculty:* 2
Courses Offered: Acting; Directing; Oral Interpretation; Speech; Theater Workshop, Theater Literature
Financial Assistance: Scholarships
Performing Groups: Drama Guild; AY Fraternity
Workshops/Festivals: Fine Arts Festival; Shakespeare Banquet

BARAT COLLEGE
700 E Westleigh Rd, Lake Forest   Illinois 60045
312 234-3000
  Private and 4 Year
  Arts Areas: Dance, Instrumental Music, Vocal Music, Theatre, Visual Arts and Studio Art
  Performing Series: Lecture Committee Events
  Performance Facilities: Drake Theatre; Hilton Theatre; Reicher Gallery

DANCE

Carol Walker, Director   **Number Of Faculty:** 5   **Number Of Students:** 130
Degrees Offered: BA in Theatre & Dance with emphasis on Dance
Courses Offered: Introduction to Dance; Dance Today; Afro-American Dance; Intermediate Dance
Techniques; Choreography; Pointe, Ballet; Advanced Dance Techniques; History of Dance; Advanced
Choreography
Technical Training: Classical; Modern
Financial Assistance: Internships, Assistantships and Work-Study Grants
Performing Groups: Barat Repertory Dance Group
Workshops/Festivals: Guest Artists Series with Master Classes & Lecture Demonstrations

MUSIC

Platon Karmeres, Chairman   **Number Of Faculty:** 2   **Number Of Students:** 71
Courses Offered: Black Music; Opera; Fundamentals of Music; Theory ; Barat College Singers;
Instrumental Ensemble and/or Lake Forest Symphony; Music History; Theory; Music Education Teaching
Methods; Conducting; The Beethoven Symphonies; Wagner's Ring; Russian & Soviet Music; Form &
Analysis; Orchestration; Musicology Seminar
Technical Training: History; Musicology; Voice; Instrumental
Teaching Certification Available
Financial Assistance: Internships, Assistantships and Work-Study Grants
Performing Groups: Barat Singers

THEATRE

James Maloon, Chairman   **Number Of Faculty:** 4   **Number Of Students:** 69
Degrees Offered: BA in Theatre & Dance with emphasis on Theatre
Courses Offered: Introduction to Theatre Arts; Production Workshop; Speech Communication; Oral
Interpretation of Literature; Participation in Theatre Arts; Acting; Scene Design; Children's Theatre;
Playwriting; Directing; History of Theatre; Costume Design; Lighting Design; Problems in Design; Theatre
Administration; Seminar in Stage Management; American Theatre History
Technical Training: Scenery; Costume & Lighting Design; Stage Management; Theatre Management
Teaching Certification Available
Financial Assistance: Internships, Assistantships and Work-Study Grants
Performing Groups: Barat Players; Children's Theatre
Artists-In-Residence/Guest Artists: Angela Del Moral; Antonios Ballet of Madrid; National Spanish Ballet
of Spain

BLACK HAWK COLLEGE
6600 34th Ave, Moline   Illinois 61265
309 796-1311
  Private and 2 Year
  Arts Areas: Instrumental Music, Vocal Music, Theatre, Film Arts, Television and Visual Arts
  Performing Series: Children's Touring Theatre; Fall & Spring Concerts; Madrigal Dinner
  Performance Facilities: College Cafeteria

MUSIC

Roger Perley, Chairman   **Number Of Faculty:** 4 Full-time, 20 Part-time
Number Of Students: 160   **Degrees Offered:** AA
Financial Assistance: Scholarships and Work-Study Grants
Performing Groups: Brass & Woodwind Ensembles; Instrumental Ensemble; College Choir; The Hawks
(Pop Vocal Group)
Workshops/Festivals: Fall & Spring Fine Arts Festival; Opera Workshop

(continued on next page)

THEATRE

Ralph Drexler, Chairman   **Number Of Faculty:** 5   **Number Of Students:** 250
Degrees Offered: AA
Financial Assistance: Scholarships and Work-Study Grants
Performing Groups: Children's Touring Theatre

BLACKBURN COLLEGE
Carlinville   Illinois 62626, 217 854-3231
Private and 4 Year
Arts Areas: Instrumental Music, Vocal Music and Theatre
Performance Facilities: Bothwell Auditorium

MUSIC

Harold S Lowe, Professor   **Number Of Faculty:** 2 Full-time, 3 Part-time
Number Of Students: 30   **Degrees Offered:** BA
Teaching Certification Available   **Financial Assistance:** Work-Study Grants
Performing Groups: Madrigals; Choir

THEATRE

Thomas Anderson, Professor   **Number Of Faculty:** 2   **Number Of Students:** 24
Degrees Offered: BA   **Financial Assistance:** Work-Study Grants
Performing Groups: Blackburn Players

BRADLEY UNIVERSITY
1501 W Bradley Ave, Peoria   Illinois 61606
309 676-7611
Private and 4 Year
Arts Areas: Instrumental Music, Vocal Music, Theatre and Visual Arts

MUSIC

Dr Allen Coannon, Chairman   **Number Of Faculty:** 18
Number Of Students: 185   **Degrees Offered:** BMus; BMusEd; BA Applied Music
Teaching Certification Available   **Financial Assistance:** Scholarships
Performing Groups: Madrigal Singers; Symphony Orchestra; Ensembles
Workshops/Festivals: Annual New Music Clinic, Opera Workshop

THEATRE

John Clifford, Chairman   **Number Of Faculty:** 10   **Number Of Students:** 140
Degrees Offered: B Speech; MA; M Speech   **Teaching Certification Available**
Financial Assistance: Scholarships   **Performing Groups:** University Theatre

---

CHICAGO CITY COLLEGE, AMUNDSEN - MAYFAIR COLLEGE
4626 N Knox Ave, Chicago   Illinois 60630
312 286-1323
City and 2 Year   **Arts Areas:** Theatre and Visual Arts
Degrees Offered: AA   **Financial Assistance:** Scholarships

CHICAGO CITY COLLEGE, MALCOLM X COLLEGE
2250 W Van Buren St, Chicago   Illinois 60612
312 942-3000
City and 2 Year   **Arts Areas:** Theatre and Visual Arts
Degrees Offered: AA   **Financial Assistance:** Assistantships
Performing Groups: Drama Group

CHICAGO CITY COLLEGE, OLIVE - HARVEY COLLEGE
6800 S Anthony Ave, Chicago   Illinois 60617
312 568-3700

City and 2 Year   *Arts Areas:* Instrumental Music, Vocal Music and Theatre

MUSIC

Judith H Cieslak, Chairman   *Degrees Offered:* AA
Financial Assistance: Scholarships   *Degrees Offered:* AA
Performing Groups: Drama Club

CHICAGO CITY COLLEGE, SOUTHWEST COLLEGE
3939 W 79th, Chicago   Illinois 60652
312 735-3000

City and 2 Year   *Arts Areas:* Theatre   *Degrees Offered:* AA
Financial Assistance: Scholarships   *Performing Groups:* Drama Club

CHICAGO CONSERVATORY COLLEGE
410 S Michigan Ave, Chicago   Illinois 60605
312 427-0500

Private and 4 Year   *Arts Areas:* Instrumental Music and Vocal Music
Performing Series: Faculty Concert Series; Guest Artists Series

MUSIC

Dr Enrique Alberto Arias, Dean   *Number Of Faculty:* 59
Number Of Students: 135
Degrees Offered: BMus in Applied, Music Education, Theory & Composition; MMus in Applied, Music Education, Theory & Composition
Performing Groups: Opera Workshop; Chicago Conservatory College Chorus, Collegiate Chorale
Workshops/Festivals: Opera Workshop

CHICAGO STATE UNIVERSITY
95th St & King Dr, Chicago   Illinois 60628
312 995-2105

State and 4 Year   *Arts Areas:* Instrumental Music and Vocal Music

MUSIC

Frank Garcia, Chairman   *Number Of Faculty:* 11   *Number Of Students:* 135
Degrees Offered: BMusEd; BMus
Courses Offered: Fundamentals; Voice; Diction; Keyboard Skills; Theory; Composition
Teaching Certification Available
Financial Assistance: Scholarships and Work-Study Grants
Performing Groups: CSU Jazz Ensemble; CSU Concert Band; Choir

THEATRE

James W Dresser, Chairman   *Degrees Offered:* BA
Teaching Certification Available
Financial Assistance: Scholarships and Work-Study Grants

UNIVERSITY OF CHICAGO
5706 S University, Chicago   Illinois 60637
312 753-3583

Private, 4 Year and Graduate   *Arts Areas:* Theatre
Performing Series: Court Theatre; Court Winter Theatre; Court Studio Theatre
Performance Facilities: Mandel Hall; Reynolds Club Theatre; New Theatre

(continued on next page)

MUSIC

Robert L Marshall, Chairman   **Number Of Faculty:** 12
Number Of Students: 100   **Degrees Offered:** BA; MA; PhD
Technical Training: Electronic Music   **Teaching Certification Available**
Financial Assistance: Scholarships and Work-Study Grants
Performing Groups: Symphony Orchestra; Chorus; Collegium Musicum; Contemporary Chamber Players
Performing Groups: Court Theatre - Summer & Winter

COLLEGE OF DU PAGE
Lambert Rd, Glen Ellyn   Illinois 60137
312 858-2800
State and 2 Year
Arts Areas: Dance, Instrumental Music, Vocal Music, Theatre, Film Arts, Television and Visual Arts
Performing Series: Colloquim Series
Performance Facilities: College of Du Page Auditorium

DANCE

Donna Oleson, Chairman   **Number Of Faculty:** 1

MUSIC

Carl Lambert, Director   **Number Of Faculty:** 2   **Number Of Students:** 500
Technical Training: Theory Instruction
Performing Groups: Swing Singer; Community Chorus; College Singers; Barbershop Quartet; Stage Band; Marching Band; Jazz Band
Workshops/Festivals: Summer Children's Creative Arts Workshop

THEATRE

Richard Holgate, Director   **Number Of Faculty:** 7   **Number Of Students:** 300
Performing Groups: Readers' Theatre; Children's Theatre; Repertory Theatre; Summer Theatre
Workshops/Festivals: Children's Creative Arts Workshop

COLLEGE OF SAINT FRANCIS
500 Wilcox St, Joliet   Illinois 60435
815 726-7311 Ext 225
Private and 4 Year
Arts Areas: Dance, Instrumental Music, Vocal Music, Theatre and Visual Arts
Performance Facilities: Walden III Theatre; Gymnasium

DANCE

Sister Eileen Bannon, Chairman   **Number Of Faculty:** 1
Number Of Students: 25
Courses Offered: Movement & Dance; Beginning Acting; Stagecraft; Directing
Teaching Certification Available
Financial Assistance: Scholarships and Work-Study Grants
Performing Groups: Dance Group

MUSIC

Sister Rosaire Schlueb, Professor   **Number Of Faculty:** 4
Number Of Students: 75   **Degrees Offered:** BMus; BA
Courses Offered: Orchestration; Composition; Chamber Music; Comprehensive Musicianship
Teaching Certification Available
Financial Assistance: Scholarships and Work-Study Grants
Performing Groups: CSF Chorus; CSF Band; Choir

THEATRE

Daniel McCarter, Associate Professor   **Number Of Faculty:** 3
Number Of Students: 50   **Degrees Offered:** BA Speech & Theatre

(continued on next page)

Technical Training: Plays; Workshops   **Teaching Certification Available**
Financial Assistance: Scholarships and Work-Study Grants
Performing Groups: Drama Club

CONCORDIA TEACHERS COLLEGE
7400 Augusta St, River Forest   Illinois 60305
312 771-8300 Ext 245
Private and 4 Year
Arts Areas: Instrumental Music, Vocal Music, Theatre and Visual Arts

MUSIC

Thomas Gieschen, Chairman   **Number Of Faculty:** 15   **Number Of Students:** 61
Degrees Offered: BA Ed; BA Mus; M Church Music
Teaching Certification Available
Financial Assistance: Assistantships, Scholarships and Work-Study Grants
Performing Groups: The Chapel Choir; College Chorus; The Kapelle; Concert Band; Jazz Band; Recorder Ensemble; Pep Band; Brass Ensemble
Workshops/Festivals: Annual Lectures in Church Music; Luther High School Band Festival; Lutheran High School Choral Festival; Choral Reading Workshop

THEATRE

Eunice Eifert, Professor   **Number Of Faculty:** 3   **Number Of Students:** 50
Degrees Offered: BA Speech   **Teaching Certification Available**
Financial Assistance: Assistantships, Scholarships and Work-Study Grants
Performing Groups: Concordia Players

DEPAUL UNIVERSITY
25 E Jackson Blvd, Chicago   Illinois 60604
312 321-7600
Private and 4 Year
Arts Areas: Dance, Instrumental Music, Vocal Music and Visual Arts
Performing Series: DePaul Artist/Faculty Series
Performance Facilities: College Theatre; Recital Hall

MUSIC

Frederick Miller, Dean   **Number Of Faculty:** 57   **Number Of Students:** 500
Degrees Offered: BMus; MMus
Courses Offered: Church Music; Music Therapy; Music Education; Composition; Theory; Performance; Conducting; Church Music; Music Education
Teaching Certification Available
Financial Assistance: Scholarships, Work-Study Grants and Tuition Grants
Performing Groups: Symphony Orchestra; Concert Band; Choir; Wind Ensemble; Jazz Band; Contemporary Music Ensemble; Chamber Music
Workshops/Festivals: Opera Workshop

THEATRE

Dr Frank Andersen, Chairman   **Number Of Faculty:** 4   **Number Of Students:** 35
Degrees Offered: BA   **Courses Offered:** Speech Arts; Drama; Communications
Technical Training: Stagecraft   **Teaching Certification Available**
Financial Assistance: Scholarships, Work-Study Grants and Tuition Grants

EASTERN ILLINOIS UNIVERSITY
Charleston   Illinois 61920, 217 581-2917
Private and 4 Year
Arts Areas: Instrumental Music, Vocal Music, Theatre and Visual Arts
Performance Facilities: Dvorak Concert Hall; Fine Arts Theatre; Fine Arts Playroom

(continued on next page)

DANCE

Dance program under auspices of Physical Education Department

MUSIC

Rhoderick E Key, Chairman   **Number Of Faculty:** 31   **Number Of Students:** 275
Courses Offered: Voice, Piano, History & Literature of Music; Music Theory & Literature; Workshop; Aural Training; Choral Conducting
Teaching Certification Available
Financial Assistance: Assistantships, Scholarships and Work-Study Grants
Performing Groups: Cecilian Singers; Mixed Chorus; Concert Choir; Concert Band; Marching Band; Pep Bands; Stage Band; String Orchestra; Symphonic Winds; Symphony Orchestra; Oratorio Chorus
Workshops/Festivals: Marching Band Festival; District V Festival; High School Chorus Festival; I H S A Band Music Contest; E I U Jazz Festival; Illinois College Choir Festival; Metropolitan Opera Audition; Piano Pedagogy Workshop; Eastern Music Camp

THEATRE

E G Gabbard, Chairperson   **Number Of Faculty:** 7   **Number Of Students:** 44
Degrees Offered: BA; BA with Teaching Certificate
Courses Offered: Practicum I, II; Voice & Phonetics; Beginning Interp; Acting; Technical Direction; Scene Design; Costuming; Directing; History
Teaching Certification Available   Performing Groups: The Players
Workshops/Festivals: Theatre and oral interpretation workshops for high school students during summer

---

ELMHURST COLLEGE
190 Prospect, Elmhurst   Illinois 60126
312 279-4100 Ext 357
Private and 4 Year
Arts Areas: Instrumental Music, Vocal Music, Theatre and Visual Arts
Performing Series: Irion Recital Series
Performance Facilities: Hammerschmidt Chapel; Irion Recital Hall; Sub - Cub; Mill Theatre

MUSIC

James Sorensen, Chairman   **Number Of Faculty:** 30   **Number Of Students:** 65
Degrees Offered: BA, BS, BM Music Ed, Music Business, Music
Teaching Certification Available
Financial Assistance: Scholarships and Work-Study Grants
Performing Groups: Band; Jazz Band; Choir; Barbershop Quartet; Men's Glee Club; Women's Choir; Ensembles; Choral Union
Workshops/Festivals: Church Music Workshop; Marching Band Festival; Suzuki Festival; Concert Band Festival; Choir Festival

THEATRE

Donald R Low, PhD, Chairperson   **Number Of Faculty:** 2
Number Of Students: 50   **Degrees Offered:** BA; BS
Courses Offered: Acting; Directing; Oral Interpretation; Development of Theatre; Independent Study; Practicum
Technical Training: Curricular & Co-Curricular
Teaching Certification Available
Financial Assistance: Scholarships and Work-Study Grants
Performing Groups: Elmhurst College Theatre

EUREKA COLLEGE
300 College Ave, Eureka   Illinois 61530
309 467-3721
Private and 4 Year
Arts Areas: Instrumental Music, Vocal Music, Theatre, Television and Visual Arts
Performance Facilities: Pritchard Fine Arts Center; Rinker Outdoor Theatre

(continued on next page)

MUSIC

Greg Upton, Director   **Number Of Faculty:** 3   **Number Of Students:** 50
Degrees Offered: BA Music   **Courses Offered:** History, Theory, Voice
Technical Training: Music Therapy   **Teaching Certification Available**
Financial Assistance: Scholarships and Work-Study Grants
Performing Groups: Eureka College Chorale; Eureka College Bell Choir

THEATRE

Bill Davis, Director   **Number Of Faculty:** 3   **Number Of Students:** 40
Degrees Offered: BA Theatre; BA Speech
Courses Offered: History, Acting, Directing, Tech Theatre; Radio/TV
Teaching Certification Available
Financial Assistance: Scholarships and Work-Study Grants
Performing Groups: Eureka College Theatre
Artists-In-Residence/Guest Artists: Margaret Beals

FELICIAN COLLEGE
3800 Peterson Ave, Chicago   Illinois 60659
312 539-1919

Private and 2 Year
Arts Areas: Instrumental Music, Vocal Music and Visual Arts
Performing Series: Christmas Program; Spring Concert
Performance Facilities: College Auditorium

MUSIC

Sister Mary Alphonsetta, Chairman   **Number Of Faculty:** 1
Degrees Offered: AA Music
Courses Offered: Voice; Piano; Organ; Chorus; Theory; History of Music; Appreciation of Music
Financial Assistance: Scholarships
Performing Groups: Vocal Ensembles; Chorus
Workshops/Festivals: Christmas Program; Spring Concert
Artists-In-Residence/Guest Artists: Diane Klema; Elizabeth Staffen; Ronalee Rand

---

GOODMAN SCHOOL OF DRAMA
A SCHOOL OF THE ART INSTITUTE OF CHICAGO
200 S Columbus Dr, Chicago   Illinois 60603
312 443-3833

Private and Special   **Arts Areas:** Theatre
Performance Facilities: Goodman Theatre; Studio Theatre
Number Of Faculty: 25   **Number Of Students:** 180   **Degrees Offered:** BFA; MFA
Technical Training: Acting; Directing; Costume Design; Scene Design; Technical Direction
Financial Assistance: Assistantships, Scholarships and Work-Study Grants

---

GREENVILLE COLLEGE
Greenville   Illinois 62246, 618 664-1840

Private and 4 Year
Arts Areas: Instrumental Music, Vocal Music and Visual Arts
Performing Series: Guest Artist Series
Performance Facilities: LaDue Auditorium

MUSIC

Dr James E Wilson, Chairman   **Number Of Faculty:** 4 Full-time, 3 Part-time
Number Of Students: 40 Majors   **Degrees Offered:** BMusEd; BA
Teaching Certification Available
Financial Assistance: Scholarships and Work-Study Grants
Performing Groups: A Cappella Choir; College Band; Madrigal Singers
Workshops/Festivals: High School - College Band Festival; High School - College Choral Festival

ILLINOIS BENEDICTINE COLLEGE
5700 College Rd, Lisle   Illinois 60532
312 968-7270

Private and 4 Year   **Arts Areas:** Instrumental Music and Vocal Music

MUSIC

Rev Alban Hrebic, Chairman   **Number Of Faculty:** 6
Degrees Offered: BA MusEd; BM Composition, Sacred Music or Performance
Courses Offered: Theoretical & Applied Music
Teaching Certification Available
Financial Assistance: Scholarships and Work-Study Grants
Performing Groups: Chorus; Symphony Orchestra; Stage Band

THEATRE

Michael Madach, Chairman   **Number Of Faculty:** 1½
Performing Groups: IBC Productions (8 shows per season)

ILLINOIS CENTRAL COLLEGE
East Peoria   Illinois 61635, 309 694-5011
2 Year
Arts Areas: Dance, Instrumental Music, Vocal Music, Theatre, Television and Visual Arts
Performing Series: Cultural Arts Series
Performance Facilities: ICC Lecture - Recital Hall; ICC Performing Arts Building

DANCE

Marc Ligon, Artistic Director   **Number Of Faculty:** 2
Number Of Students: 100   **Courses Offered:** Ballet
Performing Groups: Mid America Dance Theatre of the Peoria Civic Ballet Company
Workshops/Festivals: Winter & Spring Ballet Concerts, Mini Concerts in Peoria Public Schools; Summer
Workshop; Guest Concerts Throughout the State; ICC Fine Arts Festival; Cultural Arts Series

MUSIC

Tubal Holmes, Program Director   **Number Of Faculty:** 11
Number Of Students: 620   **Degrees Offered:** AA; AS
Courses Offered: Music Appreciation; Performing; Class Instrumental Instruction
Performing Groups: ICC Community Orchestra; Concert Band; Concert Choir; Chamber Singers; Jazz
Band; Pep Band
Workshops/Festivals: ICC Fine Arts Festival; Piano Instructors' Workshop; Concert Receptions; Cultural
Arts Series; High School Band Directors' Workshop

THEATRE

Don Marine, Program Director   **Number Of Faculty:** 3
Number Of Students: 120   **Degrees Offered:** AA; AS
Courses Offered: Introductory; Technical; Stage Design; Creative Dramatics; Acting; Directing
Technical Training: Technical Theatre
Performing Groups: Season's Major Productions; Field Touring Theatre; Readers' Theatre; Children's
Theatre
Workshops/Festivals: ICC Fine Arts Festival; High School Production & Directing Workshops; Cultural
Arts Series
Artists-In-Residence/Guest Artists: Marc Ligon

ILLINOIS COLLEGE
1101 W College, Jacksonville   Illinois 62650
217 245-7126

Private and 4 Year
Arts Areas: Instrumental Music, Vocal Music and Theatre
Performing Series: Concert Series
Performance Facilities: Chapel Auditorium; Theatre Stage

(continued on next page)

MUSIC

Rick Erickson, Chairman   **Number Of Faculty:** 1   **Number Of Students:** 25
Degrees Offered: BA Fine Arts   **Financial Assistance:** Scholarships
Performing Groups: Chorus; Band/Orchestra; Madrigal Singers; Stage Band
Workshops/Festivals: Music Tour

THEATRE

Geraldine Staley, Director   **Number Of Faculty:** 1   **Number Of Students:** 40
Degrees Offered: BA in Speech & Drama   **Financial Assistance:** Scholarships
Performing Groups: Hilltop Players
Artists-In-Residence/Guest Artists: St Louis Symphony Chamber Group

---

ILLINOIS WESLEYAN UNIVERSITY
210 E University, Bloomington   Illinois 61701
309 556-3131
Private and 4 Year
Arts Areas: Dance, Instrumental Music, Vocal Music and Theatre
Performance Facilities: Westbrook Auditorium (Presser Hall); McPherson Theatre

DANCE

Thom Cobb, Instructor, Assistant Professor   **Number Of Faculty:** 1
Courses Offered: Beginning & Intermediate Modern Dance; Folk; Square; Social; Dance for Theatre
Financial Assistance: Scholarships and Work-Study Grants
Performing Groups: Illinois Wesleyan Dance Theatre; Wesleyan Folk Song & Dance Ensemble

MUSIC

Dr Albert Shaw, Director   **Number Of Faculty:** 21   **Number Of Students:** 192
Degrees Offered: BMus; BMusEd; MSM
Financial Assistance: Assistantships, Scholarships and Work-Study Grants
Performing Groups: University Orchestra; Concert Band; Collegiate Choir; Festival Choir; Women's
Chorus; Chamber Singers; Jazz Ensemble; Woodwind, Brass, String & Percussion Ensembles; Marching
Band; Wesleyan Singers (Swing Choir)
Workshops/Festivals: Church Music Conference; Symposium of Contemporary Music; Jazz Workshop; Jazz
Festival

THEATRE

Dr Carole Brandt, Director   **Number Of Faculty:** 7   **Number Of Students:** 91
Degrees Offered: BA; BFA   **Financial Assistance:** Scholarships
Workshops/Festivals: Fine Arts Festival

UNIVERSITY OF ILLINOIS AT CHICAGO CIRCLE
601 S Morgan, Chicago   Illinois 60680
312 996-3000
State and 4 Year
Arts Areas: Instrumental Music, Vocal Music and Theatre

MUSIC

Richard Monaco, Head/Professor   **Number Of Faculty:** 11
Number Of Students: 80   **Degrees Offered:** BA
Courses Offered: Theory; History; Literature; Performance; Performing Groups
Technical Training: Piano; Voice; Woodwinds
Financial Assistance: Scholarships and Work-Study Grants
Performing Groups: Chamber Choir; Chamber Ensembles; Concert Band; Concert Choir; Jazz Ensemble;
Jazz Improvisation Group; Madrigal Singers; Wind Ensembles

THEATRE

Anthony Graham - White, Head   **Number Of Faculty:** 19
Number Of Students: 200   **Degrees Offered:** BA; MA

(continued on next page)

Courses Offered: Theatre; Communication; Mass Media
Technical Training: Acting; Directing; Set & Costume Design; Television
Teaching Certification Available
Financial Assistance: Assistantships and Talent Tuition Waiver

---

ILLINOIS STATE UNIVERSITY
Normal   Illinois 61761, 309 436-8321
State and 4 Year
Arts Areas: Dance, Instrumental Music, Vocal Music, Theatre, Film Arts, Television and Visual Arts
Performing Series: Fine Arts Festival
Performance Facilities: University Auditorium

DANCE

Dr Gwen K Smith, Program Director   **Number Of Faculty:** 5.5
Number Of Students: 65   **Degrees Offered:** BA; BS; BSEd
Courses Offered: Social; Folk; Square; Modern; Jazz; Tap; Ballet; Theory; History
Teaching Certification Available
Financial Assistance: Assistantships, Work-Study Grants and Tuition Waivers
Performing Groups: American Heritage Dancers; University Dance Theatre I & II

MUSIC

David L Shrader, Chairman   **Number Of Faculty:** 47   **Number Of Students:** 520
Degrees Offered: BA; BS; BMusEd; BMus   **Teaching Certification Available**
Financial Assistance: Assistantships, Work-Study Grants and Tuition Waivers
Performing Groups: Quartet; Quintet; Madrigal; Orchestra; Bands; Choirs
Workshops/Festivals: Fine Arts Festival

THEATRE

Calvin Lee Pritner, Chairman   **Number Of Faculty:** 22
Number Of Students: 242   **Degrees Offered:** BA; BS; MA; MS; MFA
Courses Offered: Acting; Directing; Scene & Costume Design; Playwriting
Teaching Certification Available
Financial Assistance: Assistantships, Work-Study Grants and Tuition Waivers
Performing Groups: Mainstage; Children's Theatre; Humanities Education Theatre Company;
Experimental
Workshops/Festivals: Fine Arts Festival

JOLIET JUNIOR COLLEGE
1216 Humbolt Ave, Joliet   Illinois 60436
815 729-9020
State and 2 Year
Arts Areas: Instrumental Music, Vocal Music and Theatre
Performance Facilities: Gymnasium; Recital Hall; Theatre

MUSIC

Jerry E Lewis, Chairman   **Number Of Faculty:** 5   **Number Of Students:** 75
Degrees Offered: AA
Courses Offered: Theory; Music Literature; Applied Piano, Brass, Woodwinds, Voice, Percussion;
Percussion Methods; Brass Methods; Woodwind Methods; Elementary Class Piano, Band, Choir, Jazz Band,
Music Fundamentals; Swing Choir; Brass Choir; Percussion Ensemble
Financial Assistance: Scholarships and Work-Study Grants
Performing Groups: Concert Choir; Swing Choir; Community Chorale; Concert Band; Jazz Band;
Community Orchestra; Brass Choir; Flute Quartet
Workshops/Festivals: Concert Band Clinic; Jazz Clinic   **Number Of Faculty:** 2

KASKASKIA COLLEGE
Shattuc Rd, Centralia   Illinois 62801
618 532-1981 Ext 188
State and 2 Year
Arts Areas: Instrumental Music, Vocal Music, Theatre and Visual Arts
Performance Facilities: College Auditorium

MUSIC

Don Schroeder, Director   *Number Of Faculty:* 7   *Number Of Students:* 75
Degrees Offered: AA Music
Financial Assistance: Scholarships and Work-Study Grants
Performing Groups: Band; Chorus; Jazz Band

THEATRE

D K Klein, Director   *Number Of Faculty:* 1   *Number Of Students:* 40

KENNEDY - KING COLLEGE
6800 S Wentworth Ave, Chicago   Illinois 60621
312 962-3300
City and 2 Year
Arts Areas: Instrumental Music, Vocal Music, Theatre, Television and Radio
Performance Facilities: The Theatre of the Drama Guild; The Playhouse

MUSIC

Otto Jelinek, Chairman   *Number Of Faculty:* 5   *Degrees Offered:* AA; AS
Financial Assistance: Work-Study Grants

THEATRE

Dr H Adrian Rehner, Chairman   *Number Of Faculty:* 17
Number Of Students: 1,300   *Degrees Offered:* AS; AA
Technical Training: Theatre Technology; Broadcasting Technology
Financial Assistance: Assistantships and Work-Study Grants
Performing Groups: The Drama Guild; The Professional Performing Equity Company of The Drama Guild
Workshops/Festivals: All City Chicago One - Act Play Festival; One Act Festival for the College

KISHWAUKEE COLLEGE
Malta   Illinois 60150, 815 825-2086
State and 2 Year
Arts Areas: Instrumental Music, Vocal Music, Theatre and Visual Arts
Performance Facilities: College Auditorium

MUSIC

Richard Kroeger, Instructor   *Number Of Faculty:* 2   *Number Of Students:* 80
Degrees Offered: AAS
Financial Assistance: Scholarships, Work-Study Grants and BEOG, SEOG, NOSL
Performing Groups: Chorale; Music Ensemble; Theatre Group

THEATRE

Dr Tyrone Turning, Chairman   *Number Of Faculty:* 2   *Number Of Students:* 64
Degrees Offered: AAS
Financial Assistance: Scholarships, Work-Study Grants and BEOG, SEOG, NOSL
Performing Groups: Kishwaukee College Community Theatre Group
Artists-In-Residence/Guest Artists: Richard Kroeger

KNOX COLLEGE
Galesburg   Illinois 61401, 309 343-0112
Private and 4 Year
Arts Areas: Instrumental Music, Vocal Music, Theatre and Visual Arts
Performing Series: Janet Greig Post Adventures in the Arts Series; Repertory Theatre ; Union Board Concerts
Performance Facilities: Eleanor Abbott Ford Center for the Fine Arts
Courses Offered: Offered on group-interest basis

MUSIC

Charles Farley; Robert W Murphy, Professors
Number Of Faculty: 4 Full-time, 12 Part-time   **Number Of Students:** 65
Degrees Offered: BA   **Teaching Certification Available**
Financial Assistance: Scholarships, Work-Study Grants and Loan Programs

THEATRE

Ivan H Davidson, Associate Professor   **Number Of Faculty:** 4
Number Of Students: 85   **Degrees Offered:** BA
Teaching Certification Available
Financial Assistance: Scholarships, Work-Study Grants and Loan Programs
Performing Groups: Knox Theatre; Second Stage and Repertory Theatre (every 3 years)

LAKE FOREST COLLEGE
College & Sheridan Rds, Lake Forest   Illinois 60045
312 234-3100
Private and 4 Year
Arts Areas: Instrumental Music, Vocal Music, Theatre, Film Arts, Visual Arts and Studio Arts
Performance Facilities: Hixon Hall Theater; Reid Chapel; Ravine Lodge

MUSIC

Ann D Bowen, Professor   **Number Of Faculty:** 5   **Number Of Students:** 30
Degrees Offered: BA Music
Financial Assistance: Internships, Scholarships and Work-Study Grants
Performing Groups: Various Choral Groups; Choir; Madrigal Singers

THEATRE

Russ Tutterow, Director   **Number Of Faculty:** 1   **Number Of Students:** 40
Degrees Offered: BA Art History
Courses Offered: Introduction to Theater; Art of Actor
Technical Training: Garrick Players Workshops
Financial Assistance: Internships, Scholarships and Work-Study Grants
Performing Groups: The Garrick Players
Workshops/Festivals: R A Festival of Spring; Various Pub Productions; Acting Workshops; Artist in Residence

LAKE LAND COLLEGE
US 45 South, Matoon   Illinois 61938
217 235-3131
County and 2 Year
Arts Areas: Instrumental Music, Vocal Music, Television and Visual Arts
Performing Series: Cultural Events Series
Performance Facilities: College Auditorium   **Number Of Faculty:** 2
Number Of Students: 30   **Degrees Offered:** AA
Performing Groups: Vocal & Instrumental Ensembles

LEWIS & CLARK COMMUNITY COLLEGE
Godfrey   Illinois 62035, 618 466-3411

County and 2 Year
Arts Areas: Instrumental Music, Vocal Music and Theatre
Performance Facilities: College Auditorium   *Degrees Offered:* AA Music
Performing Groups: Vocal & Instrumental Ensembles   *Degrees Offered:* AA Drama
Performing Groups: Drama Club

LEWIS UNIVERSITY
Route 53, Lockport   Illinois 60441
815 838-0500

Private and 4 Year
Arts Areas: Instrumental Music, Vocal Music, Theatre and Visual Arts
Performance Facilities: Ives Hall; Sancta Alberta Chapel; Philip Lynch Theatre

MUSIC

Daniel Binder, Chairman   *Number Of Faculty:* 8   *Number Of Students:* 562
Degrees Offered: BA
Courses Offered: Music Theory; History; Appreciation; Applied Voice; Applied Piano; Applied Guitar; Applied Woodwinds; Applied Strings; Applied Accordion; Applied Organ; Applied Percussion; Applied Brass
Teaching Certification Available   Financial Assistance: Scholarships and Work-Study Grants
Performing Groups: Chorale; Young Sounds; Concert Band; Madrigals; Stage Band

THEATRE

Chester Kondratowicz, Director   *Number Of Faculty:* 4
Number Of Students: 967   *Degrees Offered:* BA
Courses Offered: Theatre History; Drama   *Teaching Certification Available*
Financial Assistance: Scholarships and Work-Study Grants
Performing Groups: University Theatre; Children's Theatre
Workshops/Festivals: Annual Production

LINCOLN COLLEGE
300 Keokuk St, Lincoln   Illinois 62656
217 732-3155

Private and 2 Year
Arts Areas: Dance, Instrumental Music, Vocal Music, Theatre, Film Arts, Visual Arts and Broadcasting
Performing Series: Concert & Lecture Series
Performance Facilities: Johnston Center for Performing Arts houses Theatre and Hostic Studio Theatre

DANCE

Number Of Faculty: 1   *Number Of Students:* 30
Courses Offered: Introduction to Dance; Dance Performance; Private Lessons
Financial Assistance: Assistantships, Scholarships and Work-Study Grants
Performing Groups: Dance Performance Group

MUSIC

Number Of Faculty: 4   *Number Of Students:* 95   *Degrees Offered:* AA
Courses Offered: Theory; History & Literature; Piano & Voice Class; Vocal & Instrumental Ensembles; Private Lessons
Financial Assistance: Assistantships, Scholarships and Work-Study Grants
Performing Groups: Lincoln Symphony; Lincoln College Chorale; Chamber Singers; Jazz Ensemble

THEATRE

Number Of Faculty: 3   *Number Of Students:* 75   *Degrees Offered:* AA
Courses Offered: Acting; Stagecraft; Introduction to Theatre
Financial Assistance: Scholarships and Work-Study Grants   *Performing Groups:* University Theatre
Artists-In-Residence/Guest Artists: Margaret Beals; Parker Drew

LINCOLN LAND COMMUNITY COLLEGE
Shepherd Rd, Springfield   Illinois 62708
217 786-2320
County and 2 Year
Arts Areas: Instrumental Music, Vocal Music, Theatre, Film Arts and Visual Arts
Performance Facilities: Logan Hall Auditorium; Menard Hall Art Gallery; Recital Rooms; Student Union

MUSIC

Number Of Faculty: 3   *Number Of Students:* 100   *Degrees Offered:* AA
Courses Offered: Band; Jazz Band; Choir; Orchestra; Theory; Music Education; Class Piano; Class Guitar; Music History; Music Fundamentals; Music Appreciation
Financial Assistance: Work-Study Grants   *Performing Groups:* Choir; Jazz Band; Band; Orchestra
Workshops/Festivals: Jazz Band Clinic; Brass Clinic; Flute Clinic

THEATRE

Number Of Faculty: 1   *Number Of Students:* 20   *Degrees Offered:* AA
Courses Offered: Acting; Introduction to Theatre; Stagecraft; Modern Theatre; Oral Interpretation
Financial Assistance: Work-Study Grants   *Performing Groups:* Student Players
Workshops/Festivals: Arts and the Aging

LINCOLN TRAIL COLLEGE
RR 1, Robinson   Illinois 62454
618 544-8657
County and 2 Year
Arts Areas: Dance, Instrumental Music, Vocal Music and Theatre
Performance Facilities: Zwermann Arts Center

DANCE

Number Of Faculty: 1   *Number Of Students:* 15   *Courses Offered:* Jazz; Tap; Modern

MUSIC

Herbert Kuebler, Chairman, Fine Arts Department   *Number Of Faculty:* 10
Number Of Students: 220   *Degrees Offered:* AA; AS
Courses Offered: Music Appreciation; Conducting; Music History; Sight Singing & Entertaining; Piano Pedagogy; Jazz Band & Choir; Theory; Concert Choir; Music Fundamentals
Financial Assistance: Scholarships and Work-Study Grants
Performing Groups: Concert Choir; Madrigal Singers; Jazz Band & Choir
Workshops/Festivals: Choral Workshop

THEATRE

Phil Evans, Chairman   *Number Of Faculty:* 1   *Number Of Students:* 30
Courses Offered: Acting; Theatre History; Lighting; Stagecraft; Stage Make-up
Financial Assistance: Scholarships and Work-Study Grants
Performing Groups: Lincoln Trail College Theatre Department
Workshops/Festivals: Opera Workshop; Children's Theatre; Musical Theatre Workshop

LOOP COLLEGE
64 E Lake St, Chicago   Illinois 60601
312 236-8100
State and 2 Year
Arts Areas: Dance, Instrumental Music, Vocal Music, Theatre, Film Arts, Television and Visual Arts
Performance Facilities: Loop College Theatre

MUSIC

James Mack, Chairman   *Number Of Faculty:* 7   *Number Of Students:* 500
Degrees Offered: AA   *Financial Assistance:* Assistantships and Work-Study Grants

THEATRE

Sydney R Daniels, Chairman   *Number Of Faculty:* 4   *Number Of Students:* 300

(continued on next page)

Degrees Offered: AA   **Technical Training:** Technical Theatre
Financial Assistance: Assistantships and Work-Study Grants
Workshops/Festivals: Workshop Productions

LOYOLA UNIVERSITY OF CHICAGO
820 N Michigan Ave, Chicago   Illinois 60611
312 670-2900

Private and 4 Year   **Arts Areas:** Theatre, Television and Visual Arts
Performing Series: Theatre Season Subscription Series
Performance Facilities: Kathleen Mullady Memorial Theatre

THEATRE

Dr Arthur Bloom, Chairman   **Number Of Faculty:** 7 Full-time, 12 Part-time
Number Of Students: 77   **Degrees Offered:** AB Theatre
Financial Assistance: Scholarships, Work-Study Grants and University & Stage Grants
Performing Groups: Loyola University Mime Company
Workshops/Festivals: Studio Theatre; Student Directed Workshop Productions

---

MACMURRAY COLLEGE
Jacksonville   Illinois 62650, 217 245-6151

Private and 4 Year
Arts Areas: Instrumental Music, Vocal Music, Theatre and Visual Arts
Performing Series: Jacksonville - Mac Murray Music Association; Guest Lecturer Series
Performance Facilities: Annie Merner Chapel; Orr Auditorium; College Theatre; College Art Gallery

MUSIC

Dr Jay Peterson, Assistant Professor   **Number Of Faculty:** 5
Number Of Students: 60   **Degrees Offered:** BMus; BA
Courses Offered: Applied Music; Music Education
Teaching Certification Available
Financial Assistance: Scholarships and Work-Study Grants
Performing Groups: Concert Band; Stage Band; Concert Choir; Madrigal Singers; Various Instrumental Ensembles
Workshops/Festivals: Opera Workshop; High School Band Festival

THEATRE

Dr Philip Decker, Professor of Theatre Arts   **Number Of Faculty:** 3
Number Of Students: 50   **Degrees Offered:** BA
Courses Offered: Speech; Theatre   **Teaching Certification Available**
Financial Assistance: Scholarships and Work-Study Grants
Performing Groups: MacMurray College Players
Artists-In-Residence/Guest Artists: New DeCormier Singers; John Walker; American Chamber Trio; Trio Flamenco; Wilma Jensen

---

MCKENDREE COLLEGE
Lebanon   Illinois 62254, 618 537-4481

Private and 4 Year
Arts Areas: Instrumental Music, Vocal Music, Theatre and Visual Arts
Performing Series: McKendree College Fine Arts Division Series
Number Of Faculty: 3   **Degrees Offered:** BA; BMusEd
Teaching Certification Available
Financial Assistance: Internships, Scholarships and Work-Study Grants
Performing Groups: Various Ensembles; Band; Chorus
Workshops/Festivals: Spring Concert; Christmas Choral; Travelling Groups

MILLIKIN UNIVERSITY
1184 W Main St, Decatur   Illinois 62522
217 424-6211
Private and 4 Year
Arts Areas: Dance, Instrumental Music, Vocal Music, Theatre and Visual Arts
Performing Series: University Concert Series
Performance Facilities: Kirkland Fine Arts Center; Albert Taylor Hall; Kaeuper Hall

DANCE

Number Of Faculty: 2   *Courses Offered:* Ballet & Modern Dance; Eurythmics
Financial Assistance: Scholarships and Work-Study Grants

MUSIC

Dr Clayton W Henderson, Dean   *Number Of Faculty:* 34
Number Of Students: 150
Degrees Offered: BMusEd, Applied Music & Church Music; BA Mus
Courses Offered: Music Education & Church Music; Music History & Literature; Music Theory
Teaching Certification Available
Financial Assistance: Internships, Assistantships, Scholarships and Work-Study Grants
Performing Groups: Choruses; Bands; Jazz Lab Bands; Symphony Orchestra; Instrumental Ensembles
Workshops/Festivals: Paul Christianson Choral Workshop

THEATRE

Dr Arthur Hopper, Chairman   *Number Of Faculty:* 3   *Number Of Students:* 25
Degrees Offered: BA; BFA
Courses Offered: Stagecraft; Acting; Directing; Lighting; Costume; Makeup; Scene Design; Theatre History
Financial Assistance: Internships, Assistantships, Scholarships and Work-Study Grants
Performing Groups: Showcase Theatre; Experimental Theatre
Workshops/Festivals: Summer Showcase Theatre

MONMOUTH COLLEGE
700 E Broadway, Monmouth   Illinois 61462
309 457-2311
Private and 4 Year
Arts Areas: Instrumental Music, Vocal Music, Theatre, Film Arts and Television
Performance Facilities: Monmouth College Little Theatre; Monmouth College Auditorium

MUSIC

Michael Sproston, Chairman   *Number Of Faculty:* 4   *Number Of Students:* 50
Degrees Offered: BA; AA
Courses Offered: Private Performance; Techniques; Theory; Education; Conducting
Teaching Certification Available
Financial Assistance: Assistantships, Scholarships and Work-Study Grants
Performing Groups: Wind Ensemble; Jazz Band; Concert Choir; Chamber Singers; 'Sound of Five' Pop Group
Workshops/Festivals: Workshops for High School Students; Jazz Festival

THEATRE

Dr James De Young, Chairman   *Number Of Faculty:* 3   *Number Of Students:* 70
Degrees Offered: BA
Courses Offered: Speech-Communications Tract; Broadcasting Tract; Performing Arts Tract
Technical Training: Radio; Television; Set Design
Teaching Certification Available
Financial Assistance: Assistantships, Scholarships and Work-Study Grants
Performing Groups: Crimson Masque; Readers' Theatre Touring Group; Summer Resident Theatre Group
Workshops/Festivals: Summer Dinner Theatre; Organization Communication Workshop; 'Trust' Workshop

MOODY BIBLE INSTITUTE
820 N LaSalle St, Chicago   Illinois 60610
312 329-4000

Private and 4 Year   *Arts Areas:* Instrumental Music and Vocal Music

MUSIC

Wilfred L Burton, Sacred Music Director   *Degrees Offered:* BA Sacred Music
Financial Assistance: Scholarships   *Performing Groups:* Choir

MORTON COLLEGE
2500 S Austin Blvd, Cicero   Illinois 60650
312 656-2610

County and 2 Year
Arts Areas: Instrumental Music, Vocal Music and Theatre
Performing Series: Cultural Events Series *Performance Facilities:* College Auditorium

MUSIC

Degrees Offered: AA Music
Financial Assistance: Scholarships and Work-Study Grants
Performing Groups: Vocal & Instrumental Ensembles

THEATRE

Charlotte C Pillap, Chairman   *Number Of Faculty:* 6
Number Of Students: 90   *Degrees Offered:* AA
Performing Groups: Theatre Guild

MUNDELEIN COLLEGE
6363 Sheridan Rd, Chicago   Illinois 60660
312 262-8100

Private and 4 Year
Arts Areas: Dance, Instrumental Music, Vocal Music, Theatre and Film Arts
Performance Facilities: College Auditorium; Little Theatre; Galvin Hall

DANCE

Kathy Burg, Instructor
Dance program under auspices of Physical Education Department
Financial Assistance: Scholarships and Work-Study Grants
Performing Groups: Orchesis

MUSIC

Sister Eliza Kenney, Chairperson   *Number Of Faculty:* 7
Number Of Students: 45   *Degrees Offered:* BA
Courses Offered: Voice; Piano/Organ; Instrumental
Teaching Certification Available
Financial Assistance: Scholarships and Work-Study Grants
Performing Groups: MC's Chorus
Workshops/Festivals: Christmas & Spring Concerts

THEATRE

Sister Jeanelle Bergen, BVM, Associate Professor   *Number Of Faculty:* 3
Number Of Students: 28   *Degrees Offered:* BA
Financial Assistance: Scholarships and Work-Study Grants
Performing Groups: Individual Performances; Small Theatre Groups
Workshops/Festivals: One Acts - Student - produced & directed

NATIONAL COLLEGE OF EDUCATION
2840 Sheridan Rd, Evanston   Illinois 60201
312 256-5150

Private and 4 Year
Arts Areas: Dance, Instrumental Music, Vocal Music, Theatre, Television and Visual Arts
Performance Facilities: Weinstein Center for Performing Arts

DANCE

Sybil Shearer, Chairman   *Number Of Faculty:* 1

MUSIC

Lloyd Cousins, Chairman   *Number Of Faculty:* 3   *Number Of Students:* 25
Degrees Offered: BA; ME; MS; MAT   *Teaching Certification Available*
Financial Assistance: Scholarships and Work-Study Grants
Performing Groups: Chamber Orchestra; Choir

THEATRE

Richard Bagg, Chairman   *Number Of Faculty:* 3   *Number Of Students:* 25
Degrees Offered: BA; BMusEd; MS; MA   *Teaching Certification Available*
Financial Assistance: Scholarships and Work-Study Grants
Performing Groups: Children's Theatre; College Drama Group

NORTH CENTRAL COLLEGE
30 N Brainard St, Naperville   Illinois 60540
312 355-5500

Private and 4 Year
Arts Areas: Instrumental Music, Vocal Music, Theatre and Visual Arts
Performing Series: Special Events Series
Performance Facilities: Pfeiffer Hall

MUSIC

Dr Ann McKinley, Chairman   *Number Of Faculty:* 6   *Number Of Students:* 78
Degrees Offered: BMus; MBusEd   *Teaching Certification Available*
Financial Assistance: Scholarships and Work-Study Grants
Performing Groups: College Orchestra; Chamber Orchestra; Choir; Ensemble;
Workshops/Festivals: College sponsored trips to musical events

THEATRE

Donald Shanower, Chairman   *Number Of Faculty:* 4   *Number Of Students:* 52
Degrees Offered: Drama & Speech
Financial Assistance: Scholarships and Work-Study Grants
Performing Groups: Theatre Guild

NORTH PARK COLLEGE
5125 N Spaulding, Chicago   Illinois 60625
312 583-2700 Ext 228

Private, 4 Year and Seminary
Arts Areas: Instrumental Music, Vocal Music, Theatre and Visual Arts
Performing Series: Public Events Series (varied performances, 4 yearly); Film Series
Performance Facilities: Lecture Hall - Auditorium; Old Chapel; Hanson Recital Hall; Isaacson Chapel

MUSIC

Monroe B Olson, Chairman, Fine Arts Division   *Number Of Faculty:* 8
Number Of Students: 56
Degrees Offered: BA, BMusEd, BMus, BA in Music Management; BM in Church Music
Courses Offered: Theory; History; Conducting; Education; Applied; Ensemble; Composition; Church Music
Teaching Certification Available

(continued on next page)

(North Park College — cont'd)

Financial Assistance: Scholarships, Work-Study Grants and Performance Awards
Performing Groups: College Choir; College Wind Ensemble; College Chorus; Chamber Singers; Chamber Orchestra; Jazz Lab Band; Opera Workshop

THEATRE

Mickey Benson, Chairman   **Number Of Faculty:** 2   **Number Of Students:** 35
Degrees Offered: BA
Courses Offered: Acting; Oral Interpretation; Play Production; Radio & TV; Film; Independent Study for Emphasis; Directing
Teaching Certification Available
Financial Assistance: Scholarships, Work-Study Grants and Performance Awards

---

NORTHEASTERN ILLINOIS UNIVERSITY
5500 N St Louis Ave, Chicago   Illinois 60625
312 583-4050
Arts Areas: Instrumental Music, Vocal Music and Visual Arts
Performing Series: Concert Artist Series

MUSIC

Harold Berlinger, Professor   **Number Of Faculty:** 16
Number Of Students: 225
Degrees Offered: BA (All performance areas; Music Ed, Theory, History & Literature; Piano Pedagogy)
Courses Offered: Full Range of Music Curricula
Technical Training: Performance; Opera Workshop; Chorus; Jazz Band
Teaching Certification Available
Financial Assistance: Scholarships and Work-Study Grants
Performing Groups: Band; Chorus; Concert Choir; Collegium Musicum; Opera Workshop; Orchestra; Wind Band; Jazz Band; New Music; Other Instrumental Ensembles
Workshops/Festivals: Music Education & Performance Workshops

THEATRE

James W Barushok, Chairman   **Number Of Faculty:** 12
Number Of Students: 230   **Degrees Offered:** BA; MA
Courses Offered: Complete Theatre Training Program in all Theatre Arts & Crafts
Technical Training: Co - Curricular Dramatic Production
Teaching Certification Available
Financial Assistance: Scholarships and Work-Study Grants
Performing Groups: Interpretors Theatre; Stage Players
Workshops/Festivals: American College Theatre Festival (Region VIII)

NORTHERN ILLINOIS UNIVERSITY
DeKalb   Illinois 60115, 815 753-1635
State, 4 Year and Graduate work through the doctorate
Arts Areas: Dance, Instrumental Music, Vocal Music, Theatre and Visual Arts
Performing Series: NIU Artist Series
Performance Facilities: Matteo - American Ethnic Dance Theatre; Erick Hawkins Dance Company; Jean - Pierre Rampal

DANCE

Dance program under auspices of Theatre Department   **Number Of Faculty:** 2
Courses Offered: Ballet; Modern Dance; Ethnic; Choreography
Financial Assistance: Scholarships and Work-Study Grants
Performing Groups: Northern Illinois Dance Repertoire Company

MUSIC

Paul O Steg, Acting Chairman   **Number Of Faculty:** 51
Number Of Students: 350   **Degrees Offered:** BA; BMus; MA; MFA; MMus
Teaching Certification Available

(continued on next page)

Financial Assistance: Assistantships, Scholarships and Work-Study Grants
Performing Groups: Jazz Ensemble; University Symphony Orchestra; Concert Choir; Chorus; University Band; Vocal Ensembles; Opera Theatre Workshop

THEATRE

Richard Arnold, Chairman   **Number Of Faculty:** 12   **Number Of Students:** 200
Degrees Offered: BA; MA   **Teaching Certification Available**
Financial Assistance: Assistantships, Scholarships and Work-Study Grants
Performing Groups: Children's Theatre; University Theatre; Players Theatre; Theatre on Wheels

NORTHWESTERN UNIVERSITY
633 Clark St, Evanston   Illinois 60201
312 492-3741

Private and 4 Year
Arts Areas: Dance, Instrumental Music, Vocal Music, Theatre, Film Arts and Visual Arts
Performance Facilities: Cahn Auditorium; Laboratory Theatre; Norrif University Center

DANCE

Delta Bamister, Chairman of Physical Education Department
Number Of Faculty: 3   **Number Of Students:** 400   **Degrees Offered:** BEd; MEd
Technical Training: Modern; Ballet; Movement for Theatre; Conducting; Yoga; Musical Comedy
Performing Groups: Concert Group; Modern Dance
Workshops/Festivals: Orgy of the Arts

MUSIC

S W Miller, Dean   **Number Of Faculty:** 4   **Number Of Students:** 514
Degrees Offered: BMus; BMusEd;MMus; DMA; PhD
Technical Training: Areas of Concentration; Applied Music; Music Ed; Theory; Composition; Music, History & Literature; Church Music & Conducting; Comprehensive Performance Opportunities are offered in complete range of Performing Organizations
Teaching Certification Available
Financial Assistance: Assistantships, Scholarships and Work-Study Grants
Performing Groups: University Symphony Orchestra; Repertory Orchestra; Marching Band; Concert Band; University Wind Ensemble; Symphonic Band; Jazz Ensemble; Concert Choir; Mixed Chorus; University Chorus; Chamber Singers
Workshops/Festivals: Opera Workshop; Summer Workshops

THEATRE

Dr Leslie Hindericks, Chairman   **Number Of Faculty:** 24
Number Of Students: 350
Degrees Offered: BS; BFA; BA; MA; MFA; M Theatre; PhD
Technical Training: Mimes; Scene Design   **Teaching Certification Available**
Financial Assistance: Scholarships and Work-Study Grants
Performing Groups: Northwestern Mime Company; University Theatre; Children's Theatre; Creative Dramatics
Workshops/Festivals: Acting & Directing Workshop; Summer Drama Festival; Outdoor Theatre

OLIVET NAZARENE COLLEGE
Box 592, Kankakee   Illinois 60901
815 939-5011

Private and 4 Year
Arts Areas: Instrumental Music, Vocal Music, Television, Visual Arts and Dramatics
Performing Series: Culture Series; Choral & Instrumental Groups - Campus & Tour Concerts
Performance Facilities: Chalfant Hall; Wisner Hall; Reed Lecture Hall

MUSIC

Dr Harlow Hopkins, Chairman   **Number Of Faculty:** 13
Number Of Students: 200

(continued on next page)

Degrees Offered: BA or BS MusEd; BA Music Performance; BA or BS Church and Choral Music
Courses Offered: Organ, Piano, Strings, Woodwinds, Brass, Music Theory; Church Music, Music Education, Music Literature & History
Teaching Certification Available
Financial Assistance: Assistantships, Scholarships, Work-Study Grants and Basic Grant, Illinois Monetary Award
Performing Groups: Orpheus Choir, Viking Male Chorus, Treble Clef Choir, Brass Choir, Concert Singers; Choral Union, Handbell Choir
Workshops/Festivals: Summer Music Workshop for Teens; Summer Music Symposium

THEATRE

Dr David Kale, Chairman **Number Of Faculty:** 2 **Number Of Students:** 40
Teaching Certification Available
Financial Assistance: Assistantships, Scholarships, Work-Study Grants and Basic Grant, Illinois Monetary Award
Performing Groups: Drama Club

PRINCIPIA COLLEGE
Elsah Illinois 62028, 618 966-2131
Private and 4 Year
Arts Areas: Instrumental Music, Vocal Music, Theatre and Visual Arts

MUSIC

Reinhart S Ross, Chairman **Number Of Faculty:** 3 **Number Of Students:** 39
Degrees Offered: BA **Teaching Certification Available**
Financial Assistance: Scholarships and Work-Study Grants
Performing Groups: College Choir; Instrumental Groups

THEATRE

Donald Mainwarling, Chairman **Number Of Faculty:** 4
Number Of Students: 52 **Degrees Offered:** BA
Teaching Certification Available
Financial Assistance: Scholarships and Work-Study Grants
Performing Groups: College Players

QUINCY COLLEGE
1831 College Ave, Quincy Illinois 62301
217 222-8020
Private and 4 Year
Arts Areas: Instrumental Music, Vocal Music and Theatre
Performance Facilities: McHugh Theater; Solano Hall

MUSIC

Lavern Wagner, PhD, Chairman **Number Of Faculty:** 5
Number Of Students: 25 - 30 **Degrees Offered:** BS in Mus Business; BS in MusEd
Technical Training: Music Ed **Teaching Certification Available**
Financial Assistance: Scholarships and Work-Study Grants
Performing Groups: Wind Ensemble; Chorus; Jazz Band; Chamber Choir; Swing Choir; Brass Ensemble; Collegium Musicum

THEATRE

Hugh Fitzgerald, Chairman **Number Of Faculty:** 2
Courses Offered: MS; BA; BFA **Teaching Certification Available**
Financial Assistance: Scholarships and Work-Study Grants
Performing Groups: College Theater

REND LAKE COLLEGE
RR 1, Ina   Illinois 62846
618 437-5321 Ext 63
State and 2 Year
Arts Areas: Instrumental Music, Vocal Music, Theatre and Visual Arts
Performance Facilities: College Theatre   *Number Of Faculty:* 3
Number Of Students: 30   *Degrees Offered:* AA
Courses Offered: Full two year transfer curriculum
Financial Assistance: Work-Study Grants
Performing Groups: Concert Band; Jazz Band; Orchestra; Concert Choir; Community Chorus; Show Choir
Number Of Faculty: 1   *Number Of Students:* 10   *Degrees Offered:* AA
Courses Offered: Basic Introductory Theatre Courses
Financial Assistance: Work-Study Grants
Performing Groups: Rend Lake Theatre; Little Egypt Regional Theatre (community theatre group based at RLC)

ROCK VALLEY COLLEGE
3301 N Mulford Rd, Rockford   Illinois 61111
815 226-2600
County and 2 Year   *Arts Areas:* Instrumental Music and Vocal Music
Performance Facilities: College Auditorium   *Degrees Offered:* AA Music

ROCKFORD COLLEGE
5050 E State St, Rockford   Illinois 61101
815 226-4000
Private and 4 Year
Arts Areas: Dance, Instrumental Music, Vocal Music and Theatre
Performing Series: Association of Illinois Dance Company - Spring Festival; Performing Arts Series
Performance Facilities: Maddox Theatre; Cheek Theatre; Music/Dance Rehearsal Hall; Severson Auditorium

DANCE

Jayne Poor, Chairman   *Number Of Faculty:* 2   *Number Of Students:* 40
Degrees Offered: BA in Dance; BFA in Performing Arts, Dance Emphasis
Courses Offered: Modern Dance; Modern Dance Emphasis; Dance History; Ballet; Technique
Technical Training: Production Training in Theatre Department; Ballet & Technique
Teaching Certification Available   *Financial Assistance:* Scholarships
Performing Groups: Orchesis
Workshops/Festivals: Rockford Dance Company; Artist-in-Residence (Eugene Tanner, Lyric Opera Ballet); Trip to New York City to study dance

MUSIC

Walter Whipple, Assistant Professor, Chairman   *Number Of Faculty:* 5
Number Of Students: 90
Degrees Offered: BFA in Performing Arts, Music Emphasis
Courses Offered: Music Theory; Vocal; Piano; Organ; Harmony; Music History; Some Instrumental
Technical Training: Production Training in Theatre Department; Individual Lessons (Vocal & Instrumental)
Teaching Certification Available   *Financial Assistance:* Scholarships
Performing Groups: Rockford College Chorus; Rockford College Regent Singers

THEATRE

Neil Thackaberry, Assistant Professor, Chairman   *Number Of Faculty:* 3
Number Of Students: 40
Degrees Offered: BA in Theatre Arts; BFA in Performing Arts, Theatre Arts Emphasis
Courses Offered: Scene Design; Light Design; Technical Theatre; Acting; Directing; Theatre History

(continued on next page)

Technical Training: Scene & Light Design; Technical Theatre; Acting; Directing
Teaching Certification Available   Performing Groups: University Theatre
Artists-In-Residence/Guest Artists: Eric Christmas

ROOSEVELT UNIVERSITY
430 S Michigan Ave, Chicago   Illinois 60605
312 341-3500

Private and 4 Year   **Arts Areas:** Instrumental Music and Vocal Music

MUSIC

Felix Ganz, Dean, Chicago Musical College   **Number Of Faculty:** 61
Number Of Students: 925
Degrees Offered: BM Performance, Music History, Music Theory, Composition (Electronic & Traditional), Music Education; MM Performance, Musicology, Theory, Composition, Music Education, Choral Conducting; BA with concentration in Music (Applied, Theory, Music Literature); B, General Studies with concentration in Music (Applied, Theory, Music Literature)
Financial Assistance: Assistantships, Scholarships and Work-Study Grants
Performing Groups: Faculty Baroque Ensemble; Faculty Chamber Groups; Sixteen Student Ensembles (from Guitar Ensemble to Two-Piano to Jazz Lab Band)
Workshops/Festivals: Master Classes; Instrument Clinics; Music Education Workshops

THEATRE

Yolanda Lyon, Director   **Number Of Faculty:** 3 - 4   **Number Of Students:** 125
Degrees Offered: BA
Courses Offered: Acting; Directing; Speech & Body Movement
Technical Training: Stagecraft; Design   **Teaching Certification Available**
Financial Assistance: Assistantships, Scholarships and Work-Study Grants
Performing Groups: University Theatre; Workshops
Workshops/Festivals: Special Workshop/Short Courses taught by Professionals in Theatre; Guest Artist Workshops

ROSARY COLLEGE
7900 W Division, River Forest   Illinois 60305
312 369-6320

Private and 4 Year
Arts Areas: Instrumental Music, Vocal Music, Theatre and Visual Arts

MUSIC

Harold McGhee, Chairman   **Number Of Faculty:** 6   **Number Of Students:** 114
Degrees Offered: BMus; MMus   **Technical Training:** Opera
Financial Assistance: Scholarships and Work-Study Grants   **Teaching Certification Available**
Performing Groups: Glee Club; Concert Choir; Band; Chamber Ensemble
Workshops/Festivals: Opera Workshop; Arts Festival

THEATRE

Number Of Faculty: 2   **Number Of Students:** 25   **Degrees Offered:** BA Speech & Theatre
Financial Assistance: Scholarships and Work-Study Grants
Performing Groups: Rosary Hill College Players   **Workshops/Festivals:** Arts Series

SAINT XAVIER COLLEGE
3700 W 103rd St, Chicago   Illinois 60655
312 779-3300

Private and 4 Year   **Arts Areas:** Dance and Film Arts

MUSIC

Gregory Schmit, Assistant Professor
Number Of Faculty: 4 Full-time, 10 Part-time   **Number Of Students:** 20
Degrees Offered: BA in Music Literature & Performance; BA in Education

(*continued on next page*)

Courses Offered: Traditional & Inprovisatory
Technical Training: Applied Lessons in most areas
Teaching Certification Available
Financial Assistance: Scholarships and Work-Study Grants
Performing Groups: Concert Choir; Madrigal Singers; Opera Workshop; Jazz Band; Community Band

SANGAMON STATE UNIVERSITY
Shephard Rd, Springfield   Illinois 62708
217 786-6600
   State and Upper Division
   Arts Areas: Dance, Instrumental Music, Vocal Music, Theatre, Film Arts and Visual Arts
   Performing Series: University Events Series
   Performance Facilities: Brookens Auditorium; SSU Gallery; Capital Campus Ballroom (Theater)

DANCE

J Katz, Director   *Number Of Faculty:* 2   *Number Of Students:* 24
Degrees Offered: MA Community Arts Management
Financial Assistance: Internships, Assistantships, Scholarships, Work-Study Grants and National Direct
Student Loan & Tuition Waivers

MUSIC

Mark Siebert, Chairman   *Number Of Faculty:* 2   *Number Of Students:* 32
Degrees Offered: BA Creative Arts   *Technical Training:* Opera
Teaching Certification Available
Financial Assistance: Scholarships and Work-Study Grants
Performing Groups: Wind, String & Percussion Ensembles; Jazz - Rock Ensemble; Vocal Ensemble

THEATRE

Guy Romans, Director   *Number Of Faculty:* 1   *Number Of Students:* 32
Degrees Offered: BA Creative Arts   *Teaching Certification Available*
Financial Assistance: Scholarships and Work-Study Grants
Workshops/Festivals: University Theatre

SHERWOOD MUSIC SCHOOL
1014 S Michigan Ave, Chicago   Illinois 60605
312 427-6267
   Private and Special   *Arts Areas:* Instrumental Music and Vocal Music
   Performance Facilities: School Auditorium

MUSIC

Arthur Wildman, Music Director   *Number Of Faculty:* 29
Number Of Students: 300   *Degrees Offered:* BMus; BMusEd
Technical Training: Piano; Organ; Voice; Violin; Viola; Cello; Wind Instruments
Financial Assistance: Scholarships
Performing Groups: Orchestra; Chorus; Wind Ensembles
Workshops/Festivals: Summer Workshop for Keyboard Teachers

SOUTHERN ILLINOIS UNIVERSITY
Carbondale   Illinois 62901, 618 453-2121
   State and 4 Year
   Arts Areas: Instrumental Music, Vocal Music, Theatre and Visual Arts

MUSIC

Robert House, Chairman   *Number Of Faculty:* 25   *Number Of Students:* 215
Degrees Offered: BMus; BMusEd; B Applied Music; MMus; MMusEd
Teaching Certification Available
Financial Assistance: Scholarships and Work-Study Grants
Performing Groups: Marjorie Lawrence Opera Theatre; Band; Chamber Orchestra
Workshops/Festivals: Summer Opera Workshop; Mississippi River Festival; Music Theatre Workshop

(continued on next page)

THEATRE

Archibald McLeod, Chairman   **Number Of Faculty:** 10
Number Of Students: 110
Degrees Offered: B Speech & Theatre; M Theatre & Speech; D Theatre & Speech
Teaching Certification Available
Financial Assistance: Scholarships and Work-Study Grants
Performing Groups: Southern Players

SOUTHERN ILLINOIS UNIVERSITY AT EDWARDSVILLE
Edwardsville   Illinois 62026, 618 692-2771
State, 4 Year and Graduate
Arts Areas: Dance, Instrumental Music, Vocal Music, Theatre, Television and Visual Arts
Performance Facilities: Communications Building Theater; Lovejoy Auditorium; Festival Site; Quonset Theater

MUSIC

Dr William Tarwater, Chairman   **Number Of Faculty:** 25
Number Of Students: 1,691
Degrees Offered: BMusEd, Mu Performance, Mu Theory/Composition; BA; MMusEd, Mu Performance
Courses Offered: Full major - minor programs for various degrees
Teaching Certification Available
Financial Assistance: Assistantships, Scholarships and Work-Study Grants
Performing Groups: Symphonic Band; University Band; Young Artists, Lincoln String Quartet; University Symphony Orchestra; Collequium Musicum; Community Choral Society; University Chorus; Concert Chorale; Opera Workshop
Workshops/Festivals: Mississippi River Festival Institute; Dance Workshops; Theatre Workshops

THEATRE

Dr William Vilhauer, Chairman   **Number Of Faculty:** 8
Number Of Students: 662   **Degrees Offered:** BA; BS; MA
Courses Offered: Full major - minor with Performance Emphasis; Design/Technical Emphasis; Dance Emphasis
Teaching Certification Available
Financial Assistance: Assistantships, Scholarships and Work-Study Grants
Performing Groups: University Theater; Quonset Theater; Children's Theater
Workshops/Festivals: Mississippi River Festival Institute; Theater Workshops

---

SPRINGFIELD COLLEGE, ILLINOIS
1500 N 5th St, Springfield   Illinois 62702
217 525-1420
Private and 2 Year
Arts Areas: Instrumental Music, Vocal Music and Theatre
Performance Facilities: Music Hall of Springfield College, Illinois

MUSIC

Sister M Annunciate Horan, Chairman   **Number Of Faculty:** 5
Number Of Students: 40   **Degrees Offered:** A
Financial Assistance: Scholarships and Work-Study Grants
Performing Groups: Madrigals; Choir; Jazz Lab Band; Concert Band
Workshops/Festivals: Opera Workshop; Music Workshop

THORNTON COMMUNITY COLLEGE
15800 S State St, South Holland   Illinois 60473
312 596-2000 Ext 296
State and 2 Year
Arts Areas: Instrumental Music, Vocal Music and Theatre
Performance Facilities: Performing Arts Center

(continued on next page)

MUSIC

Fred L Hanzelin, Director   **Number Of Faculty:** 20   **Number Of Students:** 300
Degrees Offered: AA   **Courses Offered:** Applied; Theory; History; Band; Choir
Financial Assistance: Scholarships and Work-Study Grants
Performing Groups: Symphonic Band; Jazz Band; Concert Choir; Thornton Evening Chorale; Thornton College Singers
Workshops/Festivals: Spring Fine Arts Festival; Madrigal Dinner Conference (national)

THEATRE

Courses Offered: Introduction to Theatre I & II; Theatre Production I & II
Performing Groups: Young People's Theatre; Drama Society; Community Theatre

---

TRINITY CHRISTIAN COLLEGE
6601 W College Dr, Palos Heights   Illinois 60463
312 597-3000

Private and 4 Year
Arts Areas: Instrumental Music, Vocal Music and Visual Arts
Performing Series: Cultural Events Series; Madrigal Dinners
Performance Facilities: College Auditorium

MUSIC

Dr Gerald Hoekstra, Assistant Professor   **Number Of Faculty:** 4
Degrees Offered: BA Mus; BA MusEd; BA Applied Music
Technical Training: Opera   **Teaching Certification Available**
Financial Assistance: Scholarships and Work-Study Grants
Performing Groups: Choir; Chamber Ensemble; Early Music Ensembles
Workshops/Festivals: Organ Workshop; Fine Arts Festival

THEATRE

Number Of Faculty: 1   **Courses Offered:** The Actor's Theatre (Drama for Classroom Use)

TRINITY COLLEGE
2045 Half Day Rd, Deerfield   Illinois 60015
312 945-6700

Private and 4 Year   **Performing Series:** 2,3

MUSIC

Dr E Morris Faugerstrom, Chairman
Number Of Faculty: 5 Full-time, 5 Part-time   **Number Of Students:** 76
Degrees Offered: BA Mus
Courses Offered: Specilizations in: Applied Music, Music Theory, Church Music, Music/Secondary Education
Teaching Certification Available   **Financial Assistance:** Scholarships and Work-Study Grants
Performing Groups: Brass Ensemble; Concert Choir; Women's Chorale; Orchestra; Vocal/Instrumental Groups; Concert Band

---

TRITON COLLEGE
2000 Fifth Ave, River Grove   Illinois 60171
312 456-0300 Ext 291

State and 2 Year
Arts Areas: Instrumental Music, Vocal Music, Theatre and Visual Arts
Performance Facilities: Little Theatre; Auditorium

MUSIC

Music program under auspices of Fine Arts Department   **Number Of Faculty:** 5
Number Of Students: 200   **Degrees Offered:** AA
Performing Groups: Jazz Band; Concert Bands; College Choir; Chorale Ensemble

(continued on next page)

THEATRE

Number Of Faculty: 4   **Number Of Students:** 50   **Degrees Offered:** AA

UNIVERSITY OF ILLINOIS
College of Fine and Applied Arts, Urbana   Illinois 61801
217 333-1661
State and 4 Year
Arts Areas: Dance, Instrumental Music, Vocal Music, Theatre, Film Arts, Visual Arts and Architecture
Performing Series: Marquee Series
Performance Facilities: Krannert Center for the Performing Arts

DANCE

Patrick K Knowles, Acting Head   **Number Of Faculty:** 9
Number Of Students: 118   **Degrees Offered:** BA; BFA; MA
Technical Training: Stress Performing; Choreography
Teaching Certification Available
Financial Assistance: Internships and Assistantships
Performing Groups: Illinois Dance Theatre

MUSIC

Robert E Bays, Director   **Number Of Faculty:** 100   **Number Of Students:** 800
Degrees Offered: BMus; BS; BA; MMus; MS; EdD; PhD; DMA
Technical Training: Applied Music; Theory - Composition; Musicology; MusEd
Teaching Certification Available
Financial Assistance: Internships, Assistantships, Scholarships and Work-Study Grants
Performing Groups: Universtiy Orchestra; Chamber Orchestra; Civic Orchestra; University Bands; Wind &
Jazz Ensembles; Men's Chorus; Concert Choir; Chamber Choir; Ineluctible Modality; Contemporary
Chamber Players; Illinois Opera Theatre
Workshops/Festivals: Summer Youth Music

THEATRE

Burnet M Hobgood, Head   **Number Of Faculty:** 15   **Number Of Students:** 200
Degrees Offered: BFA; MA; MFA; PhD   **Technical Training:** Design; Theatre Tech
Financial Assistance: Assistantships, Scholarships and Work-Study Grants
Performing Groups: University Theatre
Workshops/Festivals: American College Theatre Festival

WAUBONSEE COMMUNITY COLLEGE
Sugar Grove   Illinois 60544, 312 466-4811
State and 2 Year
Arts Areas: Instrumental Music, Vocal Music, Theatre, Television and Visual Arts
Performance Facilities: Little Theatre; Auditorium; Gymnasium
Number Of Faculty: 3   **Degrees Offered:** AA
Financial Assistance: Scholarships and Work-Study Grants
Number Of Faculty: 1   **Degrees Offered:** AA

WESTERN ILLINOIS UNIVERSITY
Macomb   Illinois 61455, 309 298-1552
State and 4 Year
Arts Areas: Instrumental Music, Vocal Music, Theatre and Visual Arts
Performing Series: Young Artist Series

MUSIC

Christopher Izzo, Chairman   **Number Of Faculty:** 30
Number Of Students: 225   **Degrees Offered:** BA; BAEd; MA
Teaching Certification Available
Financial Assistance: Assistantships and Work-Study Grants
Performing Groups: Camerta Woodwind Quintet; Lydian Trio
Workshops/Festivals: Summer Music Camp

(continued on next page)

THEATRE

Jared Brown, Acting Chairman   **Number Of Faculty:** 8
Number Of Students: 100   **Degrees Offered:** BA; MA
Teaching Certification Available
Financial Assistance: Assistantships and Work-Study Grants
Performing Groups: Regional Touring Theatre Company
Workshops/Festivals: Summer Music Theatre

WHEATON COLLEGE
Wheaton   Illinois 60187, 312 682-5098

Private and 4 Year   **Arts Areas:** Instrumental Music and Vocal Music
Performing Series: Wheaton College Artist Series
Performance Facilities: Edman Memorial Chapel

MUSIC

Harold Best, Dean   **Number Of Faculty:** 30   **Number Of Students:** 180
Degrees Offered: BA; BMus; BMusEd   **Teaching Certification Available**
Financial Assistance: Scholarships and Work-Study Grants
Performing Groups: Concert Choir; Women's Glee Club; Men's Glee Club; Concert Band; Symphony Orchestra

---

WILBUR WRIGHT COLLEGE, CITY COLLEGE OF CHICAGO
3400 N Austin Ave, Chicago   Illinois 60634
312 777-7900

City and 2 Year
Arts Areas: Instrumental Music, Vocal Music, Theatre and Film Arts
Performance Facilities: Auditorium

MUSIC

John De Roule, Section Chairman   **Number Of Faculty:** 4
Number Of Students: 500   **Degrees Offered:** AA
Courses Offered: Fundamentals; Harmony; Piano; Strings; Woodwinds; Brass; Percussion; Chorus; Concert Band; Orchestra; Instrumental Ensembles
Financial Assistance: Scholarships, Work-Study Grants and BEOG
Performing Groups: Concert Band; Jazz Band; Orchestra; Choir

THEATRE

Donald Subeck, Speech Department Chairman   **Number Of Faculty:** 2
Number Of Students: 60   **Degrees Offered:** AA
Courses Offered: Oral Interpretation; Acting
Financial Assistance: Scholarships, Work-Study Grants and BEOG
Performing Groups: Drama Club

WILLIAM RAINEY HARPER COLLEGE
Algonquin & Roselle Rds, Palatine   Illinois 60067
312 397-3000

State and 2 Year
Arts Areas: Instrumental Music, Vocal Music and Visual Arts
Performance Facilities: College Center Lounge

MUSIC

Dr George Makas, Professor   **Number Of Faculty:** 27
Number Of Students: 115   **Degrees Offered:** AA
Financial Assistance: Scholarships
Performing Groups: Concert Choir; Community Orchestra; Community Chorus; Wind Ensemble; Camerata Singers; Jazz Band
Workshops/Festivals: Piano Workshop; Noon Guest Recitals

ANDERSON COLLEGE
1100 E 5th St, Anderson   Indiana 46011
317 644-0951 Ext 215
Private and 4 Year
Arts Areas: Instrumental Music, Vocal Music, Theatre, Film Arts, Television and Visual Arts
Performing Series: Performing Arts Series
Performance Facilities: Byrum Hall; O C Lewis Gymnasium

MUSIC

F Dale Bengston, Chairman   *Number Of Faculty:* 22   *Number Of Students:* 250
Degrees Offered: AB
Courses Offered: Theory; Literature & Church Music; Music Education; Applied Music
Technical Training: Opera   *Teaching Certification Available*
Financial Assistance: Scholarships and Work-Study Grants
Performing Groups: Operate Theatre; Orchestra; Jazz Lab; Chorale Ensembles

THEATRE

Robert N Smith, Chairman   *Number Of Faculty:* 5   *Number Of Students:* 100
Degrees Offered: AB
Courses Offered: Speech; Debate; Theatre; Radio; Drama (Technical)
Teaching Certification Available
Financial Assistance: Scholarships and Work-Study Grants
Performing Groups: Dramatics Club

BALL STATE UNIVERSITY
2000 University Ave, Muncie   Indiana 47306
317 289-1241
State and 4 Year
Arts Areas: Instrumental Music, Vocal Music, Theatre, Visual Arts and Radio
Performing Series: Concert & Artist Series
Performance Facilities: The Ball State Theatre

MUSIC

Dr Robert Hargreaves, Director   *Number Of Faculty:* 60
Number Of Students: 850   *Degrees Offered:* BMus; MMus
Technical Training: Opera; Organ   *Teaching Certification Available*
Financial Assistance: Internships, Assistantships, Scholarships and Work-Study Grants
Performing Groups: Instrumental Ensembles; Opera; Orchestra; String Ensembles
Workshops/Festivals: Opera Workshop; Summer Arts Festival

THEATRE

Alan W Huckleberry, Chairman   *Number Of Faculty:* 4
Number Of Students: 80
Financial Assistance: Scholarships and Work-Study Grants
Performing Groups: Ball State Theatre; Children's Theatre; Musical Theatre; Puppet Theatre
Workshops/Festivals: Summer Arts Festival

BETHEL COLLEGE
1001 W McKinley Ave, Mishawaka   Indiana 46544
219 259-8511 Ext 66
Private and 4 Year
Arts Areas: Instrumental Music, Vocal Music, Theatre and Communication
Performing Series: Annual Music - Lecture Series
Performance Facilities: Goodman Auditorium; Hall of Science Octorium

(continued on next page)

MUSIC

Elliott A Nordgre, Chairman, Division of Fine Arts   **Number Of Faculty:** 7
Number Of Students: 75   **Degrees Offered:** BA
Courses Offered: Theory; Music Education & Methods; Music Literature & History
Technical Training: Instrumental & Vocal Soloists; Groups; Choirs
Teaching Certification Available
Financial Assistance: Scholarships and Work-Study Grants
Performing Groups: Concert Choir; Chapel Choir & Ensembles; Oratorio; Orchestra
Workshops/Festivals: Opera Workshop

THEATRE

Dr Earl Reimer, Professor of English   **Number Of Faculty:** 2
Degrees Offered: BA (drama minor)
Courses Offered: Religious Drama; Dramatics I & II; Dramatics Lab
Technical Training: Plays; Musicals   **Teaching Certification Available**
Financial Assistance: Scholarships and Work-Study Grants
Performing Groups: Genesians   **Workshops/Festivals:** Annual Plays & Musicals
Artists-In-Residence/Guest Artists: Vienna Choir Boys; Truth; Jerome Hines

---

BUTLER UNIVERSITY
JORDAN COLLEGE OF MUSIC
4600 Sunset Ave, Indianapolis   Indiana 46208
317 283-9231
  Private and 4 Year
  Arts Areas: Dance, Instrumental Music, Vocal Music, Theatre and Visual Arts
  Performance Facilities: Clowes Hall

DANCE

Martha Cornick, Chairman   **Number Of Faculty:** 8   **Number Of Students:** 100
Degrees Offered: BA Dance; MA Dance
Financial Assistance: Assistantships and Scholarships
Performing Groups: Butler Ballet (Touring & Campus Companies)

MUSIC

Louis F Chenette, Chairman   **Number Of Faculty:** 45
Number Of Students: 300   **Degrees Offered:** BMus; BA; BFA; MMus
Teaching Certification Available
Financial Assistance: Assistantships and Scholarships
Performing Groups: Band; Orchestra; Chamber Music Groups; Choral Organizations; Jazz Ensemble
Workshops/Festivals: Summer Workshops for Graduate Students; Annual Romantic Festival

THEATRE

George Willeford, Chairman   **Number Of Faculty:** 5   **Number Of Students:** 30
Degrees Offered: BA   **Teaching Certification Available**
Financial Assistance: Assistantships and Scholarships

DEPAUW UNIVERSITY
Greencastle   Indiana 46135, 317 653-9721 Ext 404
  Private and 4 Year
  Arts Areas: Dance, Instrumental Music, Vocal Music, Theatre and Visual Arts
  Performing Series: Performing Arts Series
  Performance Facilities: Kresge Auditorium; The Theatre; Recital Hall

MUSIC

Donald H White, Director   **Number Of Faculty:** 32   **Number Of Students:** 160
Degrees Offered: BM & BA in Music
Courses Offered: Performance; Area Performance; Music Ed; Music/Business; Church Music; Composition
Teaching Certification Available

(continued on next page)

Financial Assistance: Scholarships and Work-Study Grants
Performing Groups: Symphony Orchestra; Chamber Symphony; Band; Symphonic Wind Ensemble; Opera/Theater; Jazz Ensemble; Chamber Music Ensembles; Strings, Brass, Woodwinds & Percussion; Concert Choir; Festival Choir; Century Singers; Faculty Ensembles: Aeolian Trio (Piano, Violin & Cello), Woodwind Quintet, Brass Ensemble
Workshops/Festivals: Annual Festival of Contemporary Music

THEATRE

Robert O Weiss, Head, Communication Arts & Sciences   *Number Of Faculty:* 2
Degrees Offered: BA
Courses Offered: Oral Interpretation; Advanced Interpretation & Acting; Rehearsal & Performance; Theatre Production; Theatrical History & Criticism; Topics in Theatre; Projects
Teaching Certification Available
Financial Assistance: Scholarships and Work-Study Grants
Performing Groups: Little Theatre; Duzer Du

EARLHAM COLLEGE
Richmond   Indiana 47374, 317 962-6561 Ext 416
Private and 4 Year
Arts Areas: Dance, Instrumental Music, Vocal Music, Theatre and Visual Arts
Performing Series: Artist Series
Performance Facilities: Wilkinson Theater; Goddard Auditorium; Leeds Gallery

MUSIC

Leonard Holvik, Professor   *Number Of Faculty:* 6   *Number Of Students:* 700
Degrees Offered: BA
Courses Offered: History; Theory & Compositon; Integrated Fine Arts (Western & Japanese); introduction for general students; Instrumental & Choral Groups
Technical Training: Applied Lessons in Voice, Keyboard, Strings, Woodwinds, Brasses
Financial Assistance: Scholarships and Work-Study Grants
Performing Groups: Oratorio Chorus; Chamber Singers; Chamber Musicians; Revelations (Afro-American); Symphony Orchestra; Brass Choir; Wind Ensemble

THEATRE

Mark Malinauskas, Assistant Professor of Drama   *Number Of Faculty:* 3
Number Of Students: 200   *Degrees Offered:* BA
Courses Offered: Introduction to Theater; Acting; Basic Stagecraft; Oral Interpretation; Theater Design; Intensive Theatre; Applied Theatre; Play Production; Interdisciplinary Courses in Theatre History and the Arts
Technical Training: Applied Dance; Dance Composition
Financial Assistance: Scholarships and Work-Study Grants
Performing Groups: Mask & Mantle Drama Society
Artists-In-Residence/Guest Artists: Mitsuo Kakutani, Japanese Artist-in-Residence

---

FORT WAYNE BIBLE COLLEGE
1025 W Rudisill Blvd, Fort Wayne   Indiana 46807
219 456-2111 Ext 204
Private and 4 Year   *Arts Areas:* Instrumental Music and Vocal Music
Performing Series: College/Community Artist Series

MUSIC

Jay D Platte, Chairman   *Number Of Faculty:* 12   *Number Of Students:* 50
Degrees Offered: BMus; BMusEd; BS in Music & Christian Education
Courses Offered: Music History & Literature; Theory; Conducting; Education; Church Music; Performance
Technical Training: Field Study Program required
Teaching Certification Available
Financial Assistance: Scholarships and Work-Study Grants
Performing Groups: Chorale; Choral Union; Concert Band; Vocal & Instrumental Ensembles

FRANKLIN COLLEGE
Franklin Indiana 46131, 317 736-8441
Private and 4 Year   *Arts Areas:* Vocal Music

MUSIC

Samuel B Hicks, Associate Professor   *Number Of Faculty:* 1
Courses Offered: Art of Listening; Music for Elementary Teachers; Theory I & II; History of Music I & II;
Choral Conducting; Voice
Teaching Certification Available
Performing Groups: The Keys; The Kites; The Gathering

GOSHEN COLLEGE
Goshen Indiana 46526, 219 533-3161 Ext 223
Private and 4 Year
Arts Areas: Instrumental Music, Vocal Music, Theatre and Visual Arts
Performing Series: The Goshen College Artists Series
Performance Facilities: Union Auditorium; John S Umble Center

DANCE

Dance program under auspices of Physical Education Department

MUSIC

Doyle Preheim, Chairman   *Number Of Faculty:* 9   *Number Of Students:* 57
Degrees Offered: BA Music
Courses Offered: Courses in Music Theory, Music Education, Music History & Literature; Piano Pedagogy;
Applied Music
Technical Training: Introductory Music Therapy; Conducting; Piano Pedagogy; Applied Music
Teaching Certification Available
Financial Assistance: Scholarships and Work-Study Grants
Performing Groups: Chamber Choir; Chorale; Orchestra; Jazz Band; Ensembles
Workshops/Festivals: Campus Religious Festivals; Handel's Messiah with the community; Music Workshop
for Piano Teachers; Music Workshop for High School Upperclassmen; Campus Music - Drama Productions

THEATRE

Roy H Umble, Professor of Communications   *Number Of Faculty:* 1
Number Of Students: 8   *Degrees Offered:* BA Communications
Courses Offered: Oral Interpretation; Studies in Drama: Theatre, Play Production; Religious Drama
Workshop
Technical Training: Play Production
Financial Assistance: Scholarships and Work-Study Grants
Performing Groups: The Goshen College Players; Student Touring Groups
Workshops/Festivals: Religious Drama Workshop
Artists-In-Residence/Guest Artists: Nicholas C Lindsay, Poet-in-Residence

GRACE COLLEGE
Winona Lake Indiana 46590, 219 267-8191 Ext 197
Private and 4 Year
Arts Areas: Instrumental Music, Vocal Music and Theatre
Performance Facilities: Rodeheaver Auditorium

MUSIC

Donald E Ogden, Chairman   *Number Of Faculty:* 5   *Number Of Students:* 40
Degrees Offered: BMusEd; BMus; BA
Courses Offered: Introduction to Music Theory
Teaching Certification Available
Financial Assistance: Scholarships and Work-Study Grants
Performing Groups: Concert Band; Brass Choir; Wind Ensemble; Percussion Ensemble; Concert Choir;
Freshman Choir; Oratorio Society

(continued on next page)

THEATRE

Mervin Ziegler, Chairman   **Number Of Faculty:** 3

HANOVER COLLEGE
Hanover   Indiana 47243, 812 866-2151 Ext 223
Private and 4 Year
Arts Areas: Dance, Instrumental Music, Vocal Music and Theatre
Performing Series: Community Artist Series
Performance Facilities: Parker Auditorium; J Graham Brown Campus Center

DANCE

Debora Ridenour, Physical Education Instructor
Dance program under auspices of Physical Education Department
Number Of Faculty: 1
Financial Assistance: Scholarships and Work-Study Grants
Workshops/Festivals: Modern Dance Concerts

MUSIC

J David Wagner, Professor   **Number Of Faculty:** 3   **Degrees Offered:** BA
Teaching Certification Available
Financial Assistance: Scholarships and Work-Study Grants
Performing Groups: Choir; Chamber Singers Band
Workshops/Festivals: Annual Christmas Concert; Annual Band Concert

THEATRE

Thomas G Evans, Professor of Speech/Drama   **Number Of Faculty:** 1
Degrees Offered: BA   **Teaching Certification Available**
Financial Assistance: Scholarships and Work-Study Grants
Performing Groups: Theatre Company

HUNTINGTON COLLEGE
2303 College Ave, Huntington   Indiana 46750
219 356-6000 Ext 44
Private and 4 Year
Arts Areas: Instrumental Music, Vocal Music, Theatre, Television and Visual Arts
Performance Facilities: Davis Auditorium

MUSIC

Dr Marlene Langosch, Chairman   **Number Of Faculty:** 3 Full-time, 8 Part-time
Number Of Students: 125   **Degrees Offered:** BA; BS
Courses Offered: Music Performance; Music Composition; Music Education; Choral; Instrumental
Teaching Certification Available
Financial Assistance: Scholarships and Work-Study Grants
Performing Groups: Choir; Wind Ensemble; Chamber Orchestra; Collegium Musicum; Brass Ensemble;
String Ensemble

THEATRE

Dr Carl D Zurcher, Chairman   **Number Of Faculty:** 1   **Number Of Students:** 20
Degrees Offered: BA or BS Speech or Communication
Performing Groups: Campus Players

INDIANA STATE UNIVERSITY
Terre Haute   Indiana 47809, 812 232-6311 Ext 2577
State and 4 Year
Arts Areas: Dance, Instrumental Music, Vocal Music, Theatre, Film Arts, Television and Visual Arts
Performing Series: Convocations-Artist Series; Theatre Series
Children's Theatre Series; Film Series; Terre Haute Symphony Orchestra Series

(continued on next page)

Performance Facilities: Tilson Music Hall; Tirey Memorial Union: Heritage Room, State Room, Sycamore Playhouse
ISU Hulman Civic University Center; ISU Conference Center; Tirey Memorial Union South

DANCE

Dr Mildren Lemen, Chairperson, Department of Women's Physical Education
Number Of Faculty: 18   **Number Of Students:** 300
Degrees Offered: BA; BS; MA; MS
Courses Offered: Modern (Beginning, Intermediate, Advanced); Folk; Square; Social
Teaching Certification Available   Financial Assistance: Assistantships
Performing Groups: Modern Dance Club   **Workshops/Festivals:** Annual Performance

MUSIC

Dr Robert L Cowden, Chairperson   **Number Of Faculty:** 33
Degrees Offered: BMus; BA; BS; MA; MS   **Teaching Certification Available**
Financial Assistance: Assistantships, Scholarships and Work-Study Grants
Performing Groups: Symphonic Band; Wind Ensemble; Varsity Band; Marching Sycamores Band;
University Symphony; Terre Haute Symphony; University Singers; Concert Choir; Sycamore Singers; Jazz Ensembles; Chamber Ensembles; Opera; Musicals
Workshops/Festivals: Contemporary Music Festival (with the Indianapolis Symphony Orchestra); Concert & Marching Bands; Orchestra; Swing Choir; Choral; Harp; Music Education

THEATRE

Dr Gary L Stewart, Director   **Number Of Faculty:** 8   **Number Of Students:** 60
Degrees Offered: BA; BS; MA; MS   **Teaching Certification Available**
Financial Assistance: Assistantships, Scholarships and Work-Study Grants
Performing Groups: Sycamore Players; Summer Theatre Company; Peppermint Stick Players
Workshops/Festivals: Summer Theatre

INDIANA UNIVERSITY - PURDUE UNIVERSITY AT FORT WAYNE
2101 E Coliseum Blvd, Fort Wayne   Indiana 46805
219 482-5121

State and 4 Year
Arts Areas: Dance, Instrumental Music, Vocal Music, Theatre, Television and Visual Arts
Performing Series: Concert Series; Theatre Season
Performance Facilities: Purdue - Indiana Theatre; Neff Recital Hall

MUSIC

James Ator, Acting Chairman   **Number Of Faculty:** 35
Number Of Students: 160
Degrees Offered: BMus, Performance, Instrumental & Choral; BS Music Therapy; BS Mus & Outside Field; MS MusEd
Courses Offered: Ensembles: Piano Accompanying, University Instrumental, University Choral, Jazz, Brass, String Instrument, Woodwind & Percussion; Applied Music ; Music Education: Class Piano Instruction & Teaching of Music in the Elementary Schools
Technical Training: Performance opportunity with the Fort Wayne Philharmonic as paid professionals; Music Therapy majors have the opportunity to work with several mental health centers in the Fort Wayne area
Financial Assistance: Scholarships
Performing Groups: University Jazz Band; Chamber Orchestra; Band; Various Choral Groups
Workshops/Festivals: Music Education Workshops; Dickens Dinner

THEATRE

Daniel Cashman, Acting Chairman   **Number Of Faculty:** 4
Number Of Students: 50   **Degrees Offered:** BA Theatre
Courses Offered: Speech for the Stage; Stage Movement I & II; Acting; Rehearsal & Performance; Stagecraft for Secondary Schools; Advanced Problems in Theatre Directing; Costume for Stage; Theatre Management; Advanced Problems in Technical Theatre; Studies in Dramatic Structure (Tradegy & Comedy); History of the Theatre I & II; Directed Study of Special Theatre Problems

(continued on next page)

Technical Training: Fencing; Stage Movement
Performing Groups: Purdue - Indiana Theatre

INDIANA UNIVERSITY - PURDUE UNIVERSITY, INDIANAPOLIS
1201 E 38th St, Indianapolis   Indiana 46205
317 635-8661
State and 4 Year
Arts Areas: Instrumental Music, Vocal Music and Theatre
Courses Offered: Piano; Introduction to Music; Music Appreciation; Music Literature; Teaching Elementary School Music
Performing Groups: Chamber Ensemble; Chorus

THEATRE

J Edgar Webb, Director   **Number Of Faculty:** 7   **Number Of Students:** 43
Degrees Offered: BA   **Teaching Certification Available**
Financial Assistance: Scholarships and Work-Study Grants
Performing Groups: Children's Theatre; Experimental Theatre; Puppet & Marionettes; Theatre Productions

INDIANA UNIVERSITY, BLOOMINGTON
Bloomington   Indiana 47401, 812 337-9053
State and 4 Year
Arts Areas: Dance, Instrumental Music, Vocal Music, Theatre, Film Arts and Visual Arts
Performing Series: Auditorium Series; Theatre Series; Dance Series
Performance Facilities: Musical Arts Center; Opera House; University Theatre; Experimental Theatre

DANCE

Marina Svetlove, Ballet Director, School of Music
Anita Aldrich Chairman, Health, Recreation & Physical Education
Degrees Offered: Ballet: BS Performance, Teaching; MS Performance, Teaching; Modern: BS Dance; MS Dance
Teaching Certification Available
Financial Assistance: Assistantships, Scholarships and Work-Study Grants
Performing Groups: Modern; UI Dance Theatre

MUSIC

Charles H Webb, Jr, Chairman   **Number Of Faculty:** 150
Number Of Students: 1,600
Degrees Offered: B Mus; BMusEd; BS; BMus; MMusEd; MS; MMusEd; MA; MA Teaching; DMusEd; PhD
Teaching Certification Available
Financial Assistance: Assistantships, Scholarships and Work-Study Grants
Performing Groups: Orchestras; Opera Theatre; Bands; Chamber Ensembles; Ethnic Music Groups; Musical Theatre; Choir; Madrigals; Baroque; Choral Ensembles
Workshops/Festivals: 35 Workshops annually for students, educators, professional artists

THEATRE

R Keith Michael, Jr, Chairman   **Number Of Faculty:** 15
Number Of Students: 403
Technical Training: Work as professionals with Brown County Playhouse; Study under outstanding educators, including Oscar G Brockett, 1974 President of American Theatre Association
Financial Assistance: Assistantships, Scholarships and Work-Study Grants
Performing Groups: Indiana Theatre Company; Brown County Playhouse Summer Professional Theatre

INDIANA UNIVERSITY, EAST
Chester Blvd, Richmond   Indiana 47374
317 966-8261
State and 4 Year
Arts Areas: Instrumental Music, Vocal Music and Theatre

(continued on next page)

Courses Offered: Music; Music Appreciation; Theatre; Acting; Theatre Appreciation

INDIANA UNIVERSITY NORTHWEST
3400 Broadway, Gary   Indiana 46408
219 980-6808

State and 4 Year   **Arts Areas:** Dance, Vocal Music and Theatre
Performing Series: University Theatre Performing Arts Series
Performance Facilities: University Theatre; Experimental Theatre.

DANCE

Garrett Cope, Assistant Professor   **Number Of Faculty:** 1
Number Of Students: 48   **Courses Offered:** Modern Dance Techniques
Technical Training: Private Teachers; Ballet, Modern, Tap, Mime
Financial Assistance: Scholarships, Work-Study Grants and BEOG
Performing Groups: University Theatre Dance Companies I & II

MUSIC

Robert Foor, Chairman   **Number Of Faculty:** 2
Courses Offered: Music History & Literature; Introduction to Music Fundamentals; University Choral Ensemble
Financial Assistance: Scholarships, Work-Study Grants and BEOG

THEATRE

Robert Foor, Chairman   **Number Of Faculty:** 4   **Number Of Students:** 55
Degrees Offered: BA in Theatre; BA in Fine Arts; Major in Studio Practice
Courses Offered: Introduction to Theatre; Acting; Stagecraft; Stage Costuming; Stage Lighting; Directing; Theatre History; Scene Design; Oral Interpretation; Readers Theatre
Teaching Certification Available
Financial Assistance: Scholarships, Work-Study Grants and BEOG
Workshops/Festivals: One Act Workshop; Experimental Student Workshop

INDIANA UNIVERSITY AT SOUTH BEND
1700 Mishawaka Ave, South Bend   Indiana 46615
219 237-4111

State and 4 Year
Arts Areas: Instrumental Music, Vocal Music, Theatre and Visual Arts
Performing Series: IUSB Philharmonic Series; Symphonic Wind Ensemble Series
Chamber Music Festival; South Bend Youth Symphony Series; Theatre Series
Performance Facilities: IUSB Main Auditorium/Theatre, Northside Hall
IUSB Little Theatre/Recital Hall, Northside West Hall

MUSIC

Robert W Demaree, Jr, Chairman   **Number Of Faculty:** 34
Number Of Students: 125
Degrees Offered: AS Jazz & Commercial Music; BSMus; BMus; BMusEd
Teaching Certification Available
Financial Assistance: Scholarships and Work-Study Grants
Performing Groups: International String Quartet

THEATRE

Warren Pepperdine, Chairman   **Number Of Faculty:** 3   **Number Of Students:** 30
Degrees Offered: AB Speech & Theatre
Artists-In-Residence/Guest Artists: The International String Quartet; The South Bend Symphonic Choir

INDIANA UNIVERSITY, SOUTHEAST
4501 Grant Line Rd, New Albany   Indiana 47150
812 945-2731
State and 4 Year
Arts Areas: Instrumental Music, Vocal Music, Theatre and Visual Arts
Performing Series: Concert - Lecture Series
Performing Groups: Chamber Ensemble; Choral Ensemble; Jazz Ensemble

MANCHESTER COLLEGE
604 College Ave, North Manchester   Indiana 46962
219 982-2141
Private and 4 Year
Arts Areas: Instrumental Music, Vocal Music, Theatre, Film Arts and Television
Performing Series: Artist/Lecture Series
Performance Facilities: College Auditorium; Winger Recital Hall; Wampler Auditorium

MUSIC

Dr R Gary Deavel, Chairman   **Number Of Faculty:** 7   **Number Of Students:** 25
Degrees Offered: BS; BA
Courses Offered: Theory; History; Woodwinds; Percussion; Brass; String; Voice; Ensembles; Choirs; Independent Study; Seminars
Teaching Certification Available
Financial Assistance: Scholarships and Work-Study Grants
Performing Groups: College/Civic Symphony Orchestra; A Cappella Choir; Concert Band; Jazz Ensemble; Chorale; Various Ensembles
Workshops/Festivals: Piano Workshop; Vocal Workshop; Jazz Ensemble Workshop

THEATRE

Dr Ronald L Aungst, Chairman   **Number Of Faculty:** 4
Number Of Students: 30   **Degrees Offered:** BS, BA & AA in Broadcast Media
Courses Offered: World Theater & Drama I & II; Acting; Creative Dramatics; Stagecraft & Design; Directing
Technical Training: Stagecraft & Design with practical experience
Teaching Certification Available
Financial Assistance: Scholarships and Work-Study Grants
Performing Groups: Kenapocomoco Players; Alpha Psi Omega
Artists-In-Residence/Guest Artists: Phyllis Curtin; The National Players; Goldovsky Grand Opera Theater; Anjani Ambegaokar & Troupe (Kathak Dances)

MARIAN COLLEGE, INDIANAPOLIS
3200 Cold Spring Rd, Indianapolis   Indiana 46222
317 924-3291
Private and 4 Year
Arts Areas: Instrumental Music, Vocal Music, Theatre and Visual Arts

MUSIC

Sister Ruth A Wirtz, Chairman   **Number Of Faculty:** 8
Number Of Students: 80   **Degrees Offered:** BMus
Technical Training: Overseas Study   **Teaching Certification Available**
Financial Assistance: Scholarships and Work-Study Grants
Performing Groups: Chorus; Drum and Bugle Corps; Wind Ensemble

THEATRE

Donald Johnson, Chairman   **Number Of Faculty:** 3   **Number Of Students:** 35
Degrees Offered: BA   **Technical Training:** Overseas Study
Teaching Certification Available
Financial Assistance: Scholarships and Work-Study Grants
Performing Groups: The Players

MARION COLLEGE
4201 S Washington St, Marion   Indiana 46952
317 674-6901

   Private and 4 Year   *Arts Areas:* Instrumental Music and Vocal Music
   Performance Facilities: Wurlitzer Auditorium; McConn Auditorium; Baldwin Center
   Number Of Faculty: 10   *Number Of Students:* 40   *Degrees Offered:* AB; BS
   Technical Training: Individual Training   *Teaching Certification Available*
   Financial Assistance: Scholarships and Work-Study Grants
   Performing Groups: Concord Players; Christian Service Teams; Jazz Ensemble; Sounds of Praise

OAKLAND CITY COLLEGE
Oakland City   Indiana 47560, 812 749-4031
   Private and 4 Year
   Arts Areas: Instrumental Music, Vocal Music and Visual Arts
   Performance Facilities: College Auditorium   *Degrees Offered:* BMus
   Technical Training: Opera   *Teaching Certification Available*
   Performing Groups: Choir; Marching Band; Vocal & Instrumental Ensembles

PURDUE UNIVERSITY
West Lafayette   Indiana 47907, 317 494-8702
   State and 4 Year
   Arts Areas: Dance, Instrumental Music, Vocal Music, Theatre, Television and Visual Arts
   Performing Series: Loeb Music Series; Purdue Festival Series; Special Convocations
   Performance Facilities: Edward C Elliott Hall of Music; Loeb Playhouse; Experimental Theatre; Fowler
   Hall

DANCE

Peggy Anderson - Lewellen, Program Instructor   *Number Of Faculty:* 3
Number Of Students: 300
Courses Offered: Folk Dance; Square Dance; Modern Dance (intermediate & advanced); Ballet
(intermediate & advanced); Jazz; Contemporary Social Dance
Performing Groups: Purdue Modern Dance Club; Purdue Dance Ensemble

MUSIC

Professor Ronald R Kidd, Chairman; Al G Wright, Director of University Bands
Number Of Faculty: 4, Band 5   *Number Of Students:* Band 750
Courses Offered: Theory; History; Literature; Elementary Education; BAND - Jazz Ensemble; Variety
Band; Symphony Orchestra
Performing Groups: "All American" Marching Band; Concert, Variety, Symphony, Ceremonial & Stage
Bands; Symphony Orchestra; Renaissance Ensemble; Jazz Groups; Wind Ensemble; Brass Chorus
Workshops/Festivals: Twirling Workshop; Jazz Workshop; Music - Reading Clinic; Band Camp

THEATRE

Dale Miller, Director   *Number Of Faculty:* 12   *Number Of Students:* 65
Degrees Offered: BA; MA
Courses Offered: Speech for Stage; Stage Movement; Acting; Rehearsal & Performance; Stagecraft; Stage
Mechanics; Technical Theatre Production; Appreciation; Makeup; Introduction to Theatre History;
Dramatic Structure
Performing Groups: High School Touring Show
Artists-In-Residence/Guest Artists: Stanley Butts III

SAINT FRANCIS COLLEGE
2701 Spring St, Fort Wayne   Indiana 46808
219 432-3551
   Private and 4 Year
   Arts Areas: Instrumental Music, Vocal Music and Visual Arts
   Performing Series: Concert - Lecture Series

(continued on next page)

MUSIC

Richard Brown, Chairman   **Number Of Faculty:** 8   **Number Of Students:** 120
Degrees Offered: BMus; BMusEd   **Teaching Certification Available**
Financial Assistance: Assistantships, Scholarships and Work-Study Grants
Performing Groups: Chorus; Orchestra; Band; Instrumental Ensembles

THEATRE

Harold Gunderson, Chairman   **Number Of Faculty:** 2   **Number Of Students:** 30
Teaching Certification Available
Financial Assistance: Assistantships, Scholarships and Work-Study Grants
Performing Groups: Dramatic Arts Club

SAINT JOSEPH'S COLLEGE
Rensselaer   Indiana 47978, 219 866-7111
Private and 4 Year
Arts Areas: Instrumental Music, Vocal Music, Theatre, Television and Visual Arts
Performance Facilities: Auditorium

MUSIC

Dr John Egan, Chairman   **Number Of Faculty:** 5   **Number Of Students:** 50
Degrees Offered: BA; BS   **Teaching Certification Available**
Financial Assistance: Work-Study Grants
Performing Groups: Chorus; Marching Band; Dance Bands

THEATRE

Dr Ralph Cappuccilli, Chairman   **Number Of Faculty:** 2
Number Of Students: 30   **Degrees Offered:** BA; BS
Financial Assistance: Work-Study Grants   **Performing Groups:** Columbian Players

---

SAINT MARY-OF-THE-WOODS COLLEGE
Saint Mary-of-the-Woods   Indiana 47876, 812 535-4141
Private and 4 Year
Arts Areas: Dance, Instrumental Music, Vocal Music, Theatre and Visual Arts
Performing Series: Artist - Lecture Series
Performance Facilities: Cecilian Auditorium; Little Theatre; Experimental Theatre

DANCE

Dance program under auspices of Physical Education Department

MUSIC

Laurette Bellamy, S P, Chairman   **Number Of Faculty:** 6
Degrees Offered: BA   **Courses Offered:** Voice; Drama
Teaching Certification Available
Financial Assistance: Assistantships, Scholarships and Work-Study Grants
Performing Groups: Orchestral Ensemble; College Chorale; Madrigal Singers

THEATRE

Joseph Klein, Chairman, Speech & Drama   **Number Of Faculty:** 4
Number Of Students: 25
Degrees Offered: BA Speech & Drama; AA Technical Theatre
Technical Training: Lighting; Set Design   **Teaching Certification Available**
Financial Assistance: Assistantships, Scholarships and Work-Study Grants
Performing Groups: Peppermint Stick Players (children's theatre troupe)
Artists-In-Residence/Guest Artists: Juan Antonio

SAINT MARY'S COLLEGE
Notre Dame   Indiana 46556, 219 232-3031
>   Private and 4 Year
>   *Arts Areas:* Dance, Instrumental Music, Vocal Music, Theatre, Film Arts, Television and Visual Arts
>   *Performing Series:* Saint Mary's College Performing Arts Series
>   *Performance Facilities:* O'Laughlin Auditorium; Moreau Hall Little Theater

DANCE

Dance program under auspices of Speech & Drama Department
Courses Offered: Classical Ballet; Modern

MUSIC

Susan Stevens, Chairman   *Number Of Faculty:* 8   *Number Of Students:* 390
Degrees Offered: BMusEd; BMus Theory & Literature; BMus Applied Music; BA in Applied Music
Courses Offered: Class Piano; Class Voice; Piano; Organ; Harpsichord; Voice; Voilin; Viola; Cello;
Percussion; Flute; Accompanying; String Bass; Oboe; Clarinet; Bassoon; Trumpet; French Horn;
Trombone; Baritone Horn; Tuba; Harp; Guitar; Theory; Collegiate Choir; Women's Chorus; Opera
Workshops; Chamber Orchestra; Introduction to Literature; Music Appreciation; Jazz, Folk & Rock; The
Musical Experience; Music History; Conducting; Mid-Renaissance
Teaching Certification Available
Financial Assistance: Internships, Scholarships and Work-Study Grants
Performing Groups: Collegiate Choir; Chamber Singers; Women's Chorus; Chamber Orchestra; Opera
Workshops
Workshops/Festivals: Departmental Concert Series; Workshops to students by visiting artists; Saint Mary's
College Summer Camp (for young people)

THEATRE

Reginald Bain, Chairman, Speech & Drama Department   *Number Of Faculty:* 7
Number Of Students: 130   *Degrees Offered:* BA Speech & Drama
Courses Offered: Speech Commmunication; Introduction to Theater; Mass Communication; Cinema; Oral
Interpretation; Stagecraft; Theatre Illumination; Introduction to Acting; Introduction to Costuming; Public
Speaking; Neo-Realism/New Wave; TV Practice; Film Production; Debate; Technical Practice;
Argumentation; Business/Professional Speech; Acting Periods, Styles; Drama Theory & Criticism; Small
Group Interactions; Theater for Young People
Teaching Certification Available
Financial Assistance: Scholarships and Work-Study Grants
Performing Groups: Notre Dame - Saint Mary's College Theatre
Workshops/Festivals: Notre Dame - Saint Mary's College Summer Theatre (productions for adults and
children); Summer High School Workshops
Artists-In-Residence/Guest Artists: Newport Jazz Festival All-Stars; The Rotterdam Philharmonic; Erick
Hawkins Dance Company; The Cartoon Opera Minstrel Theatre

TAYLOR UNIVERSITY
Upland   Indiana 46989, 317 998-2751 Ext 206
>   Private and 4 Year
>   *Arts Areas:* Instrumental Music, Vocal Music, Theatre and Visual Arts
>   *Performance Facilities:* Theatre; Chapel/Auditorium

MUSIC

Dr Philip Kroker, Chairman   *Number Of Faculty:* 16   *Number Of Students:* 53
Degrees Offered: AB; BS in Teaching   *Teaching Certification Available*
Financial Assistance: Scholarships, Work-Study Grants and Loans, Grants
Performing Groups: Taylor Singers; Chorale; Orchestra; Band; Ensembles, Choral & Instrumental

THEATRE

Dr Dale Jackson, Chairman   *Number Of Faculty:* 3   *Number Of Students:* 16
Degrees Offered: AB; BS in Teaching   *Teaching Certification Available*
Financial Assistance: Scholarships, Work-Study Grants and Loans, Grants
Performing Groups: Trojan Players

UNIVERSITY OF EVANSVILLE
PO Box 329, Evansville   Indiana 47702
812 479-2281

Private and 4 Year
Arts Areas: Instrumental Music, Vocal Music and Drama
Performing Series: Tuesday & Thursday Night Series (faculty & guest recitals)
Performance Facilities: Wheeler Concert Hall; Shanklin Theatre

MUSIC

Dr Paul Dove, Head   **Number Of Faculty:** 19   **Number Of Students:** 160
Degrees Offered: BMus; BMusEd; BA; BS Mus & Asso Studies; BS Mus
Courses Offered: Two Year Music Theory; Three Year Music History & Literature; Conducting; Management; Arranging; Form & Analysis; Counterpoint; Music Ed; Applied Music; Pedagogy; Lit of Applied
Teaching Certification Available
Financial Assistance: Internships and Scholarships
Performing Groups: Evansville String Quartet; Choral-Ayres; Jazz Ensemble; Woodwind Trio; Marching Band; UE Choir

THEATRE

Dr Dudley Thomas, Head, Department of Drama   **Number Of Faculty:** 4
Number Of Students: 55   **Degrees Offered:** BA; BS; BFA
Courses Offered: Theatre History; Costuming; Design; Acting; Directing; Dance; Playwriting
Technical Training: Stagecraft; Lighting; Makeup
Teaching Certification Available
Financial Assistance: Assistantships, Scholarships and Work-Study Grants
Performing Groups: UE Theatre; Pantomime Troupe
Workshops/Festivals: High School Institute; High School Workshop

UNIVERSITY OF NOTRE DAME
1235 Longfellow Ave, South Bend   Indiana 46615
219 283-6011

Private and 4 Year
Arts Areas: Instrumental Music, Vocal Music, Theatre and Visual Arts

MUSIC

William Cerny, Professor & Chairman   **Number Of Faculty:** 10
Number Of Students: 35   **Degrees Offered:** BA; BMus; MMus; MA
Courses Offered: Music History; Theory; Performance; Liturgical Music
Financial Assistance: Assistantships and Scholarships
Performing Groups: Chapel Choir; University Chorus; Glee Club; Chorale; Band; Orchestra; Piano Trio
Workshops/Festivals: Summer Piano Workshop; Summer Music & Liturgy Workshop

THEATRE

Reginald F Barn, Associate Professor & Chairman   **Number Of Faculty:** 6
Number Of Students: 50   **Degrees Offered:** BA
Courses Offered: History; Theory; Performance (Acting, Directing, Design)
Teaching Certification Available
Financial Assistance: Assistantships and Scholarships
Performing Groups: ND/SMC Theatre
Workshops/Festivals: Summer Theatre Company

VALPARAISO UNIVERSITY
University Pl, Valparaiso   Indiana 46383
219 462-5111

Private and 4 Year
Arts Areas: Instrumental Music, Vocal Music, Theatre and Visual Arts
Performing Series: Concert Series

(continued on next page)

MUSIC

Dr Frederick H Telschon, Chairman   **Number Of Faculty:** 20
Number Of Students: 280   **Degrees Offered:** BMus; BMusEd
Technical Training: Opera   **Teaching Certification Available**
Financial Assistance: Assistantships, Scholarships and Work-Study Grants
Performing Groups: University - Civic Orchestra; 7 Choirs; 6 Bands; Orchestras; Chamber & Choral Ensembles
Workshops/Festivals: Opera Workshop

THEATRE

Fred Sitton, Chairman   **Number Of Faculty:** 7   **Number Of Students:** 100
Degrees Offered: BA   **Teaching Certification Available**
Financial Assistance: Assistantships, Scholarships and Work-Study Grants
Performing Groups: University Players

VINCENNES UNIVERSITY
1002 N First St, Vincennes   Indiana 47591
812 882-3350 Ext 480
State and 2 Year
Arts Areas: Dance, Instrumental Music, Vocal Music, Theatre, Film Arts, Television and Visual Arts
Performance Facilities: Green Auditorium; Shircliff Center Theatre

MUSIC

Richard Ertel, Chairman   **Number Of Faculty:** 4   **Number Of Students:** 77
Degrees Offered: AS; AA
Courses Offered: Music - Fine Arts; Education (Music Major)
Financial Assistance: Scholarships, Work-Study Grants and Performing Grants
Performing Groups: Roaring Twenties Vocal Group; University Chorus; Concert Band; Pep Band; Stage Band

THEATRE

James Spurrier, Director   **Number Of Faculty:** 1   **Number Of Students:** 30
Degrees Offered: AS; AA   **Courses Offered:** Theatrical Production
Financial Assistance: Scholarships, Work-Study Grants and Performing Grants
Performing Groups: VU Theatre; VU Music Theatre; VU Summer Theatre

---

WABASH COLLEGE
301 W Wabash Ave, Crawfordsville   Indiana 47933
317 362-1400
Private and 4 Year
Arts Areas: Instrumental Music, Vocal Music and Visual Arts
Performing Series: Annual Lecture Series; Arts '77, '78
Performance Facilities: Ball Theatre; Yandes Hall; Memorial Chapel

MUSIC

Dr David Greene, Jr, Chairman   **Number Of Faculty:** 3
Number Of Students: 150   **Degrees Offered:** BA
Performing Groups: Glee Club; Band; Chamber Ensemble

THEATRE

Robert Zyromski, Chairman   **Number Of Faculty:** 2   **Number Of Students:** 70
Degrees Offered: BA   **Performing Groups:** Scarlet Masque
Artists-In-Residence/Guest Artists: Second City; Indianapolis Symphony Orchestra; The Fine Arts Quartet; Mummenschanz; Legends of Jazz; Music for Awhile

BUENA VISTA COLLEGE
Storm Lake   Iowa 50588, 712 749-2351
> Private and 4 Year
> *Arts Areas:* Instrumental Music, Vocal Music, Theatre, Film Arts, Television and Visual Arts
> *Performance Facilities:* Schaller Memorial Chapel

MUSIC

James Hejl, Chairman, Division of Fine Arts   *Number Of Faculty:* 4
Number Of Students: 30   *Degrees Offered:* BA Music
Technical Training: Voice; Piano; Organ; Instrumental & Strings
Teaching Certification Available
Financial Assistance: Scholarships and Work-Study Grants
Performing Groups: Marching & Concert Bands; Jazz Ensemble; A Cappella Choir; Vista Singers;
Buena Vista Dozen

THEATRE

Michael Whitlatch, Director   *Number Of Faculty:* 1   *Number Of Students:* 20
Degrees Offered: BA Drama & Speech   *Technical Training:* Technical Theatre
Teaching Certification Available
Financial Assistance: Scholarships and Work-Study Grants
Performing Groups: Buena Vista Players; Alpha Psi Omega
Workshops/Festivals: Guthrie Theatre Workshops

CENTRAL COLLEGE
Pella   Iowa 50219, 515 628-4151
> Private and 4 Year
> *Arts Areas:* Instrumental Music, Vocal Music, Theatre and Visual Arts
> *Performing Series:* Cultural Affairs Series
> *Performance Facilities:* College Auditorium; Recital Hall; Drama Workshop Arena

MUSIC

Davis L Folkerts, Chairman   *Number Of Faculty:* 7   *Number Of Students:* 40
Degrees Offered: BA
Courses Offered: Music Education Major - Vocal & Instrumental; Applied Music Major
Teaching Certification Available
Financial Assistance: Scholarships and Work-Study Grants
Performing Groups: Symphonic, Wind Ensemble, Marching & Jazz Bands; A Cappella & Concert Choirs;
Madrigal; Swing Choir; Orchestra
Workshops/Festivals: Band Workshop

THEATRE

Robert Schanke, Director   *Number Of Faculty:* 2   *Number Of Students:* 20
Degrees Offered: BA, Technical Theatre or Directing/Acting emphasis
Teaching Certification Available
Financial Assistance: Scholarships and Work-Study Grants
Performing Groups: Three Major Productions; Direction Class Productions; One Student Directed Major
Production; Alpha Psi Omega
Workshops/Festivals: High School Theatre Workshop; Touring Company Performances

CLARKE COLLEGE
Dubuque   Iowa 52001, 319 588-6316
> Private and 4 Year
> *Arts Areas:* Instrumental Music, Vocal Music, Theatre and Visual Arts
> *Performing Series:* Cultural Events Series
> *Performance Facilities:* College Auditorium

(continued on next page)

MUSIC

Sister M Virginia Gaume, Chairman   **Number Of Faculty:** 9
Number Of Students: 50   **Degrees Offered:** BMus; BMusEd
Financial Assistance: Scholarships and Work-Study Grants
Performing Groups: Chorus

THEATRE

Carol Blitzen, Chairman   **Number Of Faculty:** 5   **Number Of Students:** 50
Degrees Offered: BA Drama & Speech
Financial Assistance: Scholarships and Work-Study Grants
Performing Groups: Drama Group

COE COLLEGE
1220 First Ave, NE, Cedar Rapids   Iowa 52402
319 398-1600
Private and 4 Year
Arts Areas: Instrumental Music, Vocal Music and Theatre
Performing Series: Coe Artist Series; Coe Chamber Series
Performance Facilities: Sinclair Auditorium; Daehler - Kitchin Auditorium; Sutherland C Dows Fine Arts Center (two theaters)

MUSIC

Dr Thomas C Slattery, Associate Professor   **Number Of Faculty:** 7
Degrees Offered: BMus
Courses Offered: Applied Music; Music for the Elementary Teacher; Music Fundamentals; Music in America; Black Music in America; Diction for Singers; Theory of Music; Composite Materials; Advanced Counterpoint; Advanced Form & Analysis; Advanced Orchestration; Composition I, II, III; Music History & Literature; Conducting; Music Education: An Introductory Seminar; Elementary & Secondary Vocal & Instrumental Methods; Student Teaching in the Elementary & Secondary School; Advanced Seminar in Music Education
Teaching Certification Available
Financial Assistance: Scholarships and Work-Study Grants
Performing Groups: Concert & Jazz Bands; Madrigal Singers; Women's Concert Chorale; Chamber Orchestra; "College Vocal Show Ensemble"; Chamber Music Ensemble; Baroque Ensemble; Opera Workshop
Workshops/Festivals: Opera Workshop; Cedar Rapids Youth Symphony Orchestra; High School Jazz Festival; Coe Instrumental Festival Iowa Composer's Concert

THEATRE

Dr Michael Pufall, Director   **Number Of Faculty:** 2 Full-time, 2 Part-time
Degrees Offered: BA
Courses Offered: Introduction to Theatre; Theatre Skills Workshop; Fundamentals of Acting I & II; Stagecraft; Costuming; Stage Management/History of Directing; Scene Study I & II; Scene Design; Costume Design; Stage Lighting; Directing I, II, III; Styles of Acting I, II, III, IV; Advanced Projects in Design; Voice & Diction; Stage Movement; Directing IV; Independent Study in Theater
Teaching Certification Available
Financial Assistance: Assistantships, Scholarships and Work-Study Grants

---

DORDT COLLEGE
Sioux Center   Iowa 51250, 712 722-3771
Private and 4 Year
Arts Areas: Instrumental Music, Vocal Music and Theatre

MUSIC

Dale Grotenhuis, Professor   **Number Of Faculty:** 6   **Number Of Students:** 150
Degrees Offered: BA; BA MusED   **Technical Training:** Production & Performance
Teaching Certification Available
Financial Assistance: Scholarships and Work-Study Grants

(continued on next page)

Performing Groups: Concert Choir; Chorale; Concert Band; Stage Band; Brass Choir; Other Small Vocal & Instrumental Ensembles
Workshops/Festivals: Music Education Workshop; Spring Music Festival

THEATRE

James Koldenhoven, Chairman   **Number Of Faculty:** 3   **Number Of Students:** 80
Degrees Offered: AB General, Theatre Arts Major
Technical Training: Production & Performance Directed Experience
Teaching Certification Available
Financial Assistance: Scholarships and Work-Study Grants
Performing Groups: A season of five productions on main stage; Experimental Theatre Productions; Choral Theatre Group
Workshops/Festivals: New World Theatre Consortium

DRAKE UNIVERSITY
Des Moines   Iowa 50311, 515 271-3131
Private and 4 Year
Arts Areas: Dance, Instrumental Music, Vocal Music, Theatre, Film Arts, Television and Visual Arts
Performing Series: University Theatre Series; Summer Dinner Theatre; New Plays Summer Series
Performance Facilities: The Hall of the Performing Arts; Monroe Recital Hall; The Studio Theatre

DANCE

Dance program under auspices of Theatre Department & Women's PE Department

MUSIC

Paul J Jackson, Chairman   **Number Of Faculty:** 30   **Number Of Students:** 225
Degrees Offered: BMus; BMusEd; B Church Mus; MMus; MMusEd; BMus in Applied, Jazz, Theory & Composition; M History; M Business
Technical Training: Private Lessons; Techniques; Counterpoint & Theory
Teaching Certification Available
Financial Assistance: Assistantships, Scholarships and Work-Study Grants
Performing Groups: Symphony Orchestra; Chamber Ensembles; Concert Band; Marching Band; Bulldog Band; Jazz Bands; Choir; Chorus
Workshops/Festivals: The Contemporary Music Symposium; The Jazz Spectacular; Workshops by Sherrill Milnes & Ruth Slenczynska

THEATRE

Gary Hobbs, Chairperson   **Number Of Faculty:** 7   **Number Of Students:** 85
Degrees Offered: B Theatre Arts, Master of Theatre Arts
Technical Training: Acting & Directing Technique; Design; Lighting; Costuming
Teaching Certification Available
Financial Assistance: Assistantships, Scholarships and Work-Study Grants
Performing Groups: Drake University Theatre
Artists-In-Residence/Guest Artists: Sherrill Milnes; Ruth Slenczynska

---

FAITH BAPTIST BIBLE COLLEGE
1900 NW 4th St, Ankeny   Iowa 50021
515 964-0601
Private and 4 Year   **Arts Areas:** Instrumental Music and Vocal Music
Performing Series: Guest Artists; Oratorio Performance; Conference Musicians
Performance Facilities: Convocation Building; Classroom I (recital hall)

MUSIC

Charles B Bergerson, Associate Professor   **Number Of Faculty:** 5
Number Of Students: 622   **Degrees Offered:** BS; BA
Courses Offered: Applied Music; Conducting; Composition

(continued on next page)

Financial Assistance: Scholarships
Performing Groups: Chorale (mixed voices); Ladies' Chorus; Mensingers; Concert Band; Various Small Vocal & Instrumental Groups

GRACELAND COLLEGE
Lamoni   Iowa 50140, 515 784-3311
Private and 4 Year
Arts Areas: Instrumental Music, Vocal Music, Theatre, Film Arts and Visual Arts
Performing Series: Concert - Lecture Series
Performance Facilities: Memorial Student Center; Playshop

MUSIC

Donald Breshears, Associate Professor   *Number Of Faculty:* 6
Number Of Students: 60   *Degrees Offered:* BMusEd; B Mus Performance
Courses Offered: Theory; Literature; History; Methods; Applied Music; Ensemble Music
Teaching Certification Available
Financial Assistance: Scholarships, Work-Study Grants and Student Work Assignments
Performing Groups: Chapel Choir; Concert Choir; Concert Band; Orchestra; Stage Band; Chamber Singers

THEATRE

Celia Schall, Associate Professor   *Number Of Faculty:* 2
Number Of Students: 15   *Degrees Offered:* Theatre & Speech Major
Courses Offered: Acting; Play Production; History; Directing; Performance
Teaching Certification Available
Financial Assistance: Scholarships, Work-Study Grants and Student Work Assignments
Performing Groups: Graceland Players

GRINNELL COLLEGE
Grinnell   Iowa 50112, 515 236-6181
Private and 4 Year
Arts Areas: Instrumental Music, Vocal Music, Theatre and Visual Arts
Performing Series: Concert Series   *Performance Facilities:* College Auditorium

MUSIC

Number Of Faculty: 9   *Number Of Students:* 60   *Degrees Offered:* BMus
Financial Assistance: Scholarships and Work-Study Grants
Performing Groups: Choir; Orchestra   *Workshops/Festivals:* Concert Series

THEATRE

A S Moffett, Chairman   *Number Of Faculty:* 6   *Number Of Students:* 66
Degrees Offered: BA
Financial Assistance: Scholarships and Work-Study Grants
Performing Groups: Theatre Group

IOWA CENTRAL COMMUNITY COLLEGE, EAGLE GROVE
Eagle Grove   Iowa 51334, 515 448-4723
County and 2 Year
Arts Areas: Instrumental Music, Vocal Music and Visual Arts
Degrees Offered: AA   *Financial Assistance:* Scholarships
Performing Groups: Vocal & Instrumental Ensembles

IOWA CENTRAL COMMUNITY COLLEGE, FT DODGE
330 Avenue M, Fort Dodge   Iowa 50501
515 576-7201
County and 2 Year
Arts Areas: Instrumental Music, Vocal Music and Visual Arts
Performance Facilities: College Auditorium

(continued on next page)

MUSIC

J Eugene McKinely, Chairman   **Degrees Offered:** AA
Courses Offered: Transfer Program
Performing Groups: Instrumental & Vocal Ensembles

IOWA LAKES COMMUNITY COLLEGE
300 S 18th, Estherville   Iowa 51334
712 362-2604
2 Year and Area
Arts Areas: Dance, Instrumental Music, Vocal Music, Theatre and Visual Arts
Performance Facilities: Auditorium; Music Performance Room

DANCE

Number Of Faculty: 1 Part-time   **Number Of Students:** 10
Courses Offered: Introduction to Dance   **Number Of Faculty:** 2

MUSIC

Number Of Students: 12   **Degrees Offered:** AA
Courses Offered: Music Education & Performance; Transfer General Education Courses
Technical Training: Ensemble & Studio
Financial Assistance: Scholarships and Work-Study Grants
Performing Groups: Jazz Ensemble; Concert Band; Madrigal; Choir
Workshops/Festivals: Jazz Festival; Swing Choir Festival; Directors' Workshop

THEATRE

Number Of Faculty: 1   **Number Of Students:** 10   **Degrees Offered:** AA
Courses Offered: Play Production; Speech Activities, Humanities
Financial Assistance: Scholarships and Work-Study Grants
Workshops/Festivals: Musical Production

IOWA STATE UNIVERSITY
Ames   Iowa 50011, 515 294-4111
State and 4 Year
Arts Areas: Dance, Instrumental Music, Vocal Music, Theatre and Visual Arts
Performing Series: Music Council Series
Performance Facilities: C Y Stephens Auditorium; Fisher Theater; Schenman Auditorium

DANCE

Betty Toman, Director   **Number Of Faculty:** 3½   **Number Of Students:** 500
Degrees Offered: BS in Physical Education with emphasis in Dance; BS Non-certification dance option
Courses Offered: Modern; Jazz; Ballet; Social; Folk; Square; Dance Composition; Sound & Movement;
History & Philosophy of Dance; Dance Appreciation; Concert & Theater Dance; Methods of Teaching all
forms of Dance
Teaching Certification Available   **Financial Assistance:** Scholarships
Performing Groups: Orchesis I & II; ISU Tour Company
Workshops/Festivals: Barjche (annual student dance production)

MUSIC

Arthur G Swift, Head   **Number Of Faculty:** 24   **Number Of Students:** 2,000
Degrees Offered: BA; BMus
Courses Offered: History; Theory; Appreciation; Applied; Teaching Methods; Large performing groups
(band, orchestra, choral)
Teaching Certification Available
Financial Assistance: Assistantships, Scholarships and Work-Study Grants

(continued on next page)

Performing Groups: Wind Ensemble; Concert & Marching Band; Jazz Ensemble; Symphony Orchestra; Musica Antiqua; ISU Singers; Oratorio Chorus; University Chorus; Chamber Singers; Cardinal Keynotes; Various Wind, String, & Percussion Ensembles
Workshops/Festivals: American Orff Schulwerk; Kodaly Institute; Comprehensive Musicianship; Ames International Orchestra Festival

THEATRE

Patrick D Gouran, Director   *Number Of Faculty:* 9   *Number Of Students:* 150
Degrees Offered: BA; BS
Courses Offered: Acting; Directing; Lighting; Design; Makeup; Costuming
Teaching Certification Available
Financial Assistance: Assistantships, Scholarships and Work-Study Grants
Performing Groups: Iowa State Players
Workshops/Festivals: Drama Workshops - Travels the State of Iowa

IOWA WESLEYAN COLLEGE
N Main, Mt Pleasant   Iowa 52641
319 385-8021

Private and 4 Year
Arts Areas: Instrumental Music, Vocal Music, Theatre and Visual Arts
Performing Series: Performing Arts Series
Performance Facilities: College Chapel - Auditorium

MUSIC

Burton P Mahle, Head   *Number Of Faculty:* 4   *Number Of Students:* 30
Degrees Offered: BMusEd; BA; AFA
Courses Offered: Teaching Degree Courses; Church Music; Applied Majors
Teaching Certification Available   *Financial Assistance:* Scholarships
Performing Groups: Southeast Iowa Symphony Orchestra; A Cappella Choir; Jazz Band; Wind Ensemble; Pep Band; Madrigal Singers; Motet Choir
Workshops/Festivals: Robert Pace Piano Pedagogy Workshop

THEATRE

David File, Instructor   *Number Of Faculty:* 1   *Degrees Offered:* BA
Teaching Certification Available   *Financial Assistance:* Scholarships
Artists-In-Residence/Guest Artists: Charles Hiz; Gary Pedersen

KIRKWOOD COMMUNITY COLLEGE
Box 2068, Cedar Rapids   Iowa 52405
319 398-5533

County and 2 Year   *Arts Areas:* Instrumental Music and Vocal Music

MUSIC

Charles E Traylor, Head, Fine Arts Department   *Number Of Faculty:* 2
Number Of Students: 23   *Degrees Offered:* AA
Courses Offered: Applied Vocal; Applied Instrumental; Theory; Choir; Ensemble; Band
Permanent Staff: Elgen Shea   *Financial Assistance:* Work-Study Grants
Performing Groups: Choir; Band; Ensemble
Workshops/Festivals: Iowa Community College Choir Festival

LORAS COLLEGE
1450 Alta Visa, Dubuque   Iowa 52001
319 588-7100

Private and 4 Year
Arts Areas: Instrumental Music, Vocal Music, Theatre and Visual Arts
Performing Series: Concert - Lecture Series

(continued on next page)

MUSIC

J C Colaluca, Chairman   **Number Of Faculty:** 4   **Number Of Students:** 40
Degrees Offered: BMus   **Teaching Certification Available**
Financial Assistance: Scholarships and Work-Study Grants
Performing Groups: Chamber Groups; Choir; Band

THEATRE

Donald W Stribling, Chairman   **Number Of Faculty:** 3
Number Of Students: 35   **Degrees Offered:** BA
Teaching Certification Available
Financial Assistance: Scholarships and Work-Study Grants
Performing Groups: Loras Players

LUTHER COLLEGE
Decorah   Iowa 52101, 319 387-2000
Private and 4 Year
Arts Areas: Instrumental Music, Vocal Music, Theatre and Visual Arts
Performing Series: Community Concerts Series
Performance Facilities: Luther College Field House; Luther College Center for Faith & Life

DANCE

Robert J Larson, Head   **Number Of Faculty:** 1
Courses Offered: Basic beginning & intermediate courses in Modern Dance
Financial Assistance: Work-Study Grants   **Performing Groups:** Orchesis
Workshops/Festivals: Involvement with the dance touring program of the National Endowment for the Humanities

MUSIC

Maurice Monhardt, Professor   **Number Of Faculty:** 16 Full-time, 7 Part-time
Number Of Students: 342   **Degrees Offered:** BA
Courses Offered: Theory; Ear Training; Music Literature; History; Conducting; Church Music; Opera; Twentieth Century Music; Special Topics by Independent Study
Technical Training: Methods in Applied Areas; Piano Tuning; Opera - Technical
Teaching Certification Available
Financial Assistance: Scholarships and Work-Study Grants
Performing Groups: Brass Choir; Collegium Musicum; Concert Band; Lerka; Jazz Lab Band; Nordic Choir; Oratorio Chorus; Orchestra; Varsity Band; Women's Chorale
Workshops/Festivals: Junior High Vocal Workshop; Voice Workshop; Opera Workshop; Piano Workshop; Dorian Keyboard Festival; Dorian Band Festival; Dorian Vocal Festival; Dorian Orchestra Festival; Dorian Summer Camp

THEATRE

Robert J Larson, Assistant Professor of Speech & Theatre
Number Of Faculty: 2   **Number Of Students:** 30
Degrees Offered: BA in Theatre
Courses Offered: Acting; Directing; Scene & Costume Design; History; Oral Interpretation; Makeup; Stagecraft; Introduction to Theatre
Technical Training: Work on various college theatre productions
Teaching Certification Available
Financial Assistance: Scholarships and Work-Study Grants
Performing Groups: Tatterstage Players; Inter-campus Repertory; The Oneota Players
Workshops/Festivals: Workshops in Dance/Movement; Summer Theatre Workshops for High School Students

MARYCREST COLLEGE
1607 W 12th St, Davenport   Iowa 52804
319 326-9512

Private and 4 Year
Arts Areas: Dance, Instrumental Music, Vocal Music, Theatre, Film Arts, Television and Visual Arts
Performance Facilities: Marycrest College Theatre

DANCE

Betty Dalton, Chairman   *Number Of Faculty:* 2
Financial Assistance: Scholarships and Work-Study Grants
Performing Groups: Orchesis

MUSIC

Robert Farris, Chairman   *Number Of Faculty:* 4   *Number Of Students:* 35
Degrees Offered: BA   *Teaching Certification Available*
Financial Assistance: Scholarships and Work-Study Grants
Performing Groups: College Choir; MC Chamber Singers; Instrumental Ensembles
Workshops/Festivals: Jazz Band Festival; Opera Workshop

THEATRE

Leslie Schimelpfenig, Chairman   *Number Of Faculty:* 3
Number Of Students: 22   *Degrees Offered:* BA
Teaching Certification Available
Financial Assistance: Scholarships and Work-Study Grants
Performing Groups: MC Theatre; MC Children's Theatre; MC Musical Theatre

MORNINGSIDE COLLEGE
1501 Morningside Ave, Sioux City   Iowa 51106
712 277-5821

Private and 4 Year
Arts Areas: Instrumental Music, Vocal Music, Theatre, Film Arts and Radio
Performing Series: Summer Dinner Theater Series
Performance Facilities: Klinger - Neal Theatre; Eppley Auditorium

MUSIC

Dr Lawrence DeWitt, Associate Professor   *Number Of Faculty:* 10
Number Of Students: 130   *Degrees Offered:* BMusEd; BMus; BA
Teaching Certification Available
Financial Assistance: Scholarships and Work-Study Grants
Performing Groups: Faculty Trio
Workshops/Festivals: Annual Junior High Music Camp; Annual Senior High Music Camp; Jazz Festival

THEATRE

Dr Fred Phelps, Chairman, Speech, Drama & Mass Communications
Number Of Faculty: 4   *Number Of Students:* 70   *Degrees Offered:* BA
Teaching Certification Available
Financial Assistance: Scholarships and Work-Study Grants
Performing Groups: Morningside College Players
Workshops/Festivals: Annual High School Speech Contest; Guest Professional Artist Visit; Summer Theater Workshop (Dinner Theater Series)

MOUNT SAINT CLARE COLLEGE
Bluff Blvd at Springdale Dr, Clinton   Iowa 52732
319 242-4023

Private and 2 Year
Arts Areas: Instrumental Music, Vocal Music and Visual Arts
Performance Facilities: College Theater

(continued on next page)

MUSIC

S Judith McKenna, Chairman   **Number Of Faculty:** 2   **Number Of Students:** 6
Degrees Offered: AA
Courses Offered: Music Theory; Ear Training & Sight Singing; Applied Music; Chorus; Music Appreciation

THEATRE

M H Mullany, Chairman   **Number Of Faculty:** 2   **Number Of Students:** 20
Degrees Offered: AA Drama & Speech
Performing Groups: Players; Delta Psi Omega

NORTH IOWA AREA COMMUNITY COLLEGE
500 College Dr, Mason City   Iowa 50401
515 423-1264
Private and 2 Year
Arts Areas: Instrumental Music, Vocal Music, Theatre and Visual Arts
Performance Facilities College Auditorium   **Degrees Offered:** AA Music, Speech/Theatre
Courses Offered: Transfer Programs

UNIVERSITY OF NORTHERN IOWA
Cedar Falls   Iowa 50613, 319 273-2761
State and 4 Year
Arts Areas: Instrumental Music, Vocal Music, Theatre, Film Arts, Television and Visual Arts
Performing Series: Artist Series; Chamber Music Series
Performance Facilities: University Auditorium; Russell Hall; Strayer-Wood Theatre; UNI-Dome; University Hall

MUSIC

Dr Ronald D Ross, Head   **Number Of Faculty:** 38   **Number Of Students:** 325
Degrees Offered: BMus; BA; BFA; MMus; MA   **Teaching Certification Available**
Financial Assistance: Assistantships, Scholarships and Work-Study Grants
Performing Groups: Music Theater; Concert Chorale; Women's Chorus; University Chorus; Chamber Choir; Varsity Men's Glee Club; Wind Ensemble; Symphonic Band; Jazz Band; Orchestra; Percussion Ensemble; String Ensemble Tuba - Euphonium Ensemble; Harp Ensemble
Workshops/Festivals: Summer Music Camp; Summer Opera Workshop; Tallcorn Conferences (for High School Student) (1) Strings & Harp, (2) Stage Band, (3) Band, (4) Vocal/Piano, (5) Music Theater

THEATRE

Dr D Terry Williams, Director   **Number Of Faculty:** 7
Number Of Students: 70   **Degrees Offered:** BA Teaching; BA Liberal Arts; MA
Teaching Certification Available
Financial Assistance: Assistantships, Scholarships and Work-Study Grants
Performing Groups: Theatre UNI produces five major productions during school year and three in summer repertory
Workshops/Festivals: High School Drama Workshops

NORTHWESTERN COLLEGE
Orange City   Iowa 51041, 712 737-4821 Ext 69
Private and 4 Year
Arts Areas: Dance, Instrumental Music, Vocal Music, Theatre and Visual Arts
Performance Facilities: The Playhouse   **Courses Offered:** Ballet; Modern Dance

MUSIC

Dr Rodney Jiskoot, Chairman   **Number Of Faculty:** 7   **Number Of Students:** 36
Degrees Offered: BA   **Financial Assistance:** Scholarships and Work-Study Grants
Performing Groups: Band; Orchestra; Concert Choir; Chapel Choir; Heritage Singers; Chamber Opera; Stage Band
Workshops/Festivals: Piano Workshop; Voice Workshop; Instrumental Workshop; CMA Band Festival

(continued on next page)

THEATRE

Number Of Faculty: 2   **Number Of Students:** 15   **Degrees Offered:** BA
Teaching Certification Available
Financial Assistance: Scholarships and Work-Study Grants
Performing Groups: Choral Readers
Workshops/Festivals: Oral Interpretation Festival; Mime Workshop; Voice & Movements Workshop

OTTUMWA HEIGHTS COLLEGE
Grandview at Elm St, Ottumwa   Iowa 52501
515 682-4551
Private and 2 Year
Arts Areas: Dance, Instrumental Music, Vocal Music, Theatre and Visual Arts
Performance Facilities: Ottumwa Heights Auditorium

DANCE

Ms Mace, Chairman   **Number Of Faculty:** 1   **Number Of Students:** 30
Degrees Offered: AA
Financial Assistance: Internships, Scholarships and Work-Study Grants

MUSIC

John Bowitz, Chairman   **Number Of Faculty:** 5   **Number Of Students:** 100
Degrees Offered: AA
Financial Assistance: Internships, Scholarships and Work-Study Grants

THEATRE

R Spero, Chairman   **Number Of Faculty:** 1   **Number Of Students:** 25
Degrees Offered: AA
Financial Assistance: Internships, Scholarships and Work-Study Grants

SAINT AMBROSE COLLEGE
518 W Locust St, Davenport   Iowa 52803
319 324-1681
Private and 4 Year
Arts Areas: Instrumental Music, Vocal Music, Theatre and Visual Arts
Performance Facilities: Alleart Theatre; Galvin Fine Arts Center

MUSIC

Fr James Greene, Chairman   **Number Of Faculty:** 5   **Number Of Students:** 70
Degrees Offered: BMus; BMusEd   **Teaching Certification Available**
Financial Assistance: Scholarships and Work-Study Grants
Performing Groups: Choir

THEATRE

Michael Kennedy, Chairman   **Number Of Faculty:** 4   **Number Of Students:** 60
Degrees Offered: Drama & Speech   **Teaching Certification Available**
Financial Assistance: Scholarships and Work-Study Grants
Performing Groups: Theatre Three Players
Workshops/Festivals: Summer Repertory Theatre
Affilate of Iowa Arts Council; Quad Cities Arts Council; Illinois Arts Council

SIMPSON COLLEGE
Indianola   Iowa 50125, 515 961-6251
Private and 4 Year
Arts Areas: Instrumental Music, Vocal Music and Theatre
Performing Series: Guest Artist Series
Performance Facilities: The A H & Theo Blank Performing Arts Center

(continued on next page)

MUSIC

Robert L Larsen, DM, Head   **Number Of Faculty:** 9   **Number Of Students:** 95
Degrees Offered: BA; BMus
Courses Offered: Music Theory & History; Performance; Music Education; Applied Music
Technical Training: Renaissance Music; Opera
Teaching Certification Available
Financial Assistance: Scholarships, Work-Study Grants and Performance Merit Awards given for quality auditions
Performing Groups: Opera Theatre; Madrigal Singers; College Choir; Band; Small Instrumental Ensembles
Workshops/Festivals: Madrigal Clinic; Opera Workshop

THEATRE

W Keith Leonard, MA, Head, Department of Theatre Arts/Speech Communication
Number Of Faculty: 4   **Number Of Students:** 55   **Degrees Offered:** BA
Courses Offered: Dramatic Theory; History; Literature - Criticism; Directing; Design; Scene Lighting; Stage Production; Costuming; Forensics
Technical Training: Scenic Production; Lighting; Design; Costuming; Stagecraft; Prop Construction; Drafting; Oral Interpretation
Teaching Certification Available
Financial Assistance: Scholarships, Work-Study Grants and Performance Merit Awards given for quality auditions
Performing Groups: Theatre Simpson; Improv Acting Company; Children's Theatre; Dinner Theatre; Readers' Theatre
Workshops/Festivals: Alpha Psi High School Workshop; Performing Arts in Worship Workshop
Artists-In-Residence/Guest Artists: Michael Carson; Maruxa Vialta; James Avery; Marian Barnum

---

UNIVERSITY OF DUBUQUE
Dubuque   Iowa 52001, 301 557-2241
Private and 4 Year
Arts Areas: Instrumental Music, Vocal Music and Theatre
Performing Series: Concert - Lecture Series
Performance Facilities: University Auditorium   **Number Of Faculty:** 5
Number Of Students: 50   **Degrees Offered:** BMus; BMusEd; BMus Applied
Financial Assistance: Scholarships and Work-Study Grants
Performing Groups: Band; Orchestra

THEATRE

Raymond L Thompson, Chairman   **Number Of Faculty:** 3   **Number Of Students:** 5
Degrees Offered: BA Drama & Speech
Financial Assistance: Scholarships and Work-Study Grants
Performing Groups: University Theatre

THE UNIVERSITY OF IOWA
Iowa City   Iowa 52242, 319 353-2121
State and 4 Year
Arts Areas: Dance, Instrumental Music, Vocal Music, Theatre, Film Arts, Television and Visual Arts
Performing Series: Concert, Variety, Dance, Chamber Music, Piano, and Guitar Series; Young People's Concerts
Performance Facilities: Virgil M Hancher Auditorium; Clapp Recital Hall; Harper Hall; E C Mabie Theatre; Studio Theatre

DANCE

Judith Allen, Chairman   **Number Of Faculty:** 6   **Number Of Students:** 38
Degrees Offered: BA Dance; MA Dance
Courses Offered: Modern Dance; Ballet; Jazz; Pointe; History & Appreciation; Techniques; Movement; Pedagogy; Choreography; Labanotation; Dance Therapy
Teaching Certification Available
Financial Assistance: Assistantships and Scholarships

(*continued on next page*)

Performing Groups: University of Iowa Dance Company
Workshops/Festivals: Iowa Dance Council Workshop

MUSIC

Himie Voxman, Chairman   **Number Of Faculty:** 50   **Number Of Students:** 589
Degrees Offered: BA; BMus; MA; MFA; PhD; DMA
Courses Offered: Theory; Composition; History & Musicology; Sacred Music; Research & Literature; Music Ed; Applied Music; Ensemble
Teaching Certification Available
Financial Assistance: Assistantships, Scholarships and Work-Study Grants
Performing Groups: University Symphony; Symphony Band; Sinfonietta; Stradivari Quartet; Brass Quintet; Woodwind Quintet; Baroque Players; Oratorio Chorus; Opera Theater; Collegium Musicum; Woodwind Ensemble; Concert Band; Marching Band; Percussion Ensemble; Jazz/Stage Bands; Camerata Singers; University Choir; Kantorei
Workshops/Festivals: Music Education Workshops; Music Camp; Choral Clinic

THEATRE

Samuel Becker, Head, Department of Speech & Dramatic Arts
Number Of Faculty: 10   **Number Of Students:** 150
Degrees Offered: BA; MA; MFA; PhD
Courses Offered: Acting; Directing; Playwriting; Set Design; Lighting; Costumes; Technical Direction; Arts Management
Teaching Certification Available
Financial Assistance: Assistantships, Scholarships and Work-Study Grants
Performing Groups: Playwright's Ensemble; Readers' Theatre
Workshops/Festivals: High School Drama Conference; Critics Week; High School Teachers' Institute

---

UPPER IOWA UNIVERSITY
Fayette   Iowa 52142, 319 425-3311
Private and 4 Year
Arts Areas: Instrumental Music, Vocal Music, Theatre and Visual Arts
Performing Series: Artist Series

MUSIC

Dennis J Smith, Chairman   **Number Of Faculty:** 4   **Number Of Students:** 60
Degrees Offered: BMus   **Teaching Certification Available**
Financial Assistance: Scholarships and Work-Study Grants

THEATRE

Adrian Harris, Chairman   **Number Of Faculty:** 3   **Number Of Students:** 50
Degrees Offered: BA   **Teaching Certification Available**
Financial Assistance: Scholarships and Work-Study Grants
Performing Groups: University Players

WALDORF COLLEGE
Forest City   Iowa 50436, 515 582-2450 Ext 230
Private and 2 Year
Arts Areas: Instrumental Music, Vocal Music and Theatre
Performing Series: Christmas Concert; Large Group Tours
Performance Facilities: Civic Auditorium

MUSIC

Adrian Johnson, Chairman   **Number Of Faculty:** 4   **Number Of Students:** 25
Degrees Offered: AA
Courses Offered: Theory; Applied; Appreciation; Fundamentals of Music
Financial Assistance: Scholarships and Work-Study Grants
Performing Groups: Concert Choir; Concert Band; New World Singers; Minikor; Brass and other Ensembles
Workshops/Festivals: Clinic for High School Students; Piano Workshop

(continued on next page)

THEATRE

Ken Hansen, Director   **Number Of Faculty:** 1   **Number Of Students:** 11
Degrees Offered: AA   **Courses Offered:** Introduction to Theatre
Financial Assistance: Scholarships and Work-Study Grants

WARTBURG COLLEGE
Waverly   Iowa 50677, 319 352-1200
Private and 4 Year
Arts Areas: Dance, Instrumental Music, Vocal Music, Theatre, Film Arts and Visual Arts
Performing Series: Artist Series; Organizational and Individual Concerts and Recitals
Performance Facilities: Liemohn Hall of Music; Neumann Auditorium; Players Theatre

DANCE

Dance program under the auspices of the Physical Education Department

MUSIC

Dr Warren Schmidt, Chairman   **Number Of Faculty:** 11
Number Of Students: 122   **Degrees Offered:** BA; BMus; BMusEd
Courses Offered: Theory; History; Composition; Music Education; Conduction; Music Therapy; Applied Music; Private Instruction; Supervised Teaching; Performance in Piano, Organ, Voice, Instruments
Teaching Certification Available
Financial Assistance: Scholarships, Work-Study Grants and Loans
Performing Groups: Castle Singers; College Band; Community Symphony Orchestra; Chamber Orchestra; Chamber Choir; College Choir
Workshops/Festivals: Meistersinger Workshops (Five during year); Summer Music Camp

THEATRE

Joyce Birkland, Instructor in Speech & Drama   **Number Of Faculty:** 1
Number Of Students: 45   **Degrees Offered:** BA
Courses Offered: Oral Interpretation; Stagecraft; Acting; Direction; Studies in Contemporary Theatre
Technical Training: Theatre Practicum   **Teaching Certification Available**
Financial Assistance: Scholarships, Work-Study Grants and Loans
Performing Groups: Touring Theatre; Wartburg Players

WESTMAR COLLEGE
1002 Third Ave SE, Le Mars   Iowa 51031
712 546-7081
Private and 4 Year
Arts Areas: Instrumental Music, Vocal Music, Theatre and Visual Arts

MUSIC

Frank N Summerside, Chairman   **Number Of Faculty:** 6
Number Of Students: 90   **Degrees Offered:** BMus
Teaching Certification Available
Financial Assistance: Scholarships and Work-Study Grants
Performing Groups: Band; Chamber Ensembles; Choir

THEATRE

James Fletcher, Chairman   **Number Of Faculty:** 3   **Number Of Students:** 50
Degrees Offered: BA   **Teaching Certification Available**
Financial Assistance: Scholarships and Work-Study Grants
Performing Groups: College Theatre

ALLEN COUNTY COMMUNITY JUNIOR COLLEGE
1801 W Cottonwood, Iola   Kansas 66749
316 365-5116
> County and 2 Year
> **Arts Areas:** Instrumental Music, Vocal Music and Visual Arts
> **Performing Series:** Concert - Lecture Series   **Degrees Offered:** AA Music
> **Performing Groups:** Instrumental & Vocal Ensembles

BAKER UNIVERSITY
606 Eighth St, Baldwin City   Kansas 66006
913 594-6451
> Private and 4 Year
> **Arts Areas:** Instrumental Music, Vocal Music and Visual Arts
> **Performing Series:** Concert Series
> **Performance Facilities:** Baker University Theatre

MUSIC

William C Rice, Chairman   **Number Of Faculty:** 8   **Number Of Students:** 176
Degrees Offered: BMus; BMusEd   **Technical Training:** Opera
Teaching Certification Available
Financial Assistance: Scholarships and Work-Study Grants
Performing Groups: Opera Theatre; Orchestra; Chorale Ensembles; Instrumental Ensembles
Workshops/Festivals: Opera Workshop

THEATRE

Thelma R Morreale, Chairman   **Number Of Faculty:** 1   **Number Of Students:** 25
Degrees Offered: BA   **Teaching Certification Available**
Financial Assistance: Scholarships and Work-Study Grants
Performing Groups: Alpha Psi Omega; Baker Players

BARTON COUNTY COMMUNITY COLLEGE
RR 1, Great Bend   Kansas 67530
316 792-2701
> County and 2 Year
> **Arts Areas:** Instrumental Music, Vocal Music, Theatre, Television and Visual Arts
> **Performing Series:** Winter Concert; Spring Concert; Fine Arts Week; Artist & Lecture Series
> **Performance Facilities:** Fine Arts Auditorium; Little Theatre

MUSIC

J B Webster, Instructor   **Number Of Faculty:** 4   **Number Of Students:** 50
Degrees Offered: AA Music
Courses Offered: Harmony; Aural Skills I - IV; Music Literature; Sight Singing I - IV; Chorus; Band; Pep Band; Jazz Improvisation I - IV; Voice; Piano; Organ
Financial Assistance: Scholarships and Work-Study Grants
Performing Groups: Hilltop Singers; Community Orchestra; Pep Band; Jazz Ensemble
Workshops/Festivals: Fine Arts Week; Area High School Festivals & Clinics; Winter Concert; Spring Concert

THEATRE

Mary Misegadis, Instructor   **Number Of Faculty:** 2   **Number Of Students:** 25
Degrees Offered: AA Speech & Drama
Courses Offered: Introduction to Theatre; Acting I & II; Play Production Character Acting; Creative Dramatics
Financial Assistance: Scholarships and Work-Study Grants
Performing Groups: Barton Players
Workshops/Festivals: Area High School Speech & Drama Festivals; Fine Arts Week

BENEDICTINE COLLEGE
Second & Division Sts, Atchison Kansas 66002
913 367-5340

Private and 4 Year
Arts Areas: Dance, Instrumental Music, Vocal Music, Theatre, Television and Visual Arts
Performance Facilities: Benedictine College Auditorium; Little Theatre; Experimental Theatre; Presbyterian Community Theatre
Courses Offered: Beginning & Intermediate Modern Dance; Folk, Social & Square Dancing
Performing Groups: Terpsichore

MUSIC

Sister Joachin Holtaus, Chairman **Number Of Faculty:** 8
Number Of Students: 100 **Degrees Offered:** BA; BMusEd; BMus; BA Mus Marketing
Courses Offered: Harmonic Theory; Sight Singing & Ear Training; Form & Analysis; Counterpoint; Orchestration; Composition; Understanding Music; Survey of Music Literature; History of Music; String, Woodwind, Brass & Percussion Instruments; Voice & Choral Methods; Elementary Music Methods for the Classroom Teacher; Conducting; Violin, Cello, Voice Methods & Repertoire; Music Methods for the Elementary School; Piano Methods & Repertoire; Organ Methods & Repetoire; Secondary Curriculum, Media & Methods; Diction for Singers; Harp; String Bass; Viola; Violoncello; Piano; Organ; Voice; Violin; Brass & Woodwind; Guitar
Teaching Certification Available
Financial Assistance: Scholarships, Work-Study Grants and Tuition Grants; Achievement Awards
Performing Groups: Orchestra; Chamber Singers; Concert Chorale; Chamber Groups; Faculty Instrumental Trio; Faculty Piano Duo; Church Choir
Workshops/Festivals: Atchison Communtiy Concerts; Student Faculty Concerts

THEATRE

Doug McKenzie, Chairman **Number Of Faculty:** 2 **Number Of Students:** 23
Degrees Offered: BA
Courses Offered: Introduction to the Theatre; Technical Theatre Workshop; Acting Workshop; Creative Dramatics for Elementary Teachers; Oral Communication; Oral Interpretation; Voice & Diction; Reader's Theatre; Techniques of Acting; Stagecraft; Scene Design; Shakespeare; Stage Lighting & Properties; Stage Makeup; Stage Costuming; Principles of Acting; Television Workshop; Public Speaking; New York Theatre; Classic, Medieval, & Renaissance Theatre; Restoration: 18th & 19th Century Theatre; Modern Theatre; Contemporary & Avant - Garde Theatre; Secondary School Theatre; Play Direction; Theatre Practicum
Teaching Certification Available
Financial Assistance: Scholarships, Work-Study Grants and Tuition Grants; Achievement Awards
Performing Groups: Twin Campus Players - associated with Atchison Community Theatre
Workshops/Festivals: Annual Workshop
Artists-In-Residence/Guest Artists: Bhasker Dance Troupe

BETHANY COLLEGE
Box 111, Lindsborg Kansas 67456
913 227-3312

Private and 4 Year
Arts Areas: Instrumental Music, Vocal Music and Visual Arts
Performing Series: Concert - Lecture Series
Performance Facilities: Presser Auditorium; Burnett Center

MUSIC

Elmer Copley, Chairman **Number Of Faculty:** 10 **Number Of Students:** 150
Degrees Offered: BA **Teaching Certification Available**
Financial Assistance: Scholarships and Work-Study Grants
Performing Groups: College - Community Symphony Orchestra; Chorus; Chamber Orchestra; Symphonic Band; Stage Band
Workshops/Festivals: General Messiah Week Festival; Bach's "St Matthew Passion" annually

(continued on next page)

THEATRE

Piet Knetsch, Chairman   **Number Of Faculty:** 1   **Number Of Students:** 40
Degrees Offered: BA
Financial Assistance: Scholarships and Work-Study Grants
Performing Groups: Alpha Psi Omega; Bethany Players

BETHEL COLLEGE
North Newton   Kansas 67117, 316 283-2500
Private and 4 Year
Arts Areas: Instrumental Music, Vocal Music, Theatre and Visual Arts
Performance Facilities: Fine Arts Center

MUSIC

J Harold Moyer, Chairman   **Number Of Faculty:** 8   **Number Of Students:** 40
Degrees Offered: AB
Courses Offered: Music Performance; Theory; History; Education
Teaching Certification Available
Financial Assistance: Assistantships, Scholarships and Work-Study Grants
Performing Groups: College Choir; Ensemble Singers; Oratorio Chorus; Wind Ensemble; Orchestra; Jazz Band; Madrigals; Pops Singers
Workshops/Festivals: Opera Workshop each spring

THEATRE

Arlo Kasper, Chairman   **Number Of Faculty:** 3   **Number Of Students:** 20
Degrees Offered: AB
Courses Offered: Acting; Theater Practice; Costume & Stage Design; Mime; Directing; History
Teaching Certification Available
Financial Assistance: Assistantships, Scholarships and Work-Study Grants
Workshops/Festivals: Summer Community Theater

BUTLER COUNTY COMMUNITY JUNIOR COLLEGE
El Dorado   Kansas 67042, 316 321-5083
County and 2 Year
Arts Areas: Instrumental Music, Vocal Music, Theatre and Visual Arts
Performance Facilities: College Auditorium

MUSIC

Robert Chism, Chairman   **Number Of Faculty:** 3   **Number Of Students:** 70
Degrees Offered: AA Music   **Technical Training:** Opera
Financial Assistance: Work-Study Grants
Performing Groups: Vocal & Instrumental Ensembles

THEATRE

Number Of Faculty: 1   **Number Of Students:** 25   **Degrees Offered:** AA Drama
Performing Groups: Drama Fraternity

CENTRAL COLLEGE
McPherson   Kansas 67460, 316 241-0723
Private and 2 Year
Arts Areas: Instrumental Music, Vocal Music and Visual Arts
Performance Facilities: Pyle Chapel

MUSIC

Tom Walker, Chairman   **Number Of Faculty:** 3   **Degrees Offered:** AA; AGS
Courses Offered: Fundamentals of Music; Music Appreciation; Seminar in Church Music; Elementary School Music; Voice; Piano; Organ; Orchestral Instruments
Technical Training: Music Theory; Survey Musical Thought; Percussion Techniques; Basic Conducting; Applied Music; Music Ensembles
Financial Assistance: Scholarships and Work-Study Grants

(*continued on next page*)

Performing Groups: Choir; Band; Piano Ensemble; Chorale; String Ensemble; Three small performing vocal groups (Joyful Praise, Heartsong, Brighter Day); The Living Faith (Summer traveling team)
Workshops/Festivals: Band Festival; Trombone Workshop
Artists-In-Residence/Guest Artists: Salvador Estrada

CLOUD COUNTY COMMUNITY COLLEGE
2221 Campus Dr, Concordia   Kansas 66901
913 243-1435
County and 2 Year
Arts Areas: Instrumental Music, Vocal Music and Theatre
Performance Facilities: College Auditorium

MUSIC

Everett Miller, Chairman   **Number Of Faculty:** 3
Degrees Offered: AA Music, Drama, Music Education
Courses Offered: Theory & Applied Music Courses
Financial Assistance: Scholarships, Work-Study Grants and BEOG
Performing Groups: Jazz Instrumental Group "Jazz '78"; The Great Society (Select Vocal Group)
Workshops/Festivals: Youth for Music (Regional, County Vocal & Instrumental Groups

THEATRE

Mrs Peggy Doyen, Chairman   **Number Of Faculty:** 2
Degrees Offered: AA Drama
Courses Offered: Introduction Courses; Acting I & II; Play Production
Financial Assistance: Scholarships, Work-Study Grants and BEOG
Performing Groups: CCCC Players

COFFEYVILLE COMMUNITY JUNIOR COLLEGE
11th & Willow, Coffeyville   Kansas 67337
316 251-7700 Ext 47
City and 2 Year
Arts Areas: Instrumental Music, Vocal Music, Theatre, Television and Visual Arts
Performance Facilities: Auditorium

MUSIC

James Criswell, Director of Instrumental Music   **Number Of Faculty:** 4
Number Of Students: 200   **Degrees Offered:** AA
Courses Offered: Band; Stage; Jazz Band; All Instruments; Comprehensive Musicanship; Vocal
Financial Assistance: Scholarships and Work-Study Grants
Performing Groups: Marching & Stage Jazz Bands; Concert Choir; Collegiates (small jazz vocal)
Workshops/Festivals: Stage Band Workshop; Marching Band Workshop

THEATRE

Kenneth H Burchinal, Director   **Number Of Faculty:** 1
Number Of Students: 75   **Degrees Offered:** AA
Courses Offered: Acting; Stage Production; History of Theatre
Technical Training: Theatre Scenery
Financial Assistance: Scholarships and Work-Study Grants
Workshops/Festivals: Workshop in Movement; Technique; Lighting; National Shakespeare Company
Artists-In-Residence/Guest Artists: Jack Carraher

COLBY COMMUNITY COLLEGE
1255 S Range, Colby   Kansas 67701
913 462-3984 Ext 222
County and 2 Year
Arts Areas: Instrumental Music, Vocal Music, Theatre, Television and Visual Arts
Performing Series: Western Plains Arts Council Series (co-sponsor)
Performance Facilities: Northwest Kansas Cultural Arts Center Theater; Robert Burnett Memorial Student Union

(continued on next page)

MUSIC

Number Of Faculty: 3   **Number Of Students:** 50   **Degrees Offered:** AA
Courses Offered: Introduction to Music; Recital Attendance, Music Literature; Harmony; Ear Training; Chorus; Concert Band; Voice; Chorale; Jazz Ensemble; Pep Band; Barbershop Chorus; Instrumental Ensemble; Applied Music
Financial Assistance: Scholarships, Work-Study Grants and Federal Grants
Performing Groups: College Choir, Sunflower Singers, Barbershop Chorus; Concert Band, Jazz Ensemble, Pep Band, Dixieland Band

THEATRE

Number Of Faculty: 2   **Number Of Students:** 15   **Degrees Offered:** AA
Courses Offered: Oral Interpretation; Introduction to Theatre
Technical Training: Performance; Stagecraft; Makeup; Theatre Practicum
Financial Assistance: Scholarships, Work-Study Grants and Student Grants
Performing Groups: Readers' Theatre Groups; Players of the Golden Plains (summer theatre company); Touring Children's Theatre Company
Workshops/Festivals: Children's Theatre Workshop; Community Theatre Workshop
Artists-In-Residence/Guest Artists: The Company (guest artist, Broadway music); Legends of Jazz; Omaha Opera Company

---

COLLEGE OF EMPORIA
1300 W 12th Ave, Emporia   Kansas 66801
316 342-3670
Private and 4 Year
Arts Areas: Instrumental Music, Vocal Music, Theatre and Visual Arts
Performing Series: Performing Artist Series

MUSIC

Roger H Johnson, Chairman   **Number Of Faculty:** 8   **Number Of Students:** 120
Degrees Offered: BMus; BMusEd   **Teaching Certification Available**
Financial Assistance: Scholarships and Work-Study Grants
Performing Groups: Band; Orchestra; Chorale Ensemble

COWLEY COUNTY COMMUNITY COLLEGE
125 E Second St, Arkansas City   Kansas 67005
316 442-0430
County and 2 Year
Arts Areas: Instrumental Music, Vocal Music, Theatre and Visual Arts
Performance Facilities: Auditorium

MUSIC

Sydney W Pratt, Head   **Number Of Faculty:** 2   **Number Of Students:** 30
Degrees Offered: AA
Courses Offered: Private Lessons; Theory; Performing Groups; Music Appreciation
Financial Assistance: Scholarships and Work-Study Grants
Performing Groups: Band; Chorus; Stage Chorus; Stage Band; Music Theatre

THEATRE

Number Of Faculty: 1   **Number Of Students:** 8   **Courses Offered:** Drama
Financial Assistance: Scholarships and Work-Study Grants
Performing Groups: Drama Workshop

DONNELLY COLLEGE
1236 Sandusky, Kansas City   Kansas 66102
913 621-6070

Private and 2 Year
Arts Areas: Dance, Vocal Music, Theatre and Film Arts
Performance Facilities: Bennett Auditorium

DANCE

Number Of Faculty: 1 Part-time   *Number Of Students:* 15   *Courses Offered:* Modern Dance; Folk Dancing
Financial Assistance: Scholarships, Work-Study Grants and Kansas Tuition Grants; BEOG; SEOG

MUSIC

Number Of Faculty: 1 Part-time   *Technical Training:* Chorus; Guitar
Financial Assistance: Scholarships, Work-Study Grants and Kansas Tuition Grants; BEOG; SEOG

EMPORIA STATE UNIVERSITY
1200 Commercial St, Emporia   Kansas 66801
316 343-1200

State and 4 Year
Arts Areas: Instrumental Music, Vocal Music, Theatre, Visual Arts and Merchandising & Oral
Interpretation
Performing Series: Emporia Arts Council Series; Visiting Artists Series
Performance Facilities: Albert Taylor Hall; Beach Music Hall; Opera Theatre Workshop
Pocket Playhouse; Thymele, University Theatres

MUSIC

Dr Peter L Ciurczak, Chairperson   *Number Of Faculty:* 20
Number Of Students: 175   *Degrees Offered:* BMus; BMusEd; MA; MMus
Courses Offered: Music Reading & Hearing; Composition; Music History; Orchestra; Marching Band;
Jazz; Chamber Music; Conducting; Orchestration; Vocal Performing Groups; Applied Music: Voice, Piano,
Organ, Violin, Viola, Cello, String Bass, Flute, Oboe, Clarinet, Bassoon, Saxophone, Trumpet, French Horn,
Trombone, Baritone, Tuba, Percussion, Classical Guitar
Technical Training: Music Merchandising   *Teaching Certification Available*
Financial Assistance: Assistantships, Scholarships and Work-Study Grants
Performing Groups: Symphonic Band; Symphonic Orchestra; Jazz Workshop; Symphonic Choir; Treble
Clef; E - State Chorale; Mid - American Woodwind Quintet; Great Plains Trio

THEATRE

Laura J Barrett, Director   *Number Of Faculty:* 6   *Number Of Students:* 120
Degrees Offered: BA; BFA (performance & technical - design); BSE; MA
Courses Offered: Stage Movement; Acting; Directing; Oral Interpretation; Stagecraft; Stage Lighting;
Costuming; Scenography; Children's Theatre
Technical Training: Opportunities for the execution of student creative projects in directing and/or design
as well as experience in management and practicum credit
Teaching Certification Available
Financial Assistance: Scholarships and Work-Study Grants
Performing Groups: Educational Theatre Company; Emporia State Players
Workshops/Festivals: Flint Hills Oral Interpretation Festival
Artists-In-Residence/Guest Artists: Fred Sherry; Kees Cooper; Eugene Bosart; Klara Barton; Donald
Senta; Gary Carton; "Cabaret" (tour group)

FORT HAYS STATE UNIVERSITY
Hays   Kansas 67601, 913 628-4226

State and 4 Year
Arts Areas: Dance, Instrumental Music, Vocal Music, Theatre, Film Arts, Television and Visual Arts
Performing Series: Special Events Series; Chamber Music Series; Memorial Union Activities Board Series
Performance Facilities: Malloy Hall; Sheridan Coliseum; Gross Memorial Coliseum; Memorial Union

(continued on next page)

DANCE

Marilyn Brightman, Instructor
Dance program under auspices of Physical Education Department
Number Of Faculty: 3   **Number Of Students:** 60
Courses Offered: Social; Folk; Modern; Square; Methods of Teaching Dance
Teaching Certification Available   Financial Assistance: Work-Study Grants
Performing Groups: Fort Hays State Dancers

MUSIC

Leland Bartholomew, Chairman   **Number Of Faculty:** 17
Number Of Students: 150
Degrees Offered: BMusEd, Performance; Theory/Comprehensive; BA Mus; MM MusEd, Performance,
Theory/Comprehensive; Music History & Literature
Teaching Certification Available
Financial Assistance: Scholarships and Work-Study Grants
Performing Groups: Band; Orchestra; Choir; Chamber Music; Jazz Ensemble; Small Instrumental & Vocal
Choirs
Workshops/Festivals: High Plains Band Camp; Marching Festival; Workshops for: Elementary Music,
Piano Teachers, Church Musicians; Band Directors; Orchestra; Jazz Improvisation

THEATRE

Suzanne Trauth, Director   **Number Of Faculty:** 3   **Number Of Students:** 40
Degrees Offered: BS Speech - Theatre Emphasis
Courses Offered: Acting; Directing; History; Literature; Creative Drama
Technical Training: Scene Design; Costuming; Lighting; Makeup; Stagecraft
Teaching Certification Available
Financial Assistance: Scholarships and Work-Study Grants
Performing Groups: Touring Children's Theatre; Fort Hays State Players

---

FORT SCOTT COMMUNITY JUNIOR COLLEGE
2108 Harton, Fort Scott   Kansas 66701
316 233-2700

County and 2 Year
Arts Areas: Instrumental Music, Vocal Music and Visual Arts
Performance Facilities: College Auditorium   **Degrees Offered:** AA Music
Performing Groups: Vocal & Instrumental Ensembles

FRIENDS UNIVERSITY
2100 University, Wichita   Kansas 67213
316 263-9131

Private and 4 Year
Arts Areas: Instrumental Music, Vocal Music, Theatre and Visual Arts
Performing Series: Fine Arts Series
Performance Facilities: Alexander Auditorium

MUSIC

Dr Cecil J Riney, Chairman   **Number Of Faculty:** 15
Number Of Students: 150   **Degrees Offered:** BMus; BMusEd; BMus; Church Music
Technical Training: Opera   **Teaching Certification Available**
Financial Assistance: Scholarships and Work-Study Grants
Performing Groups: Opera Theatre; Musical Theatre; University - Community Orchestra; Chamber
Ensembles; Chorus; Symphonic Choir; Orchestra; String Ensembles

THEATRE

James C Abrell, Chairman   **Number Of Faculty:** 1   **Number Of Students:** 20
Degrees Offered: BA Drama - Speech   **Teaching Certification Available**
Financial Assistance: Scholarships and Work-Study Grants
Performing Groups: Black Masquers; Musical Theatre

GARDEN CITY COMMUNITY COLLEGE
801 Campus Dr, Garden City   Kansas 67846
316 276-7611
State and 2 Year
Arts Areas: Dance, Instrumental Music, Vocal Music, Theatre and Visual Arts
Performance Facilities: Fine Arts Auditorium

MUSIC

Number Of Faculty: 1   *Number Of Students:* 25
Courses Offered: Modern Dance; Jazz; Tap; Interpretive Dance; Modern Rhythms; Choreography; Dance Production
Financial Assistance: Assistantships, Scholarships and Work-Study Grants
Performing Groups: "The Bustlines"

MUSIC

Norman Raoke, Chairman   *Number Of Faculty:* 3   *Number Of Students:* 125
Degrees Offered: Associate Degree   *Courses Offered:* Vocal; Instrumental
Financial Assistance: Assistantships, Scholarships and Work-Study Grants
Performing Groups: Stage Band; Pep Band; Juco Singers; College Choir; Several Ensembles

THEATRE

Gretchen Tiberghien, Director   *Number Of Faculty:* 1
Number Of Students: 30   *Degrees Offered:* Associate Degree
Courses Offered: Acting I & II; Scene Design; Makeup; Fundamentals of Directing; Community Theatre; Introduction to Theatre History I & II; Stagecraft I & II; Children's Theatre
Financial Assistance: Assistantships, Scholarships and Work-Study Grants
Performing Groups: Groups from College Drama Classes

HESSTON COLLEGE
Hesston   Kansas 67062, 316 327-4221
Private and 2 Year
Arts Areas: Instrumental Music, Vocal Music, Theatre and Visual Arts
Performing Series: Concert - Lecture Series
Performance Facilities: College Auditorium

MUSIC

Randall Zercher, Chairman   *Degrees Offered:* AA Music
Courses Offered: Year Abroad Program   *Financial Assistance:* Work-Study Grants
Performing Groups: Choirs; Instrumental Ensembles

THEATRE

Arlo Kasper, Chairman   *Performing Groups:* Drama Group

HUTCHINSON COMMUNITY COLLEGE
1300 N Plum, Hutchinson   Kansas 67501
316 663-5781
County and 2 Year
Arts Areas: Dance, Instrumental Music, Vocal Music, Theatre, Television and Visual Arts
Performance Facilities: Lockman Hall Auditorium

DANCE

Ruby Munzer, Chairman, Health, PE & Recreation
Dance program under auspices of Physical Education Department
Number Of Faculty: 1   *Number Of Students:* 169   *Degrees Offered:* AA
Courses Offered: Folk Dance; Rhythms III & IV; Beginning & Advanced Social Dance
Financial Assistance: Work-Study Grants   *Performing Groups:* The Dragon Dolls

(continued on next page)

MUSIC

Leo Ashcraft, Instrumental Music
Russell Dickenson - Vocal Music; Bryce Luty - Jazz Studies
Number Of Faculty: 5   **Number Of Students:** 580   **Degrees Offered:** AA
Financial Assistance: Scholarships and Work-Study Grants
Performing Groups: Concert & Varsity Bands; Jazz Ensembles I & II; Concert Choir; HCJC Singers; The Dragonnaires
Workshops/Festivals: Celebrity Concert (Jazz)

THEATRE

Erlene Hendrix, Director   **Number Of Faculty:** 1   **Number Of Students:** 12
Degrees Offered: AA   **Courses Offered:** Theory; Design; Production
Financial Assistance: Scholarships and Work-Study Grants
Performing Groups: The Lockman Players
Artists-In-Residence/Guest Artists: Bob Montgomery; Ed Shaughnessy

---

INDEPENDENCE COMMUNITY JUNIOR COLLEGE
Box 708, Independence   Kansas 67301
316 331-4100
County and 2 Year
Arts Areas: Instrumental Music, Vocal Music, Theatre and Visual Arts
Performing Series: Concert - Lecture Series
Performance Facilities: College Auditorium

MUSIC

Number Of Faculty: 4   **Degrees Offered:** AA
Financial Assistance: Scholarships and Work-Study Grants
Performing Groups: Vocal & Instrumental Ensembles

THEATRE

Margaret Doheen, Chairman   **Number Of Faculty:** 2
Performing Groups: ICJC Players

KANSAS CITY KANSAS COMMUNITY COLLEGE
7250 State Ave, Kansas City   Kansas 66112
913 334-1100
City and 2 Year   **Arts Areas:** Instrumental Music, Vocal Music and Theatre
Performing Series: Wyandotte County Community Players
Performance Facilities: Performing Arts Center

MUSIC

Ann Standefer, Chairman, Humanities   **Number Of Faculty:** 3
Number Of Students: 55   **Degrees Offered:** AA Music
Financial Assistance: Scholarships and Work-Study Grants
Performing Groups: Concert Choir; Flint Tones; Jazz Band; Concert Band

THEATRE

Ann Standefer, Chairman, Humanities   **Number Of Faculty:** 2
Number Of Students: 30   **Degrees Offered:** AA Music
Financial Assistance: Scholarships and Work-Study Grants
Performing Groups: Drama Group

KANSAS NEWMAN COLLEGE
3100 McCormick Ave, Wichita   Kansas 67213
316 942-4291 Ext 65
Private and 4 Year
Arts Areas: Instrumental Music, Vocal Music, Theatre and Visual Arts

(continued on next page)

Performing Series: Fine Arts Guild
Performance Facilities: Wichita's Century II Little Theatre; Kansas Newman College's Chapel Auditorium

MUSIC

Sr Betty Adams, Chairman   **Number Of Faculty:** 11   **Number Of Students:** 50
Degrees Offered: BA   **Technical Training:** Internships; Practicum
Teaching Certification Available
Financial Assistance: Internships, Scholarships and Work-Study Grants
Performing Groups: Chorale; Madrigals

THEATRE

Prof Patrick Schiarra, Chairman   **Number Of Faculty:** 1
Number Of Students: 25   **Technical Training:** Theatre Practicum
Teaching Certification Available

KANSAS STATE UNIVERSITY
Eisenhower Hall, Manhattan   Kansas 66506
913 532-6900

State, 4 Year and Graduate University
Arts Areas: Dance, Instrumental Music, Vocal Music, Theatre, Film Arts, Television and Visual Arts
Performance Facilities: Danforth Chapel; McCain Auditorium; Purple Masque Theatre

DANCE

Ronnie J Mahler, Assistant Professor   **Number Of Faculty:** 3
Number Of Students: 350   **Degrees Offered:** BA and BS, Dance major
Courses Offered: Methods & Materials of Dance; Dance Composition; Dance Workshop; History of Dance;
Social, Folk, Square Dance; Stage Movement; Movement Exploration; Kinesiology
Technical Training: Ballet 1 & 2, Intermediate & Advanced; Modern Dance 1 & 2, Intermediate &
Advanced; Jazz Dance
Financial Assistance: Assistantships and Work-Study Grants
Performing Groups: Kansas State University Dance Workshop
Workshops/Festivals: Master Class Series; Lecture - Demonstration Series; Student Composition Series;
Concert Series

MUSIC

Robert A Steinbauer, Chairman   **Number Of Faculty:** 21
Number Of Students: 250   **Degrees Offered:** BA MusEd; BMus; MMus
Courses Offered: Professional Music Courses in Music Education & Applied Music
Technical Training: Opera   **Teaching Certification Available**
Financial Assistance: Internships, Assistantships, Scholarships and Work-Study Grants
Performing Groups: Opera Theatre; Symphony Orchestra; Musical Theatre; Symphonic Wind Ensembles;
Concert Band; Marching Band; Concert Choir; Collegiate Chorale; Men's & Women's Glee Clubs
Workshops/Festivals: Music Workshops for all phases of instrumental and choral music, plus music
practicum workshops

THEATRE

Harold J Nichols, Administrative Director of Theatre   **Number Of Faculty:** 11
Number Of Students: 110   **Degrees Offered:** BA; BS; MA
Courses Offered: Acting; Directing; Playwriting; Technical Production; Dramatic Literature; Theatre
History
Teaching Certification Available
Financial Assistance: Internships, Assistantships, Scholarships and Work-Study Grants
Performing Groups: K - State Players; Musical Theatre; Opera Theatre; Playwright's Workshop
Artists-In-Residence/Guest Artists: Elizabeth Sewell; Mme Maria Yurieva Swoboda; Marion McPartland;
Gary Grafmann

KANSAS WESLEYAN UNIVERSITY
S Santa Fe, Salina   Kansas 67401
913 827-5541 Ext 217
Private and 4 Year
Arts Areas: Instrumental Music, Vocal Music and Theatre
Performance Facilities: Sams Chapel; Fitzpatrick Auditorium

MUSIC

Harry Huber, Chairman   *Number Of Faculty:* 4   *Degrees Offered:* BA
Teaching Certification Available
Financial Assistance: Scholarships and Work-Study Grants
Performing Groups: Philharmonic Choir; Wesleyan Singers

THEATRE

Richard Crouse, Associate Professor   *Number Of Faculty:* 2
Degrees Offered: BA   *Teaching Certification Available*
Financial Assistance: Scholarships and Work-Study Grants
Performing Groups: Wesleyan Players

UNIVERSITY OF KANSAS
Lawrence   Kansas 66045, 913 864-3421
State and 4 Year
Arts Areas: Dance, Instrumental Music, Vocal Music, Theatre, Film Arts, Television and Visual Arts
Performing Series: Concert Series; Chamber Music Series
Performance Facilities: Hoch Auditorium; University Theatre; Swarthout Recital Hall; Inge Memorial Theatre

DANCE

Wayne Osness, Chairman, Physical Education   *Number Of Faculty:* 3
Number Of Students: 500
Degrees Offered: BS with Dance Major, Options in Dance Education - Dance Performance; MS in Education, Dance Specialty
Teaching Certification Available
Financial Assistance: Assistantships and Scholarships
Performing Groups: University Dance Company; Tau Sigma Fraternity
Workshops/Festivals: About three or four per year in a variety of areas

MUSIC

Kenneth Smith, Chairman, Music Performance
James Ralston, Chairman, Music Ensembles
Number Of Faculty: 50   *Number Of Students:* 500
Degrees Offered: BMus; BMusEd; BS; BA; MMus; MMusEd; PhD; DMA
Teaching Certification Available
Financial Assistance: Assistantships, Scholarships and Work-Study Grants
Performing Groups: Symphony Orchestra, Symphonic Band, Concert Band, Varsity Band, Jazz Ensembles, Chamber Choir, Concert Chorale, University Chorus, University Singers, Collegium Musicum, Percussion Ensemble, Opera and Opera Workshop
Workshops/Festivals: Midwestern Music and Art Camp; Institute for Organ and Church Music; Piano, Organ, Winds, Strings, and Voice Master Classes

THEATRE

Dr Ronald A Willis, Director   *Number Of Faculty:* 14
Number Of Students: 200   *Degrees Offered:* BA; BGS; MA; PhD
Teaching Certification Available
Financial Assistance: Assistantships, Scholarships and Work-Study Grants
Performing Groups: Main Stage Series; Inge Theatre Series; Kansas University Theatre for Young People Series; Kansas Repertory Theatre
Artists-In-Residence/Guest Artists: Leon Fleischer; Gary Graffman; Catharine Crozier; Michael Schneider

LABETTE COMMUNITY JUNIOR COLLEGE
200 S 14th, Parsons   Kansas 67357
316 421-6700

County and 2 Year
Arts Areas: Instrumental Music, Vocal Music, Theatre, Film Arts and Visual Arts
Performance Facilities: Thiebaud Theatre

MUSIC

Dana J Saliba, Instructor   *Number Of Faculty:* 2   *Number Of Students:* 95
Degrees Offered: AA
Courses Offered: Music Theory; Appreciation; Class Piano; Orchestra; Choir; Class Guitar; Voice Class;
Applied Music in all media
Financial Assistance: Scholarships
Performing Groups: Chamber Orchestra; Cardinal Choir

THEATRE

Jim Benson, Instructor   *Number Of Faculty:* 1   *Degrees Offered:* AA

MARYMOUNT COLLEGE
E Iron Ave, Salina   Kansas 67401
913 825-2101 Ext 200

Private and 4 Year
Arts Areas: Dance, Instrumental Music, Vocal Music, Theatre and Visual Arts
Performance Facilities: Fine Arts Theatre; Experimental Theatre; Ballroom/Theatre
Number Of Faculty: 1 Part-time   *Performing Groups:* Maymont Dance Company

MUSIC

James Braswell, Chairman   *Number Of Faculty:* 5   *Number Of Students:* 30
Degrees Offered: BMus; BA; BMusEd   *Teaching Certification Available*
Financial Assistance: Scholarships, Work-Study Grants and Fine Arts Grants; State Tution Grants
Performing Groups: Chamber Singers; Marymount Choir; Marymount Band; Jazz Ensemble; Early Music
Ensemble; Marymount String Quartet
Workshops/Festivals: Elementary Music Education; Chamber Music; Recitals Series; Strings Workshop;
Artist Series

THEATRE

Dr Dennis Denning, Chairman   *Number Of Faculty:* 3   *Number Of Students:* 35
Degrees Offered: BA; BS   *Teaching Certification Available*
Financial Assistance: Scholarships, Work-Study Grants and Fine Arts Grants; State Tution Grants
Performing Groups: Marymount Players
Workshops/Festivals: High School Summer Workshop; Experimental Theatre Festival for Colleges &
Universities

MC PHERSON COLLEGE
1600 E Euclid, McPherson   Kansas 67460
316 241-0731

Private and 4 Year
Arts Areas: Instrumental Music, Vocal Music, Theatre, Television and Visual Arts
Performing Series: Programs on Cable TV
Performance Facilities: Brown Auditorium

MUSIC

Paul V Sollenberger, Chairman   *Number Of Faculty:* 4
Number Of Students: 100   *Degrees Offered:* BA Instrumental, Vocal & Education
Teaching Certification Available
Financial Assistance: Assistantships, Scholarships and Work-Study Grants
Performing Groups: College Choir; Band; Community Orchestra; Several Small Ensembles
Workshops/Festivals: Host for State Music Festival

(continued on next page)

THEATRE

Rick Tyler, Assistant Professor of Drama   **Number Of Faculty:** 1
Number Of Students: 25   **Degrees Offered:** BA Speech & Theatre
Teaching Certification Available
Financial Assistance: Scholarships and Work-Study Grants
Performing Groups: McPherson College Players

OTTAWA UNIVERSITY
10th & Cedar St, Ottawa   Kansas 66067
913 242-5200 Ext 218
Private and 4 Year
Arts Areas: Dance, Instrumental Music, Vocal Music and Visual Arts
Performance Facilities: University Chapel; Administration Building Auditorium; Tauy Jones Recital Hall

MUSIC

Stanley DeFries, PhD, Chairman   **Number Of Faculty:** 5
Number Of Students: 50   **Degrees Offered:** BA
Courses Offered: Performance; Church Music; Music Education; Music Therapy
Technical Training: Suzuki Teacher Education
Teaching Certification Available
Financial Assistance: Scholarships and Work-Study Grants
Performing Groups: Chorale; Concert Choir; Jazz Ensemble; Wind Ensemble; Symphonette
Workshops/Festivals: Suzuki Workshop; Church Music Workshop; Samuel Barber Festival; Clark Terry Jazz Festival

THEATRE

Rufus Cadigan, Chairman   **Number Of Faculty:** 2   **Number Of Students:** 25
Degrees Offered: BA   **Courses Offered:** Drama Education & Performance
Teaching Certification Available
Financial Assistance: Scholarships and Work-Study Grants
Performing Groups: Alpha Psi Omega
Artists-In-Residence/Guest Artists: Samuel Barber

PITTSBURGH STATE UNIVERSITY
Pittsburgh   Kansas 66762, 316 231-7000
State and 4 Year
Arts Areas: Instrumental Music, Vocal Music, Theatre and Visual Arts
Performing Series: Solo & Chamber Music Series; Summer Artist Series

MUSIC

Millard M Laing, Chairman   **Number Of Faculty:** 20   **Number Of Students:** 375
Degrees Offered: BMus; MMus; BMusEd; MMusEd
Teaching Certification Available
Financial Assistance: Internships, Assistantships, Scholarships and Work-Study Grants
Performing Groups: Chorale Ensemble; Band; Instrumental Ensembles; Orchestra; Opera
Workshops/Festivals: Opera Workshop

THEATRE

Harold W Lay, Chairman   **Number Of Faculty:** 7   **Number Of Students:** 140
Degrees Offered: BA; MA   **Teaching Certification Available**
Financial Assistance: Internships, Assistantships, Scholarships and Work-Study Grants
Performing Groups: College Theatre

PRATT COMMUNITY COLLEGE
Hwy 61, Pratt   Kansas 67124
316 672-5641

County and 2 Year
Arts Areas: Instrumental Music, Vocal Music, Theatre, Television and Visual Arts
Performance Facilities: College Auditorium

MUSIC

Floyd Carpenter, Instructor   *Number Of Faculty:* 1
Degrees Offered: AA Mus; AA Applied Music; AA MusEd
Courses Offered: Instrumental; Vocal; Theory; Appreciation
Technical Training: Opera
Financial Assistance: Scholarships, Work-Study Grants and BEOG; NDSL; SEOG
Performing Groups: Vocal & Instrumental Groups, Student & Community

THEATRE

Edwin Gorsky, Instructor   *Number Of Faculty:* 1
Degrees Offered: AA Drama, Speech, Radio & Cable TV
Courses Offered: Introduction to Acting; Directing; Interpretation; Radio & TV
Technical Training: Technical Theatre; Radio & TV
Performing Groups: Blue Masque; All school & community productions

SAINT JOHN'S COLLEGE
7th & College, Winfield   Kansas 67156
316 221-4000

Private and 2 Year   *Arts Areas:* Instrumental Music and Vocal Music
Performance Facilities: Meyer Hall Activity/Workshop Center

MUSIC

Lee Stocker, Coordinator   *Number Of Faculty:* 3   *Number Of Students:* 100
Courses Offered: Keyboard; Voice
Financial Assistance: Scholarships and Work-Study Grants
Performing Groups: A Cappella Choir; Chapel Choir; Several Vocal Ensembles
Workshops/Festivals: Annual presentation of the "Elijah" in cooperation with Southwestern College & City of Winfield

SAINT MARY COLLEGE
Leavenworth   Kansas -6048, 913 682-5151

Private and 4 Year
Arts Areas: Dance, Instrumental Music, Vocal Music, Theatre and Visual Arts
Performing Series: Fine Arts Series
Performance Facilities: Xavier Theatre; St Joseph Hall

DANCE

Sister Jean Clare Bachle, Instructor   *Number Of Faculty:* 2
Number Of Students: 85   *Degrees Offered:* Minor in Dance
Financial Assistance: Scholarships and Work-Study Grants
Performing Groups: Concert Dance Ensemble

MUSIC

Sister Anne Callahan, Chairman   *Number Of Faculty:* 5
Number Of Students: 30
Degrees Offered: BMusEd; BA; BMus (Piano, Violin, Voice)
Courses Offered: Theory & Practice (Piano, Violin, Voice)
Technical Training: Performances   *Teaching Certification Available*
Financial Assistance: Scholarships and Work-Study Grants

(continued on next page)

Performing Groups: Saint Mary Singers; Concert Choir; Stage Band; Sounds of Praise
Workshops/Festivals: Spring Musical

THEATRE

Sr Mary Dolonta Flynn, Chairman   **Number Of Faculty:** 5
Number Of Students: 30   **Degrees Offered:** BA Drama
Courses Offered: Production & Performance
Technical Training: Available through program with Theatre for Young America
Teaching Certification Available
Financial Assistance: Scholarships and Work-Study Grants
Performing Groups: Xavier Theatre Group
Workshops/Festivals: Theatre for Young America; KC Equity Theatre Group; Interim
Artists-In-Residence/Guest Artists: Alvin Ailey Dancers; National Players

---

SAINT MARY OF THE PLAINS COLLEGE
Dodge City   Kansas 67801, 316 225-4171
Private and 4 Year
Arts Areas: Instrumental Music, Vocal Music, Theatre and Visual Arts
Performing Series: Artist - Lecture Series

MUSIC

Dr Frank Boehnien, Chairman   **Number Of Faculty:** 7   **Number Of Students:** 70
Degrees Offered: BS MusEd; BMus   **Technical Training:** Opera
Teaching Certification Available
Financial Assistance: Scholarships and Work-Study Grants
Performing Groups: Opera Theatre; Band; Choir; Orchestra; Instrumental Ensembles

THEATRE

Sister M Christian, Chairman   **Number Of Faculty:** 3
Number Of Students: 30   **Degrees Offered:** BA Speech - Drama
Teaching Certification Available
Financial Assistance: Scholarships and Work-Study Grants
Performing Groups: Plains Players

SEWARD COUNTY COMMUNITY COLLEGE
Box 1137, Liberal   Kansas 67901
316 624-1951
State and 2 Year
Arts Areas: Instrumental Music, Vocal Music, Theatre and Visual Arts
Performance Facilities: Theatre   **Number Of Faculty:** 2
Number Of Students: 150   **Degrees Offered:** AA
Courses Offered: Theory & Performance
Financial Assistance: Scholarships and Work-Study Grants
Performing Groups: "Our Gang", Choir; Community Chorus; Pep Band; Community Orchestra
Workshops/Festivals: High School Band Festival   **Number Of Faculty:** 1
Number Of Students: 25   **Degrees Offered:** AA
Courses Offered: Theory & Performance
Financial Assistance: Scholarships and Work-Study Grants
Performing Groups: Drama & Musicals

SOUTHWESTERN COLLEGE
100 College St, Windfield   Kansas 67156
316 221-4150 Ext 69
Private and 4 Year
Arts Areas: Instrumental Music, Vocal Music, Theatre and Visual Arts
Performing Series: Cultural Arts Series   **Number Of Faculty:** 7
Number Of Students: 100   **Degrees Offered:** BMus   **Technical Training:** Organ
Teaching Certification Available

(continued on next page)

Financial Assistance: Scholarships and Work-Study Grants
Performing Groups: Orchestra; Instrumental Ensembles; Band; Chorale Ensemble

THEATRE

Norman D Callison, Chairman   *Number Of Faculty:* 2   *Number Of Students:* 30
Degrees Offered: BA   *Teaching Certification Available*
Financial Assistance: Scholarships and Work-Study Grants
Performing Groups: Southwestern College Drama Productions

STERLING COLLEGE
Sterling   Kansas 67579, 316 278-2173 Ext 217
Private and 4 Year
Arts Areas: Dance, Instrumental Music, Vocal Music, Theatre and Visual Arts
Performing Series: Artist - Lecture Series; Rice County Arts Council Series
Performance Facilities: Theatre; Auditorium

DANCE

Dance courses offered in Theatre Department

MUSIC

Robert Gordon, Chairman   *Number Of Faculty:* 3 Full-time, 3 Part-time
Number Of Students: 40   *Degrees Offered:* BSMusEd
Courses Offered: Vocal & Instrumental Elementary & Secondary Teacher Preparation; Theory
Teaching Certification Available
Financial Assistance: Scholarships and Work-Study Grants
Performing Groups: Marching & Concert Band; Stage Band; Select Choir; Campus Chorus
Workshops/Festivals: District Music Festival; Local Invitational Festival for High School Students; College
Consortium sponsors Workshops each year in music - related subjects

THEATRE

Gordon King, Chairman   *Number Of Faculty:* 3   *Number Of Students:* 25
Degrees Offered: AB
Technical Training: Makeup; Costume; Stage Design & Construction
Teaching Certification Available
Financial Assistance: Scholarships and Work-Study Grants
Performing Groups: Children's Theatre; Musical Theatre
Workshops/Festivals: District Speech/Theatre festival for High School Students; Occasional workshop for
college students co-sponsored with six - college consortium

TABOR COLLEGE
400 S Jefferson, Hillsboro   Kansas 67063
316 947-3121
Private and 4 Year
Arts Areas: Instrumental Music, Vocal Music and Visual Arts
Performing Series: Lecture - Concert Series

MUSIC

Dr Jonah C Kliewer, Chairman   *Number Of Faculty:* 5
Number Of Students: 60   *Degrees Offered:* BMus; BMusEd
Teaching Certification Available
Financial Assistance: Scholarships and Work-Study Grants
Performing Groups: Concert Choir; Chamber Choir; Women's Glee Club; Concert Band; Jazz Band; String
Ensemble; Brass Choir

WASHBURN UNIVERSITY OF TOPEKA
17th St, Topeka   Kansas 66621
913 295-3600
City and 4 Year
Arts Areas: Dance, Instrumental Music, Vocal Music, Theatre, Film Arts, Television and Visual Arts
Performing Series: Fall Chamber Music Festival
Performance Facilities: White Concert Hall; University Theater

DANCE

Belinda McPherson, Instructor/Director   *Number Of Faculty:* 2
Number Of Students: 90   *Degrees Offered:* BAEd Dance Emphasis
Financial Assistance: Scholarships and Work-Study Grants
Performing Groups: Modern Dance Club
Workshops/Festivals: Spring Dance Festival

MUSIC

Dr John L Iltis, Chairman   *Number Of Faculty:* 12   *Number Of Students:* 75
Degrees Offered: BMus, Applied Music, BMusEd; BA Music
Technical Training: Vocal; Instrumental; Directing; Teaching
Teaching Certification Available
Financial Assistance: Scholarships and Work-Study Grants
Performing Groups: Band; Symphonette; Jazz Ensemble; String Ensemble; Choir; Concert Choir; Singers; Clarinet Chorus; Brass Ensemble
Workshops/Festivals: Fine Arts Festival String Workshop; Summer Music Program for High School Students; Faculty & Student Recital Series

THEATRE

Hugh McCausland, Director   *Number Of Faculty:* 2   *Number Of Students:* 200
Degrees Offered: BA
Technical Training: Acting; Stage Makeup; Directing; Stagecraft; Lighting
Teaching Certification Available
Financial Assistance: Scholarships and Work-Study Grants
Performing Groups: Washburn Players
Workshops/Festivals: Four fall & spring semester plays and musicals; Washburn Summer Theater
Artists-In-Residence/Guest Artists: James Rivers; Chapman Kelley; Kato Havas

WICHITA STATE UNIVERSITY
1845 Fairmount, Wichita   Kansas 67208
316 689-3456
State and 4 Year
Arts Areas: Instrumental Music, Vocal Music and Visual Arts
Performing Series: Guest Artist Series

MUSIC

Howard Ellis, Chairman   *Number Of Faculty:* 43   *Number Of Students:* 1,300
Degrees Offered: BMus; BMusEd; MMus; MMusEd
Technical Training: Opera; Theory   *Teaching Certification Available*
Financial Assistance: Assistantships, Scholarships and Work-Study Grants
Performing Groups: Opera Theatre; Symphony Orchestra; Choral Ensemble; Jazz Ensemble; Strings Ensembles; Wind Ensembles
Workshops/Festivals: Opera Workshop

THEATRE

Richard Welsbacher, Chairman   *Number Of Faculty:* 5
Number Of Students: 150   *Degrees Offered:* BA Speech
Teaching Certification Available
Financial Assistance: Assistantships, Scholarships and Work-Study Grants
Performing Groups: University Theatre

ALICE LLOYD COLLEGE
Pippa Passes   Kentucky 41844, 606 368-2101
>Private and 2 Year
>*Arts Areas:* Dance, Instrumental Music, Vocal Music, Theatre and Visual Arts
>*Performing Series:* Our Appalachia Day; Cultural Convocation Series; Fine Arts Festival
>*Performance Facilities:* Cushing Hall

MUSIC

Paul Tse, Director of Voices of Appalachia Choir, Assistant Professor of Music
Number Of Faculty: 1   *Number Of Students:* 60   *Degrees Offered:* AA
Courses Offered: Music Appreciation; Elements of Music; Chorus
Technical Training: Voice; Piano; Organ
Financial Assistance: Scholarships and Work-Study Grants
Performing Groups: Voices of Appalachia Choir

THEATRE

Terry Cornett, Professor of English/Drama   *Number Of Faculty:* 1
Number Of Students: 25   *Degrees Offered:* AA
Courses Offered: Playwriting Sources; Public Speaking; Play Production
Technical Training: Production; Design; Acting; Directing
Financial Assistance: Scholarships and Work-Study Grants
Performing Groups: Appalachian Summer Theatre
Artists-In-Residence/Guest Artists: Louisville Ballet

ASBURY COLLEGE
Lexington Ave, Wilmore   Kentucky 40390
606 585-3511 Ext 244
>Private and 4 Year   *Arts Areas:* Instrumental Music and Vocal Music
>*Performing Series:* Artist Series
>*Performance Facilities:* Akers Recital Auditorium; Hughes Auditorium

MUSIC

Jack A Rains, Chairman, Division of Fine Arts
Number Of Faculty: 1 Full-time, 10 Part-time   *Number Of Students:* 190
Degrees Offered: BA Mus; BS Mus
Courses Offered: Performance; Church Music; Music Education; Art; Art Education
Technical Training: Voice; Organ; Piano; All Instruments
Teaching Certification Available
Financial Assistance: Scholarships and Work-Study Grants
Performing Groups: Concert Choir; Concert Band; Chamber Orchestra; Oratorio Chorus; Brass Choir; Stage Band I & II

BELLARMINE COLLEGE
Newburg Rd, Louisville   Kentucky 40205
502 452-8300
>Private and 4 Year   *Arts Areas:* Instrumental Music and Vocal Music
>*Performance Facilities:* New Science Theater

MUSIC

Gus Coin, Professor   *Number Of Faculty:* 12   *Number Of Students:* 50
Degrees Offered: BA Mus & Jazz
Courses Offered: Applied Music; Music Theory & History; Ensembles
Technical Training: Ensembles   *Teaching Certification Available*
Financial Assistance: Scholarships and Work-Study Grants
Performing Groups: Jazz Ensemble; Bellarmine College Singers; Bellarmine Pep Band; Vocal Ensemble
Workshops/Festivals: Jazz Clinic

BEREA COLLEGE
Berea   Kentucky 40404, 606 986-9341
   Private and 4 Year
   Arts Areas: Dance, Instrumental Music, Vocal Music, Theatre, Television and Visual Arts

DANCE

John Ramsay, Director of Recreation Extension   *Number Of Faculty:* 1
Degrees Offered: Independent majors offered in Recreation and Dance
Financial Assistance: Assistantships and Work-Study Grants
Performing Groups: Berea College Country Dancers
Workshops/Festivals: Several workshops & festivals are held each year

MUSIC

Robert Lewis, Chairman   *Number Of Faculty:* 8
Degrees Offered: BA MusEd, Organ, Piano, Voice
Teaching Certification Available
Financial Assistance: Scholarships and Work-Study Grants
Performing Groups: Berea College Band; Berea College Chapel Choir

THEATRE

Paul Power, Chairman   *Number Of Faculty:* 1   *Number Of Students:* 45
Degrees Offered: Independent majors in Communications or Theater Arts
Teaching Certification Available
Financial Assistance: Scholarships and Work-Study Grants
Performing Groups: Berea College Players

BRESCIA COLLEGE
120 W Seventh St, Owensboro   Kentucky 42301
502 685-3131
   Private and 4 Year
   Arts Areas: Instrumental Music, Vocal Music, Theatre and Visual Arts
   Performing Series: Sack Lunch Concerts
   Performance Facilities: Brescia College Auditorium; Le Petit Theatre

MUSIC

James D White, Director   *Number Of Faculty:* 5 Full-time, 5 Part-time
Number Of Students: 500   *Degrees Offered:* BMus; BMusEd
Courses Offered: Piano; Voice; Organ; Violin; Other String Instruments
Teaching Certification Available
Financial Assistance: Assistantships, Scholarships and Work-Study Grants
Performing Groups: Brescia Singers; Brescia Chamber Orchestra; Brescia Student Trio; Brescia Faculty Trio; Brescia Boy Choir
Workshops/Festivals: Annual Spring Fine Arts Festival

THEATRE

Ray McIntosh, Chairman   *Number Of Faculty:* 1   *Number Of Students:* 10 - 15
Financial Assistance: Assistantships, Scholarships and Work-Study Grants
Performing Groups: Brescia

CAMPBELLSVILLE COLLEGE
Campbellsville   Kentucky 42718, 502 465-8158 Ext 41
   Private and 4 Year
   Arts Areas: Instrumental Music, Vocal Music, Theatre and Visual Arts
   Performing Series: Central Kentucky Arts Series; Exchange concerts with other college faculties
   Performance Facilities: College Chapel; Recital Hall; Local Church & School Facilities

(continued on next page)

MUSIC

Larry W Reed, Major Professor   **Number Of Faculty:** 12
Number Of Students: 90   **Degrees Offered:** BMus; BA; BS
Courses Offered: Performance; Music Education (major & minor); Church Music (major & minor)
Teaching Certification Available
Financial Assistance: Assistantships, Scholarships and Church Matching Scholarships
Performing Groups: Collegiate Chorale; Concert Chorus; Concert Band; Jazz Ensemble
Workshops/Festivals: Choral Reading Clinics; Music Education Workshops; Band Camps - Junior High &
Senior High; Church Music Workshops - Vocal & Instrumental; Master Classes - All Areas

THEATRE

Russell Mobley, Major Professor   **Number Of Faculty:** 1
Number Of Students: 10   **Courses Offered:** Minor in Drama
Teaching Certification Available
Financial Assistance: Scholarships, Work-Study Grants and Church Matching Scholarships
Performing Groups: Harlequins

CATHERINE SPAULDING COLLEGE
851 S 4th St, Louisville   Kentucky 40203
502 585-9911
Private and 4 Year
Arts Areas: Instrumental Music, Vocal Music, Theatre and Visual Arts

MUSIC

Degrees Offered: BA MusEd; Mus
Financial Assistance: Scholarships and Work-Study Grants
Performing Groups: Chorus; Orchestra

THEATRE

Sister Gertrude, Chairman   **Degrees Offered:** BA Drama - Speech
Financial Assistance: Scholarships and Work-Study Grants
Performing Groups: Roswitha Players

CENTRE COLLEGE OF KENTUCKY
Walnut St, Danville   Kentucky 40422
606 236-5211
Private and 4 Year
Arts Areas: Instrumental Music, Vocal Music, Theatre and Visual Arts
Performing Series: Music Series; Subscription Series
Performance Facilities: Newlin Hall; Weisiger Theatre

MUSIC

Robert L Weaver, PhD, Program Chairman   **Number Of Faculty:** 3
Number Of Students: 50   **Degrees Offered:** BA
Courses Offered: Applied Music; Survey of Music History; Structure & Style of Medieval Music
Technical Training: Private Instruction in Composition, Voice, Piano, Organ, Harpsichord
Teaching Certification Available
Financial Assistance: Scholarships, Work-Study Grants and Loans, Grants
Performing Groups: Centre Singers; Centre Chamber Singers; Centre; Centre College - Community
Orchestra; Early Music Group

THEATRE

West T Hill, Jr, PhD, Program Chairman   **Number Of Faculty:** 4
Number Of Students: 70   **Degrees Offered:** BA
Courses Offered: Applied Theatre; Scene Design; Stage Lighting Design; Acting; Directing; Theatre
History; Drama; Renaissance Drama
Technical Training: Scene Design; Stage Lighting; Acting; Directing
Teaching Certification Available   **Performing Groups:** Centre College Players

CUMBERLAND COLLEGE
Williamsburg   Kentucky 40769, 606 549-2030
   Private and 4 Year
   Arts Areas: Instrumental Music, Vocal Music, Theatre and Visual Arts
   Performing Series: Fine Arts Association of Southeastern Kentucky Concert Series; Cumberland College
   Convocation Series
   Performance Facilities: Gatliff Auditorium

MUSIC

Harold R Wortman, Head   *Number Of Faculty:* 8   *Number Of Students:* 50
Degrees Offered: BA; BMusEd; BMus Choral Music
Teaching Certification Available
Financial Assistance: Assistantships, Scholarships and Work-Study Grants
Workshops/Festivals: Church Music Workshop

THEATRE

Michael Waiters, Director   *Number Of Faculty:* 1
Degrees Offered: BA (English & Theatre)   *Teaching Certification Available*
Financial Assistance: Scholarships   *Performing Groups:* Circle Theatre

EASTERN KENTUCKY UNIVERSITY
Richmond   Kentucky 40475, 606 622-0111
   State and 4 Year
   Arts Areas: Dance, Instrumental Music, Vocal Music, Theatre, Television, Visual Arts and Performing Arts
   Performing Series: Center Board Concert, Lecture & Fine Arts
   Performance Facilities: Brock Auditorium; Gifford Theatre; Buchanan Theatre; Van Peursem Pavilion;
   Edwards Auditorium

DANCE

Dr Ann Uhlir, Chairman, Department of Physical Education for Women
Number Of Faculty: 1
Financial Assistance: Assistantships, Scholarships and Work-Study Grants
Performing Groups: Eastern Dance Theatre
Workshops/Festivals: Fall & Spring Concerts

MUSIC

Dr George Muns, Chairman   *Number Of Faculty:* 24   *Number Of Students:* 300
Degrees Offered: BA; BMus; BMusEd; MMus; MMusEd; MA in Ed
Teaching Certification Available
Financial Assistance: Assistantships, Scholarships and Work-Study Grants
Performing Groups: Various Vocal & Instrumental Groups
Workshops/Festivals: Stephen Foster Music Camp; KMEA Festivals; Marching Band Camps

THEATRE

Dr Richard Benson, Chairman, Department of Speech & Theatre Arts
Number Of Faculty: 8   *Number Of Students:* 50   *Degrees Offered:* BA; BFA
Technical Training: Set Design & Lighting   *Teaching Certification Available*
Financial Assistance: Assistantships, Scholarships and Work-Study Grants
Performing Groups: University Players

HAZARD COMMUNITY COLLEGE
Hazard   Kentucky 41701, 606 436-5721
   State and 2 Year   *Arts Areas:* Vocal Music and Theatre
   Performance Facilities: Hazard Community College Auditorium

MUSIC

J Brown, Chairman   *Number Of Faculty:* 1   *Degrees Offered:* AA

(continued on next page)

Number Of Faculty: 2   **Number Of Students:** 10   **Degrees Offered:** AA
Performing Groups: Black Gold Players

KENTUCKY STATE UNIVERSITY
Frankfort   Kentucky 40601, 502 223-2052
State and 4 Year
Arts Areas: Instrumental Music, Vocal Music, Theatre and Television

MUSIC

Warren C Swindell, Chairman   **Number Of Faculty:** 12
Number Of Students: 90   **Degrees Offered:** BMus; BMusEd
Financial Assistance: Scholarships and Work-Study Grants
Performing Groups: KSU Choir; Concert Band; Chamber Ensemble

THEATRE

John M Williams, Chairman   **Number Of Faculty:** 3   **Number Of Students:** 160
Degrees Offered: BA   **Teaching Certification Available**
Financial Assistance: Scholarships and Work-Study Grants
Performing Groups: The Kentucky Players

KENTUCKY WESLEYAN COLLEGE
3000 Frederica St, Owensboro   Kentucky 42301
502 926-3111
Private and 4 Year
Arts Areas: Instrumental Music, Vocal Music, Theatre, Television and Visual Arts
Performance Facilities: Theatre Playhouse

MUSIC

J Jerome Redfearn, Chairperson   **Number Of Faculty:** 4
Number Of Students: 43   **Degrees Offered:** BMus; BMusEd
Courses Offered: Sacred Music; Instrumental Music; Vocal Music; Music Education
Teaching Certification Available
Financial Assistance: Assistantships, Scholarships and Work-Study Grants
Performing Groups: Band; Ensembles; Choir

THEATRE

Robert R Pevitts, Chairman   **Number Of Faculty:** 3   **Number Of Students:** 49
Degrees Offered: AA; APS; BA
Courses Offered: Speech; Theatre; Communications; Radio; Television
Technical Training: Theatre; Radio & Television
Teaching Certification Available
Financial Assistance: Assistantships, Scholarships and Work-Study Grants
Performing Groups: Theatre Production Company
Workshops/Festivals: Six plays per year

UNIVERSITY OF KENTUCKY
Lexington   Kentucky 40506, 606 257-2797
State and 4 Year
Arts Areas: Instrumental Music, Vocal Music, Theatre and Visual Arts
Performance Facilities: Guignol Theatre; Laboratory Theatre

MUSIC

Joe B Buttram, Director   **Number Of Faculty:** 34   **Number Of Students:** 265
Degrees Offered: BA Mus; BMusEd; BM in Applied; MM in Applied; MM in Theory, Composition; MM
in MusEd; MA; PhD; DMA
Teaching Certification Available
Financial Assistance: Scholarships, Work-Study Grants and Grants-in-Aid
Performing Groups: Percussion Ensemble; Chamber Singers; Jazz Ensemble I & II; Piano Ensemble;
Concert Band; Symphonic Band; Wind Ensemble; Orchestra; Choristers; Chorus; Opera Workshop;

(continued on next page)

Collegium Musicum
Workshops/Festivals: Summer Institutes - Jazz Ensemble; Kentucky Summer Wind Ensemble; Strings & Chamber Music; Keyboard; Choral Workshop; Opera Workshop

THEATRE

Wallace N Briggs, Acting Chairman   ***Number Of Faculty:*** 8
Number Of Students: 90   ***Degrees Offered:*** BA; MA
Financial Assistance: Assistantships, Scholarships and Work-Study Grants
Performing Groups: The Theatre

UNIVERSITY OF KENTUCKY, HENDERSON COMMUNITY COLLEGE
2660 S Green St, Henderson   Kentucky 42420
502 827-1867 Ext 33

State and 2 Year
Arts Areas: Instrumental Music, Vocal Music and Television
Performance Facilities: Auditorium (Student Center)

MUSIC

Mrs Patricia E Turner, Assistant Professor   ***Number Of Faculty:*** 1
Number Of Students: 20   ***Degrees Offered:*** AS; AA
Financial Assistance: Scholarships
Performing Groups: Choristers; Madrigal; Community Chorus; Band

---

UNIVERSITY OF LOUISVILLE
9001 Shelbyville Rd, Louisville   Kentucky 40208
502 636-4307

State and 4 Year
Arts Areas: Instrumental Music, Vocal Music, Theatre and Visual Arts

MUSIC

Jerry W Ball, Dean   ***Number Of Faculty:*** 35   ***Number Of Students:*** 250
Degrees Offered: AA; BA; BMus; BMus Composition; BMus History; MMus; MMus History; MMus Composition; joint PhD in Music History with University of Kentucky
Technical Training: Preparatory School for Music & Dance
Teaching Certification Available
Financial Assistance: Assistantships, Scholarships and Work-Study Grants
Performing Groups: Chorus; Orchestra; Various Ensembles; Band; Choir; Recitals

THEATRE

Albert J Harris, Chairman   ***Number Of Faculty:*** 12   ***Number Of Students:*** 150
Degrees Offered: BA; BS; MA; MAT   ***Teaching Certification Available***
Financial Assistance: Assistantships, Scholarships and Work-Study Grants
Performing Groups: Belknap Theatre; University of Louisville Repertory Company; Laboratory Theatre; Black Theatre Workshop
Workshops/Festivals: Metroversity Summer Theatre; Shakespeare in Central Park

---

MOREHEAD STATE UNIVERSITY
Morehead   Kentucky 40351, 606 783-2221

State and 4 Year
Arts Areas: Instrumental Music, Vocal Music, Theatre, Film Arts, Television and Visual Arts
Performing Series: MSU Theatre Series; Concert & Lecture Series; Recital Hall Series
Performance Facilities: Duncan Recital Hall; Fulbright Auditorium; Button Auditorium; Kibbey Theatre

MUSIC

Glenn Fulbright, Chairman   ***Number Of Faculty:*** 33   ***Number Of Students:*** 350
Degrees Offered: BMus; BMusEd; MMus   ***Teaching Certification Available***
Financial Assistance: Internships, Assistantships, Scholarships and Work-Study Grants
Performing Groups: Bands; Orchestra; Concert Choir; Chamber Singers; Jazz Ensembles; Small Ensembles in all areas

(*continued on next page*)

Workshops/Festivals: Summer Music Camp; Band Clinic; Choral Festival; Jazz Festival; Composer Symposium; Blue/Gold Marching Band Contest

THEATRE

Dr William Layne, Coordinator   **Number Of Faculty:** 4
Number Of Students: 50   **Degrees Offered:** BA
Teaching Certification Available
Financial Assistance: Internships, Assistantships, Scholarships and Work-Study Grants
Performing Groups: Morehead Theatre; Theatre Ensemble
Workshops/Festivals: Theatre Contest Festival; Summer Theatre

---

MURRAY STATE UNIVERSITY
Murray   Kentucky 42071, 502 762-3750
State and 4 Year
Arts Areas: Instrumental Music, Vocal Music, Theatre and Visual Arts

MUSIC

Richard W Farrell, Chairman   **Number Of Faculty:** 25
Number Of Students: 280   **Degrees Offered:** BMus; BMusEd; MMus; MMusEd
Teaching Certification Available
Financial Assistance: Scholarships and Work-Study Grants
Performing Groups: Band; Orchestra

THEATRE

Robert E Johnson, Chairman   **Number Of Faculty:** 2   **Number Of Students:** 25
Degrees Offered: BS   **Teaching Certification Available**
Financial Assistance: Scholarships and Work-Study Grants
Performing Groups: Sock & Buskin

PIKEVILLE COLLEGE
Sycamore St, Pikeville   Kentucky 41501
606 432-3161 Ext 249
Private and 4 Year
Arts Areas: Instrumental Music, Vocal Music and Theatre
Performing Series: Co - sponsor series with Pikeville Concert Association
Performance Facilities: Faith Chapel; Chrisman Auditorium

MUSIC

Russell Patterson, Chairman, Department of Fine Arts   **Number Of Faculty:** 5
Degrees Offered: BME; MA
Courses Offered: Music Theory, Literature & History; Conducting; Class Piano; Form & Analysis; Private Applied Instruction; Ensemble Participation
Teaching Certification Available
Financial Assistance: Scholarships, Work-Study Grants and BEOG; SEOG; Loans
Performing Groups: Concert Choir; Symphonic Wind Ensemble; Pep Band; Jazz Band; Pops Ensemble
Workshops/Festivals: Kentucky Music Educators' High School Music Festival

THEATRE

Russell Patterson, Chairman, Department of Fine Arts
Courses Offered: Drama Practicum
Financial Assistance: Scholarships, Work-Study Grants and BEOG; SEOG; Loans
Performing Groups: Peach Orchard Players
Workshops/Festivals: High School Speech Tournament

SOUTHERN BAPTIST THEOLOGICAL SEMINARY SCHOOL OF CHURCH MUSIC
2825 Lexington Rd, Louisville   Kentucky 40206
502 897-4115

Private and 2 Year   *Arts Areas:* Instrumental Music and Vocal Music
Performance Facilities: Heeren Recital Hall   *Number Of Faculty:* 30
Number Of Students: 305
Degrees Offered: Master of Church Music; Doctor of Musical Arts
Courses Offered: Complete music curriculum covering graduate studies leading toward the master's or doctor's degree
Financial Assistance: Assistantships, Scholarships and Work-Study Grants
Performing Groups: Oratorio Chorus; Seminary Choir; Male Chorale; Chapel Choir; Seminary Winds; Seminary Strings; String Quartet; Brass Quintet; Woodwind Quintet
Workshops/Festivals: Church Music Institute

THOMAS MORE COLLEGE
Covington   Kentucky 41017, 606 341-5800

Private and 4 Year   *Arts Areas:* Theatre and Visual Arts
Performance Facilities: Thomas More Theatre

THEATRE

Ronald A Mielech, Chairman   *Number Of Faculty:* 2   *Number Of Students:* 12
Degrees Offered: BA   *Teaching Certification Available*
Financial Assistance: Scholarships and Work-Study Grants
Performing Groups: Mann Theatre

TRANSYLVANIA UNIVERSITY
300 N Broadway, Lexington   Kentucky 40508
606 233-8141

Private and 4 Year
Arts Areas: Dance, Instrumental Music, Vocal Music and Theatre
Performance Facilities: Mitchell Fine Arts Center contains Haggin Auditorium, Carrick Theater and Recital Hall

MUSIC

Number Of Faculty: 8   *Number Of Students:* 25   *Degrees Offered:* BA
Technical Training: Piano; Organ; Voice; Strings; Woodwinds; Brass; Percussion
Teaching Certification Available
Financial Assistance: Work-Study Grants and Activity
Performing Groups: Transylvania University Choir; Choral Union; Madrigal Singers; Chamber Ensemble; Jazz Ensemble; Ensembles in Strings, Piano, Woodwinds, Brass; Transylvania University Band
Workshops/Festivals: Contemporary Music Week; Kentucky Regional High School Music Contest

THEATRE

Number Of Faculty: 3   *Number Of Students:* 10   *Degrees Offered:* BA
Technical Training: Theater; Acting; Voice & Interpretation; Design; Lighting; Stagecraft; Costuming; Directing
Teaching Certification Available
Financial Assistance: Work-Study Grants and Activity
Performing Groups: Transylvania University Theater
Artists-In-Residence/Guest Artists: Daniel Pinkham

UNION COLLEGE
Barbourville   Kentucky 40906, 606 546-4151 Ext 145

Private and 4 Year
Arts Areas: Instrumental Music, Vocal Music and Theatre
Performing Series: Southwestern Kentucky Fine Arts Concert Series (Co-Sponsor)
Performance Facilities: Rector Little Theatre

(continued on next page)

MUSIC

Number Of Faculty: 6   **Number Of Students:** 35   **Degrees Offered:** BA; BS; BMus
Teaching Certification Available
Financial Assistance: Scholarships and Work-Study Grants
Performing Groups: Choir; Chorus; Wind Ensemble; Stage Band; Chamber Music Ensembles
Workshops/Festivals: Fine Arts Workshop

THEATRE

Number Of Faculty: 1   **Number Of Students:** 10   **Degrees Offered:** BS; BA
Teaching Certification Available
Financial Assistance: Scholarships and Work-Study Grants
Performing Groups: Union College Drama Department
Workshops/Festivals: Fine Arts Workshop

WESTERN KENTUCKY UNIVERSITY
Bowling Green   Kentucky 42101, 502 745-2344
State and 4 Year
Arts Areas: Dance, Instrumental Music, Vocal Music, Theatre, Film Arts and Television
Performing Series: Fine Arts Festival
Performance Facilities: Van Meter Russell Miller Theatre; Recital Hall

DANCE

Dr Burch Oglesby, Head, Physical Education & Recreation
Number Of Faculty: 1   **Number Of Students:** 250
Degrees Offered: BFA in Performing Arts; BA Dance Minor
Courses Offered: Ballet; Modern; Jazz; Tap; Dance Composition
Financial Assistance: Assistantships   **Performing Groups:** WKU Dance Company
Workshops/Festivals: Dance Educators of America Training School

MUSIC

Dr Wayne Hobbs, Head   **Number Of Faculty:** 19   **Number Of Students:** 150
Degrees Offered: BMus; BA; MMus; MA MusEd
Courses Offered: Performance; Music Education; Theory/Composition; Music History; Musical Theatre
Teaching Certification Available
Financial Assistance: Assistantships, Scholarships and Work-Study Grants
Performing Groups: University Symphony Orchestra; Concert Band; Choral Union; University Choir;
Chamber Singers; Opera Theatre; Jazz Ensemble; Jazz/Swing Choir; Brass Choir
Workshops/Festivals: Summer Youth Music; Summer Workshops; Faculty Recital Series

THEATRE

Dr Randall Capps, Head   **Number Of Faculty:** 7   **Number Of Students:** 250
Degrees Offered: BA; MA; BFA   **Courses Offered:** All phases of theatre
Teaching Certification Available
Financial Assistance: Assistantships, Scholarships and Work-Study Grants
Performing Groups: Western Players; Western Kentucky Children's Theatre
Workshops/Festivals: Summer Theatre Workshop
Artists-In-Residence/Guest Artists: Sylvia Kersenbaum; Beverly Leonard

CENTENARY COLLEGE OF LOUISANA
2911 Centenary Blvd, Shreveport   Louisiana 71104
318 869-5011
Private and 4 Year
Arts Areas: Dance, Instrumental Music, Vocal Music and Theatre

DANCE

Ginger Folmer, Chairman   *Number Of Faculty:* 1   *Number Of Students:* 80
Courses Offered: Jazz; Tap; Ballet

MUSIC

Dr Harlan C Snow, Dean, Hurley School of Music   *Number Of Faculty:* 24
Number Of Students: 110   *Degrees Offered:* BMus; BA
Courses Offered: Performance; Applied; Sacred Music; Composition
Teaching Certification Available
Financial Assistance: Scholarships and Work-Study Grants
Performing Groups: College Choir; Chamber Singers; Chamber Orchestra; Symphony Chorale; Symphony Orchestra; Wind Ensemble; Stage Band; Opera Theatre; Small Ensembles
Workshops/Festivals: Annual Piano Competition; Piano Workshops; Church Music Institute; Voice Workshops; District High School Solo & Ensemble Festival; District High School Choral Festival

THEATRE

Robert Boseick, Chairman, Theatre/Speech   *Number Of Faculty:* 3
Number Of Students: 35 - 45   *Degrees Offered:* BA
Teaching Certification Available
Financial Assistance: Scholarships and Work-Study Grants
Performing Groups: Rivertown Players

DILLARD UNIVERSITY
2601 Gentilly Blvd, New Orleans   Louisiana 70122
504 944-8751 Ext 233
Private and 4 Year
Arts Areas: Instrumental Music, Vocal Music and Theatre
Performing Series: Lyceum Guest Artist Series

MUSIC

Mrs Violet G Bowers, Coordinator   *Number Of Faculty:* 7
Number Of Students: 25   *Degrees Offered:* BA
Courses Offered: Piano; Music Ed; Voice; Organ; Instrumental
Teaching Certification Available
Financial Assistance: Scholarships and Work-Study Grants
Performing Groups: Concert Choir; University Choir; Male Quartet; Stage Band

THEATRE

Earl D A Smith, Acting Chairman   *Number Of Faculty:* 2
Number Of Students: 25   *Degrees Offered:* BA   *Courses Offered:* Drama/Speech
Technical Training: Technical Theatre   *Teaching Certification Available*
Financial Assistance: Scholarships and Work-Study Grants
Performing Groups: Drama Guild; Theatre Dance Performance Workshop
Workshops/Festivals: Christmas Festival; Theatre Dance Performance Workshop; Spring Concert (Co-Sponsored by the Music Area)

GRAMBLING COLLEGE OF LOUISIANA

Grambling   Louisiana 71245, 318 247-3761

State and 4 Year
Arts Areas: Instrumental Music, Vocal Music, Theatre and Visual Arts
Performing Series: Performing Artist Series

MUSIC

Theodore Jennings, Chairman   *Number Of Faculty:* 12
Number Of Students: 250   *Degrees Offered:* BA
Teaching Certification Available
Financial Assistance: Scholarships and Work-Study Grants
Performing Groups: Grambling College Marching Band; Concert Band; Orchestra; Jazz Ensembles; Chamber Ensembles; Choir; Chorale; Brass Ensembles; Wind Ensemble; Percussion Ensemble; String Ensemble

THEATRE

George Wesley, Chairman   *Number Of Faculty:* 8   *Number Of Students:* 200
Degrees Offered: BA   *Teaching Certification Available*
Financial Assistance: Scholarships and Work-Study Grants
Performing Groups: Little Theatre Guild

LOUISANA STATE UNIVERSITY

Baton Rouge   Louisiana 70803, 504 388-3261

State and 4 Year
Arts Areas: Dance, Instrumental Music, Vocal Music, Theatre, Visual Arts and Opera
Performing Series: Chamber Music Series; LSU Union Series; Artists & Lecture Series
Performance Facilities: LSU Union Theater, Colonnade Theater; University Theater, Greek Theater; Assembly Center; Lab School

DANCE

Terry Worthy, Chairman   *Number Of Faculty:* 3   *Degrees Offered:* BS; MA
Teaching Certification Available   *Financial Assistance:* Assistantships
Performing Groups: Dance Theatre
Workshops/Festivals: Louisiana State Dance Symposium

MUSIC

Everett Timm, Dean, School of Music   *Number Of Faculty:* 40
Number Of Students: 300   *Degrees Offered:* BMus; BMusEd; MMusEd; MA; DMA; PhD
Teaching Certification Available
Financial Assistance: Assistantships, Scholarships and Work-Study Grants
Performing Groups: LSU Orchestra; Band; A Cappella Choir; Opera; Women's Chorus; Timm Woodwind Quintet; Festival Arts Trio
Workshops/Festivals: Contemporary Music Festival

THEATRE

Bill Harbin, Chairman   *Number Of Faculty:* 24   *Number Of Students:* 200
Teaching Certification Available

LOUISIANA COLLEGE

1140 College Dr, Pineville   Louisiana 71360
318 487-7601

Private and 4 Year
Arts Areas: Instrumental Music, Vocal Music and Theatre
Performing Series: Lyceum Series   *Performance Facilities:* Guinn Auditorium

MUSIC

Jet E Turner, Chairman   *Number Of Faculty:* 7   *Number Of Students:* 75
Degrees Offered: BA   *Teaching Certification Available*

(continued on next page)

Financial Assistance: Scholarships and Work-Study Grants
Performing Groups: Mixed Chorus; Male Chorus; Mixed Choir; Jazz Band; Informal Groups
Workshops/Festivals: Vocal Clinic; Church Music Workshop; Piano Workshop; Organ Workshop; Choral Workshop

THEATRE

Frank D Bennett, Chairman   *Number Of Faculty:* 2   *Number Of Students:* 30
Degrees Offered: BA
Financial Assistance: Scholarships and Work-Study Grants

LOUISIANA POLYTECHNIC INSTITUTE
Ruston   Louisiana 71270, 318 257-0211
State and 4 Year
Arts Areas: Instrumental Music, Vocal Music, Theatre and Television

MUSIC

Raymond G Young, Chairman
Degrees Offered: BA Mus; BA MusEd; MA MusEd; MA Mus
Teaching Certification Available
Financial Assistance: Scholarships and Work-Study Grants

THEATRE

Arthur Stone, Chairman   *Degrees Offered:* BA; MA
Teaching Certification Available   *Financial Assistance:* Scholarships
Performing Groups: Tech Theatre Players

LOUISIANA TECHNICAL UNIVERSITY
Ruston   Louisiana 71270, 318 257-2641
State and 4 Year
Arts Areas: Instrumental Music, Vocal Music, Theatre, Television, Visual Arts and Radio
Performance Facilities: Howard Auditorium

MUSIC

Raymond J Young, Chairman   *Number Of Faculty:* 16   *Number Of Students:* 200
Degrees Offered: BA; MA   *Technical Training:* Opera
Teaching Certification Available
Financial Assistance: Scholarships and Work-Study Grants
Performing Groups: Chamber Ensemble; Symphony; Band; Orchestra; Chorale Ensemble; Musical Theatre; Instrumental Ensembles
Workshops/Festivals: Opera Workshop; Summer Music Camp

THEATRE

Arthur W Stone, Chairman   *Number Of Faculty:* 2
Degrees Offered: BA Speech - Drama   *Teaching Certification Available*
Financial Assistance: Scholarships and Work-Study Grants
Performing Groups: Musical Theatre; Tech Theatre Players

LOYOLA UNIVERSITY
6363 St Charles Ave, New Orleans   Louisiana 70118
504 865-2011
Private and 4 Year
Arts Areas: Dance, Instrumental Music, Vocal Music, Theatre, Television, Visual Arts and Fine Arts
Performance Facilities: Marquette Theatre; Nunemaker Hall

DANCE

Ernest J Ferlita, S J, Contractor
Dance program under auspices of Music College

(continued on next page)

Degrees Offered: BFA
Financial Assistance: Assistantships, Scholarships and Work-Study Grants

MUSIC

Dr David P Swanzy, Dean, College of Music
Number Of Faculty: 15 Full-time, 27 Part-time   *Number Of Students:* 265
Degrees Offered: BMus Harpsichord, Instrumental, Jazz Studies, Organ, Piano, Piano Pedagogy, Theory &
Composition, Voice, Music Therapy; BMusEd, Instrumental, Instrumental & Vocal, Piano, Vocal; MMus,
Instrumental, Piano, Vocal; MMusEd, Instrumental, Piano, Vocal; MMus in Music Therapy, Instrumental,
Piano, Vocal
Courses Offered: Recital; Theory I, II, III, IV; Piano; Major Instrument; Major Ensemble; Music as Value
I, II; Introduction to Music Literature; Junior Recital; Counterpoint I, II; Music History I, II; Essentials of
Conducting; Instrumental Conducting; Senior Recital; Form & Analysis I, II; Orchestration I, II;
Pre-Baroque History; Contemporary History; Perspectives of Jazz I, II; Improvisation; Evolution of Jazz
Styles; Jazz Counterpoint; 18th Century Counterpoint; Advanced Improvisation I, II; Music Therapy I, II,
III, IV; Guitar; Clinical Training (music therapy); Functional Music Barrier; Accompanying; Piano
Pedagogy & Literature; Choral Conducting; Italian Diction; Vocal Repertoire; Voice; Opera Workshop;
French Diction; German Diction; Strings; Brass & Percussion; Woodwinds
Technical Training: Music Therapy; Student Teaching
Teaching Certification Available
Financial Assistance: Assistantships, Scholarships and Work-Study Grants
Performing Groups: University Band; University Chamber Orchestra; University Chorus; University
Chorale; University Training Orchestra; University Wind Ensemble; Opera Workshop; Madrigal Singers;
Brass Ensemble; Percussion Ensemble; String Ensemble; Woodwind Ensemble; Jazz/Lab Band; Loyola
Ballet
Workshops/Festivals: Guitar Festival; Jazz Festival; Choral Festival; Summer Music Camp (Junior & High
School Students); Opera Workshop

THEATRE

Rev Ernest Ferlita, S J, Chairman, Drama & Speech   *Number Of Faculty:* 4
Number Of Students: 20
Degrees Offered: BA Drama & Speech; BFA Drama & Dance; Drama Therapy Program
Courses Offered: Fundamentals of Speech; Principles of Production; Introduction to Arts in Therapy;
Colloquium; Actor's Voice; The Actor's Art; Body Movement for the Theatre; Mime & Pantomime; Drama
Therapy I, II; Theatre Workshop; Play Production; The Director's Art; Child Drama; Directing &
Teaching Drama in High School; Lighting in the Theatre; Beginning & Advanced Set Design; Advanced
Technical Theatre; Principles of Playwriting; Theatre Experiments; Theatre Management
Financial Assistance: Assistantships, Scholarships and Work-Study Grants
Performing Groups: Loyola University Players; Experimental Theatre
Workshops/Festivals: Summer Workshop in Child Drama

MC NEESE STATE UNIVERSITY

Lake Charles   Louisiana 70609, 318 477-2520
State and 4 Year
Arts Areas: Instrumental Music, Vocal Music, Theatre and Visual Arts

Number Of Faculty: 17   *Number Of Students:* 275
Degrees Offered: BMus; BMusEd; MMus; MMusEd
Teaching Certification Available
Financial Assistance: Scholarships and Work-Study Grants
Performing Groups: Orchestra; Chamber Ensemble; Chorale Ensemble; Band
Workshops/Festivals: Opera Workshop

THEATRE

Dr Richard Levardsen, Head, Speech Department   *Number Of Faculty:* 7
Number Of Students: 130   *Degrees Offered:* BA; MA
Teaching Certification Available
Financial Assistance: Scholarships and Work-Study Grants
Performing Groups: Debate Club; Theatre

NEW ORLEANS BAPTIST THEOLOGICAL SEMINARY

3939 Gentilly Blvd, New Orleans   Louisiana 70126
504 282-4455 Ext 226

Private and 4 Year   *Arts Areas:* Instrumental Music and Vocal Music
Performance Facilities: Leavell Chapel; Martin Chapel; Choral Classroom

MUSIC

Clinton C Nichols, Chairman   *Number Of Faculty:* 8
Degrees Offered: MMus; MMusEd; DMus
Financial Assistance: Assistantships, Scholarships and Work-Study Grants
Performing Groups: The Seminarians; The Seminary Chorale; The Ladies' Choir; The Instrumental Ensemble
Workshops/Festivals: Music Symposium; Choral; Handbells; Music Reading; Music Admin in Church
Artists-In-Residence/Guest Artists: Mona Goff Bond

UNIVERSITY OF NEW ORLEANS

Lakefront, New Orleans   Louisiana 70122
504 283-0600

State and 4 Year
Arts Areas: Dance, Instrumental Music, Vocal Music, Theatre, Film Arts, Television and Visual Arts
Performance Facilities: University Theatres East & South; Recital Hall; Lab Theater

MUSIC

Mary Ann Bulla, Professor & Chairman   *Number Of Faculty:* 10
Number Of Students: 180
Degrees Offered: BA Applied Music, Music Theory & Composition, Music History; BA MusEd, Vocal & Instrumental
Technical Training: Piano; Voice; All Orchestral & Band Instruments
Teaching Certification Available
Financial Assistance: Scholarships, Work-Study Grants and Departmental Student Work
Performing Groups: University Chorus; University Chorale; University Chamber Singers; University Marching Band; University Concert Band; Wind Ensemble; Jazz Band; Lab Band

THEATRE

William Harlan Shaw, Professor   *Number Of Faculty:* 15
Number Of Students: 220   *Degrees Offered:* BA; MA; MFA
Courses Offered: Acting; Costume; Dance; Directing; Film; History; Playwriting; Scene Design; Tech Theater; Television; Theory of Drama
Technical Training: Performance; Design; Film; TV; Production
Teaching Certification Available
Financial Assistance: Assistantships and Work-Study Grants
Performing Groups: Resident Acting Company; Performance Group; University Theatre; Children's Theater; Readers' Theater

NICHOLLS STATE UNIVERSITY

Highway I, Thibodaux   Louisiana 70301
504 446-8111

State and 4 Year
Arts Areas: Instrumental Music, Vocal Music, Theatre, Television and Visual Arts
Performing Series: Concert - Artist Series
Performance Facilities: Two Auditoriums; Theatre

MUSIC

Timothy R Lindsley, Jr, Chairman   *Number Of Faculty:* 10
Number Of Students: 200   *Degrees Offered:* BMusEd; BMus
Courses Offered: Theory; History; Literature; Applied Instruments; Piano; Recitals
Teaching Certification Available

(continued on next page)

Financial Assistance: Scholarships and Work-Study Grants
Performing Groups: Chorus; Ensembles; Band   **Workshops/Festivals:** Band

THEATRE

Dr Melvin H Berry, Chairman   **Number Of Faculty:** 6   **Number Of Students:** 20
Degrees Offered: BA
Courses Offered: History, Costuming; Design; Children's Theatre; Directing; Acting; Television
Teaching Certification Available
Financial Assistance: Scholarships and Work-Study Grants
Performing Groups: Nicholls Players

NORTHEAST LOUISIANA UNIVERSITY
700 University Ave, Monroe   Louisiana 71209
318 342-2011
State and 4 Year
Arts Areas: Dance, Instrumental Music, Vocal Music, Theatre and Television
Performing Series: Arts Festival   **Performance Facilities:** Brown Auditorium

DANCE

Dr Earl D Speights, Head, Department of Health & Physical Education
Dance program under auspices of Health & Physical Education Department
Number Of Faculty: 12   **Number Of Students:** 274   **Degrees Offered:** BSEd; MEd
Courses Offered: Rhythmic Activities; Modern Dance; Social Dance; Folk Dance; Advanced Modern Dance
Technical Training: Methods in Rhythmic Activities, Organization & Administration of Dance in Schools; Dance Workshop
Teaching Certification Available
Financial Assistance: Assistantships and Work-Study Grants
Performing Groups: NLU Dance Company
Workshops/Festivals: Dance Concert (each Spring Semester)

MUSIC

Richard A Worthington, Director, School of Music   **Number Of Faculty:** 25
Number Of Students: 230
Degrees Offered: BA; BM in Performance, History & Literature, Theory & Composition; BMusEd; MMus; MMusEd
Courses Offered: Comprehensive   **Teaching Certification Available**
Financial Assistance: Assistantships, Scholarships and Work-Study Grants
Performing Groups: Band; Orchestra; University Chorus; University Chorale; Concert Choir; Electones; Jazz Ensemble; Contemporary Wind Quintet; Chamber Arts Brass Quintet

THEATRE

Dr James W Parkerson, Head, Department of Communication Arts
Number Of Faculty: 15   **Number Of Students:** 281
Degrees Offered: BA; MA; MEd   **Courses Offered:** All aspects of theatre
Technical Training: Technical Theatre   **Teaching Certification Available**
Financial Assistance: Assistantships, Scholarships and Work-Study Grants
Performing Groups: Annual High School Speech & Drama Festival; Annual Fine Arts Festival; Annual Summer Children's Theatre Festival

---

NORTHWESTERN STATE UNIVERSITY OF LOUISIANA
Natchitoches   Louisiana 71457, 318 357-6171
State and 4 Year
Arts Areas: Dance, Instrumental Music, Vocal Music, Theatre and Visual Arts
Performance Facilities: Fine Arts Building; Little Theatre

DANCE

Dr Coleen B Nelken, Chairman, College of Education
Dance program under auspices of Physical Education Department

(continued on next page)

Number Of Faculty: 3   **Degrees Offered:** BS
Teaching Certification Available
Financial Assistance: Scholarships and Work-Study Grants
Workshops/Festivals: High School & Junior High School Dance Camp

MUSIC

Dr J Robert Smith, Chairman   **Number Of Faculty:** 15
Number Of Students: 400   **Degrees Offered:** BA; BS Education; MMus; MMusEd
Teaching Certification Available
Financial Assistance: Scholarships and Work-Study Grants
Performing Groups: Opera Theatre; Band; Orchestra; Chorus; Ensembles
Workshops/Festivals: High School & Junior High School Music Camp

THEATRE

E Robert Black, Chairman   **Number Of Faculty:** 2   **Number Of Students:** 45
Degrees Offered: BA; MA   **Teaching Certification Available**
Financial Assistance: Scholarships and Work-Study Grants
Performing Groups: Summer Repertory Theatre

SAINT MARY'S DOMINICAN COLLEGE
New Orleans   Louisiana 70118, 504 866-8651
Private and 4 Year   **Arts Areas:** Dance and Visual Arts
Performing Series: Dance Ensemble

DANCE

Jon Von Erb, Director   **Number Of Faculty:** 4   **Number Of Students:** 30
Technical Training: Work - Study Abroad
Financial Assistance: Scholarships and Work-Study Grants

SOUTHEASTERN LOUISIANA UNIVERSITY
Box 767, Univ Sta, Hammond   Louisiana 70401
504 549-2101
State and 4 Year
Arts Areas: Dance, Instrumental Music, Vocal Music, Theatre and Visual Arts
Performance Facilities: Humanities Theater

DANCE

Dr Walter Russell, Chairman   **Number Of Faculty:** 2
Number Of Students: 18 - 20   **Degrees Offered:** BA
Teaching Certification Available   **Financial Assistance:** Work-Study Grants
Performing Groups: Modern Dance
Workshops/Festivals: Modern Dance Group Recitals

MUSIC

Dr David McCormick, Chairman   **Number Of Faculty:** 15
Number Of Students: 201
Degrees Offered: BA; BMusEd; BMus; MMus, Theory, Composition, Applied Music; MMusEd
Teaching Certification Available
Financial Assistance: Assistantships, Scholarships and Work-Study Grants
Performing Groups: Symphonic & Varsity Bands; Jazz Band; Orchestra; Concert Choir; Chamber Choir;
University Chorus; Chamber Groups
Workshops/Festivals: Louisiana Music Educators Association High School Band & Choral Festivals; Jazz
Workshops; Marching Band Workshops; Numerous Music Workshops

THEATRE

Luther I Wade, Chairman   **Number Of Faculty:** 6   **Number Of Students:** 55
Degrees Offered: BA Theatre; BA Speech with Theatre Emphasis
Technical Training: Scene Design; Costuming; Stagecraft

(continued on next page)

Teaching Certification Available **Financial Assistance:** Work-Study Grants
Performing Groups: Southeastern Theatre Proscenium Players
Workshops/Festivals: High School One Play Festival

SOUTHERN UNIVERSITY, BATON ROUGE
Baton Rouge   Louisiana 70813, 504 771-4500
State and 4 Year
Arts Areas: Instrumental Music, Vocal Music, Theatre and Visual Arts

MUSIC

Aldrich Adkins, Chairman   **Number Of Faculty:** 2   **Number Of Students:** 34
Degrees Offered: BMusEd; MMusEd   **Teaching Certification Available**
Financial Assistance: Scholarships and Work-Study Grants
Performing Groups: Chorus; Band; Chorale; Ensembles

THEATRE

George Whitfield, Chairman   **Number Of Faculty:** 6   **Number Of Students:** 110
Degrees Offered: BA   **Teaching Certification Available**
Financial Assistance: Scholarships and Work-Study Grants
Performing Groups: Riberband Players

UNIVERSITY OF SOUTHWESTERN LOUISANA
University Ave, Lafayette   Louisiana 70504
318 233-3850 Ext 410
State, 4 Year and Master's Programs in Music & Speech
Arts Areas: Dance, Instrumental Music, Vocal Music, Theatre, Film Arts, Television and Visual Arts
Performing Series: Concert Series; Opera Society; Reader's Theatre;
Willis Ducrest Festival of Visual & Performing Arts; The Deep South Writers & Artists Conference
Performance Facilities: Main Stage Theatre; Laboratory Theatre; Angelle Hall Auditorium; USL Union
Theatre

DANCE

Muriel Moreland, Head   **Number Of Faculty:** 3   **Number Of Students:** 100
Degrees Offered: BFA
Courses Offered: Performance; Ballet; Contemporary Dance Techniques; Creative Dance & Ballet for
Children; Philosophy & History of Dance; Choreography & Related Media
Financial Assistance: Assistantships and Scholarships
Performing Groups: Dance Repertoire Theatre; Choreotheatre; Choreodancers
Workshops/Festivals: State Dance Symposium; Artists-in-Residence Workshop

MUSIC

Nolan Sahuc, Director   **Number Of Faculty:** 23
Number Of Students: 190 - 225
Degrees Offered: BA Applied Music or Music History & Literature; BMus in Music or Theory &
Comprehension; BMusEd, M or Arts in Music, M of Music, MMusEd
Courses Offered: Theory; Ensemble; Instrument; Piano; History of Music; Form & Analysis; Counterpoint;
Orchestration; Mixed Chorus; Keyboard Harmony; Voice; Conducting; Choral Arranging
Teaching Certification Available
Financial Assistance: Assistantships, Scholarships and Work-Study Grants
Performing Groups: Concert Band; Wind Ensemble; Chamber Orchestra; Chaorale; Men's Chorus;
Women's Chorus; Opera Guild; Stage (Jazz) Band
Workshops/Festivals: LMEA Piano Festival; Band; Chorus; Vocal - Solo & Small Ensemble; Instrumental;
Solo & Small Ensemble Festivals; USL Piano Technique Festival; Ducrest French Festival of Performing
Arts; Mouton Keyboard Festival; Opera Institute; Flag Corps Contest; Marching Band Contest; Symphonia
Stage Band Festival

THEATRE

Ronald C Kern, Head, Theatre Area of the Department of Speech
Number Of Faculty: 5   **Number Of Students:** 25

(continued on next page)

Degrees Offered: BA; MS in Speech Communication
Courses Offered: Introduction to Theatre; Theatre Workshop; Acting Fundamentals; Play Production; Stage Direction; Theatre History; Stage Lighting; Stage Design; Stage Makeup; Costume Design; Readers' Theatre; Creative Dramatics; Directing
Teaching Certification Available   **Financial Assistance:** Work-Study Grants
Performing Groups: Alpha Psi Omega; Readers' Theatre Performers; USL Players; Children's Theatre Group; Lab Theatre Groups
Workshops/Festivals: Literary Rally; One Act Play Contest for secondary school students; High School Acting Workshop

TULANE UNIVERSITY
New Orleans   Louisiana 70118, 504 865-4011

Private and 4 Year
Francis L Lawrence Acting Dean, Sophie Newcomb College
Arts Areas: Dance, Instrumental Music, Vocal Music, Theatre and Visual Arts
Performing Series: First Monday (Contemporary Music Series)
Performance Facilities: Playhouse; Arena Theatre; Dixon Hall; McAlister Auditorium

DANCE

Elizabeth B Delery, Head, Department of Physical Education
Dance program under auspices of Physical Education Department
Number Of Faculty: 3   **Number Of Students:** 394
Performing Groups: Modern Dance Club; Ballet Dance Club
Workshops/Festivals: Dance Concert Annually; Spring Arts Festival

MUSIC

Francis L Monachino, Professor & Chairman   **Number Of Faculty:** 11
Number Of Students: 150   **Degrees Offered:** BA; BFA; MA; MFA
Teaching Certification Available
Financial Assistance: Assistantships, Scholarships and Work-Study Grants
Performing Groups: Band; Opera Workshop; Chorus; Orchestra; Woodwind Ensemble
Workshops/Festivals: Guitar Workshops; High School Music Theatre

THEATRE

M S Barranger, University Chairman   **Number Of Faculty:** 7.25
Number Of Students: 450   **Degrees Offered:** BA; BFA; MA; MFA
Courses Offered: Acting; Directing; Theatre History; Theory & Criticism; Technical Production; Costume Design; Scene Design; Lighting
Technical Training: Lighting & Technical Production
Financial Assistance: Assistantships, Scholarships and Work-Study Grants
Performing Groups: Tulane University Theatre; Tulane Center Stage
Workshops/Festivals: Workshops & Lecturers are sponsored during the academic year

XAVIER UNIVERSITY OF LOUISANA
7325 Palmetto St, New Orleans   Louisiana 70125
504 486-7411

Private and 4 Year
Arts Areas: Instrumental Music, Vocal Music, Theatre and Television

MUSIC

Dr Malcolm Breda, Chairman   **Number Of Faculty:** 9 Full-time, 5 Part-Time
Number Of Students: 80   **Degrees Offered:** BMus; BMusEd; BA
Technical Training: Opera   **Teaching Certification Available**
Financial Assistance: Scholarships and Work-Study Grants
Performing Groups: Chapel Choir; University Chorus; Concert Choir; Symphonic Band; Jazz Lab Band
Workshops/Festivals: Opera Workshop

(continued on next page)

THEATRE

Dr Joe A Melcher, Chairman, Communication & Theatre
Number Of Faculty: 7 Full-time, 1 Part-time   **Number Of Students:** 110
Degrees Offered: BA; BS   **Courses Offered:** Drama; Speech; Communications
Teaching Certification Available

BATES COLLEGE
Lewiston   Maine 04240, 207 782-5533
   Private and 4 Year
   Arts Areas: Instrumental Music, Vocal Music, Theatre and Visual Arts
   Performing Series: Concert - Lecture Series
   Performance Facilities: Little Theatre

MUSIC

D Robert Smith, Chairman   *Number Of Faculty:* 3   *Number Of Students:* 38
Degrees Offered: BA   *Teaching Certification Available*
Financial Assistance: Scholarships and Work-Study Grants

THEATRE

Bill Beard, Chairman   *Number Of Faculty:* 3   *Number Of Students:* 42
Courses Offered: Introduction; Play Production; Acting
Performing Groups: Bates College Theatre

BOWDOIN COLLEGE
Brunswick   Maine 04011, 207 725-8731
   Private and 4 Year
   Arts Areas: Dance, Instrumental Music, Vocal Music, Theatre, Film Arts, Television and Visual Arts
   Performing Series: Curtis - Zimbalist Concert Series
   Performance Facilities: Pickard & Experimental Theaters; Kresge & Smith Auditoriums;
   Sills Hall; Daggett Lounge; Bowdoin Senior Center; Gibson Hall of Music

DANCE

June A Vail, Director   *Number Of Faculty:* 1   *Number Of Students:* 40
Financial Assistance: Scholarships and Work-Study Grants
Performing Groups: Bowdoin Dance Group
Workshops/Festivals: Annual Spring Dance Festival

MUSIC

Elliott S Schwartz, Professor   *Number Of Faculty:* 4
Number Of Students: 150   *Degrees Offered:* AB
Courses Offered: Introduction to Music; World Music; Contemporary Music; Introduction to
Ethomusicology; Electronic Music; Studies in Music Literature: The Classical & Romantic Symphony, The
Symphony in the Twentieth Century; Introduction to the Structure of Music; Advanced Materials of Music;
Music History & Literature; Orchestration; Composition; Collegium Musicum; Form & Analysis; Advanced
Topics in Music Literature; The Concerto in the Baroque & Classical Perids; The Art Song; Applied Music
& Ensemble
Technical Training: Applied Music Instruction including ensemble training
Financial Assistance: Scholarships and Work-Study Grants
Performing Groups: Glee Club; Chorale; Chamber Orchestra; Brass Ensemble; Meddiebempsters &
Miscellania (undergraduate singing groups); Marching Band; Stage Band
Workshops/Festivals: Summer Music School; Annual Contemporary Music Festival

THEATRE

A Raymond Rutan, Director   *Number Of Faculty:* 2   *Number Of Students:* 50
Degrees Offered: AB
Courses Offered: Playwriting; Acting & Directing; Set Design
Financial Assistance: Scholarships and Work-Study Grants
Performing Groups: Masque & Gown
Workshops/Festivals: Annual One-Act Play Contest

COLBY COLLEGE
Waterville   Maine 04901, 207 873-1131
   Private and 4 Year
   Arts Areas: Dance, Instrumental Music, Vocal Music and Theatre
   Performing Series: Colby Music Series
   Performance Facilities: Given Auditorium; Strider Theater

DANCE

Number Of Faculty: 1   *Performing Groups:* Colby Dancers
Workshops/Festivals: Visiting Artist Groups

MUSIC

James F Armstrong, Professor   *Number Of Faculty:* 5
Number Of Students: 30
Performing Groups: Colby Glee Club; Colby Band; Colby Community Symphony Orchestra; A Cappella
Singers

THEATRE

Professor F Celand Witham, Coordinator   *Number Of Faculty:* 5
Performing Groups: Powder & Wig Dramatic Society; Performing Arts Production

---

UNIVERSITY OF MAINE AT PORTLAND - GORHAM
College Ave, Gorham   Maine 04038
207 839-6771
   State and 4 Year
   Arts Areas: Instrumental Music, Vocal Music, Theatre and Visual Arts

MUSIC

Dr Ronald F Cole, Chairman   *Number Of Faculty:* 10   *Number Of Students:* 85
Degrees Offered: BA; BS   *Courses Offered:* Music; Music Education
Teaching Certification Available
Financial Assistance: Scholarships and Work-Study Grants
Performing Groups: A Cappella Chorus; Chamber Orchestra; University Band; Chamber Singers; Chorale;
Workshops/Festivals: Summer Workshops in Music Education

THEATRE

William P Steele, Chairman   *Number Of Faculty:* 5   *Number Of Students:* 55
Degrees Offered: BA   *Courses Offered:* Theater History & Practicum
Technical Training: Scene Design & Construction
Financial Assistance: Scholarships and Work-Study Grants
Performing Groups: University Players; Children's Theater of Maine; Performing Arts Ensemble

---

UNIVERSITY OF MAINE, ORONO
123 Lord Hall, Orono   Maine 04473
207 581-7534
   State and 4 Year
   Arts Areas: Dance, Instrumental Music, Vocal Music, Theatre, Film Arts and Television
   Performance Facilities: Hauck Auditorium   *Number Of Faculty:* 1 Part-time
   Courses Offered: Beginning & Intermediate Dance (Flamenco & Ballet); Jazz Fundamentals

MUSIC

Murray North, Acting Coordinator   *Number Of Faculty:* 17
Number Of Students: 115   *Degrees Offered:* BA Mus; BSMusEd; BMus Applied; MM
Courses Offered: Counterpoint; History; Conducting; Music Lit; Appreciation; Theory; Composition;
Teaching Certification Available   *Financial Assistance:* Assistantships
Performing Groups: Marching Band; Concert Band; Pep Band; Symphony Band; University Orchestra;

(continued on next page)

University Singers; University Chorus; Chamber Singers; Oratorio Society; 20th Century Music Ensemble; Karl Mellon Clarinet Choir; Two Graduate String Quartets
Workshops/Festivals: Maine Summer Youth Music Camp; Summer Chamber Music School

THEATRE

Arnold Colbath, Coordinator   *Number Of Faculty:* 4
Number Of Students: 300   *Degrees Offered:* BA; MA
Technical Training: Stage Design; Costume & Lighting Design; Stagecraft; Play Production
Performing Groups: Maine Masque Theatre
Workshops/Festivals: High School Theatre Workshop

MASSON COLLEGE
Springvale   Maine 04083, 207 324-5340
Private and 4 Year   *Arts Areas:* Dance and Theatre
Performing Series: Concert - Lecture Series; Film Series
Performance Facilities: Little Theatre; Hilltop House; Student Activity Center; Coffee House

DANCE

Number Of Faculty: 1   *Number Of Students:* 30
Courses Offered: Dance I & II; Modern Jazz
Financial Assistance: Internships, Assistantships, Scholarships and Work-Study Grants
Performing Groups: Ram Island Dance Company

MUSIC

Number Of Faculty: 1   *Number Of Students:* 35
Financial Assistance: Internships, Assistantships, Scholarships and Work-Study Grants

THEATRE

Leonard D Whittier, Chairman   *Number Of Faculty:* 3
Number Of Students: 25   *Degrees Offered:* BA
Financial Assistance: Internships, Assistantships, Scholarships and Work-Study Grants
Performing Groups: Footlighters; Touring Company

RICKER COLLEGE
Houlton   Maine 04730, 207 532-2223
Private and 4 Year
Arts Areas: Instrumental Music, Vocal Music and Theatre

MUSIC

Number Of Faculty: 2   *Number Of Students:* 24
Performing Groups: Vocal and Instrumental Ensembles

THEATRE

Number Of Faculty: 2   *Number Of Students:* 30   *Degrees Offered:* BA
Teaching Certification Available
Financial Assistance: Scholarships and Work-Study Grants
Performing Groups: College Theatre

MARYLAND

ANNE ARUNDEL COMMUNITY COLLEGE
Arnold   Maryland 21012, 301 647-7100
County and 2 Year   **Arts Areas:** Theatre
Performance Facilities: College Auditorium   **Degrees Offered:** AA
Performing Groups: Drama Group

BOWIE STATE COLLEGE
Bowie   Maryland 20715, 301 262-3350 Ext 303
State and 4 Year
Arts Areas: Dance, Instrumental Music, Vocal Music, Theatre, Film Arts and Visual Arts
Performing Series: Bowie Fine Arts Society
Performance Facilities: Martin Luther King Jr Communications Arts Center

DANCE

Dance program under auspices of Physical Education Department
Performing Groups: The Bowie Dancers
Workshops/Festivals: Annual Fine Arts Festival

MUSIC

Number Of Faculty: 13   **Number Of Students:** 50   **Degrees Offered:** BS Mus Ed
Technical Training: Concentration in Piano, Voice, Organ, Guitar, Orchestral Instruments
Teaching Certification Available
Financial Assistance: Assistantships, Scholarships and Work-Study Grants
Performing Groups: Bowie State College Chorale, Bowie Chamber Choir, Jazz Band, and Concert Band
Workshops/Festivals: Annual Fine Arts Festival, Graduate Choral Workshop, Black Music Workshop

THEATRE

Sister M G Donovan, Chairman   **Number Of Faculty:** 5
Number Of Students: 20   **Degrees Offered:** BA
Teaching Certification Available
Financial Assistance: Assistantships and Work-Study Grants
Performing Groups: Theatre Group
Workshops/Festivals: Annual Fine Arts Festival

CECIL COMMUNITY COLLEGE
Bayview, North East   Maryland 21901
301 287-6060
County and 2 Year
Arts Areas: Dance, Instrumental Music, Vocal Music, Theatre, Film Arts and Visual Arts
Performance Facilities: Three Auditoriums; Little Theatre

THEATRE

John Jay Jackson, Associate Professor   **Number Of Faculty:** 1
Number Of Students: 40   **Degrees Offered:** Transfer Programs
Technical Training: Stagecraft; Theatre Practica
Performing Groups: Alpha Ensemble Theatre of Delta Psi Omega
Workshops/Festivals: Summer Workshop

COLUMBIA UNION COLLEGE
7600 Flower Ave, Takoma Park   Maryland 20012
301 270-9200 Ext 252
Private and 4 Year
Arts Areas: Instrumental Music, Vocal Music and Visual Arts
Performance Facilities: Recital Hall; Sligo Seventh - Day Adventist Church

(continued on next page)

MUSIC

Van Knauss, DMA, Chairman   **Number Of Faculty:** 11   **Number Of Students:** 30
Degrees Offered: BA; BS Performance; BSMusEd
Courses Offered: History & Literature; Theory; Performance
Teaching Certification Available
Financial Assistance: Scholarships and Work-Study Grants
Performing Groups: Pro Musica (Choral); College Choir; Concert Band; Orchestra; Bell Choir; Brass Choir
Workshops/Festivals: Vocal Clinic; Two Piano Workshops
Artists-In-Residence/Guest Artists: Sontraud Speide; Richard Collins; Leslie Riskowitz

---

COMMUNITY COLLEGE OF BALTIMORE
2901 Liberty Heights Ave, Baltimore   Maryland 21215
301 396-0400
City and 2 Year
Arts Areas: Dance, Vocal Music, Theatre, Film Arts, Television and Visual Arts
Performance Facilities: Campus Theatre

MUSIC

Jaap van Opstal, Chairperson   **Degrees Offered:** AA
Financial Assistance: Work-Study Grants
Performing Groups: Choral Group; Instrumental Ensemble

THEATRE

Clarence Gregory, Liaison, Department of Speech, Drama & TV
Financial Assistance: Work-Study Grants   **Performing Groups:** CCB Players

---

EASTERN CHRISTIAN COLLEGE
Bel Air   Maryland 21014, 301 734-6222
Private and 2 Year   **Arts Areas:** Instrumental Music and Vocal Music
Degrees Offered: AA Church Music   **Financial Assistance:** Scholarships
Performing Groups: Choir, Instrumental Ensembles

ESSEX COMMUNITY COLLEGE
Ridge Rd, Baltimore   Maryland 21014
301 682-6000
County and 2 Year   **Arts Areas:** Vocal Music and Theatre
Performing Series: Concert Series   **Performance Facilities:** College Auditorium

MUSIC

Arno Drucker, Chairman   **Degrees Offered:** AA   **Technical Training:** Opera
Financial Assistance: Scholarships
Performing Groups: Vocal and Instrumental Ensembles

FROSTBURG STATE COLLEGE
E College Ave, Frostburg   Maryland 21532
301 689-6621
State and 4 Year
Arts Areas: Instrumental Music, Vocal Music, Theatre and Visual Arts
Performing Series: Artist - Lecture Series

MUSIC

Huot Fisher, Chairman   **Number Of Faculty:** 9   **Number Of Students:** 145
Degrees Offered: BA, BA MusEd   **Technical Training:** Opera
Teaching Certification Available   **Financial Assistance:** Work-Study Grants
Performing Groups: Orchestra, String Ensembles, Wind Ensembles, Choir, Bands

(continued on next page)

THEATRE

Betsy Ross Rankin, Chairman   **Number Of Faculty:** 3   **Number Of Students:** 50
Degrees Offered: BA Speech - Theatre   **Teaching Certification Available**
Financial Assistance: Work-Study Grants   **Performing Groups:** Little Theatre

---

GOUCHER COLLEGE
1021 Dulaney Valley Rd, Towson   Maryland 21204
301 825-3300
Private and 4 Year
Arts Areas: Instrumental Music, Vocal Music, Theatre and Visual Arts
Performing Series: Concert Series

MUSIC

Dr Elliott W Galkin, Chairman   **Number Of Faculty:** 12
Number Of Students: 145   **Degrees Offered:** BA
Teaching Certification Available
Financial Assistance: Internships, Assistantships, Scholarships and Work-Study Grants
Performing Groups: Orchestra, Choir, String Ensembles, Bands

THEATRE

George B Dowell, Chairman   **Number Of Faculty:** 4   **Number Of Students:** 50
Degrees Offered: BA   **Teaching Certification Available**
Financial Assistance: Internships, Assistantships, Scholarships and Work-Study Grants
Performing Groups: Masks & Faces

HOOD COLLEGE
Frederick   Maryland 21701, 301 663-3131 217
Private and 4 Year
Arts Areas: Instrumental Music, Vocal Music and Visual Arts
Performing Series: Community Forum Performing Artist Series
Performance Facilities: Brodbeck Auditorium; Coffman Chapel

MUSIC

William Sprigg, Chairman   **Number Of Faculty:** 3 Full-time, 5 Part-time
Number Of Students: 208   **Degrees Offered:** AB
Financial Assistance: Scholarships and Work-Study Grants
Performing Groups: Orchestra; Band; Ensembles; Chorus
Artists-In-Residence/Guest Artists: Noel Lester

UNIVERSITY OF MARYLAND
College Park   Maryland 20742, 301 454-2740
State, 4 Year and Graduate Studies
Arts Areas: Dance, Instrumental Music, Vocal Music, Theatre, Film Arts and Television
Performance Facilities: Theater; Recital Hall

DANCE

Elizabeth Ince, Chairperson   **Number Of Faculty:** 22
Number Of Students: 115   **Degrees Offered:** BA
Courses Offered: Dance Technique; Ethnic & Jazz; Modern & Ballet, Dance Production; Dance History; Theory & Philosophy; Music for Dance; Kinesiology for Dance
Teaching Certification Available
Financial Assistance: Internships and Scholarships
Performing Groups: Maryland Dance Theater
Workshops/Festivals: Maryland Arts Council Dance Festival; Summer Performance Series

MUSIC

Eugene W Troth, Chairman   **Number Of Faculty:** 50 Full-time, 10 Part-time
Number Of Students: 500

(*continued on next page*)

Degrees Offered: BA; BMus; BS; MMus; MA; MEd; DMA; PhD; EdD
Courses Offered: Performance; Theory; Composition; Music Education; Musicology
Teaching Certification Available
Financial Assistance: Assistantships, Scholarships and Work-Study Grants
Performing Groups: Symphony Band; Concert Band; Marching Band; Jazz Band; Chorale; Chapel Choir; Symphony Orchestra; Collegium Musicum; Opera Theater; 20th Century Ensemble; Miscellaneous Chamber Music Ensembles; Gospel Choir
Workshops/Festivals: International Piano Festival & Competition; Mid - Winter Music Conference; Great variety of Instrumental, Vocal & Music Education Workshops & Master Classes

THEATRE

Dr Rudolph E Pugliese, Professor   ***Number Of Faculty:*** 15
Number Of Students: 250   ***Degrees Offered:*** BA; MA
Courses Offered: Introduction to the Theatre; Acting Fundamentals; Creative Expression; Stagecraft; Makeup; Speech for the Stage; Scenographic Techniques; Historic Costuming for the Stage; Costume Crafts; Play Production; Intermediate Acting; Play Directing; Stage Decor; Stage Design; Styles & Theories of Acting; Actor's Studio; Advanced Directing for the Stage; Children's Dramatics; Directing Plays for Children's Theatre; American Musical Comedy; Theatre Management I & II; Advanced Scenic Design; Principles & Theories of Stage Lighting; Advanced Lighting Design; Theatre Workshop; Stage Costume Design I & II; Advanced Makeup; History of the Theatre II; History of Theatrical Theory & Criticism; Independent Study
Financial Assistance: Assistantships, Scholarships and Work-Study Grants
Performing Groups: University Theatre; Children's Workshop; Experimental Theatre

---

UNIVERSITY OF MARYLAND, EASTERN SHORE
PO Box 1014, Princess Anne   Maryland 21853
301 651-2200
County and 4 Year

State and 4 Year
Arts Areas: Instrumental Music, Vocal Music, Theatre and Visual Arts
Performance Facilities: Ella Fitzgerald Center for the Performing Arts

MUSIC

Dr Gerald W Johnson, Chairman   ***Number Of Faculty:*** 6
Number Of Students: 40   ***Degrees Offered:*** BA
Teaching Certification Available
Financial Assistance: Scholarships and Work-Study Grants
Performing Groups: Choir, Bands, Ensembles

THEATRE

Della Dameron, Director   ***Performing Groups:*** Stagecrafters

---

MONTGOMERY COLLEGE
51 Mannakee St, Rockville   Maryland 20850
301 762-7400 Ext 360
County and 2 Year
Arts Areas: Dance, Instrumental Music, Vocal Music, Theatre, Television and Visual Arts
Performing Series: Theatre Subscription; Faculty - Artist,, Collegiate Concert Series
Summer Musical Theatre; Montgomery Performing Arts Society
Performance Facilities: Fine Arts Theatre; Recital Hall

DANCE

Dance program under auspices of Physical Education, Speech & Drama
Number Of Faculty: 1½   ***Number Of Students:*** 50
Courses Offered: Ballet; Modern Dance; Body Movement
Technical Training: Ballet
Financial Assistance: Assistantships, Scholarships and Work-Study Grants
Performing Groups: Modern Dance Group
Workshops/Festivals: Dance Workshop Performance

(continued on next page)

MUSIC

Gerald Muller, Chairman   *Number Of Faculty:* 34   *Number Of Students:* 2,200
Degrees Offered: AA   *Courses Offered:* Full two year Music & Music Theatre
Teaching Certification Available
Financial Assistance: Internships, Assistantships, Scholarships and Work-Study Grants
Performing Groups: Music Theatre Production; College Chorus; Chamber Singers; Ensembles for Pianists & Singers; Light Opera Chorus; MCR Orchestra; Wind Ensemble; String & Guitar Ensemble; Woodwind & Saxaphone Ensemble; Brass Ensemble; Collegium Musicum; Trombone Ensemble; Percussion Ensemble; Jazz Ensemble; Improvisational Ensemble
Workshops/Festivals: Piano Workshop; Jazz Workshop; Brass Workshop; String Workshop; Music Theatre Workshop

THEATRE

Martin Brodey, Professor, Chairman   *Number Of Faculty:* 7
Number Of Students: 500   *Degrees Offered:* AA
Financial Assistance: Internships, Assistantships, Scholarships and Work-Study Grants
Performing Groups: Youth Shakespeare Theatre; Drama Workshop; Student Experimental Theatre
Workshops/Festivals: Active participation in Regional American College Theatre Festival

---

MORGAN STATE COLLEGE
Baltimore   Maryland 21239, 301 323-2270 Ext 294
State and 4 Year
Arts Areas: Dance, Instrumental Music, Vocal Music, Theatre, Film Arts, Television and Visual Arts
Performance Facilities: Murphy Auditorium, Murphy Theatre

DANCE

Number Of Faculty: 3
Dance Department under auspices of Health & Physical Education Department
Financial Assistance: Work-Study Grants
Workshops/Festivals: Black Arts Festival

MUSIC

Nathan Carter, Chairman   *Number Of Faculty:* 12   *Degrees Offered:* BA
Teaching Certification Available   *Financial Assistance:* Work-Study Grants
Performing Groups: Choir, Band, Jazz Ensembles
Workshops/Festivals: Black Arts Festival

THEATRE

Dr Lucia S Hawthorne, Chairman   *Number Of Faculty:* 7
Number Of Students: 94   *Degrees Offered:* BA
Teaching Certification Available   *Financial Assistance:* Work-Study Grants
Performing Groups: Ira Aldridge Players, Alpha Psi Omega
Workshops/Festivals: Black Arts Festival

COLLEGE OF NOTRE DAME OF MARYLAND
4701 N Charles St, Baltimore   Maryland 21210
301 435-0100
Private and 4 Year
Arts Areas: Instrumental Music, Vocal Music, Theatre and Visual Arts
Performing Series: Performing Artists Series
Performance Facilities: Little Theatre

MUSIC

Christy Izdebski, Chairman   *Number Of Faculty:* 9   *Number Of Students:* 100
Degrees Offered: BA   *Teaching Certification Available*
Financial Assistance: Scholarships and Work-Study Grants
Performing Groups: Band, Chorus, Orchestra

(continued on next page)

THEATRE

Sister Kathleen M Engers, Chairman   **Number Of Faculty:** 3
Number Of Students: 35   **Degrees Offered:** BA English/Drama
Teaching Certification Available
Financial Assistance: Scholarships and Work-Study Grants
Performing Groups: Merrie Masquers

PEABODY INSTITUTE OF THE JOHNS HOPKINS UNIVERSITY
1 E Mount Vernon Place, Baltimore   Maryland 21202
Private and 4 Year   **Arts Areas:** Instrumental Music and Vocal Music
Performing Series: Evening Concert Series; Wednesday Noon Series
Performance Facilities: Peabody Concert Hall; North Hall; East Hall; Leakin Hall

MUSIC

James Hustic, Dean of the Conservatory   **Number Of Faculty:** 90
Number Of Students: 500
Degrees Offered: BMus; MMus; DMA; BMus, MusEd; Artist Diploma
Financial Assistance: Assistantships, Scholarships, Work-Study Grants and NDSL; SEOG; BEOG
Performing Groups: Orchestra; Chamber Orchestra; Wind Ensemble; Contemporary Music Ensemble; Percussion Ensemble; Guitar Ensemble; String Ensemble; Chorus; Opera Chorus; Concert Singers; Opera Workshop; Woodwind Quintet; Brass Ensemble; Double Bass Ensemble; Harpsichord Ensemble; Recorder Ensemble

---

PRINCE GEORGES COMMUNITY COLLEGE
301 Largo Rd, Largo   Maryland 20870
301 336-6000
County and 2 Year   **Arts Areas:** Instrumental Music and Vocal Music

MUSIC

Frank Schinonelli, Chairman   **Number Of Faculty:** 3 Full-time, 25 Part-time
Number Of Students: 200   **Degrees Offered:** AA
Financial Assistance: Work-Study Grants
Performing Groups: Stage Band; Concert Band; Jazz Ensemble; Chorus; Madrigals
Workshops/Festivals: Dimensions in Music

THEATRE

John Handley, Associate Dean & Director   **Number Of Faculty:** 11
Number Of Students: 150   **Degrees Offered:** AA
Performing Groups: Hallam Players; Experimental Theatre

SAINT MARY'S COLLEGE OF MARYLAND
St Mary's City   Maryland 20686, 301 994-1600 Ext 286
State and 4 Year
Arts Areas: Dance, Instrumental Music, Vocal Music, Theatre and Visual Arts
Performing Series: Music Concert Series
Performance Facilities: St Mary's Hall; Art Gallery (Anne Arundel Hall); Theatre/Dance Room

DANCE

Number Of Faculty: 1/2   **Number Of Students:** 60
Financial Assistance: Scholarships and Work-Study Grants
Workshops/Festivals: One Fall & One Spring Concert

MUSIC

Number Of Faculty: 5   **Number Of Students:** 60   **Degrees Offered:** BA
Technical Training: Vocal & Instrumental Performance
Teaching Certification Available

(continued on next page)

Financial Assistance: Scholarships and Work-Study Grants
Performing Groups: Choir; Madrigal Singers; Wind Ensemble; Jazz Ensemble
Workshops/Festivals: Tidewater Music Festival (Summers)   *Number Of Faculty:* 3

THEATRE

Number Of Students: 25
Courses Offered: Introduction; History; Acting; Directing

SALISBURY STATE COLLEGE
Camden Ave, Salisbury   Maryland 21801
301 749-7191
State and 4 Year
Arts Areas: Instrumental Music, Vocal Music, Theatre and Visual Arts
Performing Series: Salisbury Artist Series

MUSIC

Jessie L Fleming, Chairman   *Number Of Faculty:* 6 Full-time, 5 Part-time
Number Of Students: 45   *Degrees Offered:* BS; BA   *Technical Training:* Voice
Teaching Certification Available
Financial Assistance: Scholarships and Work-Study Grants
Performing Groups: Chorus; Band; Jazz Ensemble; Chamber Ensembles

THEATRE

Robert Wesley, Chairman   *Number Of Faculty:* 3   *Number Of Students:* 50
Degrees Offered: BA Speech/Theatre; MEd   *Teaching Certification Available*
Financial Assistance: Scholarships and Work-Study Grants
Performing Groups: Sophanes Players; Readers' Theatre; Children's Theatre

---

TOWSON STATE UNIVERSITY
Baltimore   Maryland 21204, 301 321-2000
State and 4 Year
Arts Areas: Dance, Instrumental Music, Vocal Music, Theatre, Film Arts, Television, Visual Arts and Radio
Performing Series: Public Program Series
Performance Facilities: Fine Arts Center; Towson Center

DANCE

Dr Helene Breazeale, Chairman   *Number Of Faculty:* 4
Number Of Students: 70   *Degrees Offered:* BS; BA
Teaching Certification Available   *Financial Assistance:* Work-Study Grants
Performing Groups: Towson State University Dance Company
Workshops/Festivals: Summer Dance Workshop; January Workshop; Department also sponsors a professional company-in-residence each year

MUSIC

Dr Golden E Arrington, Chairman   *Number Of Faculty:* 48
Number Of Students: 550   *Degrees Offered:* BA; BS; MMusEd
Courses Offered: Vocal; General, Instrumental, Performance; Music Literature, Theory
Teaching Certification Available
Financial Assistance: Assistantships, Scholarships and Work-Study Grants
Performing Groups: Concert Band; Orchestra; Wind Ensemble; Jazz Ensemble; Chorale; Glee Club; Women's Chorus; Community Chorus; Brass Ensemble; Clarinet Choir; Flute Ensemble; Percussion Ensemble; Saxophone Ensemble; String Ensemble; Woodwind Ensemble; Chamber Singers; Octet
Workshops/Festivals: Opera Workshop; Stan Kenton Jazz Workshop

THEATRE

Dr Paul Berman, Chairperson   *Number Of Faculty:* 12
Number Of Students: 130   *Degrees Offered:* BA; BS
Financial Assistance: Assistantships, Scholarships and Work-Study Grants
Performing Groups: The Electric Shakespeare Company
Workshops/Festivals: High School Theatre Workshop

VILLA JULIE COLLEGE
Valley Rd, Stevenson   Maryland 21153
301 486-7000
> Private and 2 Year
> *Arts Areas:* Dance, Vocal Music, Theatre, Television and Visual Arts
> *Performance Facilities:* Inscape Theatre

DANCE

Eddie Stewart, Chairman   **Number Of Faculty:** 1   **Number Of Students:** 50
Courses Offered: Ballet

MUSIC

C Marc Tardue, Chairman   **Number Of Faculty:** 2   **Number Of Students:** 30
Financial Assistance: Work-Study Grants

THEATRE

Sally Harris, Chairman   **Number Of Faculty:** 3   **Degrees Offered:** AA
Courses Offered: Improvisation; Acting Styles; Interpersonal Communication; Creative Drama; Theatre
Promotion; Stage Design; Makeup & Costuming
Financial Assistance: Work-Study Grants   **Performing Groups:** Inscape Ensemble
Workshops/Festivals: Fine Arts Festival
Artists-In-Residence/Guest Artists: Living Stage

WASHINGTON COLLEGE
Chestertown   Maryland 21620, 301 778-2800
> Private and 4 Year
> *Arts Areas:* Dance, Instrumental Music, Vocal Music, Theatre and Visual Arts
> *Performing Series:* Washington College Concert Series
> *Performance Facilities:* Gibson Fine Arts Center; William Smith Auditorium

DANCE

Karen Smith, Assistant Professor   **Number Of Faculty:** 1
Number Of Students: 15   **Degrees Offered:** BA
Courses Offered: Ballet; Modern Dance; Jazz; Tap
Financial Assistance: Assistantships, Scholarships and Work-Study Grants
Performing Groups: Washington College Dancers
Workshops/Festivals: Washington College Dance Company Concert

MUSIC

Garry E Clarke, Associate Professor   **Number Of Faculty:** 5
Number Of Students: 50   **Degrees Offered:** BA
Courses Offered: Intro; Theory; History of Western Music; Counterpoint; Analytical Technique; American
Music; Medieval & Renaissance Music; Opera; Music in 20th Century; Instrumental Methods; Conducting
& Orchestration; Applied Music; Instruction in Voice, Piano, Woodwinds, Brass
Teaching Certification Available
Financial Assistance: Scholarships and Work-Study Grants
Performing Groups: Choir; Wind Ensemble; Chorale; Chamber Groups

THEATRE

Timothy Maloney, Associate Professor   **Number Of Faculty:** 2
Number Of Students: 25   **Degrees Offered:** BA
Courses Offered: History of the Theatre; Acting I, II, III; Directing I, II; Theatre Technology; Scenic
Design; Elements of Theatrical Production; Dramatic Theory
Technical Training: Drama Workshop; Apprentice Semester
Teaching Certification Available
Financial Assistance: Scholarships and Work-Study Grants

(continued on next page)

Performing Groups: Washington Players
Artists-In-Residence/Guest Artists: Concerto Soloists of Philadelphia; Tedd Joselson; Annapolis Brass Quintet; Music for Awhile; Mandala International Folk Dance Company

---

WESTERN MARYLAND COLLEGE
College Hill, Westminster   Maryland 21157
301 848-7000
Private and 4 Year
Arts Areas: Instrumental Music, Vocal Music, Theatre and Visual Arts

MUSIC

Gerald E Cole, Chairman   **Number Of Faculty:** 8   **Number Of Students:** 110
Degrees Offered: BA, MA MusEd, MEd   **Teaching Certification Available**
Financial Assistance: Scholarships and Work-Study Grants
Performing Groups: Orchestra, Choir, Bands, Ensembles

THEATRE

William L Tribby, Chairman   **Number Of Faculty:** 4   **Number Of Students:** 55
Degrees Offered: BA, MEd   **Teaching Certification Available**
Financial Assistance: Scholarships and Work-Study Grants
Performing Groups: College Players

ALL NEWTON MUSIC SCHOOL
321 Chestnut St, West Newton   Massachusetts 02165
617 527-4553
> Private and Special
> *Arts Areas:* Dance, Instrumental Music and Vocal Music

DANCE

> Katherine Ostrovsky, Chairman   *Financial Assistance:* Scholarships
> *Number Of Faculty:* 60   *Number Of Students:* 1,200
> *Financial Assistance:* Scholarships

AMERICAN CENTER FOR THE PERFORMING ARTS
551 Tremont, Boston   Massachusetts 02116
617 423-3629
> Private and 2 Year   *Arts Areas:* Theatre
> *Performance Facilities:* American Center for the Performing Arts

THEATRE

> Alan Kennedy, Director   *Number Of Faculty:* 9   *Number Of Students:* 40
> *Financial Assistance:* Scholarships and Work-Study Grants
> *Performing Groups:* American Center Theatre, Professional Theatre Arts

AMHERST COLLEGE
Amherst   Massachusetts 01002, 413 542-2000
> Private and 4 Year
> *Arts Areas:* Instrumental Music, Vocal Music, Theatre and Visual Arts
> *Performing Series:* Concert Series
> *Performance Facilities:* Kirby Memorial Theatre; Buckley Recital Hall

MUSIC

> Lewis Spratlan, Chairman   *Number Of Faculty:* 5   *Number Of Students:* 30
> *Degrees Offered:* BA   *Teaching Certification Available*
> *Financial Assistance:* Scholarships
> *Performing Groups:* Chamber Orchestra, Vocal Ensemble

THEATRE

> Walter L Boughton, Chairman   *Number Of Faculty:* 5   *Number Of Students:* 45
> *Degrees Offered:* BA
> *Technical Training:* National Theatre Institute participation offered
> *Teaching Certification Available*   *Financial Assistance:* Scholarships

ANNA MARIA COLLEGE
Sunset Lane, Paxton   Massachusetts 01612
617 757-4586
> Private and 4 Year
> *Arts Areas:* Instrumental Music, Vocal Music and Visual Arts
> *Performance Facilities:* Foundress Hall Auditorium; Miriam Hall - Recital Hall

MUSIC

> Robert Goepfert, Chairman   *Number Of Faculty:* 14   *Number Of Students:* 63
> *Degrees Offered:* BA; BMus in Applied; BMus
> *Courses Offered:* Applied Music; Music Education; Sacred Music; Music Therapy
> *Teaching Certification Available*

(continued on next page)

(Anna Maria College — cont'd)

Financial Assistance: Scholarships and Work-Study Grants
Performing Groups: Women's Chorus; Mixed Chorus; Instrumental Ensembles
Workshops/Festivals: Orff Workshop; Voice Workshop

ATLANTIC UNION COLLEGE
THAYER CONSERVATORY OF MUSIC
Main St, S Lancaster   Massachusetts 01561
617 365-4561 Ext 65

Private and 4 Year
Arts Areas: Instrumental Music, Vocal Music and Visual Arts

MUSIC

Arthur R Starnes, Chairman   **Number Of Faculty:** 20   **Number Of Students:** 30
Degrees Offered: BA Mus; BMus; BMusEd   **Teaching Certification Available**
Financial Assistance: Scholarships and Work-Study Grants
Performing Groups: Atlantic Union College Brass Ensemble; Thayer Conservatory Orchestra; Choirs:
Jubilate, Cantus

BAY PATH JUNIOR COLLEGE
588 Longmeadow St, Longmeadow   Massachusetts 01106
413 567-0621 Ext 35

Private and 2 Year
Arts Areas: Dance, Instrumental Music, Vocal Music, Theatre and Visual Arts

DANCE

John P Gaffney, Chairman, Theatre Arts Department   **Number Of Faculty:** 1

MUSIC

Charles E Page, Chairman   **Number Of Faculty:** 3
Courses Offered: Theory & Harmony; Music of the Romantic Era; Music History & Appreciation;
Twentieth Century Music
Technical Training: Applied Piano, Organ & Voice
Financial Assistance: Scholarships and Work-Study Grants
Performing Groups: Keynotes/Chamber Singers; College Glee Club

THEATRE

John P Gaffney, Chairman   **Number Of Faculty:** 2   **Degrees Offered:** AA
Courses Offered: Theatre Workshop; History & Appreciation of Modern Theatre; Speech; Introduction to
Theatre; Acting I & II; History & Appreciation of Musical Theatre
Technical Training: Acting
Financial Assistance: Scholarships and Work-Study Grants
Performing Groups: Two Annual Productions

BELMONT MUSIC SCHOOL
582A Pleasant St, Belmont   Massachusetts 02178
617 484-4696

Lessons by the Semester   **Arts Areas:** Instrumental Music and Vocal Music
Performing Series: Home Concert Series
Performance Facilities: Unitarian Church; Belmont High School
Number Of Faculty: 48   **Number Of Students:** 569
Courses Offered: Instrumental Study; Musicianship; Eurhythmics; Ensemble
Technical Training: Instrumental   **Financial Assistance:** Scholarships
Performing Groups: Wind Octet; String Trio; Baroque Groups; Renaissance Consort; Various Chamber
Music Combinations
Workshops/Festivals: Keyboard Improvisation Workshops; String Workshops; Relaxation Workshops

BERKLEE COLLEGE OF MUSIC
1140 Boylston St, Boston   Massachusetts 02215
617 266-1400

Private and 4 Year   **Arts Areas:** Instrumental Music and Vocal Music
Performing Series: Jazz Masters Series
Performance Facilities: Berklee Performance Center

MUSIC

Robert Share, Administrator   **Number Of Faculty:** 200
Number Of Students: 2,500   **Degrees Offered:** BMus; Majors in Composition
Courses Offered: Music Education; Applied Music
Technical Training: Special Professional Diploma Program
Teaching Certification Available
Financial Assistance: Work-Study Grants and Loans, BEOG
Performing Groups: Variety of Faculty or Student Performing Groups
Workshops/Festivals: High School Jazz Festival; Summer Music Educator Workshops

BERKSHIRE CHRISTIAN COLLEGE
200 Stockbridge Rd, Lenox   Massachusetts 01240
413 637-0838

Private and 4 Year   **Arts Areas:** Instrumental Music and Vocal Music
Number Of Faculty: 2   **Number Of Students:** 10
Degrees Offered: BA in Theology   **Courses Offered:** Church Music
Financial Assistance: Scholarships and Work-Study Grants
Performing Groups: Chorale

BERKSHIRE COMMUNITY COLLEGE
West St, Pittsfield   Massachusetts 01201
413 499-0886

State and 2 Year   **Arts Areas:** Theatre and Visual Arts
Performance Facilities: Koussevitsky Arts Center

THEATRE

Robert M Boland, Chairman of Fine Arts
Number Of Faculty: 1 Full-time, 1 Part-time   **Number Of Students:** 7
Degrees Offered: AS
Courses Offered: Theatre Practicum; Fundamentals of Acting; Stagecraft I & II; Acting II; Costume Design
Technical Training: Stagecraft; Production, Management; Performance
Performing Groups: Berkshire Community College Players; Departmental Productions

BERKSHIRE MUSIC CENTER, TANGLEWOOD
c/o Symphony Hall, Boston   Massachusetts 02115
617 255-1492

Private and Special   **Arts Areas:** Instrumental Music and Vocal Music

MUSIC

Joseph Silverstein, Chairman of Faculty   **Number Of Faculty:** 45
Number Of Students: 440
Courses Offered: Composition, Conducting, Orchestral Study and Performance
Financial Assistance: Internships
Performing Groups: Chamber and Orchestral Music, Vocal Music
Workshops/Festivals: Berkshire Music Center runs concurrently with the Berkshire Festival

BOSTON COLLEGE
140 Commonwealth Ave, Chestnut Hill   Massachusetts 02167
617 969-0100

> Private and 4 Year   **Arts Areas:** Theatre
> **Performing Series:** Humanities Series

MUSIC

Dr Olga Stone, Chairman
Technical Training: Baroque Music, Music of the Theatre, History of Music of the Americas
Performing Groups: University Chorale of Boston College, Marching Band, Concert Band
Workshops/Festivals: Arts Festival, Religion in Arts

THEATRE

Dr Paul Marcoux, Chairman   **Degrees Offered:** BA
Teaching Certification Available   Financial Assistance: Scholarships
Performing Groups: Boston College Dramatic Society

BOSTON CONSERVATORY OF MUSIC
8 The Fenway, Boston   Massachusetts 02215
617 536-6340

> Private and 4 Year
> **Arts Areas:** Dance, Instrumental Music, Vocal Music and Theatre

DANCE

Ruth Sandholm Ambrose, Artistic Advisor   **Number Of Faculty:** 12
Degrees Offered: BFA   **Teaching Certification Available**
Financial Assistance: Scholarships   **Performing Groups:** Senior Dance Groups
Workshops/Festivals: Choreography workshops

MUSIC

Number Of Faculty: 96   **Degrees Offered:** B Mus, MMus   **Teaching Certification Available**
Financial Assistance: Scholarships
Performing Groups: Stage Band, Orchestra, Wind Ensemble, Chorus, Chorale, String Ensemble, Brass
Ensemble, Percussion Ensemble
Workshops/Festivals: Opera Workshop

THEATRE

Robert Owczarek, Acting Chairman   **Number Of Faculty:** 11
Degrees Offered: BFA   **Teaching Certification Available**
Financial Assistance: Scholarships
Performing Groups: BCM Theatre, Musical Theatre

BOSTON UNIVERSITY SCHOOL FOR THE ARTS
855 Commonwealth Ave, Boston   Massachusetts 02214
617 353-3334

> Private and 4 Year
> **Arts Areas:** Instrumental Music, Vocal Music, Theatre, Visual Arts and Music Composition and History
> **Performing Series:** Boston University Celebrity Series
> **Performance Facilities:** Boston University Theatre, Boston University Concert Hall

MUSIC

Wilbur D Fullbright, Chairman   **Number Of Faculty:** 91
Number Of Students: 633   **Degrees Offered:** BMus, MMus, DMA
Teaching Certification Available
Financial Assistance: Assistantships, Scholarships and Work-Study Grants
Performing Groups: Orchestra, Wind Ensemble, Chorus, Chamber Ensemble, Recitalists

(continued on next page)

THEATRE

Mouzon Law, Chairman   **Number Of Faculty:** 26   **Number Of Students:** 283
Degrees Offered: BFA, MFA   **Teaching Certification Available**
Financial Assistance: Internships, Assistantships, Scholarships and Work-Study Grants

---

BRADFORD COLLEGE
Bradford   Massachusetts 01830, 617 372-7161
Private and 2 Year
Arts Areas: Dance, Instrumental Music, Vocal Music, Theatre and Visual Arts
Number Of Faculty: 1   **Courses Offered:** Modern Dance

MUSIC

Charles Ludington, Department Head   **Number Of Faculty:** 3
Degrees Offered: AA   **Financial Assistance:** Work-Study Grants

THEATRE

Mark Waistuck, Department Head   **Number Of Faculty:** 3   **Degrees Offered:** AA
Financial Assistance: Work-Study Grants   **Performing Groups:** Masqueraders

---

BRANDEIS UNIVERSITY
South St, Waltham   Massachusetts 02154
617 647-2000
Private and 4 Year
Arts Areas: Instrumental Music, Vocal Music, Theatre and Visual Arts
Performance Facilities: Slosberg Center; Spingold Theatre

MUSIC

Robert L Koff, Professor   **Number Of Faculty:** 22   **Number Of Students:** 80
Degrees Offered: BA; MFA; PhD
Courses Offered: Musicology; Theory & Composition
Financial Assistance: Assistantships and Scholarships
Performing Groups: University Chorus; Early Music Ensemble; Symphony Orchestra; Music Club

THEATRE

Charles W Moore, Professor   **Number Of Faculty:** 13
Number Of Students: 125   **Degrees Offered:** BA; MFA
Courses Offered: Acting; Directing; Design/Technical; Playwriting
Financial Assistance: Assistantships and Scholarships
Workshops/Festivals: Expressions Dance Series; Brandeis Playwrights Festival
Artists-In-Residence/Guest Artists: Charles Marowitz

BRIDGEWATER STATE COLLEGE
Grove St, Bridgewater   Massachusetts 02324
617 697-6161
State and 4 Year
Arts Areas: Instrumental Music, Vocal Music, Theatre and Visual Arts
Performance Facilities: College Auditorium

MUSIC

Dr Kenneth Falkner, Chairman   **Financial Assistance:** Scholarships

THEATRE

Robert J Barnett, Chairman   **Degrees Offered:** BA Speech/Theatre
Teaching Certification Available
Financial Assistance: Scholarships and Work-Study Grants
Performing Groups: Drama Club

BUNKER HILL COMMUNITY COLLEGE

Rutherford Ave, Charlestown   Massachusetts 02129
617 241-8600
2 Year
Arts Areas: Dance, Instrumental Music, Vocal Music, Theatre, Film Arts, Television and Visual Arts
Performance Facilities: Bunker Hill Auditorium

MUSIC

Linda Ostrander, Chairman   *Number Of Faculty:* 1   *Number Of Students:* 100
Degrees Offered: AA
Technical Training: Music for Early Childhood, Music Theory
Financial Assistance: Assistantships and Work-Study Grants
Performing Groups: Jazz Ensemble, Choral Ensemble
Workshops/Festivals: Faculty Arts Festival, Students' Art Festival, Children's Arts Workshop

THEATRE

Susan Rosenbaum, Chairman   *Number Of Faculty:* 1   *Number Of Students:* 50
Degrees Offered: AA
Financial Assistance: Assistantships and Work-Study Grants
Performing Groups: Improvisation Ensemble
Workshops/Festivals: Faculty Arts Festival; Students' Arts Festival; Children's Arts Workshop; Theatre Performance Workshop

CAPE COD CONSERVATORY OF MUSIC AND ARTS

Route 6A & Hyannis Rd, Barnstable   Massachusetts 02630
617 362-2772
Private and Special
Arts Areas: Dance, Instrumental Music and Vocal Music

DANCE

Sandra Faxon, Chairman   *Number Of Faculty:* 2   *Number Of Students:* 30

MUSIC

Richard Casper, Chairman   *Number Of Faculty:* 31   *Number Of Students:* 480

CLARK UNIVERSITY

950 Main St, Worcester   Massachusetts 01610
617 793-7711
Private and 4 Year
Arts Areas: Instrumental Music, Vocal Music, Theatre, Film Arts and Visual Arts
Performance Facilities: Little Center; Atwood Hall

MUSIC

Wesley M Fuller, Associate Professor   *Number Of Faculty:* 9
Degrees Offered: BA with Music Major
Courses Offered: Theory; Composition; History; Performance; Electronic Music; World Music; Jazz
Technical Training: Piano; Flute; Guitar; Voice; Violin; Viola
Financial Assistance: Internships, Assistantships, Scholarships and Work-Study Grants
Performing Groups: Clark University Chamber Players; Jazz Workshop; Clark Choral Society;
Clark-Consortium Instrumental Performers
Workshops/Festivals: Jazz Workshop; Worcester Consortium Choral Festival; Various Yearly Workshops
(Piano, Electronic, Composition)

THEATRE

Carol Sica, Associate Professor of Theatre Art
Number Of Faculty: 3 Full-time, 1 Part-time
Degrees Offered: BA with Theatre Arts Major

(continued on next page)

Courses Offered: Acting; Directing; Technical/Design; History; Drama Literature; Movement
Technical Training: American Musical; Voice & Diction; Stage Management
Financial Assistance: Internships, Assistantships, Scholarships and Work-Study Grants
Workshops/Festivals: Major Productions - produced & directed by faculty; Faculty workshops - acting; Faculty Performance

CURRY COLLEGE
Milton Massachusetts 02186, 617 333-0500 Ext 143
Private and 4 Year
Arts Areas: Dance, Instrumental Music, Vocal Music, Theatre and Visual Arts
Performing Series: Fine Arts Series

DANCE

Dr Ronald Warners, Coordinator for Fine Arts **Number Of Faculty:** 2
Number Of Students: 60 **Degrees Offered:** BA
Financial Assistance: Internships and Work-Study Grants

MUSIC

Dr Ronald H Warners, Coordinator for Fine Arts **Number Of Faculty:** 9
Number Of Students: 190 **Degrees Offered:** BA
Courses Offered: Theory; History; Education; Performance
Technical Training: Private study in all instruments and voice
Teaching Certification Available
Financial Assistance: Internships and Work-Study Grants
Performing Groups: Curry College Choir; Curry College Chamber Choir; Instrumental Ensembles
Workshops/Festivals: Orff - Schulwerk Workshops; Guitar Master Classes; Piano Master Classes

THEATRE

Dr Ronald Warners, Coordinator for Fine Arts **Number Of Faculty:** 3
Number Of Students: 150 **Degrees Offered:** BA
Courses Offered: Full Complement of Undergraduate Theater Courses
Technical Training: Technical Theater **Teaching Certification Available**
Financial Assistance: Internships and Work-Study Grants
Performing Groups: Three - Four Major Productions per year
Workshops/Festivals: Mime Workshops
Artists-In-Residence/Guest Artists: Pocket Mime; Frances Wildeboor; Rebekah Buchman Zak; James Lanzillotta; Marlene Francel

DEAN JUNIOR COLLEGE
99 Main St, Franklin Massachusetts 02038
617 528-9100
Private and 2 Year
Arts Areas: Dance, Instrumental Music, Vocal Music, Theatre and Visual Arts
Performing Series: Franklin - Dean Community Concert Series; Dean Dept of Visual Arts Theatre Productions
Performance Facilities: Center for Performing Arts

DANCE

Joan P Palladino, Director, Dean Dance Company **Number Of Faculty:** 1
Number Of Students: 10
Degrees Offered: AA in Musical Theatre (Dance Emphasis)
Courses Offered: Creative Movement; Dance Theory - Delsarte Method; Modern Dance; Rhythms, Square Dancing, Folk Dancing for Men & Women
Technical Training: Modern Dance I, II, III
Financial Assistance: Scholarships, Work-Study Grants and BEOG
Performing Groups: Dean Dance Company

(continued on next page)

MUSIC

Lawry N Reid, Chairman, Department of Visual & Performing Arts
Number Of Faculty: 8   **Number Of Students:** 17
Degrees Offered: AA in Music, Musical Theatre, Music Therapy
Courses Offered: Introduction to Music; Vocal Ensembles; Instrumental Ensemble; Applied Music I, II, III, IV; American Musical Theatre; History of Jazz; Creative Music; Fundamentals of Music; Music Theory I, II, III, Class Piano I, II
Financial Assistance: Scholarships, Work-Study Grants and BEOG
Performing Groups: Glee Club; Chamber Choir; Choraliers; Chamber Ensembles; Pit Orchestra; Jazz Ensemble
Workshops/Festivals: New England Community & Junior College Choral Festival

THEATRE

Lawry N Reid, Chairman, Department of Visual & Performing Arts
Number Of Faculty: 3   **Number Of Students:** 10
Degrees Offered: AA in Theatre Arts
Courses Offered: Introduction to Theatre; Fundamentals of Acting I, II; Introduction to Technical Production; Creative Dramatics; Rehearsal & Performance
Financial Assistance: Scholarships, Work-Study Grants and BEOG
Workshops/Festivals: Faculty/Student Productions

EASTERN NAZARENE COLLEGE
23 E Elm Ave, Wollaston   Massachusetts 02170
617 773-6350

Private and 4 Year   **Arts Areas:** Instrumental Music and Vocal Music
Number Of Faculty: 5   **Number Of Students:** 40
Degrees Offered: BA MusEd, BA Applied   **Teaching Certification Available**
Financial Assistance: Scholarships
Performing Groups: Vocal Ensembles, Chorus, Instrumental Ensembles, Orchestra

---

EMERSON COLLEGE
148 Beacon St, Boston   Massachusetts 02116
617 262-2010

Private and 4 Year
Arts Areas: Dance, Instrumental Music, Vocal Music, Theatre, Film Arts, Television and Visual Arts
Performance Facilities: Emerson College Carriage House Theatre

DANCE

Leonidas Nickole, Chairman, Department of Theatre Education
Dance program under auspices of Theatre Education Department
Number Of Faculty: 3   **Number Of Students:** 20   **Degrees Offered:** BFA
Courses Offered: Beginning, Intermediate & Advanced Dance Technique
Technical Training: Choreography; Practicum in Dance Education; Graduate Study in Dance Education
Teaching Certification Available
Financial Assistance: Assistantships and Work-Study Grants
Performing Groups: Emerson Dance Company

MUSIC

Steve Wilson, Chairman   **Number Of Faculty:** 3   **Number Of Students:** 12
Degrees Offered: BM through Longy School of Music
Courses Offered: History of Jazz; Directed Study, History; Directed Study, Theory; Basic Musicanship; Foundations of Music; Pop Music since 1950; Chorus, Voice I & II; Practical Beginning Theory; Music in Western Culture I & II; Music Programming
Technical Training: Chorus; Voice I & II; Practical Beginning Theory; Basic Musicianship; Music Programming
Teaching Certification Available   **Financial Assistance:** Scholarships
Performing Groups: Choir; Chorus; Jazz Ensemble
Workshops/Festivals: Spring Concert

(continued on next page)

THEATRE

William Sharp, Chairman, Dramatic Arts Department
Leonidas Nichole, Chairman, Theatre Education Department
Number Of Faculty: 11   **Number Of Students:** 348
Degrees Offered: BS; BS; BFA; MS; MA
Courses Offered: Fundamentals of Acting; Movement; Dramatic Theory & Criticism; History of American Theatre; Stage Design; Scenic Design; Stage Makeup; Creative Dramatics; Children's Theatre
Teaching Certification Available   **Financial Assistance:** Scholarships
Performing Groups: Emerson Theatre Company; Strolling Players; Youtheatre Creative Dramatics Experimental Workshop; Education Theatre Repertory Company
Workshops/Festivals: Theatre Educational Festival for High School Students
Artists-In-Residence/Guest Artists: Jack Stein

EMMANUEL COLLEGE
400 The Fenway, Boston   Massachusetts 02115
617 277-9340
Private and 4 Year
Arts Areas: Instrumental Music, Vocal Music and Visual Arts

MUSIC

Sister Therese Julie Fitzmaurice, Chairman   **Number Of Faculty:** 7
Number Of Students: 70   **Degrees Offered:** BA Mus, BA Applied
Teaching Certification Available
Financial Assistance: Scholarships and Work-Study Grants
Performing Groups: Instrumental Ensembles, Choir

ENDICOTT COLLEGE
Beverly   Massachusetts 01915, 617 927-0585
Private and 2 Year
Arts Areas: Instrumental Music, Vocal Music, Television and Visual Arts
Performance Facilities: Auditorium; Little Theater; Audio - Visual Auditorium; Television Studio

MUSIC

Edward Avedisian, Chairman   **Number Of Faculty:** 1
Courses Offered: Music History; Music Appreciation; Chorus
Performing Groups: Endicott Chorale

GOLDOVSKY OPERA INSTITUTE
183 Clinton Rd, Brookline   Massachusetts 02146
617 734-5255
Private and Special   **Arts Areas:** Vocal Music and Theatre
Technical Training: Post graduate instruction
Performing Groups: Goldovsky Opera Theatre Touring Company
Workshops/Festivals: Summer Workshops, University of South Eastern Massachusetts; Ogleby Park, in Wheeling, West Virginia

GORDON COLLEGE
255 Grapevine Rd, Wenham   Massachusetts 01984
617 927-2300
Private and 4 Year   **Arts Areas:** Instrumental Music and Vocal Music

MUSIC

Alton Byrum, Chairman   **Number Of Faculty:** 2   **Number Of Students:** 24
Degrees Offered: BA Mus, BA MusEd   **Teaching Certification Available**
Financial Assistance: Scholarships   **Performing Groups:** Orchestra, Choir

GRAHM JUNIOR COLLEGE
632 Beacon St, Boston   Massachusetts 02215
617 536-2050

Private and 2 Year   *Arts Areas:* Theatre
Performance Facilities: Soep Hall   *Number Of Faculty:* 7
Number Of Students: 25   *Degrees Offered:* AA
Financial Assistance: Work-Study Grants

HARVARD UNIVERSITY
64 Brattle St, Cambridge   Massachusetts 02138
617 495-2668

Private and 4 Year
Arts Areas: Dance, Instrumental Music, Vocal Music, Theatre, Film Arts and Visual Arts
Performing Series: Special Series   *Performance Facilities:* Loeb Drama Center

DANCE

Dance program offered through Radcliffe College
Courses Offered: Afro-American Dance, Russian Conditioning; Ballet, Modern Dance, Jazz Dance
Performing Groups: Summer School program of Special Study

MUSIC

Prof Elliot Forbes, Chairman   *Number Of Faculty:* 16
Degrees Offered: BMus, MMus, PhD
Financial Assistance: Internships, Assistantships and Scholarships
Courses Offered: Acting, Kabuki, Mime, Directing, Lighting, Set Design, Stage Management, Voice, Costuming, Management

HOLY CROSS COLLEGE
College St, Worcester   Massachusetts 01610
617 793-2011

Private and 4 Year
Arts Areas: Instrumental Music, Theatre and Visual Arts
Performing Series: Fenwick Theatre Season
Performance Facilities: Fenwick Theatre

MUSIC

Joan Nylen Italiano, Associate Professor   *Number Of Faculty:* 4
Number Of Students: 250   *Courses Offered:* Music History; Theory; Composition
Financial Assistance: Scholarships and Work-Study Grants
Workshops/Festivals: Concert Series; Consortium for Higher Education Music Activities; Choral Concerts

THEATRE

Edward J Herson, Director, Division of Theatre Art   *Number Of Faculty:* 3
Number Of Students: 50
Courses Offered: Acting; Design; Technical Theatre; Theatre Criticism; Play Theory; Tutorials
Financial Assistance: Scholarships and Work-Study Grants
Performing Groups: The Fenwick Theatre Company

HOLYOKE COMMUNITY COLLEGE
303 Homestead Ave, Holyoke   Massachusetts 01040
413 538-7000

State and 2 Year
Arts Areas: Instrumental Music, Vocal Music, Theatre and Music Education
Performing Series: Concert Series; Cultural Affairs Series; Drama Series
Performance Facilities: Theatre

(continued on next page)

MUSIC

Sidney B Smith, Director **Number Of Faculty:** 2 Full-time, 16 Part-time
Number Of Students: 100 **Degrees Offered:** AA Arts, Music Education
Courses Offered: Music Literature; Theory; Counterpoint; Dictation & Sight Singing; Classes in Piano, Woodwinds, Voice, Brass & Strings; Applied Music
Financial Assistance: Scholarships and Work-Study Grants
Performing Groups: Chorale; Stage Band; Wind Ensemble; College - Civic Orchestra; Handbell Choir; Accordion Ensemble; Percussion Ensemble; Guitar Ensemble
Workshops/Festivals: Vocal Workshop

THEATRE

Leslie Phillips, Director of Drama **Number Of Faculty:** 4
Number Of Students: 125 **Degrees Offered:** AA with option in Speech/Drama
Courses Offered: Introduction to Theatre; Playwriting; Play Production; Modern Drama; Creative Dramatics; Shakespeare; Speech; Oral Interpretation
Financial Assistance: Scholarships and Work-Study Grants
Performing Groups: Holyoke Community College Players
Workshops/Festivals: Weekly Workshops in Improvisation; Yearly competition for original one - act plays

---

THE JOY OF MOVEMENT CENTER
536 Massachusetts Ave, Cambridge Massachusetts 02139
617 492-4680

Private and Special **Arts Areas:** Dance and Theatre

DANCE

Andrienne Hawkins, Assistant Director **Number Of Faculty:** 45
Number Of Students: 3,000
Courses Offered: Traditional & Contemporary Dance; Ethnic; Creative Movement
Financial Assistance: Scholarships and Work-Study Grants
Performing Groups: Impulse Dance Company; Expansions
Artists-In-Residence/Guest Artists: Merce Cunningham

KODALY CENTER OF AMERICA
15 Denton Rd, Wellesley Massachusetts 02181
617 237-2744

Private and 2 Year **Arts Areas:** Vocal Music
Courses Offered: Teacher training in Kodaly method of musical training
Technical Training: One year certificate course; One month summer course; Classroom Teacher's course at Boston University School of Education; Master's Degree through Cincinnati College Conservatory of Music and other affiliated universities & institutions
Financial Assistance: Scholarships and Teaching Fellowships

LELAND POWERS SCHOOL
70 Brookline Ave, Boston Massachusetts 02115
617 247-1300

Private and Special **Arts Areas:** Theatre and Television and Radio
Performance Facilities: Leland Powers Mini-Theatre

THEATRE

Richard C Swan, Chairman **Number Of Faculty:** 4 **Number Of Students:** 20
Technical Training: Mime, Pantomime, Makeup, Speech, Body Movement, Interpretation
Financial Assistance: Scholarships
Workshops/Festivals: Weekly creative workshops

LESLEY COLLEGE
29 Everett St, Cambridge   Massachusetts 02138
617 868-9600

Private and 4 Year   *Arts Areas:* Instrumental Music and Vocal Music
Degrees Offered: BS MusEd   *Teaching Certification Available*
Financial Assistance: Scholarships

LONGY SCHOOL OF MUSIC
1 Follen St, Cambridge   Massachusetts 02138
617 876-0956

Private and 4 Year
Arts Areas: Instrumental Music, Vocal Music and Theory
Performance Facilities: Edward Pickman Concert Hall

MUSIC

Margaret Rohde, Interim Director   *Number Of Faculty:* 75
Number Of Students: 600
Degrees Offered: BMus; Longy Senior Diploma; Soloists Diploma
Courses Offered: Solfege; Harmony; Music History; Counterpoint; Orchestration
Technical Training: Private lessons in most instruments & voice
Teaching Certification Available
Financial Assistance: Scholarships and Work-Study Grants
Performing Groups: Chamber Ensembles; Early Music Ensembles; Chorus

UNIVERSITY OF LOWELL
1 University Ave, Lowell   Massachusetts 01854
617 454-8011 Ext 250

State and 4 Year   *Arts Areas:* Instrumental Music and Vocal Music
Performance Facilities: William R Fisher Recital Hall; Durgin Hall; Concert Hall

MUSIC

Antone Holevas, Chairman, Department of Performance
John Ogasapian, Chairman, Department of Academic Studies
Number Of Faculty: 20 Full-time, 25 Part-time   *Number Of Students:* 520
Degrees Offered: BA; BMus; MMus; BM in Music Ed, Music Theory, Music History, Performance
Teaching Certification Available   *Financial Assistance:* Work-Study Grants
Performing Groups: Workshop Chorus; Concert Choir; Collegiate Chorale; Opera Workshop; Symphony
Orchestra; String Orchestra; Wind Sinfonia; Wind Orchestra; String Ensemble; Consortium Artis Musicae;
Vocal Chamber Ensemble; Piano Ensemble; Woodwind Ensemble; Brass & Percussion Ensembles; Studio
Orchestra; French Horn Choir; Collegium Musicum; Chamber Ensemble; Woodwind Quintet;
Contemporary Music Ensemble
Workshops/Festivals: Massachusetts All - State; Northeast District Festival; New England Solo Festival;
Opera New England

UNIVERSITY OF MASSACHUSETTS
Amherst   Massachusetts 01003, 413 545-0111

State and 4 Year
Arts Areas: Dance, Instrumental Music, Vocal Music, Theatre, Film Arts, Television and Visual Arts
Performing Series: Faculty Recitals
Performance Facilities: Bowker Auditorium; Fine Arts Center Auditorium; Recital Hall; Fine Arts Center
Theater

DANCE

Marilyn Patton, Director   *Number Of Faculty:* 4   *Number Of Students:* 50
Degrees Offered: PE Degree with concentration in Dance; Bachelor's Degree with Individual
Concentration
Courses Offered: Modern Dance I, II, III, IV, V; Ballet I, II, III; Jazz Dance I, II, III; University

(continued on next page)

Dancers; Analysis of Rhythm; Dance Improvisation; Dance Composition; Dance History; Dance Production
Technical Training: Technique in Modern Ballet & Jazz
Teaching Certification Available
Financial Assistance: Scholarships and Work-Study Grants
Performing Groups: University Dance Group; Concert Dance Group; Beginning Dance Group
Workshops/Festivals: Dance Workshop for High School Students; Dance Workshop for Dance Teachers

MUSIC

Dr Charles L Bestor, Head, Music & Dance Department   *Number Of Faculty:* 38
Number Of Students: 190   *Degrees Offered:* BA; BMus; MMus
Courses Offered: Introduction to Music; Literature of Music; Afro - American Music & Musicians;
Historical Survey of Music; Music from Monteverdi to Bach; Gothic & Renaissance Music; Music of the
20th Century; History of Jazz; Haydn, Mozart & Beethoven; Music from Schubert to Debussy; History of
Opera; Elementary, Intermediate & Advanced Music Theory; Contemporary Techniques; Jazz Theory and
Improvisation I & II; Composition; Jazz Arranging & Composition; Instrumental Techniques; Practicum in
Music Education; Instrumental Music in the Public Schools; Music in Elementary Education; Choral
Music in Secondary Education; Classroom Music in Secondary Education; Vocal Pedagogy; Marching Band
Technical Training: Piano Technology & Tuning; Performance; Vocal & MusEd; Theory Composition;
Music History
Teaching Certification Available
Financial Assistance: Assistantships, Scholarships and Work-Study Grants
Performing Groups: University Chorale; University Chorus; Women's Choir; Chamber Singers; Madrigal
Singers; University Orchestra; Marching Band; Symphony Band; Concert Band; Various Ensembles
Workshops/Festivals: Band & Orchestra Festival; Solo & Ensemble Festival; Choral Music Festival;
Summer Workshop; Jazz Workshop

THEATRE

David M Knauf, Chairman   *Number Of Faculty:* 16   *Number Of Students:* 140
Degrees Offered: BA; MFA
Courses Offered: Introduction to Theater; Theater Practices; Dramaturgy; Performance; Scenography;
Rehearsal & Production; Theatrical Makeup; Theater Management; Conventions of the Classical Theater;
Conventions of the Modern Theater; Convention of the Avantgarde Theatre; American Theater; Black
Theater; Concert Theater; Stage Diction; Stage Movement; Acting; Scenic Design; Lighting Design;
Costume Design; Playwriting; Projects in Dramaturgy; Speech Styles & Dialects; Styles of Stage Movement;
Acting Study; Directing; Concert Theater Ensemble; Senior Ensemble Projects in Performance
Technical Training: Scene Design; Costuming; Lighting
Financial Assistance: Scholarships and Work-Study Grants
Performing Groups: University Ensemble Theater

UNIVERSITY OF MASSACHUSETTS, BOSTON
Boston   Massachusetts 02116, 617 542-6500
State and 4 Year
Arts Areas: Instrumental Music, Vocal Music and Visual Arts

MUSIC

Number Of Faculty: 2   *Number Of Students:* 30   *Degrees Offered:* BMus
Performing Groups: Chorus, Instrumental Ensemble

MASSASOIT COMMUNITY COLLEGE
290 Thatcher St, Brockton   Massachusetts 02402
617 588-9100 Ext 115
State and 2 Year   *Arts Areas:* Theatre
Performing Series: Coordinated Residency Touring Program for Dance
Performance Facilities: Student Center

THEATRE

Michael Pevzner, Chairman   *Number Of Faculty:* 3   *Number Of Students:* 50
Performing Groups: Little Theatre Company

MOUNT HOLYOKE COLLEGE

South Hadley   Massachusetts 01075, 413 538-2000

Private and 4 Year

Arts Areas: Dance, Instrumental Music, Vocal Music, Theatre and Visual Arts

Performing Series: Arts in Performance; Warbeke Chamber Music Concerts

Performance Facilities: Kendall Hall; Richard Glenn Gettell Amphitheater; Laborary Theatre; Chapin & Pratt Auditoriums

DANCE

Ruth L Evedt, Professor of Physical Education   **Number Of Faculty:** 3

Degrees Offered: AB

Courses Offered: Dance Theory & Composition; Notation; History; Choreography; Dance Techniques

Financial Assistance: Scholarships   **Performing Groups:** Concert Dance Group

MUSIC

Irving R Eisley, Professor of Music   **Number Of Faculty:** 23

Degrees Offered: AB; AM

Courses Offered: Instrument & Vocal Music; Theory; Harmony; Choral Conducting; Works of the Great Composers; Classical & Modern

Financial Assistance: Scholarships

Performing Groups: Concert Choirs I & II; Coro Mount Holyoke; Glee Club; University of Massachusetts - Mount Holyoke College Orchestra; Chamber Singers

THEATRE

Oliver E Allyn, Professor of Theatre Arts   **Number Of Faculty:** 7

Degrees Offered: AB; AM

Courses Offered: History of the Theatre; Scene Design; Lighting Design; Costume (History & Design); Technical Directing; Styles of Acting; Directing

Financial Assistance: Scholarships   **Performing Groups:** Readers' Theatre

THE MUSIC SCHOOL OF NORTH SHORE COMMUNITY COLLEGE

395 Bay Rd, South Hamilton   Massachusetts 01982

617 468-1201

State and 2 Year   **Arts Areas:** Instrumental Music and Vocal Music

Performing Series: Student Recitals; Faculty Recitals   **Number Of Faculty:** 18

Number Of Students: 250   **Degrees Offered:** AA

Courses Offered: Applied Music (Vocal & Instrumental)

Technical Training: Theory of Music

Financial Assistance: Scholarships and Work-Study Grants

Performing Groups: Student Ensembles

NEW ENGLAND CONSERVATORY OF MUSIC

290 Huntington Ave, Boston   Massachusetts 02115

617 262-1120

Private and 4 Year

Arts Areas: Instrumental Music, Vocal Music and Theatre

Performance Facilities: Jordan Hall; Brown Hall; Williams Recital Hall

MUSIC

J Stanley Ballinger, President   **Number Of Faculty:** 120

Number Of Students: 700   **Degrees Offered:** BMus; MMus; Artist Diploma

Courses Offered: Applied Music; Theory; Opera; Composition; Music Education; Jazz; Performance of Early Music; Conducting; Voice; Music Literature

Teaching Certification Available

Financial Assistance: Scholarships and Work-Study Grants

Performing Groups: Faculty Chamber Music; Faculty Recital Series; Symphony Orchestra; Contemporary Music Ensemble; Chorus; Opera Theater; Ragtime; Wind Ensemble; Jazz Orchestras; Swing Orchestra;

(continued on next page)

Third Stream; Collegium Musicium
Workshops/Festivals: Summer School Workshops and Course Study available at the Conservatory

NORTHEASTERN UNIVERSITY
360 Huntington Ave, Boston   Massachusetts 02115
617 437-2000

Private and 4 Year   *Arts Areas:* Vocal Music, Theatre and Visual Arts

MUSIC

Roland Nadeau, Chairman   *Number Of Faculty:* 3   *Number Of Students:* 23
Teaching Certification Available   *Financial Assistance:* Scholarships
Performing Groups: Chorus

THEATRE

Eugene Blackman, Chairman   *Number Of Faculty:* 6   *Number Of Students:* 60
Degrees Offered: BA   *Teaching Certification Available*
Financial Assistance: Scholarships and Work-Study Grants
Performing Groups: Silver Masque

PINE MANOR COLLEGE
400 Heath St, Chestnut Hill   Massachusetts 02167
617 731-7000

Private, 4 Year and 2 Year
Arts Areas: Dance, Instrumental Music, Vocal Music, Theatre and Visual Arts
Performance Facilities: Ellsworth Hall

DANCE

Christie Nichols, Instructor   *Number Of Faculty:* 1
Courses Offered: Modern Dance - Elementary & Intermediate/Advanced Technique; Ballet; Dance
Composition; Directed Studies
Financial Assistance: Scholarships and Work-Study Grants
Workshops/Festivals: Two Dance Recitals per year

MUSIC

David Hicks, Instructor   *Number Of Faculty:* 2
Courses Offered: Voice; Private Study of Instrument; Music History; Theory Courses
Financial Assistance: Scholarships and Work-Study Grants
Workshops/Festivals: Faculty Recitals

THEATRE

Thomas B Pegg, Instructor   *Number Of Faculty:* 2
Courses Offered: Stagecraft; Design; Children's Theatre; American Musical Theatre
Financial Assistance: Scholarships and Work-Study Grants
Performing Groups: Mimes & Masques
Workshops/Festivals: In conjunction with other performing arts departments, musical and dramatic
performances are given two or three times a year

PITTSFIELD COMMUNITY MUSIC SCHOOL
30 Wendell Ave, Pittsfield   Massachusetts 01201
413 442-1411

Private and Non - profit   *Arts Areas:* Instrumental Music and Vocal Music
Performing Series: Pittsfield Chamber Music Society Concert Series
Performance Facilities: Recital Hall; "House Concert" area; Outdoor Stage
Number Of Faculty: 22   *Number Of Students:* 180
Degrees Offered: Diploma (high school graduates meeting performance & theory requirements)
Courses Offered: Theory; Music History/Appreciation; Carl Orff; Dalcroze
Technical Training: Instrumental & Voice Study
Financial Assistance: Scholarships   *Performing Groups:* New England Arts Trio

RADCLIFFE COLLEGE
10 Garden St, Cambridge   Massachusetts 02138
617 495-8601
> Private and 4 Year
> *Arts Areas:* Dance, Instrumental Music, Vocal Music, Theatre and Visual Arts

DANCE

Courses Offered: Russian Conditioning, Ballet, Modern, Jazz, Afro - American
Harvard facilty of Arts & Sciences is responsible for the education of Radcliffe undergraduates
Performing Groups: Radcliffe Creative Performing Arts Program
Workshops/Festivals: Workshops with professionals, Dance Film Series

MUSIC

Myra Mayman, Coordinator   *Degrees Offered:* BA (Harvard)
Number Of Students: 400   *Technical Training:* Musical Theatre
Performing Groups: Gilbert & Sullivan Players

REGIS COLLEGE
235 Wellesley St, Wheaton   Massachusetu 02193
617 893-1820 Ext 261
> Private and 4 Year
> *Arts Areas:* Instrumental Music, Vocal Music, Theatre, Film Arts, Television and Visual Arts
> *Performing Series:* Regis Cultural Series
> *Performance Facilities:* Regis Foyer; Regis Multi - Purpose Room; Regis Gymnasium; Regis Studio Theatre

MUSIC

S Margaret W McCarthy, Associate Professor   *Number Of Faculty:* 5
Number Of Students: 110   *Degrees Offered:* AB   *Courses Offered:* History; Theory; Performance
Teaching Certification Available   *Financial Assistance:* Work-Study Grants
Performing Groups: Regis College Glee Club; Regis College Ensembles
Workshops/Festivals: Choral Concerts; Chamber Music Concerts

THEATRE

S Gretchen Bogan, Associate Professor of Drama   *Number Of Faculty:* 2
Number Of Students: 160   *Degrees Offered:* AB
Financial Assistance: Work-Study Grants   *Performing Groups:* Regis Drama Club
Workshops/Festivals: Regis Summer Theatre

SCHOOL OF CONTEMPORARY MUSIC
2001 Beacon St, Brookline   Massachusetts 02146
617 734-7174
> Private and 2 Year
> *Arts Areas:* Dance, Instrumental Music, Vocal Music, Theatre and Visual Arts
> *Performance Facilities:* School of Contemporary Music Auditorium

MUSIC

Jeffrey D Furst, Chairman   *Number Of Faculty:* 50   *Number Of Students:* 380
Degrees Offered: Two-year diploma, applicable to two years credit at university
Technical Training: Piano Tuning and Technology
Financial Assistance: Scholarships and Work-Study Grants

SIMON'S ROCK EARLY COLLEGE
Alford Rd, Great Barrington   Massachusetts 01230
413 528-0771
> Private and 4 Year
> *Arts Areas:* Dance, Instrumental Music, Vocal Music, Theatre, Visual Arts and Creative Writing
> *Performance Facilities:* A R C Auditorium; Dance Studio; Lecture Center

(continued on next page)

DANCE

Phyllis Richmond, Head   **Number Of Faculty:** 35
Degrees Offered: BA in Arts & Aestietics; AA
Courses Offered: Modern Dance; Ballet; Dance Therapy; Choreography; Improvisation
Financial Assistance: Scholarships

MUSIC

Thom Lipiczky, Head   **Number Of Faculty:** 2 Full-time, 5 Part-time
Number Of Students: 42   **Degrees Offered:** BA
Courses Offered: Musicianship & Theory; Music History; World Music; Performance Classes
Technical Training: Private Instrumental & Vocal Instruction
Financial Assistance: Scholarships and Work-Study Grants
Performing Groups: Simon's Rock Chorus; Sedentary Marching Band; Recorder Ensemble; Chamber Music Ensemble
Workshops/Festivals: Jazz Workshop; Community Music School Concerts

THEATRE

James Hardy, Head   **Number Of Faculty:** 1   **Number Of Students:** 20
Degrees Offered: BA; AA
Courses Offered: Theatre Practicum; Theatre Techniques; Acting; Orientation to Theatre
Technical Training: Lighting; Set Design

SMITH COLLEGE
Northampton   Massachusetts 01060, 413 584-2700
Private and 4 Year
Arts Areas: Dance, Instrumental Music, Vocal Music, Theatre, Television and Visual Arts
Performance Facilities: Theatre 14, Hollie Flanagan Studio Theatre
Courses Offered: various, through Theatre Department

MUSIC

Vernon Gotwals, Chairman   **Number Of Faculty:** 30   **Number Of Students:** 178
Degrees Offered: BA, MA, MMus   **Teaching Certification Available**
Financial Assistance: Scholarships
Performing Groups: Various ensembles, chorus

THEATRE

Denton McCoy Snyder, Chairman   **Number Of Faculty:** 14
Number Of Students: 152   **Degrees Offered:** BA, MFA, MA
Teaching Certification Available   **Financial Assistance:** Scholarships
Performing Groups: Smith Theatre Club

THE SOUTH SHORE CONSERVATORY OF MUSIC, INC
At "Cedar Hill", Off 19 Fort Hill St, Hingham   Massachusetts 02043
617 749-5348
Private and Community Music School
Arts Areas: Dance, Instrumental Music, Vocal Music and Visual Arts
Performing Series: Concerts by Guest Artists
Performance Facilities: The Summer Wind Ensemble Rehearsal Barn; The Conservatory Recital Hall

DANCE

Paula Finkler & Lydia Yardley Rowe, Instructors   **Number Of Faculty:** 2
Number Of Students: 70
Courses Offered: Ballet; Modern Dance; Creative Movement; Jazz Dance
Financial Assistance: Scholarships and Work-Study Grants
Workshops/Festivals: MJT Movement Theatre Concerts; Ballet Demonstrations

(continued on next page)

MUSIC

James C Simpson, Jr, Director   **Number Of Faculty:** 39
Number Of Students: 998
Courses Offered: Private Instrumental Lessons; Ensemble; Theory; History
Technical Training: Preparation for college level work
Financial Assistance: Scholarships and Work-Study Grants
Performing Groups: Arts Antiqua Trombone Trio, plus performances by many of our teachers who are freelance musicians in the Boston area, and perform with the Boston Symphony & Pops, Handel & Hydn Society
Workshops/Festivals: Workshops by well - known professionals and performing groups
Artists-In-Residence/Guest Artists: Rolf Smedvig Trumpet Recital; The Empire Brass Quintet Concert; The New England String Trio; The Delalande Harp Trio

SOUTHEASTERN MASSACHUSETTS UNIVERSITY
North Dartmouth   Massachusetts 02747, 617 997-9321
State and 4 Year
Arts Areas: Instrumental Music, Vocal Music, Theatre, Film Arts and Visual Arts
Performance Facilities: Auditorium Building

MUSIC

Dr Josef Cobert, Chairman   **Number Of Faculty:** 7
Technical Training: Opera   **Financial Assistance:** Work-Study Grants
Performing Groups: Faculty Trio
Workshops/Festivals: Summer Music Festival, Opera Performers/Conductor Workshop

THEATRE

No degree program in Theatre
Workshops/Festivals: American Theatre Institute under the direction of Paul Mann

SPRINGFIELD COLLEGE
263 Alden St, Springfield   Massachusetts 01109
413 787-2100
Private and 4 Year
Arts Areas: Dance, Instrumental Music, Vocal Music and Theatre
Performing Series: The William T Simpson Cultural Affairs Series

DANCE

Louis J Ampolo; Mary Noble (Assistant Professor of Physical Education)
Number Of Faculty: 2
Degrees Offered: BS in Physical Education (concentration in dance)
Financial Assistance: Assistantships
Performing Groups: Springfield College Dancers; Springfield College Exhibition Dancers

MUSIC

Gilbert T Vickers, Director   **Number Of Faculty:** 1
Performing Groups: Springfield College Singers; Chapel Choir; Picardilly IIIrd; Springfield College Band

THEATRE

Carroll P Britch, Associate Professor   **Number Of Faculty:** 1
Performing Groups: Attica Players; ANTA (American National Theatre & Academy)

SUFFOLK UNIVERSITY
41 Temple St, Boston   Massachusetts 02114
617 723-4700
Private and 4 Year   **Arts Areas:** Theatre, Television and Visual Arts
Performing Series: Concert - Lecture Series
Performance Facilities: University Auditorium   **Number Of Faculty:** 3

(continued on next page)

Number Of Students: 50   **Degrees Offered:** BA
Teaching Certification Available   Financial Assistance: Scholarships
Performing Groups: University Theatre

WALNUT HILL SCHOOL OF PERFORMING ARTS
912 Highland St, Natick   Massachusetts 01760
617 653-4312
Private and Special
Arts Areas: Dance, Instrumental Music, Vocal Music, Theatre and Visual Arts
Performance Facilities: Walnut Hill School Auditorium; Poole Memorial Library

DANCE

Sydelle Gomberg, Dean for the Arts   **Number Of Faculty:** 10
Number Of Students: 48
Technical Training: Ballet, Modern; Pointe; Choreography; Improvisation; Modern; Repertory; Jazz; Variations; Royal Academy of Dancing Syllabus; Dance Notation (Sutton Movement); History of Dance; Music for Dancers; Bournonville Technique
Financial Assistance: Scholarships   **Performing Groups:** Concert Dance Company
Workshops/Festivals: Dance Extension Program

MUSIC

David Seaton, Chairman   **Number Of Faculty:** 6   **Number Of Students:** 30
Technical Training: Theory I, II, III (Form & Analysis), IV (Independent Study Seminar); The Classic Period; Recorder Workshop
Financial Assistance: Scholarships
Performing Groups: Greater Boston Youth Symphony Orchestra; New England Conservatory Youth Chamber Ensemble; Young Artist Program; Walnut Hill Chamber Players; Chamber Ensembles
Workshops/Festivals: Summer Workshop for Strings & Piano

THEATRE

Mark Lindberg, Chairman   **Number Of Faculty:** 2   **Number Of Students:** 36
Technical Training: Theatre Arts, I, II, III; Speech
Financial Assistance: Scholarships   **Performing Groups:** Walnut Hill Players
Artists-In-Residence/Guest Artists: Frank Ohman of the New York City Ballet

WELLESLEY COLLEGE
Wellesley   Massachusetts 02181, 617 235-0320 Ext 418
Private and 4 Year
Arts Areas: Instrumental Music, Vocal Music, Theatre and Film Arts
Performing Series: Wellesley College Cultural Events Series
Performance Facilities: Jewett Auditorium; Alumnae Hall; Houghton Chapel

DANCE

Christine Temin, Head of Dance Activities   **Number Of Faculty:** 2
Number Of Students: 100
Courses Offered: Dance I, II, III, Afro - American Dance
Technical Training: Ballet; Modern Dance
Performing Groups: Wellesley College Dance Group
Workshops/Festivals: Master classes by professional companies

MUSIC

Evelyn Barry, Associate Professor
Number Of Faculty: 22 Part-time, 6 Full-time   **Number Of Students:** 194
Degrees Offered: BA
Courses Offered: Music Theory; Literature; Composition; Performance
Financial Assistance: Scholarships and Work-Study Grants
Performing Groups: Choir; Madrigals; Collegium; Chamber Music Society; Chamber Orchestra

(continued on next page)

THEATRE

Paul R Barstow, Professor   **Number Of Faculty:** 2   **Number Of Students:** 60
Degrees Offered: BA with major in Theatre Studies
Courses Offered: Plays, Production & Performance; Theatre History; Scene Study; Contemporary Theatre; Shakespeare in the Theatre; Design for the Stage; Theatre Lighting Design; Independent Study; Honors Program in connection with Production
Financial Assistance: Scholarships and Work-Study Grants
Performing Groups: Wellesley College Theatre; Experimental Theatre; Lunchtime Theatre; Wellesley Mime Troupe
Artists-In-Residence/Guest Artists: Mary Sadovnikoff; Daniel Stepner; The Waverly Constort; Concord String Quartet; Castle Hill Festival; Suzanne Cleverdon; Adrienne Hartzell; Christopher Krueger; Jeff Stoughton; Bethany Beardslee; 5 x 2 Dance Company; Merce Cunning Dance Company

WESTFIELD STATE COLLEGE
Western Ave, Westfield   Massachusetts 01085
413 568-3311 Ext 213
State and 4 Year
Arts Areas: Dance, Instrumental Music, Vocal Music, Theatre, Film Arts, Television and Visual Arts
Performance Facilities: College Auditorium; College Little Theatre

MUSIC

Donald Bastarache, Chairman   **Number Of Faculty:** 8
Number Of Students: 110   **Degrees Offered:** BA
Courses Offered: Performance; Musicology; Theory
Teaching Certification Available
Financial Assistance: Scholarships and Work-Study Grants
Performing Groups: Symphony; Jazz Band; Chorale; Chamber Orchestra
Workshops/Festivals: Student Arts Festival; Workshops with outside famous performing musicians

THEATRE

Frank Mello, Coordinator   **Number Of Faculty:** 3   **Number Of Students:** 20
Degrees Offered: BA English   **Courses Offered:** Theatre
Teaching Certification Available
Financial Assistance: Scholarships and Work-Study Grants
Performing Groups: Footlighters
Workshops/Festivals: Student Art Festivals; Several Theatrical Productions during year

WHEATON COLLEGE
Norton   Massachusetts 02766, 617 285-7722
Private and 4 Year
Arts Areas: Instrumental Music, Vocal Music and Visual Arts
Performing Series: Concert and Lecture Series
Performance Facilities: Watson Hall

MUSIC

Carleton T Russell, Chairman   **Number Of Faculty:** 9
Number Of Students: 46   **Degrees Offered:** BA
Teaching Certification Available
Performing Groups: Chorus, College Choir, Band, Wheaton Trio

WILLIAMS COLLEGE
Williamstown   Massachusetts 01267, 413 597-3131
Private and 4 Year
Arts Areas: Dance, Instrumental Music, Vocal Music, Theatre and Visual Arts
Performance Facilities: Chapin Hall; Thompson Chapel; Adams Memorial Theatre

(continued on next page)

DANCE

Joy Dewey, Director, Dance Activities
Dance program under auspices of Physical Education Department
Number Of Faculty: 3   **Number Of Students:** 110
Financial Assistance: Scholarships and Work-Study Grants
Performing Groups: Dance Society
Workshops/Festivals: Special production jointly of Lehar's Merry Widow with Choral Society

MUSIC

Kenneth Roberts, Professor, Chairman   **Number Of Faculty:** 11
Number Of Students: 400   **Degrees Offered:** BA
Courses Offered: Full range of Theory; Musicianship; History & Literature courses with independent study in instruments, ensemble participation
Technical Training: Private lessons and participation in small and large ensembles under direction
Financial Assistance: Scholarships and Work-Study Grants
Performing Groups: Berkshire Symphony; Chamber Players - Music-in-the-Round; Student Woodwind; Brass Ensembles; Williams Choral Society; Chamber Singers; Chapel Choir; Student Orchestra; Two Student String Quartets; Marching Band

THEATRE

J B Bucky, Director, Williams College Theatre   **Number Of Faculty:** 3½
Number Of Students: 60   **Degrees Offered:** BA
Courses Offered: History of Theatre; Design; Lighting; Acting
Technical Training: On-Job training with productions
Financial Assistance: Scholarships and Work-Study Grants
Performing Groups: Williams College Theatre
Workshops/Festivals: Williamstown Summer Theatre; Festival
Artists-In-Residence/Guest Artists: Merce Cunningham; Meredith Monk; Dan Wagoner; The Orford String Quartet of Canada; Musica Viva of Boston; Charles Rosen; Benite Valente

ADRIAN COLLEGE
100 S Madison St, Adrian   Michigan 49221
313 265-5161

> Private and 4 Year
> **Arts Areas:** Instrumental Music, Vocal Music, Theatre and Visual Arts
> **Performing Series:** Celebrity Series

MUSIC

Arthur J Jones, Chairman   **Number Of Faculty:** 10   **Number Of Students:** 100
Degrees Offered: BA   **Technical Training:** Individual Study, Opera
Teaching Certification Available
Financial Assistance: Scholarships and Work-Study Grants
Performing Groups: Orchestra, Chorus, Band

THEATRE

Alan Jorgensen, Chairman   **Number Of Faculty:** 5   **Number Of Students:** 55
Degrees Offered: BA Speech/Theatre   **Teaching Certification Available**
Financial Assistance: Scholarships and Work-Study Grants
Performing Groups: Adrian College Players

ALBION COLLEGE
Albion   Michigan 49224, 517 629-5511

> Private and 4 Year
> **Arts Areas:** Instrumental Music, Vocal Music, Theatre and Visual Arts
> **Performing Series:** Concert Series

MUSIC

Melvin S Larimer, Chairman   **Number Of Faculty:** 16   **Number Of Students:** 90
Degrees Offered: BA   **Technical Training:** New York Fine Arts Semester; Opera
Teaching Certification Available
Financial Assistance: Scholarships and Work-Study Grants
Performing Groups: Chorus; Opera; Bands; Orchestra
Workshops/Festivals: High School Choral Festival

THEATRE

Helen Manning, Chairman   **Number Of Faculty:** 6   **Number Of Students:** 30
Degrees Offered: BA Speech/Theatre
Technical Training: New York Fine Arts Semester
Teaching Certification Available
Financial Assistance: Scholarships and Work-Study Grants
Performing Groups: Albion College Players
Workshops/Festivals: High School Speech/Theatre Day

ALMA COLLEGE
Alma   Michigan 48801, 517 463-2141

> Private and 4 Year
> **Arts Areas:** Instrumental Music, Vocal Music, Theatre and Visual Arts
> **Performing Series:** Lecture/Fine Arts Series

MUSIC

Ernest G Sullivan, Chairman   **Number Of Faculty:** 6   **Number Of Students:** 96
Degrees Offered: BMus   **Technical Training:** Independent Study
Teaching Certification Available
Financial Assistance: Scholarships and Work-Study Grants
Performing Groups: Orchestra, Instrumental Ensembles

(continued on next page)

THEATRE

Robert W Smith, Chairman   **Number Of Faculty:** 3   **Number Of Students:** 48
Degrees Offered: BA Speech/Drama   **Technical Training:** Independent Study
Teaching Certification Available
Financial Assistance: Scholarships and Work-Study Grants
Performing Groups: Alma Players

ALPENA COMMUNITY COLLEGE
666 Johnson St, Alpena   Michigan 49707
517 356-9021
County and 2 Year
Arts Areas: Instrumental Music, Vocal Music, Theatre and Visual Arts

MUSIC

Robert G Hein, Instructor   **Number Of Faculty:** 1   **Number Of Students:** 80
Degrees Offered: AA   **Courses Offered:** Theory; Appreciation; Performing Groups
Financial Assistance: Scholarships and Work-Study Grants
Performing Groups: Collegiate Singers; Alpena Choral Society; Alpena Civic Orchestra

THEATRE

Keith Titus, Instructor   **Number Of Faculty:** 1   **Number Of Students:** 120
Degrees Offered: AA
Courses Offered: Speech; History of Theatre; Interpretative Reading

---

ANDREWS UNIVERSITY
Berrien Springs   Michigan 49104, 616 471-7771
Private and 4 Year
Arts Areas: Instrumental Music, Vocal Music, Television and Visual Arts
Performing Series: Concert - Picture Series

MUSIC

Paul E Hamel, Chairman   **Number Of Faculty:** 12   **Number Of Students:** 80
Degrees Offered: BMus; BMusEd; MMus   **Teaching Certification Available**
Financial Assistance: Internships, Assistantships, Scholarships and Work-Study Grants
Performing Groups: Concert Band; Symphony Orchestra; Four Choral Organizations; Numerous Chamber
Music Ensembles

AQUINAS COLLEGE
1607 Robinson Rd, SE, Grand Rapids   Michigan 49506
616 459-8281
Private and 4 Year   **Arts Areas:** Instrumental Music and Vocal Music
Performance Facilities: Wege Center Auditorium

MUSIC

Sister Henry Lerczak, Chairman   **Number Of Faculty:** 6
Number Of Students: 89   **Degrees Offered:** BMus; BMusEd
Courses Offered: Majors in Music Theory; Voice; Piano Organ; Other Instruments; Music Education;
Choral Supervision & Instrumental Supervision Majors
Teaching Certification Available
Financial Assistance: Scholarships and Work-Study Grants
Performing Groups: Aquinas College Chorus; Aquinas Collegium Musicum; Aquinas College Orchestra;
Jazz Ensemble; Instrumental Ensemble
Workshops/Festivals: Intercollegiate Jazz Festival

BAY DE NOC COMMUNITY COLLEGE
Danforth Rd, Escanaba   Michigan 49829
906 786-5802
   County and 2 Year   *Arts Areas:* Theatre and Visual Arts
   Degrees Offered: AA   *Financial Assistance:* Scholarships

CALVIN COLLEGE
Burton St & East Beltline, Grand Rapids   Michigan 49506
616 949-4000
   Private and 4 Year
   Arts Areas: Dance, Instrumental Music, Vocal Music, Theatre, Film Arts and Visual Arts
   Performing Series: Calvin Artists Series; Summer Theater; Thespians; Departmental Arts Series
   Performance Facilities: Fine Arts Auditorium

MUSIC

Dr Dale Topp, Chairman   *Number Of Faculty:* 10   *Number Of Students:* 100
Degrees Offered: AB; BA   *Courses Offered:* All Vocal & Instrumental Work
Teaching Certification Available
Financial Assistance: Scholarships and Work-Study Grants
Performing Groups: Concert Band; Studio Lab Band; Orchestra; Oratorio Society; Cappella Choir; Campus Choir
Workshops/Festivals: Church Music Workshop; Summer Music Camp; Choral Festival; Band Festival; String Orchestra Festival; Student Recitals

THEATRE

Dr Martin Vande Guchte, Chairman, Speech Department   *Number Of Faculty:* 2
Number Of Students: 20   *Degrees Offered:* AB; BD Education
Teaching Certification Available
Financial Assistance: Scholarships and Work-Study Grants
Performing Groups: Thespians; Workshop Groups

CENTRAL MICHIGAN UNIVERSITY
Mount Pleasant   Michigan 48858, 517 774-3151
   State and 4 Year
   Arts Areas: Instrumental Music, Vocal Music, Theatre, Television and Visual Arts
   Performing Series: Artists Course Series

MUSIC

Rex Hewlett, Chairman   *Number Of Faculty:* 32   *Number Of Students:* 300
Degrees Offered: BMus, BMusEd, MMus, MMusEd
Teaching Certification Available   *Permanent Staff:* Opera
Financial Assistance: Internships, Assistantships, Scholarships and Work-Study Grants
Performing Groups: Concerts, Orchestra, Chorale Ensemble, Instrumental Groups
Workshops/Festivals: Opera Workshop

THEATRE

Edwin Cohen, Chairman   *Number Of Faculty:* 5   *Number Of Students:* 100
Degrees Offered: BA Drama/Speech, MA Drama/Speech
Teaching Certification Available
Financial Assistance: Internships, Assistantships, Scholarships and Work-Study Grants
Performing Groups: University Theatre

DELTA COLLEGE
University Center   Michigan 48710, 517 686-0400
   Private and 4 Year
   Arts Areas: Dance, Instrumental Music and Vocal Music
   Performing Series: Lecture/Concert Series

(continued on next page)

DANCE

Jean Treadway, Chairman   **Number Of Faculty:** 1
Workshops/Festivals: Summer School of Ballet and Modern Dance

MUSIC

Loren Cady, Chairman   **Number Of Faculty:** 3   **Degrees Offered:** AA Music
Financial Assistance: Scholarships
Workshops/Festivals: Summer Conservatory of Music

THEATRE

Jim Leffew, Chairman   **Number Of Faculty:** 1
Workshops/Festivals: Summer Festival of Arts

DETROIT BIBLE COLLEGE
27800 Franklin Rd, Southfield   Michigan 48034
313 356-8200

Private and 4 Year   **Arts Areas:** Instrumental Music and Vocal Music
Performance Facilities: Small Recital Hall   **Number Of Faculty:** 3
Number Of Students: 40   **Degrees Offered:** BMus; B Religious Ed
Performing Groups: Chorus; Instrumental Ensembles; Handbell Choir

---

EASTERN MICHIGAN UNIVERSITY
Ypsilanti   Michigan 48197, 313 487-1849

State and 4 Year
Arts Areas: Dance, Instrumental Music, Vocal Music, Theatre, Film Arts, Television and Visual Arts
Performance Facilities: Pease Auditorium; Rynearson Stadium; Bowen Field House; Roosevelt Auditorium

MUSIC

James B Hause, Department Head   **Number Of Faculty:** 48
Number Of Students: 320
Degrees Offered: BA, BS Music; B in MusEd, Mus Performance; Mus Therapy; MA Mus
Teaching Certification Available
Financial Assistance: Internships, Assistantships, Scholarships, Work-Study Grants and Service Awards
Performing Groups: University Bands; University Choirs; EMU Madrigal Ensemble; EMU Collegium Musicum; Jazz Band
Workshops/Festivals: Opera & Musical Production; Guitar; Percussion; Special Education

THEATRE

Thomas J Murray, Head of Speech & Dramatic Arts   **Number Of Faculty:** 10
Number Of Students: 83   **Degrees Offered:** BA; MA
Technical Training: Costume Design; Stagecraft
Teaching Certification Available
Performing Groups: Portable Players; EMU Players; Little Theater of the Young; Caravan Players
Workshops/Festivals: High School Dramatic Workshop; Play Production Workshop; Mime Workshop

---

FERRIS STATE COLLEGE
Big Rapids   Michigan 49307, 616 296-9971 Ext 462

State and 4 Year
Arts Areas: Instrumental Music, Vocal Music, Theatre, Television and Visual Arts
Performing Series: General Education Convocation Council
Performance Facilities: Ferris Auditorium; Starr Auditorium; Rankin Center Dome Room; Music Center

MUSIC

Dr Dacho Dachoff, Director of Music Histories
Financial Assistance: Scholarships and Work-Study Grants
Performing Groups: Men & Women's Glee Club; Symphonic Band; Concert Band; Collegiate Singers; Orchestra; Stage Band; Jazz Lab Band
Workshops/Festivals: Festival of the Arts

(continued on next page)

THEATRE

Dr Lyle Mayer, Chairman   **Number Of Faculty:** 2
Financial Assistance: Scholarships and Work-Study Grants
Performing Groups: Theatre Productions

GLEN OAKS COMMUNITY COLLEGE
Centreville   Michigan 49032, 616 467-9945
County and 2 Year   **Arts Areas:** Instrumental Music and Vocal Music

MUSIC

Robert A Gray, Director   **Degrees Offered:** AA
Performing Groups: Instrumental and Vocal Groups

GRAND RAPIDS BAPTIST COLLEGE
1001 E Beltline, NE, Grand Rapids   Michigan 49505
616 949-5300 Ext 271
Private and 4 Year
Arts Areas: Instrumental Music, Vocal Music, Theatre and Visual Arts
Performance Facilities: Two Auditoriums

MUSIC

Henry Osborn, Fine Arts Division Chairman   **Degrees Offered:** BA Mus, BMus
Courses Offered: Theory; Conducting; Literature; Composition
Technical Training: Applied   **Teaching Certification Available**
Financial Assistance: Internships, Scholarships and Work-Study Grants
Performing Groups: Chorus, Instrumental Ensembles

THEATRE

Henry Osborn, Fine Arts Division Chairman   **Number Of Faculty:** 1
Number Of Students: 45   **Degrees Offered:** BA
Courses Offered: Survey; Production; History; Church Drama; Acting
Technical Training: Lighting; Costume; Makeup; Scenery
Teaching Certification Available
Performing Groups: Touring Players; Major Players

GRAND RAPIDS JUNIOR COLLEGE
143 Bostwick NE, Grand Rapids   Michigan 49502
616 456-4891
City and 2 Year
Arts Areas: Instrumental Music, Vocal Music and Film Arts
Number Of Faculty: 9   **Number Of Students:** 300   **Degrees Offered:** AA Mus
Financial Assistance: Work-Study Grants

HENRY FORD COMMUNITY COLLEGE
5101 Evergreen, Dearborn   Michigan 48128
313 271-2750 Ext 278
City and 2 Year
Arts Areas: Instrumental Music, Vocal Music, Theatre, Film Arts, Television and Visual Arts

MUSIC

Donald Lupp, Department Head   **Number Of Faculty:** 5
Number Of Students: 450   **Degrees Offered:** AA
Courses Offered: Choral; Men's Glee Club; Women's Glee Club; Concert Band; Instrumental Ensemble; Jazz Lab Band; Jazz Workshop
Performing Groups: Men's & Women's Glee Clubs; Concert Band; Jazz Band
Workshops/Festivals: Solo Ensemble; District Travel Festival; Michigan Band; Orchestra Association

(*continued on next page*)

THEATRE

Ronald Worsely, Director   **Number Of Faculty:** 1   **Degrees Offered:** AA
Courses Offered: Theatre Fundamental; Acting & Directing; Technical Theatre; Summer Theatre Workshop
Performing Groups: Collegiate Players

HILLSDALE COLLEGE
33 E College St, Hillsdale   Michigan 49242
517 437-7341
Private and 4 Year
Arts Areas: Dance, Instrumental Music, Vocal Music and Visual Arts
Performing Series: Adventures Series
Performance Facilities: Phillips Auditorium

DANCE

Carol Rynbrandt, Chairman   **Number Of Faculty:** 1

MUSIC

Dr Harold Lowe, Chairman   **Number Of Faculty:** 4   **Number Of Students:** 10
Degrees Offered: BA   **Teaching Certification Available**
Financial Assistance: Assistantships and Scholarships
Performing Groups: Hillsdale College - Community Orchestra; College Choir; Chorale

THEATRE

David Kelley, Director   **Number Of Faculty:** 1½   **Number Of Students:** 8
Degrees Offered: BA   **Courses Offered:** Speech; Theatre
Teaching Certification Available
Performing Groups: Hillsdale College Tower Players

HOPE COLLEGE
Holland   Michigan 49423, 616 392-5111 Ext 2205
Private and 4 Year
Arts Areas: Dance, Instrumental Music, Vocal Music, Theatre, Film Arts, Television and Visual Arts
Performance Facilities: Wichers Auditorium; Snow Auditorium; Dimnent Memorial Chapel

DANCE

Maxine DeBruyn, Coordinator   **Number Of Faculty:** 7
Number Of Students: 230
Courses Offered: Period Styles; Dance Improvisation; Eurhythmics; Anatomy; Kinesiology; Dance Composition; Teaching of Dance; History of Dance
Technical Training: Modern; Ballet; Jazz; Tap; Folk; Square
Teaching Certification Available

MUSIC

Dr Stuart Sharp, Chairman   **Number Of Faculty:** 25   **Number Of Students:** 220
Degrees Offered: BA Music, History; BA Theory; BM Vocal Music Ed; BM Instrumental Music Ed; BM Performance
Courses Offered: Theory; History; Music Ed Performances
Teaching Certification Available
Performing Groups: Orchestra; Symphonette; Concert Band; Wind & Jazz Ensembles; College Chorus; Chapel Choir; Collegium Musicum; Opera Workshop
Workshops/Festivals: NSOA Summer Workshop

THEATRE

George Ralph, Chairman   **Number Of Faculty:** 7   **Number Of Students:** 20
Degrees Offered: BA
Courses Offered: Acting; Directing; Theatre History; Stage Movement; Voice for Theatre; Introduction to

(continued on next page)

Theatre; Film Appreciation; Oral Interpretation; Stage Make-up
Technical Training: Stagecraft; Stage Lighting; Costuming; Scene Design
Performing Groups: Hope College Theatre; Hope Summer Repertory Theatre; Children's Performing Troupe (summer)
Workshops/Festivals: Symposium of Creative Expression (for high school students & teachers)
Artists-In-Residence/Guest Artists: Kathy Lowenaar; William Parker; Jay Wilkey; Maurence Heinon; Daniel Admi; Danile Phillips; Benning Dexter; Ellis Julian

INTERLOCHEN ARTS ACADEMY
Interlochen   Michigan 49643, 616 276-9221
Private and 4 Year
Arts Areas: Dance, Instrumental Music, Vocal Music, Theatre, Visual Arts and Creative Writing
Performing Series: Special Concert Series; "Festival '78"; Saturday Night Concerts
Performance Facilities: Grand Travese Performing Arts Center; Fine Arts Building-Recital Hall Grunow Theatre; Jessie V Stone Building

DANCE

Su Burns, Head   **Number Of Faculty:** 3   **Number Of Students:** 46
Degrees Offered: High School Diploma with classification as Dance Major
Courses Offered: Beginning, Intermediate & Advanced Modern Dance & Ballet, including point, improvisation, composition, repertory & choreography
Technical Training: Dance Study   **Financial Assistance:** Scholarships
Performing Groups: Ballet and modern dance groups perform approximately three times during the school year
Workshops/Festivals: Week-long tour of Michigan cities under the "Interlochen Outreach" program, supported by the Michigan Council for the Arts

MUSIC

Jon Petersen, Head   **Number Of Faculty:** 28   **Number Of Students:** 300
Degrees Offered: High School Diploma with classification as a Music Major
Courses Offered: Theory; Composition; Music History; Solfeggio; Piano Technology
Financial Assistance: Scholarships
Performing Groups: Orchestra; Band; Jazz Band; Brass Ensemble; Percussion Ensemble; Choir; Chorale
Workshops/Festivals: Master Classes by Guest Instructors; Annual Composer-on-the-Campus Workshops & Performances; A regular schedule of Recitals & Concerts by student groups; Tours of state under "Interlochen Outreach" program, supported by Michigan Council for the Arts

THEATRE

Melvin L Mrochinski, Head   **Number Of Faculty:** 3   **Number Of Students:** 56
Degrees Offered: High School Diploma with classification as Theatre Arts Major
Courses Offered: Introduction to Drama; Stagecraft; Acting; Theatre History; Stage Movement; Play Production; Voice & Diction; Oral Interpretation; Play Reading; Lighting; Technical Theatre; State Management; Directing; Studio Theatre; Special Studies
Financial Assistance: Scholarships
Performing Groups: Approximately two major productions staged during school year; Small troupes do one-act plays or children's theatre on - campus or on tour
Artists-In-Residence/Guest Artists: Krzystof Penderecki; Ballet Folklorico Mexicano de Graciella Tapia; Alvin Ailey Repertory Company; Chamber Music Society of Lower Basin St; Joffrey II Company; The Romeros

JACKSON COMMUNITY COLLEGE
2111 Emmons Rd, Jackson   Michigan 49201
517 787-0800
County and 2 Year
Arts Areas: Instrumental Music, Vocal Music and Theatre

MUSIC

David Zielinbki, Chairman   **Degrees Offered:** AA

(continued on next page)

Financial Assistance: Scholarships
Performing Groups: Vocal and Instrumental Ensembles

THEATRE

G L Blanchard, Chairman   **Number Of Faculty:** 1   **Degrees Offered:** AA
Performing Groups: The Players Club

KALAMAZOO COLLEGE
1200 Academy, Kalamazoo   Michigan 49007
616 383-8400 Ext 38511
Private and 4 Year
Arts Areas: Dance, Instrumental Music, Vocal Music, Theatre, Film Arts, Television and Visual Arts
Performance Facilities: Recital Hall; Dalton Theatre; The Playhouse; Stetson Chapel; Dungeon Theatre

DANCE

Dance program under auspices of Physical Education Department

MUSIC

Lawrence R Smith, Professor   **Number Of Faculty:** 4   **Number Of Students:** 50
Degrees Offered: BA Mus; BA MusEd
Courses Offered: History Literature & Style; Vocabulary & Materials; Composition; Conducting; Music Education; Choral, Vocal Techniques; Instrumental Methods
Teaching Certification Available
Financial Assistance: Internships, Scholarships and Work-Study Grants
Performing Groups: College Singers; Motet Choir; Wind Ensemble; Chamber Orchestra, Jazz Lab Band; Ensembles
Workshops/Festivals: Master Class Workshops by Visiting Musicians; Bach Festival; Piano & Voice Seminars

THEATRE

Nelda K Balch, Professor, Theatre Arts & Speech   **Number Of Faculty:** 4
Number Of Students: 60
Degrees Offered: BA Theatre Arts; BA Theatre Education or Communications
Courses Offered: Speech; Acting; Lighting Design; Scene Design; Theatre History; Direction; History & Aesthetics of Film; Communications; Applied Theatre; Costume Design
Technical Training: Lighting & Stage Design
Teaching Certification Available
Financial Assistance: Internships, Scholarships and Work-Study Grants
Performing Groups: Quarterly Play by students; Faculty Readers' Theatre; Dungeon Productions; Festival Playhouse (semi-professional company) in tandem with students

---

KELLOGG COMMUNITY COLLEGE
450 North Ave, Battle Creek   Michigan 49016
616 965-3931 Ext 235
County and 2 Year
Arts Areas: Instrumental Music, Vocal Music, Theatre, Television and Visual Arts

MUSIC

Gordon J Smith, Chairman   **Number Of Faculty:** 2   **Degrees Offered:** AA
Courses Offered: Theory I, II, III, IV; Music Fundamentals; Piano Class I, II; Choral; Music Appreciation; Voice, Brass & Percussion Classes
Technical Training: Opportunities for basis two year program for transfer in Music Ed & Music Theory
Financial Assistance: Scholarships and Work-Study Grants
Performing Groups: Kellogg Singers; Ecclectic Chorale; Concert Band; Jazz Lab Band; Madrigal Singers
Workshops/Festivals: Mini Concert Series that, this year, includes a Trumpet Workshop, Madrigal & Rennaisance Workshop with various performances throughout the year

(continued on next page)

THEATRE

William Wallace, Coordinator of Theatre   **Number Of Faculty:** 2
Degrees Offered: AA
Courses Offered: Acting; Directing; Introduction to Theatre; Costume and Makeup; Children's Theatre; Scene Design; Oral Intrepretation; Reader's Theatre; Voice & Diction; Exploration in Performing; Play Production
Technical Training: Opportunities for Scene Shop Assistant; Student Designing
Performing Groups: College Players

KIRTLAND COMMUNITY COLLEGE
Route 4, Box 59A, Roscommon   Michigan 48653
517 275-5121
County and 2 Year
Arts Areas: Instrumental Music, Vocal Music and Theatre

MUSIC

Barbara Hess, Instructor   **Number Of Faculty:** 1   **Number Of Students:** 25
Courses Offered: Piano; Music Appreciation; Choral Ensemble; Music Theory; Instrument Ensemble; Guitar
Financial Assistance: Scholarships and Work-Study Grants

THEATRE

Val Johnson, Instructor   **Number Of Faculty:** 1   **Number Of Students:** 20
Degrees Offered: AA   **Financial Assistance:** Scholarships and Work-Study Grants

---

LAKE MICHIGAN COLLEGE
Benton Harbor   Michigan 49022, 616 927-3571
County and 2 Year
Arts Areas: Instrumental Music, Vocal Music, Theatre and Radio Journalism

MUSIC

Number Of Faculty: 18   **Number Of Students:** 50 - 70   **Degrees Offered:** AA
Courses Offered: Performance; Classroom; Private
Financial Assistance: Scholarships and Work-Study Grants
Performing Groups: Symphonic Wind Ensemble; College Choir; Brass Ensemble; Jazz Lab Band; Swing Choir; Madrigal Choir; Woodwind Ensemble; Faculty Brass Quintet; Faculty Woodwind Quintet
Workshops/Festivals: Senior and Junior High Solo & Ensemble District Festival

THEATRE

Number Of Faculty: 1   **Number Of Students:** 20 - 30   **Degrees Offered:** AA
Courses Offered: Acting; Directing; Stagecraft; Theatre Survey & Practicum
Technical Training: Involvement in productions

LANSING COMMUNITY COLLEGE
419 N Capitol, Lansing   Michigan 48914
517 373-7400 Ext 3714
City and 2 Year
Arts Areas: Dance, Instrumental Music, Vocal Music, Theatre and Visual Arts
Performing Series: Local Art, Music, Dance

DANCE

Teri Gouze, Coordinator   **Number Of Faculty:** 20   **Number Of Students:** 600
Degrees Offered: AA   **Courses Offered:** Ballet; Ballroom; Tap; Modern; Ethnic
Technical Training: Choreography   **Financial Assistance:** Scholarships and Work-Study Grants
Performing Groups: Lansing Ballet Theater; Lansing Dance Theater, International Dances
Workshops/Festivals: Spring Festival

MUSIC

Linda Griswold, Coordinator   **Number Of Faculty:** 25
Number Of Students: 600   **Degrees Offered:** AA

(continued on next page)

Courses Offered: Choral; Instrumental; Vocal
Technical Training: Applied Instrumental
Financial Assistance: Scholarships and Work-Study Grants
Performing Groups: LanSwingers; Vocal & Instrumental Groups
Workshops/Festivals: Spring Festival

THEATRE

Steven Gilles, Production Manager   **Number Of Faculty:** 15
Number Of Students: 100   **Degrees Offered:** AA
Courses Offered: Acting; Technical Theater
Technical Training: Lighting; Design; Stage Setting
Financial Assistance: Scholarships and Work-Study Grants
Performing Groups: Boarshead Theater   **Workshops/Festivals:** Summer Festival

---

MACOMB COUNTY COMMUNITY COLLEGE - CENTER CAMPUS
16500 Hall Rd, Mount Clements   Michigan 48043
313 286-8000
County and 2 Year
Arts Areas: Dance, Instrumental Music, Vocal Music, Theatre, Film Arts, Television and Visual Arts

DANCE

John Orris, Associate Dean of Physical Education & Social Science
Number Of Faculty: 1   **Number Of Students:** 32
Degrees Offered: AA; A in General Studies; A in Applied Science; Certificate in General Education

MUSIC

Dr John Krnacik, Associate Dean, Humanities & Communications
Number Of Faculty: 1   **Number Of Students:** 140
Financial Assistance: Scholarships by audition ($200)
Performing Groups: Jazz Band; Band & Wind Ensemble; Macombers Choir; Concert Choir; Chamber Orchestra
Workshops/Festivals: Choir Directory Workshops; Jazz Clinics sponsored by the Cultural Advisory Committees

THEATRE

John Krnacik, Associate Dean of Communications & Humanities
Number Of Faculty: 1   **Number Of Students:** 80
Financial Assistance: Scholarships

MACOMB COUNTY COMMUNITY COLLEGE - SOUTH CAMPUS
14500 E Twelve Mile Rd, Warren   Michigan 48093
313 779-7000
County and 2 Year
Arts Areas: Dance, Instrumental Music, Vocal Music, Theatre, Film Arts, Television, Visual Arts and Humanities
Performing Series: Broadway Productions; Educational - Cultural Series
Performance Facilities: Student Union; South Campus Auditorium, TV Studio

DANCE

Daniel A Jaksen, Associate Dean, Humanities & Physical Education
Number Of Faculty: 2   **Number Of Students:** 80
Degrees Offered: AA; A in General Education; A in Applied Science; Certificate in General Studies
Financial Assistance: Financial Aid Office

MUSIC

Daniel Jaksen, Associate Dean, Humanities & Physical Education
Number Of Faculty: 3   **Number Of Students:** 450
Degrees Offered: AA; A in General Education; A in Applied Science; Certificate in General Studies

(continued on next page)

Financial Assistance: Financial Aid Office
Performing Groups: Jazz Band; Band & Wind Ensemble; Macombers Choir; Concert Choir; Chamber Orchestra
Workshops/Festivals: Choir Directory Workshops sponsored by the college; Jazz Clinics sponsored by the Cultural Advisory Committee

THEATRE

Donald Wing, Associate Dean, Communications   **Number Of Faculty:** 1
Number Of Students: 95
Degrees Offered: AA; A in General Education; A in Applied Science; Certificate in General Studies
Financial Assistance: Financial Aid Office

MADONNA COLLEGE
36600 Schoolcraft Rd, Livonia   Michigan 48150
313 425-8000
Private and 4 Year
Arts Areas: Instrumental Music, Vocal Music and Television
Performing Series: Cultural Performing Series
Performance Facilities: Proscenium Stage & Auditorium

MUSIC

Sister Edith Marie, Chairman   **Number Of Faculty:** 4
Number Of Students: 35   **Degrees Offered:** BA MusEd
Courses Offered: Theory; Applied Music; Performance
Teaching Certification Available
Financial Assistance: Assistantships, Scholarships and Work-Study Grants
Artists-In-Residence/Guest Artists: The Detroit Sign Company - deaf theatrical group

---

MERCY COLLEGE OF DETROIT
8200 W Outer Drive, Detroit   Michigan 48219
393 531-7820
Private and 4 Year
Arts Areas: Instrumental Music, Vocal Music and Theatre

MUSIC

Joel Ebersole, Director   **Number Of Faculty:** 2 Full-time, 2 Part-time
Number Of Students: 150
Courses Offered: Liberal Arts electives only - Applied Music & Literature; Ensembles
Performing Groups: Small Choral & Instrumental Ensembles

THEATRE

Albert Zolton, Chairman   **Number Of Faculty:** 2 Full-time, 2 Part-time
Number Of Students: 160   **Degrees Offered:** BA
Teaching Certification Available   **Performing Groups:** Mercy Players

---

MICHIGAN CHRISTIAN JUNIOR COLLEGE
800 W Avon Rd, Rochester   Michigan 48063
313 651-5800
Private and 2 Year
Arts Areas: Instrumental Music, Vocal Music and Visual Arts
Degrees Offered: AA   **Technical Training:** Opera
Financial Assistance: Scholarships
Performing Groups: Chorus, Vocal and Instrumental Ensembles

MICHIGAN STATE UNIVERSITY
East Lansing   Michigan 48824, 517 355-4597
State and 4 Year
Arts Areas: Dance, Instrumental Music, Vocal Music, Theatre, Film Arts, Television, Visual Arts and Arts Management
Performance Facilities: Michigan State Auditorium; Fairchild Theatre; Music Bldg; Auditorium

DANCE

Dixie Durr, Associate Professor - Dance Coordinator   *Number Of Faculty:* 2½
Number Of Students: 350   *Degrees Offered:* BA
Courses Offered: Social, Folk & Square Dance; Modern Dance; Ballet ; Rhythmic Form & Analysis; Methods of Teaching Dance; Dance History; Advanced Modern ; Practicum - Choreography; Dance Production
Teaching Certification Available   Financial Assistance: Assistantships
Performing Groups: MSU Repertory Dance Company; MSU Elementary Lecture Demonstration Dance Team;

MUSIC

James Niblock, Professor & Chairman   *Number Of Faculty:* 52
Number Of Students: 610   *Degrees Offered:* BA; BMus; MMus; PhD
Courses Offered: Applied Music; Music Education; Music Theory - Composition; Musicology
Teaching Certification Available
Financial Assistance: Assistantships, Scholarships and Work-Study Grants
Performing Groups: Orchestras; Bands; Choral; Chamber Music; Jazz
Workshops/Festivals: Summer Youth Music; Music for Exceptional Children; Church Music; Piano Teachers

THEATRE

Frant Rutledge, Chairman/Producer   *Number Of Faculty:* 11
Number Of Students: 257   *Degrees Offered:* BA; MA; MFA; PhD
Technical Training: Acting; Design; Directing
Teaching Certification Available
Financial Assistance: Assistantships, Scholarships and Work-Study Grants
Performing Groups: Performing Arts Company
Workshops/Festivals: Summer Circle Free Festival

THE UNIVERSITY OF MICHIGAN
Ann Arbor   Michigan 48104, 313 764-1817
State and 4 Year
Arts Areas: Dance, Instrumental Music, Vocal Music, Theatre, Film Arts, Television and Visual Arts
Performing Series: Professional Theatre Program; Ann Arbor Chamber Music Celebration; Music at Midday
Performance Facilities: Hill Auditorium; Power Center for the Performing Arts;
Lydia Mendelssohn Theatre; Rackham Auditorium; Schorling Theatre; Residential College Auditorium; School of Music Recital Hall; Arena Theatre; Trueblood Theatre; Pendelton Arts Center; Stearns Building - Cady Music Room

DANCE

Elizabeth Bergmann, Chairman; Vera Embree, Acting Chairman
Number Of Faculty: 10   *Number Of Students:* 60   *Degrees Offered:* BFA; MFA
Courses Offered: Modern Dance; Ballet; Jazz; Afro-American Dance; Dance Composition; Movement Improvisation; History of Dance; Dance Production; Methods of Teaching Dance; Labanotation
Technical Training: Techniques in Composition: Emphasis on Modern, Ballet, Afro - American, Jazz
Teaching Certification Available
Financial Assistance: Assistantships, Scholarships and Work-Study Grants
Performing Groups: The University Dance Company
Workshops/Festivals: Workshops & Festival throughout the year with professional artists such as Alvin Ailey, Pearl Lang, & Christine Dakin

(continued on next page)

MUSIC

Allen P Britton, Dean   **Number Of Faculty:** 118   **Number Of Students:** 920
Degrees Offered: BMus; BMA; MMus; MMusEd; PhD; DMA
Teaching Certification Available
Financial Assistance: Assistantships, Scholarships, Work-Study Grants and NDSEO
Performing Groups: String, Wind & Vocal Ensembles; Glee Club; Collegium Musicum; Opera Production; Opera Workshop; Four Bands; Three Jazz Bands; Four Symphony Orchestras; Three Choirs; Chamber Choir; Javanese Gamelan Ensemble; Japanese Music Study Group
Workshops/Festivals: May Festival; Summer Session at Interlochen; Summer Festival; Miscellaneous workshops throughout the year; Over 65 professional concerts annually & over 350 concerts by the School of Music

THEATRE

Jack E Bender, Interim Director   **Number Of Faculty:** 11
Number Of Students: 400
Degrees Offered: BA; MA; PhD; MFA Technical Design; MA Theatre Management
Courses Offered: Graduate & Undergraduate Acting, Directing, Technical & Design Courses
Teaching Certification Available
Financial Assistance: Assistantships, Scholarships, Work-Study Grants and NDSEO
Performing Groups: The University Theatre Program; Black Theatre Program
Workshops/Festivals: Work with resident professional companies such as The Acting Company
Artists-In-Residence/Guest Artists: George Shirley; Elisabeth Schwarzkopf; Byron Janis; John Wustman; Nafe Katter; Fred Coffin; George Pentecost; Maureen Anderman; Nicholas Pennell

---

UNIVERSITY OF MICHIGAN, FLINT
1321 E Court, Flint   Michigan 48503
313 767-4000

State and 4 Year
Arts Areas: Instrumental Music, Vocal Music, Theatre and Visual Arts
Performing Series: Concert Series

MUSIC

A Raymond Roth, Chairman   **Number Of Faculty:** 5 Full-time, 14 Part-time
Number Of Students: 300   **Degrees Offered:** BMusEd; BA (Music Major)
Teaching Certification Available
Financial Assistance: Scholarships and Work-Study Grants
Performing Groups: University Chamber Choir; University Orchestra; University Choir; University Band; Wind Ensemble; University Jazz Ensemble; Renaissance Ensemble
Workshops/Festivals: Vocal, Instrumental & Jazz Workshops

THEATRE

Marianne Fearn, Chairman   **Number Of Faculty:** 5   **Degrees Offered:** BA; BGS
Teaching Certification Available
Financial Assistance: Scholarships and Work-Study Grants
Workshops/Festivals: Genesee County Secondary Drama Teachers' Association One-Act Play Festival

---

MONROE COUNTY COMMUNITY COLLEGE
1555 S Raisinville Rd, Monroe   Michigan 48161
313 242-7300

County and 2 Year
Arts Areas: Instrumental Music, Vocal Music and Theatre
Performance Facilities: MCCC Cafetorium; Theatrical Lecture - Auditorium

MUSIC

Dr Paul Ross, Division Chairman for Humanities   **Number Of Faculty:** 2
Number Of Students: 50   **Degrees Offered:** AA
Courses Offered: Theory; Band; Choir; Applied Music; Music Ed; Literature; Jazz
Financial Assistance: Scholarships and Work-Study Grants

(continued on next page)

Performing Groups: College - Community Band; Agora Chorale; Jazz Ensemble
Workshops/Festivals: County Choral Festival; Area Solo & Ensemble Festival

THEATRE

Dr Paul Ross, Division Chairman for Humanieies   **Number Of Faculty:** 1
Financial Assistance: Scholarships and Work-Study Grants

MUSKEGON COMMUNITY COLLEGE
221 S Quarterline Rd, Muskegon   Michigan 49443
616 773-9191 Ext 323
State and 2 Year
Arts Areas: Dance, Instrumental Music, Vocal Music, Theatre, Film Arts, Television and Visual Arts
Performance Facilities: Frauenthal Foundation Art Center

MUSIC

Lee Collet, Chairman   **Number Of Faculty:** 4   **Number Of Students:** 150
Degrees Offered: AA
Financial Assistance: Scholarships and Work-Study Grants
Performing Groups: Overbrook Singers, Overbrook Concert Band, Jazz Ensemble, Collegiates
Workshops/Festivals: Spring Arts Festival, Theater Festival Day

THEATRE

Carlo V Spataro, Director   **Number Of Faculty:** 3   **Number Of Students:** 50
Degrees Offered: AA   **Technical Training:** Set Contruction, Technical Theatre
Financial Assistance: Work-Study Grants
Performing Groups: Overbrook Players; Children's Touring Theatre
Workshops/Festivals: Theater Festival Day

NATIONAL MUSIC CAMP
Interlochen   Michigan 49643, 616 276-9221
Private and Summer Program
Arts Areas: Dance, Instrumental Music, Vocal Music, Theatre and Visual Arts
Performance Facilities: Interlochen Bowl; Kresge Auditorium; Grand Traverse Performing Arts Center;
Grunow Theatre

DANCE

William Hug, Director, Modern Dance; Sheila Reilly, Director, Ballet Department
Number Of Faculty: 10   **Number Of Students:** 59
Degrees Offered: Undergraduate and graduate credit offered through the University of Michigan for
modern dance and ballet
Courses Offered: Modern Dance; Ballet; Choreography; Improvisation; Repertory
Technical Training: Extensive training in all facets of Ballet & Modern Dance
Financial Assistance: Scholarships and Work-Study Grants

MUSIC

Dr George C Wilson, Director   **Number Of Faculty:** 130
Number Of Students: 1,200
Degrees Offered: Undergraduate and graduate credit offered through the University of Michigan
Courses Offered: All Band & Orchestral Instruments; Jazz; Theory; Composition; Conducting; Guitar;
Opera; Operetta; Vocal Music; Piano; Organ; Harpsichord
Technical Training: Private and class lessons offered at all levels
Financial Assistance: Scholarships and Work-Study Grants
Performing Groups: Orchestras; Bands; Jazz Bands; Choirs; Ensembles (divided by grade level - grade
school, junior high, high school, university)
Workshops/Festivals: Operetta, Opera & Festival Choir Performances

THEATRE

Robert C Burroughs, Director   **Number Of Faculty:** 18
Number Of Students: 177

(continued on next page)

Degrees Offered: University of Michigan credit offered for Fundaments of Acting course
Courses Offered: Drama Production; Radio Production; Oral Interpretation; Readers' Theatre; Musical Theatre; Movement & Staging; Stagecraft; Costuming; Acting Technique; Make-up; Theatre History
Financial Assistance: Scholarships and Work-Study Grants
Performing Groups: Plays; Shakespearean Production; Musical
Artists-In-Residence/Guest Artists: Van Cliburn Benefit Performance; Cleveland String Quartet; U S Marine Band; Robert Shaw conducting Festival Choir

NORTHERN MICHIGAN UNIVERSITY
Marquette   Michigan 49855, 906 227-2720
State and 4 Year
Arts Areas: Dance, Instrumental Music, Vocal Music, Theatre, Film Arts, Television and Visual Arts
Performing Series: Community Concerts
Performance Facilities: Forest Roberts Theatre; Dance Studio

DANCE

Roberta Verley, Assistant Professor, Chairman   **Number Of Faculty:** 1
Number Of Students: 22   **Financial Assistance:** Work-Study Grants

MUSIC

Dr Robert Stephenson, Chairman   **Number Of Faculty:** 20
Number Of Students: 127
Degrees Offered: BMusEd; BMus Performance; BA & BS Music
Teaching Certification Available
Financial Assistance: Assistantships, Scholarships and Work-Study Grants
Performing Groups: Arts Chorale; Concert Choir; Wind Ensemble; Concert Band; Chamber Orchestra; Chamber Groups; Stage Band; Jazz Band; Percussion Ensemble
Workshops/Festivals: Solo & Ensemble Festival; High School Band Camp (Workshop); Various Clinics

THEATRE

Dr James Panowski, Director   **Number Of Faculty:** 4   **Number Of Students:** 63
Degrees Offered: BA in Liberal Arts Curriculum
Courses Offered: Introduction to Theatre; Theatre Management
Technical Training: Costuming & Sets   **Teaching Certification Available**
Financial Assistance: Scholarships and Work-Study Grants
Performing Groups: Points North Summer Theater; Children's Theater
Workshops/Festivals: Summer Theater

NORTHWESTERN MICHIGAN COLLEGE
1701 E Front St, Traverse City   Michigan 49684
616 946-5650
County and 2 Year
Arts Areas: Dance, Instrumental Music, Vocal Music, Theatre, Film Arts and Visual Arts
Performance Facilities: Fine Arts Building Recital Hall; Small Theatre; Physical Education Building

DANCE

Robert Inglis, Physical Education Department Head   **Number Of Faculty:** 5
Number Of Students: 75
Courses Offered: Beginning & Intermediate Modern Dance; Creative Dance; Social Dance
Financial Assistance: Scholarships and Work-Study Grants

MUSIC

Walter Ross, Chairman   **Number Of Students:** 300 - 350   **Degrees Offered:** AA
Courses Offered: Fundamentals of Music; Music Appreciation - Standard Literature & Jazz; Survey of Choral Literature; Ensembles in Applied Music; Madrigal Singers; Introduction to Music Literature; Theory of Music; Sight Singing & Ear Training; Applied Music; Ensembles in Applied Music; Survey of Wind Ensemble; Jazz Lab Band; Symphony Orchestra
Financial Assistance: Scholarships and Work-Study Grants
Performing Groups: Band; Lab Band; Choir; Madrigals

(continued on next page)

THEATRE

Harry Oliver, Chairman   *Number Of Faculty:* 1   *Number Of Students:* 40
Degrees Offered: AA
Courses Offered: Play Production; Introduction to the Theatre
Financial Assistance: Scholarships and Work-Study Grants
Performing Groups: NMC Players
Workshops/Festivals: Two full-length plays each year

OAKLAND COMMUNITY COLLEGE
2480 Opdyke Rd, Bloomfield Hills   Michigan 48013
313 647-6200
County and 2 Year
Arts Areas: Instrumental Music, Vocal Music and Visual Arts

MUSIC

Theordore H Mann, Associate Professor   *Degrees Offered:* AA
Financial Assistance: Scholarships and Work-Study Grants
Performing Groups: Vocal and instrumental groups

OAKLAND UNIVERSITY
Rochester   Michigan 48063, 313 377-2030
State and 4 Year
Arts Areas: Instrumental Music, Vocal Music and Theatre
Performing Series: International Series; Music Drama Series
Performance Facilities: Varner Recital Hall

MUSIC

Dr Raynold Allvin, Chairman   *Number Of Faculty:* 10 Full-time, 30 Part-time
Number Of Students: 300   *Degrees Offered:* BA; BMusEd; BMus
Courses Offered: Music Appreciation; History & Literature; Theory; Ear Training; Composition; Early Music; Jazz History; Applied Music Instruction; Music Education
Teaching Certification Available
Financial Assistance: Assistantships and Work-Study Grants
Performing Groups: OU Chorus; Oakland Singers OU Orchestra; Wind Ensemble; Collegium Musicum; The Meadow Brook Estate; Afram Lab Bands; Opera Workshop; American Musical Theatre
Workshops/Festivals: Jazz Institutes; Orff - Schulwerk Institutes; Swing Choir Camp; Oakland Youth Symphony; Electronic Music Workshop; Music for Children's Choruses
Artists-In-Residence/Guest Artists: Flavio Varani

OLIVET COLLEGE
Olivet   Michigan 49076, 616 749-7000
Private and 4 Year
Arts Areas: Instrumental Music, Vocal Music, Theatre and Visual Arts
Performing Series: Film Series; Special Events; Vocal & Instrumental Series
Performance Facilities: Mott Auditorium Upton Recital Hall; MacKay Gym

MUSIC

David McCoy, Chairman   *Number Of Faculty:* 9 Full-time, 15 Part-time
Number Of Students: 250   *Degrees Offered:* BA; BMus; BMusEd
Courses Offered: Teacher Certificate; Vocal & Instrumental Music; Performance Major; Theory - Composition Major; Theory - History Major; Church Music Major; Piano Proficiency
Teaching Certification Available
Financial Assistance: Internships, Assistantships, Scholarships, Work-Study Grants and Performance Grants
Performing Groups: Marching Band; Wind Ensemble; Symphony Band; Jazz Ensemble; Small Performing Ensembles; College Orchestra; Symphonic Choir; Varsity Chorus; Conservatory Chorale; Collegium Musicum; Musica Nova; Opera Workshop; Encore (pops)
Workshops/Festivals: Fine Arts Festival; Jazz; Opera

(continued on next page)

THEATRE

Lee A McGaan, Chairman, Communication Department   **Number Of Faculty:** 2½
Number Of Students: 70
Degrees Offered: BA; Elementary & Secondary Teaching Certificate
Courses Offered: Introduction to Film & Theatre; Oral Interpretation; Acting I & II; History & Development of Dramatic Art; Theatre Workshop; Drama; Stage Design; Play Direction; Theatre Practicum; Independent Study
Teaching Certification Available
Financial Assistance: Internships, Assistantships, Scholarships, Work-Study Grants and Performance Grants
Performing Groups: Student - produced play; College produced play; Opera; Musical play; Alpha Psi Omega Chapter

---

SAGINAW VALLEY COLLEGE
2250 Pierce Rd, Saginaw   Michigan 48710
517 793-9800
State and 4 Year
Arts Areas: Instrumental Music, Vocal Music, Theatre and Visual Arts
Performing Series: Concert/Lecture Series

MUSIC

Degrees Offered: BA Mus   **Financial Assistance:** Scholarships and Work-Study Grants
Performing Groups: Chorus, Orchestra, Instrumental groups

THEATRE

Degrees Offered: BA Dramatics   **Financial Assistance:** Scholarships and Work-Study Grants
Performing Groups: SVC Theater

SCHOOLCRAFT COLLEGE
18600 Haggerty Rd, Livonia   Michigan 48152
313 591-6400
2 Year and District
Arts Areas: Dance, Instrumental Music, Vocal Music, Theatre and Visual Arts
Performing Series: Cultural & Public Affairs Series
Performance Facilities: Liberal Arts Theater; Waterman Campus Center

DANCE

Marvin Gans, Assistant Dean, Arts & Sciences
Number Of Faculty: 4 Part-time   **Number Of Students:** 170
Courses Offered: Beginning & Intermediate Modern, Folk Square & Social Dance; Community Services courses: Ballet, Ballet Exercise, Mid - Eastern, Beginning & Intermediate Ballroom Dancing
Financial Assistance: Scholarships and Work-Study Grants

MUSIC

Robert W Jones, Instructor & Department Representative
Number Of Faculty: 3   **Number Of Students:** 110   **Degrees Offered:** AA
Courses Offered: Music Appreciation; Theory; History; Education
Technical Training: Applied Music   **Teaching Certification Available**
Financial Assistance: Scholarships, Work-Study Grants and Student Aid Opportunities
Performing Groups: Band; Orchestra; Jazz Ensemble; Choir; Madrigals
Workshops/Festivals: Michigan Music Teachers Association Workshop; Orff Music Workshop

THEATRE

Larry Rudick, Instructor, Speech - Theater   **Number Of Faculty:** 1   **Number Of Students:** 20
Degrees Offered: AA   **Courses Offered:** Theater Activities; Stagecraft & Lighting; Acting; History
Financial Assistance: Scholarships, Work-Study Grants and Student Aid Opportunities
Performing Groups: Little Theatre Company

SIENA HEIGHTS COLLEGE
1247 E Siena Heights Dr, Adrian   Michigan 49221
313 263-0831

Private and 4 Year
Arts Areas: Instrumental Music, Vocal Music, Theatre and Visual Arts
Performing Series: Performing Artists Series
Degrees Offered: BA, MA MusEd, MA MusEd, MA Teaching
Technical Training: Opera   *Teaching Certification Available*
Financial Assistance: Scholarships and Work-Study Grants
Performing Groups: Orchestra, Band, Chorus, Instrumental Ensembles

THEATRE

Sister Therese Craig, Chairman   *Number Of Faculty:* 4
Degrees Offered: BA Speech/Drama   *Teaching Certification Available*
Financial Assistance: Scholarships and Work-Study Grants
Performing Groups: Little Theatre

SPRING ARBOR COLLEGE
Spring Arbor   Michigan 49283, 517 750-1200 Ext 265

Private and 4 Year
Arts Areas: Instrumental Music, Vocal Music and Theatre
Performing Series: Fine Arts Series; Local Artist Series; Town & Gown Cultural Series
Performance Facilities: E P Hart Auditorium; Free Methodist Church

MUSIC

Kennistan Bauman, Chairman   *Number Of Faculty:* 4   *Number Of Students:* 54
Degrees Offered: BA   *Courses Offered:* Performance; Theory; History; Education
Technical Training: Piano Tuning   *Teaching Certification Available*
Financial Assistance: Scholarships, Work-Study Grants and Fellowship
Performing Groups: Concert Band; Orchestra; Jazz Ensemble; Concert Choir; Chamber Singers; Festival Choir; Commond Bond

THEATRE

Ester Lee Maddox, Chairman   *Number Of Faculty:* 14
Courses Offered: Play Producting; Directing
Financial Assistance: Scholarships, Work-Study Grants and Fellowship

UNIVERSITY OF DETROIT, MARYGROVE COLLEGE
8425 W McNichols, Detroit   Michigan 43221
313 341-1838

Private and 4 Year
Arts Areas: Dance, Instrumental Music, Vocal Music, Theatre, Film Arts, Television and Visual Arts
Performing Series: Artists and Lecture Series
Performance Facilities: The Theatre

DANCE

Dominic Missimi, Acting Chairman   *Number Of Faculty:* 6
Number Of Students: 50
Degrees Offered: BFA, MA with Specialization in Dance
Technical Training: Up to 80 hours of elementary, intermediate, and advanced dance technique offered
Financial Assistance: Scholarships and Work-Study Grants
Performing Groups: Dance Detroit
Workshops/Festivals: Dance Power Workshop, Summer School of Performing Arts

MUSIC

John Guinn, Chairman   *Number Of Faculty:* 5   *Number Of Students:* 40
Degrees Offered: BA   *Technical Training:* Voice and Operatic Training
Teaching Certification Available

(continued on next page)

Financial Assistance: Scholarships and Work-Study Grants
Performing Groups: Glee Club, Instrumental Ensembles

THEATRE

Dominic Missimi, Chairman   *Number Of Faculty:* 7   *Number Of Students:* 45
Degrees Offered: BA, BFA, MA   *Technical Training:* Acting, Directing, Design
Teaching Certification Available
Financial Assistance: Scholarships and Work-Study Grants
Performing Groups: Touring Company, Children's Theatre Company, Performing Theatre Company
Workshops/Festivals: Summer Festival for Performing Arts

WAYNE STATE UNIVERSITY
1400 Chrysler Freeway, Detroit   Michigan 48202
313 961-7302
State and 4 Year
Arts Areas: Instrumental Music, Vocal Music, Theatre, Television, Visual Arts and Radio
Performing Series: Performing Artist Series

MUSIC

Robert F Lawson, Chairman   *Number Of Faculty:* 65   *Number Of Students:* 500
Degrees Offered: BMus, BMusEd, MMus, MMusEd   *Technical Training:* Composition
Teaching Certification Available
Financial Assistance: Internships, Assistantships, Scholarships and Work-Study Grants
Performing Groups: Lyric Theatre, Orchestra, Sympony, String Ensembles, Wind Ensembles, Brass Ensembles, Percussion Groups, Chorus, Band

THEATRE

Leonard Leone, Chairman   *Number Of Faculty:* 20   *Number Of Students:* 170
Degrees Offered: BA Speech/Theatre, MA Speech/Theatre, PhD Speech/Theatre
Teaching Certification Available
Financial Assistance: Internships, Assistantships, Scholarships and Work-Study Grants
Performing Groups: University Theatre

WESTERN MICHIGAN UNIVERSITY
Kalamazoo   Michigan 49008, 616 383-1600
State and 4 Year
Arts Areas: Dance, Instrumental Music, Vocal Music and Theatre
Performing Series: Lecture & Music Series; Celebrity Series; Broadway Series

DANCE

Dr Elisabeth Hetherington, Chairperson   *Number Of Faculty:* 7
Degrees Offered: BA; BS; BFA; MA
Courses Offered: Dance Education; Performance Dance - Ballet or Contemporary; Jazz Dance; Theatrical Dance; Fine Arts - Dance
Teaching Certification Available   *Performing Groups:* University Dancers

MUSIC

Dr Robert R Find, Chairperson   *Number Of Faculty:* 40
Number Of Students: 450   *Degrees Offered:* BA; BS; BMus; BMusEd; MMus; MMusEd
Courses Offered: Performance; Music Education; Music Therapy; Music History; Music Theatre; Composition
Technical Training: Opera   *Teaching Certification Available*
Financial Assistance: Assistantships, Scholarships and Work-Study Grants
Performing Groups: Choral Ensembles; Orchestra; Opera Theatre; Bands; Wind Ensembles; New Music Ensemble; Renaissance Band; Chamber Ensemble
Workshops/Festivals: Opera Workshop; Spring Conference on Wind Persussion Music; Vocal Clinic

(continued on next page)

THEATRE

Dr Zack York, Chairperson   ***Number Of Faculty:*** 7   ***Degrees Offered:*** BA
Courses Offered: Theatre; Music Theatre; Fine Arts; Teaching Theatre
Teaching Certification Available
Financial Assistance: Assistantships, Scholarships and Work-Study Grants
Performing Groups: University Theatre

AUGSBURG COLLEGE
731 21st Ave S, Minneapolis   Minnesota 55454
612 332-5181

> Private and 4 Year
> **Arts Areas:** Instrumental Music, Vocal Music, Theatre and Visual Arts
> **Performing Series:** Celebrate Series   **Performance Facilities:** Little Theatre

MUSIC

> Robert Karlen, Chairman   **Number Of Faculty:** 20   **Number Of Students:** 185
> **Degrees Offered:** BA Mus; BMusEd; BMus; BSMus Therapy
> **Courses Offered:** History of Music; Theory; Applied Music
> **Teaching Certification Available**
> **Financial Assistance:** Scholarships and Work-Study Grants
> **Performing Groups:** Augsburg Choir & Chorale; Augsburg Concert Band; Augsburg College Orchestra; Augsburg Jazz Ensemble I & II; Augsburg Jazz Combo I & II; String & Woodwind Quartet; Brass Ensemble
> **Workshops/Festivals:** Augsburg Select Band Day

THEATRE

> Ailene Cole, Director, Drama   **Number Of Faculty:** 4
> **Number Of Students:** 60   **Degrees Offered:** BA
> **Courses Offered:** Acting; Directing; Creative Dramatics; Interpretative Reading; Stagecraft; Lighting & Design
> **Technical Training:** Lighting & Design; Production Work
> **Teaching Certification Available**
> **Financial Assistance:** Scholarships and Work-Study Grants
> **Performing Groups:** Augsburg College Players

BEMIDJI STATE COLLEGE
Bemidji   Minnesota 56601, 218 755-3990

> State and 4 Year
> **Arts Areas:** Dance, Instrumental Music, Vocal Music, Theatre, Film Arts, Television and Visual Arts
> **Performing Series:** Performing Artist Series
> **Performance Facilities:** Bangsberg Fine Arts Building

DANCE

> Myrtie Hunt, Chairman   **Number Of Faculty:** 1   **Number Of Students:** 50
> **Degrees Offered:** BS
> **Financial Assistance:** Scholarships and Work-Study Grants
> **Workshops/Festivals:** Annual Dance Program

MUSIC

> Dr Fulton Gallagher, Chairman   **Number Of Faculty:** 24
> **Number Of Students:** 250   **Degrees Offered:** BA; BS; MMusEd
> **Technical Training:** Piano Tuning   **Teaching Certification Available**
> **Financial Assistance:** Internships, Assistantships, Scholarships and Work-Study Grants
> **Performing Groups:** Concert Choir; Concert Wind Ensemble; Orchestra; Madrigal Singers; Music Theatre
> **Workshops/Festivals:** Electronic Music; Summer Music Clinic; Christiansen Choral School

THEATRE

> Dr Joan Reynolds, Chairman   **Number Of Faculty:** 5   **Number Of Students:** 100
> **Degrees Offered:** BA; BS   **Teaching Certification Available**
> **Financial Assistance:** Internships, Assistantships, Scholarships and Work-Study Grants
> **Performing Groups:** Children's Theatre

BETHANY LUTHERAN COLLEGE
734 Marsh St, Mankato Minnesota 56001
507 625-2977
> Private and 2 Year
> *Arts Areas:* Instrumental Music, Vocal Music, Theatre and Visual Arts
> *Performance Facilities:* College Chapel; College Auditorium

MUSIC

Arlene Hilding, Professor *Number Of Faculty:* 2 *Number Of Students:* 40
Degrees Offered: AA
Courses Offered: Music Appreciation; Fundamentals of Music; Forms & Music of Christian Worship; Music Theory & History; Organ History & Literature
Technical Training: Piano; Organ; Voice; Instrumental Private Lessons
Financial Assistance: Scholarships and Work-Study Grants
Performing Groups: Choirs; Enembles
Workshops/Festivals: Pre - Organ Workshop

THEATRE

Sig Lee, Chairman *Number Of Faculty:* 1½ *Number Of Students:* 12
Degrees Offered: AA *Courses Offered:* Theatre; Acting; Drama in Performance
Financial Assistance: Scholarships and Work-Study Grants
Performing Groups: Readers' Theatre; Children's Theatre; Campus Theatre

BETHEL COLLEGE
St Paul Minnesota 55101, 612 641-6400
> Private and 4 Year
> *Arts Areas:* Instrumental Music, Vocal Music, Theatre and Visual Arts

MUSIC

Julius Whitinger, Chairman *Number Of Faculty:* 3 *Number Of Students:* 12
Degrees Offered: BA *Financial Assistance:* Scholarships
Performing Groups: Belthoir Choir; Chapel Choir; Orchestra

THEATRE

Calvin Mortenson, Chairman *Number Of Faculty:* 4 *Degrees Offered:* BA
Financial Assistance: Scholarships *Performing Groups:* Royal Players

BRAINERD COMMUNITY COLLEGE
College Dr, Brainerd Minnesota 56401
612 829-1791
> State and 2 Year
> *Arts Areas:* Dance, Instrumental Music, Vocal Music, Theatre, Television and Visual Arts
> *Performing Series:* Lakes Area Music (Civic Music) Series
> *Performance Facilities:* Concert Hall & Theatre House

MUSIC

Dr A R Johnson, Chairman *Number Of Faculty:* 1 *Number Of Students:* 40
Degrees Offered: AA *Performing Groups:* Choir; Pop Folk Group
Workshops/Festivals: District High School Music Festival

THEATRE

Bob Dryden, Chairman *Number Of Faculty:* 1 *Number Of Students:* 40
Workshops/Festivals: District One-Act Play Contest (high school)

CARLETON COLLEGE
Northfield   Minnesota 55057, 507 645-4431 Ext 528
> Private and 4 Year
> **Arts Areas:** Dance, Instrumental Music, Vocal Music, Theatre and Visual Arts
> **Performing Series:** Concert Series
> **Performance Facilities:** Carleton Arena Theater & Concert Hall

MUSIC

William Wells & Anne Mayer, Chairmen   **Number Of Faculty:** 20
Degrees Offered: BA, Music History, Literature, Theory, Composition, Applied Music, Conducting
Performing Groups: Choir; Orchestra; Band; Chamber Singers; Pro Musica
Workshops/Festivals: Carleton Summer Music Festival

COLLEGE OF SAINT BENEDICT
St Joseph   Minnesota 56374, 612 363-5777
> Private and 4 Year
> **Arts Areas:** Dance, Instrumental Music, Vocal Music, Theatre and Visual Arts
> **Performing Series:** College of Saint Benedict Performance Series
> **Performance Facilities:** Auditorium; Forum; Dance Studio; Small Recital/Multi-Purpose Hall

DANCE

Kerry Lafferty, Chairperson   **Number Of Faculty:** 1   **Number Of Students:** 40
Degrees Offered: BA
Courses Offered: Classican & Contemporary Dance; Movement
Financial Assistance: Internships, Scholarships, Work-Study Grants and Loans, Grants
Performing Groups: A Company of Dancers
Workshops/Festivals: Minnesota Dance Theatre

MUSIC

S Firmin Escher, Dean, Administrator
Number Of Faculty: 10 Full-time, 3 Part-time   **Number Of Students:** 110
Degrees Offered: BA Mus
Courses Offered: Piano; Voice; All other Instruments; Symphonic Band; Jazz Ensemble
Technical Training: Basic undergraduate music skills including Opera & Electronic Music
Teaching Certification Available
Financial Assistance: Internships, Scholarships, Work-Study Grants and Loans, Grants
Performing Groups: Symphonic Band; Chamber Orchestra; Wind Ensemble; Mixed Choir; Concert Choir; Men's Choir; All-College Choir; Opera; Campus Singers; Jazz Ensemble; Liturgical Choir; Chamber Music; Old Music Consort

THEATRE

Kerry Lafferty, Chairperson   **Number Of Faculty:** 4 Full-time, 1 Part-time
Number Of Students: 40   **Degrees Offered:** BA
Courses Offered: Acting; Directing; Costuming; Lighting; Set Construction
Technical Training: Set/Costume Design & Construction; Scene Shop Methods; Lighting
Financial Assistance: Internships, Scholarships, Work-Study Grants and Loans, Grants
Workshops/Festivals: Guthrie Theater

COLLEGE OF SAINT CATHERINE
2004 Randolph Ave, St Paul   Minnesota 55105
612 698-5571
> Private and 4 Year
> **Arts Areas:** Dance, Instrumental Music, Vocal Music, Theatre, Television and Visual Arts
> **Performing Series:** Concerto Aria; Private College Series (KTCA-TV)
> **Performance Facilities:** Frey Studio Theatre, Jeanne d'Arc Auditorium; Music Recital Hall; O'Shaughnessy Auditorium

(continued on next page)

DANCE

Allys Swanson, Chairman   **Number Of Faculty:** 1   **Number Of Students:** 300
Technical Training: Modern Dance   **Financial Assistance:** Work-Study Grants
Workshops/Festivals: Fine Arts Festival

MUSIC

Albert Biales, Chairman   **Number Of Faculty:** 8   **Number Of Students:** 35
Degrees Offered: BA Mus, MusEd   **Teaching Certification Available**
Financial Assistance: Scholarships and Work-Study Grants
Performing Groups: Collegium Musicum; Opera Workshop; Women's Chorus; Chamber Singers; Chorale; Orchestra; Concert Band
Workshops/Festivals: Opera Workshop; Voice and Piano Master Classes and Workshops; Annual Fine Arts Festival

THEATRE

George Poletes, Chairman   **Number Of Faculty:** 8
Number Of Students: 75 majors   **Degrees Offered:** BA, Theatre - Speech
Technical Training: Speech Pathology; Audiology
Teaching Certification Available   **Financial Assistance:** Work-Study Grants
Performing Groups: Children's Theatre; Chapel Players
Workshops/Festivals: Fine Arts Festival

COLLEGE OF SAINT TERESA
1130 W Broadway, Winona   Minnesota 55987
507 452-1000
Private and 4 Year
Arts Areas: Dance, Instrumental Music, Vocal Music, Theatre, Film Arts and Television
Performing Series: Lee & Rose Warner Concert & Lecture Series; Tri - College Concert & Lecture Series
Performance Facilities: College of Saint Teresa Auditorium; College of Saint Teresa Bonaventure Room

DANCE

Martha LeValley, Chairperson   **Number Of Faculty:** 3   **Degrees Offered:** BA
Courses Offered: Modern; Ballet
Financial Assistance: Scholarships and Work-Study Grants
Performing Groups: Minnesota Dance Repertory Company
Workshops/Festivals: Fine Arts Workshop for High School Students

MUSIC

Elizabeth Hollway, Chairperson   **Number Of Faculty:** 10
Degrees Offered: BA
Courses Offered: Music Education; Performance; Music Theory
Teaching Certification Available
Financial Assistance: Scholarships and Work-Study Grants
Performing Groups: Triple Trio; College of Saint Teresa Orchestra; Chamber Singers; Ars Antiqua Renaisance Ensemble; Woodwind Ensemble
Workshops/Festivals: Fine Arts Workshop for High School Students

THEATRE

Eileen Whalen, Chairperson   **Number Of Faculty:** 3   **Degrees Offered:** BA
Courses Offered: Theatre Arts   **Teaching Certification Available**
Financial Assistance: Scholarships and Work-Study Grants
Workshops/Festivals: Fine Arts Workshop for High School Students

---

COLLEGE OF SAINT THOMAS
St Paul   Minnesota 55105, 612 647-5265
Private and 4 Year
Arts Areas: Instrumental Music, Vocal Music, Theatre and Visual Arts

(continued on next page)

(College of St Thomas — cont'd)

DANCE

Dr Anthony Chiuminatto, Chairman   **Number Of Faculty:** 4
Number Of Students: 20   **Degrees Offered:** BA
Financial Assistance: Scholarships and Work-Study Grants

THEATRE

James M Symons, Chairman   **Number Of Faculty:** 2   **Number Of Students:** 50
Degrees Offered: BA
Financial Assistance: Scholarships and Work-Study Grants
Performing Groups: Saint Thomas Theatre

CONCORDIA COLLEGE
901 8th St, S, Moorhead   Minnesota 56560
218 299-4321

Private and 4 Year
Arts Areas: Dance, Instrumental Music, Vocal Music, Theatre, Television and Visual Arts
Performing Series: Annual Artist Series Season
Performance Facilities: Memorial Auditorium; Knutson Center Centrum; Hvidsten Recital Hall
Humanities Theatre/Lab Theatre 300

DANCE

Lise Greer, Chairman   **Number Of Faculty:** 1

MUSIC

Dr Paul J Christiansen, Chairman   **Number Of Faculty:** 36
Number Of Students: 500   **Degrees Offered:** BMus; BA Mus
Courses Offered: Introduction to the Art of Music; Basic Musicianship I, II, III; Form & Analysis;
Fundamentals of Music for Classroom Teachers; Counterpoint I, II, III; Composition I , II;
Instrumentation; History & Literature of Music I, II; Period courses in Baroque, Classic, Romantic & 20th
Century Music; Choral Conducting I, II; Instrumental Conducting I, II; Voice Repertoire; Voice Class
Methods; Diction Class; Methods & Materials for Teaching Piano; Piano Repertoire
Technical Training: Private instruction in Voice, Brass, Woodwinds, Strings, Organ, Piano, Percussion
Teaching Certification Available   Financial Assistance: Scholarships
Performing Groups: Concordia Choir, Trio, & Orchestra; Chapel, Freshman, & Oratorio Choirs; Women's
Chorus; Concert Band; Repertory Band; Jazz, Brass, Woodwind, String, & Percussion Ensembles
Workshops/Festivals: Fall/Winter Tours; Annual Christmas Concerts; Spring Festivals

THEATRE

Dr Clair O Haugen, Chairman   **Number Of Faculty:** 7   **Number Of Students:** 75
Degrees Offered: BA
Courses Offered: Analysis for Production; Directing; Voice for Performance; The Actor's Resources;
Production Organization & Procedure; Appreciating Film; Summer Theatre Practicum; Theatre and Its
Cultures; Television Production; Senior Production Process
Teaching Certification Available   Financial Assistance: Scholarships
Performing Groups: Concordia Theatre Company
Artists-In-Residence/Guest Artists: Berl Senofshy; Jan DeGaetani; Menahem Pressler; Abbey Minstrels

---

GOLDEN VALLEY LUTHERAN COLLEGE
6125 Olson Hwy, Minneapolis   Minnesota 55422
612 542-1205

Private and 2 Year
Arts Areas: Instrumental Music, Vocal Music, Theatre and Visual Arts
Performing Series: Performing Arts Series

MUSIC

John Seagard, Division Chairperson   **Number Of Faculty:** 8
Number Of Students: 150   **Degrees Offered:** AA
Financial Assistance: Scholarships and Work-Study Grants

(continued on next page)

(*Golden Valley Lutheran College — cont'd*)

THEATRE

Richard Harrison, Chairperson   *Number Of Students:* 30
Degrees Offered: AA
Financial Assistance: Scholarships and Work-Study Grants

GUSTAVUS ADOLPHUS COLLEGE
Saint Peter   Minnesota 56082, 507 931-4300
   Private and 4 Year   *Arts Areas:* Instrumental Music and Vocal Music

MUSIC

Myron R Faick, Chairman   *Number Of Faculty:* 12   *Number Of Students:* 50
Degrees Offered: BA   *Teaching Certification Available*
Financial Assistance: Scholarships and Work-Study Grants
Performing Groups: Chamber Orchestra; Choir; Ensembles

THEATRE

Mrs E E Anderson, Chairman   *Number Of Faculty:* 2   *Number Of Students:* 33
Degrees Offered: BA   *Teaching Certification Available*
Financial Assistance: Scholarships and Work-Study Grants
Performing Groups: Drama Production Series

HAMLINE UNIVERSITY
1536 Hewitt Ave, St Paul   Minnesota 55104
612 641-2207
   Private and 4 Year
Arts Areas: Instrumental Music, Vocal Music, Theatre and Visual Arts
Performing Series: Concert Series
Performance Facilities: Bridgman Hall; Drew Fine Arts Theatre; Student Center Ballroom
Number Of Faculty: 1 Part-time
Courses Offered: Beginning & Intermediate Social Dance
Financial Assistance: Internships, Scholarships and Work-Study Grants
Workshops/Festivals: Choeogram Workshop (contemporary, professional group)

MUSIC

Russell Harris, Professor, Chairman
Number Of Faculty: 5 Full-time, 11 Part-time   *Number Of Students:* 60
Degrees Offered: BA
Courses Offered: Performance Classes; Theory; History & Literature; Education; Special Studies
Teaching Certification Available
Financial Assistance: Internships, Assistantships, Scholarships and Work-Study Grants
Performing Groups: A Cappella Choir; Newell Knoll Singers; Madrigals; Orchestra; Concert Band; Jazz Lab Band; University Women's Chorus

THEATRE

William Kimess, Assistant Professor, Chairman
Number Of Faculty: 4 Full-time 1 Part-time   *Number Of Students:* 25
Degrees Offered: BA
Courses Offered: Public Speaking/Communications; Stage Direction/Design; History & Literature; Direction
Teaching Certification Available
Financial Assistance: Internships, Assistantships, Scholarships and Work-Study Grants
Workshops/Festivals: Four department productions during the academic year; Ten student productions

MACALESTER COLLEGE
1600 Grand Ave, St Paul   Minnesota 55105
612 647-6221

Private and 4 Year
Arts Areas: Instrumental Music, Vocal Music and Theatre
Performance Facilities: Janet Wallace Fine Arts Center

MUSIC

Donald Betts, Acting Chairman   *Number Of Faculty:* 5
Number Of Students: 68   *Degrees Offered:* BA
Courses Offered: Music Theory, Literature, Appreciation; Conducting; Electronic Music Composition; Orchestration; Methods; Vocal Pedagogy
Technical Training: Arts Management; Conducting
Teaching Certification Available
Financial Assistance: Assistantships, Scholarships and Work-Study Grants
Performing Groups: Concert Choir; Orchestra; Festival Chorale; Chamber Music; Pipe Band; Early Music Ensemble; Band

THEATRE

Dr R K Mosvick, Chairman   *Number Of Faculty:* 7   *Number Of Students:* 50
Degrees Offered: BA Speech & Theatre
Technical Training: Lights; Scenic Design; Costume Design; Makeup; Acting; Directing; Creative Dramatics; Voice; Voice Diction
Teaching Certification Available
Financial Assistance: Assistantships, Scholarships and Work-Study Grants
Performing Groups: Student Studio Productions
Workshops/Festivals: Forensic & Debate Workshops

MANKATO STATE UNIVERSITY
Mankato   Minnesota 56001, 507 389-2119

State and 4 Year
Arts Areas: Dance, Instrumental Music, Vocal Music, Theatre and Visual Arts
Performance Facilities: Fine Arts Building (Concert Hall & Theatre)

MUSIC

Dr Barbara H McMurtry, Chairman
Number Of Faculty: 16 Full-time, 12 Part-time   *Number Of Students:* 200
Degrees Offered: BA; BMus; BS   *Teaching Certification Available*
Financial Assistance: Internships, Assistantships, Scholarships and Work-Study Grants
Performing Groups: Orchestra; Concert Wind Ensemble; Pep & Service Bands; Jazz Ensembles; University Choir; University Chorus; Chamber Singers

MESABI COMMUNITY COLLEGE
905 W Chestnut St, Virginia   Minnesota 55792
218 741-9200

State and 2 Year
Arts Areas: Instrumental Music, Vocal Music and Theatre
Performance Facilities: Theatre

MUSIC

Jay Carlstaard, Head   *Number Of Faculty:* 2   *Number Of Students:* 75
Degrees Offered: AA
Financial Assistance: Scholarships and Work-Study Grants
Performing Groups: Now and Then Singers
Workshops/Festivals: Bi-annual Fine Arts Festival

(continued on next page)

THEATRE

Charles D Rowland, Head   **Number Of Faculty:** 1   **Number Of Students:** 50
Degrees Offered: AA
Courses Offered: Oral Interp; Beginning Speech; Intro to Theatre; Acting; Directing; Choral Reading
Performing Groups: Theatre Mesabi
Workshops/Festivals: Bi-annual Fine Arts Festival

METROPOLITAN COMMUNITY COLLEGE
50 Willow St, Minneapolis   Minnesota 55403
612 339-9441
State and 2 Year
Arts Areas: Dance, Instrumental Music, Vocal Music, Theatre, Television, Visual Arts and Film Arts
Performance Facilities: Memorial Auditorium

DANCE

Marianne P Marr, Chairman   **Number Of Faculty:** 1.5   **Number Of Students:** 30
Courses Offered: Contemporary Dance   **Financial Assistance:** Work-Study Grants

MUSIC

James Durham, Chairman   **Number Of Faculty:** 2   **Number Of Students:** 34
Degrees Offered: AA
Financial Assistance: Scholarships and Work-Study Grants
Performing Groups: College Chorale; Vocal Ensemble

THEATRE

Keith Jones, Chairman   **Number Of Faculty:** 2   **Number Of Students:** 28
Degrees Offered: AA
Financial Assistance: Scholarships and Work-Study Grants
Workshops/Festivals: Minnesota Fine Arts Festival; Theatre Arts Workshop

---

UNIVERSITY OF MINNESOTA, MORRIS
Morris   Minnesota 56267, 612 589-2211 Ext 227
State and 4 Year
Arts Areas: Instrumental Music, Vocal Music, Theatre and Visual Arts
Performing Series: Performing Arts Series; UMM Theatre Season
Performance Facilities: Humanities Fine Arts Center (Proscenium Theatre, Black Box Theatre, Recital Hall); Edson Auditorium

MUSIC

Clyde E Johnson, Music Discipline Coordinator
Number Of Faculty: 4 Full-time, 5 Part-time   **Number Of Students:** 40
Degrees Offered: BA
Courses Offered: Theory; History & Literature; Related Courses
Technical Training: Instrumental Techniques; Choral & Instrumental Conducting; Applied Music
Teaching Certification Available
Financial Assistance: Scholarships, Work-Study Grants and Fee Waiver (in applied)
Performing Groups: Concert & Stage Bands; Chamber Singers; University Choir; Orchestra
Workshops/Festivals: Master Classes & Residencies

THEATRE

Raymond J Lammers, Speech/Theatre Discipline Coordinator
Number Of Faculty: 3   **Number Of Students:** 35 - 40   **Degrees Offered:** BA
Courses Offered: Acting; Directing; Design; Technical; History
Teaching Certification Available
Financial Assistance: Scholarships and Work-Study Grants
Performing Groups: UMM Theatre; UMM Children's Theatre; Morris Meiningens
Workshops/Festivals: District 21 High School Theatre Festival; Voice; Acting; High School Workshops
Artists-In-Residence/Guest Artists: Stan Kenton Orchestra; Minnesota Dance Theatre; Mordine & Company (Dance Company)

UNIVERSITY OF MINNESOTA, DULUTH - SCHOOL OF FINE ARTS
Humanities 212, Duluth   Minnesota 55812
218 726-7261

State and 4 Year
Arts Areas: Dance, Instrumental Music, Vocal Music, Theatre and Visual Arts
Performance Facilities: Marshall Performing Arts Center   **Number Of Faculty:** 1
Number Of Students: 30   **Degrees Offered:** Minor
Courses Offered: Ballroom; Modern; Jazz; Folk; Square; Dance History; Dance Composition; Dance
Repertory Theatre

MUSIC

Dr David E Price, Head   **Number Of Faculty:** 15   **Number Of Students:** 130
Degrees Offered: BMus
Courses Offered: Applied Music; Ensembles; Music Ed; Pedagogy & Conducting; Theory & Composition;
General
Teaching Certification Available
Financial Assistance: Assistantships and Scholarships
Performing Groups: Concert & Varsity Bands; Elizabethan & University Singers; Choruses; Jazz &
Instrumental Ensembles; Opera Workshop
Workshops/Festivals: Jazz Festivals; String Clinic; Honor Band Clinic; Choral Clinic

THEATRE

Dr Richard C Graves, Head   **Number Of Faculty:** 4   **Number Of Students:** 40
Degrees Offered: BFA
Courses Offered: Acting; History & Dramatic Literature; Costume Design; Design & Technical; Directing;
Dance; General
Teaching Certification Available
Financial Assistance: Assistantships and Scholarships
Performing Groups: UMD Theatre; Summer Theatre

NORMANDALE COMMUNITY COLLEGE
Bloomington   Minnesota 55431, 612 831-5001

State and 2 Year
Arts Areas: Instrumental Music, Vocal Music, Theatre, Television and Visual Arts
Performance Facilities: Theatre House; Concert Hall

MUSIC

Carlo Minnetti, Chairman   **Number Of Faculty:** 5   **Number Of Students:** 60
Degrees Offered: AA   **Financial Assistance:** Work-Study Grants

THEATRE

Linda Putnam, Chairman   **Number Of Faculty:** 3   **Number Of Students:** 20
Degrees Offered: AA   **Financial Assistance:** Work-Study Grants

NORTH CENTRAL BIBLE COLLEGE
910 Elliot Ave, S, Minneapolis   Minnesota 55404
612 332-3491

Private and 4 Year   **Arts Areas:** Instrumental Music and Vocal Music
Performance Facilities: F J Lindquist Chapel

MUSIC

Rev Gary D Lewis, Chairman   **Number Of Faculty:** 8   **Number Of Students:** 225
Degrees Offered: BA, BS in Sacred Music
Courses Offered: Sacred Music with emphasis on Vocal & Instrumental
Financial Assistance: Internships, Scholarships and Work-Study Grants
Performing Groups: NCBC Chorale; The Concert Choir; NCBC Instrumental Ensemble

RAINY RIVER COMMUNITY COLLEGE
International Falls   Minnesota 56649, 218 283-8491
> State and 2 Year
> *Arts Areas:* Instrumental Music, Vocal Music, Theatre, Television and Visual Arts
> *Performance Facilities:* Theater; Gymnasium

MUSIC

Benhard Niemi, Instructor   **Number Of Faculty:** 1   **Number Of Students:** 45
Financial Assistance: Scholarships and Work-Study Grants
Performing Groups: Sunshine; String Ensemble; Band

THEATRE

Arthur Przybilla, Instructor   **Number Of Students:** 40
Financial Assistance: Scholarships and Work-Study Grants

SAINT CLOUD STATE UNIVERSITY
Saint Cloud   Minnesota 56301, 612 255-0121
> State and 4 Year
> *Arts Areas:* Dance, Instrumental Music, Vocal Music, Theatre, Film Arts, Television, Visual Arts and Arts Administration
> *Performing Series:* Major Events Council Series; Student Activities Council Series; Atwood Center Series
> *Performance Facilities:* Recital Hall & Stage I, II in Performing Arts Center; Stewart Hall Auditorium; Halenbeck Hall

DANCE

Carol Brink, Instructor   **Number Of Faculty:** 3
Degrees Offered: BA; BS (Minor)
Courses Offered: Folk & Square Dancing; Modern
Financial Assistance: Scholarships, Work-Study Grants and Loans
Performing Groups: Folkdancers
Workshops/Festivals: Annual Folk Dance Festival

MUSIC

Dr David Ernest, Professor   **Number Of Faculty:** 19
Degrees Offered: BA; BMus; BS; MS
Courses Offered: Theory; Instrumental & Vocal Music; History of Music; Music Education
Teaching Certification Available
Financial Assistance: Internships, Assistantships, Scholarships, Work-Study Grants and Loans
Performing Groups: Wind & Jazz Ensembles; Concert Band; Orchestra; Women's Choir; Concert Choir; Marching & Ragime Bands
Workshops/Festivals: High School Workshops; Various Festivals

THEATRE

Dr Ronald Perrier, Assistant Professor   **Number Of Faculty:** 6
Degrees Offered: BA; BS
Courses Offered: Acting; Makeup; Costume; Cinema; Scenery Design
Teaching Certification Available
Financial Assistance: Assistantships, Scholarships, Work-Study Grants and Loans
Performing Groups: Theatre; Theatre L'Homme Dieu (summer); Readers' Theatre
Workshops/Festivals: High School Workshop

SAINT OLAF COLLEGE
Northfield   Minnesota 55057, 507 663-2222
> Private and 4 Year
> *Arts Areas:* Dance, Instrumental Music, Vocal Music, Theatre, Film Arts and Visual Arts
> *Performing Series:* St Olaf Artist Series
> *Performance Facilities:* Skoglund Auditorium; Boe Memorial Chapel; Urness Recital Hall; Theatre

(continued on next page)

DANCE

Susan Bauer, Instructor
Dance program under auspices of Physical Education Department
Number Of Faculty: 1½   **Number Of Students:** 46
Courses Offered: Technique Classes - Beginning & Intermediate Modern & Ballet
Teaching Certification Available   Financial Assistance: Work-Study Grants
Performing Groups: St Olaf Dance Company; St Olaf Apprentice Dance Company

MUSIC

Adolph White, Chairman   **Number Of Faculty:** 23 Full-time, 20 Part-time
Number Of Students: 235   **Degrees Offered:** BA; BMus
Courses Offered: Applied Music; Church Music; Music Ed; History & Literature; Theory & Composition
Teaching Certification Available
Financial Assistance: Scholarships, Work-Study Grants and Student Loans
Performing Groups: Concert & Norsemen Bands; Symphony & Chamber Orchestras; St Olaf, Chapel, Campus Choirs; Women's Chorus (Manitou Singers); Men's Chorus (Viking Chorus); Repertory Singers
Workshops/Festivals: Christmas Festival; Fine Arts Festival; Teenage Organist Workshop; Vocal Camp for High School students; Piano Workshop; Choral Conducting Workshop; Organ & Choir Workshop; Bach/Mozart Workshop & Festival

THEATRE

Dr Ralph H Haugen, Professor of Speech/Theatre, Chairman
Number Of Faculty: 6   **Number Of Students:** 2,800   **Degrees Offered:** BA; BMus
Courses Offered: Introduction to Theatre; Oral Interpretation of Literature; Voice & Diction; History of Theatre; Acting; Theatre Production; Direction; Selected Seminars
Teaching Certification Available
Financial Assistance: Scholarships, Work-Study Grants and Loans
Performing Groups: St Olaf College Theatre
Workshops/Festivals: Opera Workshops; Children's Theatre Workshops
Artists-In-Residence/Guest Artists: Paul Winter Consort; Jan De Gaetani; Abbey Simon

---

SAINT PAUL BIBLE COLLEGE
County Roads 30 & 92, Bible College   Minnesota 55375
612 446-1411
Private and 4 Year   **Arts Areas:** Instrumental Music and Vocal Music
Performance Facilities: College Auditorium

MUSIC

Dwight A Gardstrom, Chairman   **Number Of Faculty:** 9
Number Of Students: 580   **Degrees Offered:** BA Mus
Courses Offered: Theory; Applied; Composition; Church Music; Conducting
Financial Assistance: Scholarships and Work-Study Grants
Performing Groups: Choral Club; Women's Choral; Orchestra; Vocal & Instrumental Ensembles
Workshops/Festivals: Church Music Festival

UNIVERSITY OF MINNESOTA
Minneapolis   Minnesota 55455, 612 373-2851
Private and 4 Year
Arts Areas: Vocal Music, Instrumental Music and Theatre
Performing Series: Concert & Lecture Series
Performance Facilities: Scott Hall; Rarig Theatre

DANCE

Nadine Jette, Chairman   **Number Of Faculty:** 3   **Number Of Students:** 350
Degrees Offered: BA   **Technical Training:** Modern; Ballet
Financial Assistance: Assistantships   **Performing Groups:** Modern Dance Group
Workshops/Festivals: Perform at the Guild of Performing; Viola Farber & Company for 3 week residency in summer

(continued on next page)

MUSIC

Roy A Schuessler, Chairman   **Number Of Faculty:** 56
Number Of Students: 850   **Degrees Offered:** BA; MA; PhD
Teaching Certification Available
Financial Assistance: Internships, Assistantships, Scholarships and Work-Study Grants
Performing Groups: University Band; University Orchestra

THEATRE

Kenneth L Graham, Chairman   **Number Of Faculty:** 14
Number Of Students: 100   **Degrees Offered:** BA; MA; MFA; PhD
Teaching Certification Available
Financial Assistance: Internships, Assistantships, Scholarships and Work-Study Grants
Performing Groups: Theatre of the Word; Young People's Theatre; Centennial Showboat; Peppermint Tent; Rarig Summer Season
Workshops/Festivals: University of Minnesota Theatre Workshop

WILLMAR COMMUNITY COLLEGE
PO Box 797, Willmar   Minnesota 56201
612 235-2131

State and 2 Year
Arts Areas: Dance, Instrumental Music, Vocal Music, Theatre and Visual Arts
Performing Series: Willmar Community College Artists Series
Performance Facilities: Theatre; Gymnasium

MUSIC

Number Of Faculty: 2   **Number Of Students:** 10   **Degrees Offered:** AA
Financial Assistance: Work-Study Grants and Federal Programs
Performing Groups: Choir; Band; Orchestra; Small Groups
Workshops/Festivals: Choral Festival; Voice Workshop

THEATRE

Number Of Faculty: 2   **Number Of Students:** 5   **Degrees Offered:** AA
Financial Assistance: Work-Study Grants and Federal Programs
Performing Groups: Drama Production Group
Workshops/Festivals: District One-Act Play Contest

WINONA STATE UNIVERSITY
Johnson & Sanborn, Winona   Minnesota 55987
507 457-2109

State and 4 Year
Arts Areas: Instrumental Music, Vocal Music, Theatre, Film Arts, Television and Visual Arts

MUSIC

Richard Sovinec, Chairperson   **Number Of Faculty:** 9
Number Of Students: 80   **Degrees Offered:** BA; BS; MS
Courses Offered: Music Theory; Music History; Music Education; Ensembles
Teaching Certification Available
Financial Assistance: Scholarships and Work-Study Grants
Performing Groups: Concert Band; Concert Choir; Winona Symphony; Brass Ensemble; Jazz Ensemble
Workshops/Festivals: Elementary & Secondary School Music Workshops

THEATRE

Jacque Reidelberger, Chairperson   **Number Of Faculty:** 6
Number Of Students: 45   **Degrees Offered:** BA; BS
Courses Offered: Communication; Speech Correction; Theatre; History of Theatre; Speech Classes
Teaching Certification Available
Financial Assistance: Scholarships and Work-Study Grants
Performing Groups: Children's Theatre; Wenonah Players

ALCORN AGRICULTURAL & MECHANICAL COLLEGE
Lorman   Mississippi 39096, 601 437-5151

State and 4 Year

Arts Areas: Instrumental Music, Vocal Music and Visual Arts

MUSIC

Joyce Bolden, Chairman   *Degrees Offered:* BMus
Financial Assistance: Scholarships   *Performing Groups:* Band, Chorus, Ensemble

---

BELHAVEN COLLEGE
Jackson   Mississippi 39202, 601 352-0013

Private and 4 Year

Arts Areas: Instrumental Music, Vocal Music and Visual Arts

MUSIC

Virginia Hoogenakker, Chairman   *Number Of Faculty:* 10
Number Of Students: 50   *Degrees Offered:* BMus
Teaching Certification Available
Financial Assistance: Scholarships and Work-Study Grants
Performing Groups: Ensembles

BLUE MOUNTAIN COLLEGE
Box 338, Blue Mountain   Mississippi 38610
601 685-5711 Ext 30

Private and 4 Year

Arts Areas: Instrumental Music, Vocal Music and Theatre

MUSIC

Dr Stanley Richison, Chairman   *Number Of Faculty:* 4
Number Of Students: 45   *Degrees Offered:* BMus; BMusEd
Teaching Certification Available   *Financial Assistance:* Scholarships
Performing Groups: Chorus; Ensemble

THEATRE

Miss Marcia Hansen, Chairman   *Number Of Faculty:* 2
Number Of Students: 20   *Degrees Offered:* BA Drama - Speech
Teaching Certification Available   *Financial Assistance:* Scholarships
Performing Groups: Mountain Masqueraders

CLARKE COLLEGE
Box 440, Newton   Mississippi 39345
601 683-2061

Private and 2 Year   *Arts Areas:* Vocal Music and Visual Arts
Performance Facilities: Lott Fine Arts Auditorium

MUSIC

Clark Adams, Chairman   *Number Of Faculty:* 3   *Degrees Offered:* AA
Courses Offered: Music Theory; Music History & Literature; Church Music Courses
Technical Training: Private Voice, Organ & Piano
Financial Assistance: Scholarships and Work-Study Grants
Performing Groups: College Chorus; Singers; Ensembles
Workshops/Festivals: Church Music Workshop
Artists-In-Residence/Guest Artists: Mary Vermillion; Jackson Symphony - Bethoven Piano Trio, Jackson State String Quartet; Jan Douglas; Clark Measler & Clark Adams

DELTA STATE UNIVERSITY
Cleveland   Mississippi 38733, 601 846-6664
   State and 4 Year
   Arts Areas: Instrumental Music, Vocal Music and Theatre
   Performing Series: Special Programs Series; University Union Program
   Performance Facilities: Broom Auditorium; Jobe Auditorium; Zeigel Auditorium; The Union

MUSIC

Dr William James Craig, Chairman   **Number Of Faculty:** 17
Number Of Students: 120   **Degrees Offered:** BMusEd; BA; BMus; MMusEd
Teaching Certification Available
Financial Assistance: Assistantships, Scholarships and Work-Study Grants
Performing Groups: Chorus; Band; Instrumental Ensembles (Jazz, Percussion, Woodwinds, Brass); Music
Theatre Workshop
Workshops/Festivals: A variety of Clinics & Workshops for Faculty, Students, High School Faculty &
Students, and private Teachers

THEATRE

Dr Will Booth, Chairman, Speech Department   **Number Of Faculty:** 2
Number Of Students: 20   **Degrees Offered:** BSE; BA; BSGS
Teaching Certification Available
Financial Assistance: Assistantships, Scholarships and Work-Study Grants
Performing Groups: Delta Playhouse; Delta Readers
Workshops/Festivals: Workshops for Public School Teachers in Play Production & such Techniques as Role
- Playing
Artists-In-Residence/Guest Artists: New Orleans Symphony; New Shakespeare Company of San Francisco;
Alex Haley

EAST CENTRAL JUNIOR COLLEGE
Decatur   Mississippi 39327, 601 635-2111
   State and 2 Year
   Arts Areas: Instrumental Music, Vocal Music, Theatre and Visual Arts

MUSIC

R G Fick, Chairman   **Degrees Offered:** AA
Financial Assistance: Scholarships
Performing Groups: Instrumental and Vocal Ensembles
Degrees Offered: AA Drama   **Financial Assistance:** Scholarships
Performing Groups: ECJC Players

EAST MISSISSIPPI JUNIOR COLLEGE
Scooba   Mississippi 39358, 601 476-3421
   State and 2 Year
   Arts Areas: Instrumental Music, Vocal Music, Theatre and Visual Arts
   Degrees Offered: AA   **Financial Assistance:** Scholarships
   Performing Groups: Vocal and Instrumenta; Groups

THEATRE

Dayna Anderson, Chairman   **Degrees Offered:** AA
Performing Groups: EMJC Theatre, Delta Psi Omega

GULF PARK COLLEGE
Long Beach   Mississippi 39560, 601 863-6852
   Private and 2 Year
   Arts Areas: Dance, Instrumental Music, Vocal Music, Theatre and Film Arts
   Degrees Offered: AA   **Financial Assistance:** Scholarships

(continued on next page)

Performing Groups: Modern Dance Company   *Degrees Offered:* AA
Financial Assistance: Scholarships
Performing Groups: Vocal and Instrumental Groups

THEATRE

Charles F Lembright, Chairman   *Degrees Offered:* AA in Speech & Theatre
Financial Assistance: Scholarships   *Performing Groups:* Jet Maskers

---

HINDS JUNIOR COLLEGE
Raymond   Mississippi 39154, 601 857-5261
   Private and 2 Year
   Arts Areas: Instrumental Music, Vocal Music, Theatre and Visual Arts

MUSIC

James L Reeves, Chairman
Degrees Offered: AA, Cert Diploma in Applied Music
Financial Assistance: Scholarships
Performing Groups: Instrumental and Vocal Ensembles
Performing Groups: The Lendon Players

HOLMES JUNIOR COLLEGE
Goodman   Mississippi 39079, 601 472-2531
   Private and 2 Year
   Arts Areas: Instrumental Music, Vocal Music and Visual Arts

MUSIC

David W Young, Chairman   *Degrees Offered:* AA
Financial Assistance: Scholarships
Performing Groups: Local and Instrumental Ensembles

ITAWAMBA JUNIOR COLLEGE
Fulton   Mississippi 38843, 601 862-3101
   County and 2 Year   *Arts Areas:* Instrumental Music and Vocal Music

MUSIC

Marian Abel, Chairman   *Degrees Offered:* AA
Financial Assistance: Scholarships
Performing Groups: Instrumental and Vocal Groups

JACKSON STATE COLLEGE
Jackson   Mississippi 39217, 601 948-8533
   State and 4 Year
   Arts Areas: Instrumental Music, Vocal Music, Theatre and Visual Arts

MUSIC

Dollye M E Robinson, Chairman   *Number Of Faculty:* 14
Degrees Offered: BMus, BMusEd, BMus Applied Music
Teaching Certification Available
Financial Assistance: Scholarships and Work-Study Grants
Performing Groups: Concerts

THEATRE

Edward Fisher, Chairman   *Number Of Faculty:* 3   *Degrees Offered:* B Speech
Teaching Certification Available
Financial Assistance: Scholarships and Work-Study Grants
Performing Groups: Dunbar Dramatic Guild

JONES COUNTY JUNIOR COLLEGE
Ellisville   Mississippi 39437, 601 477-3347

County and 2 Year   *Arts Areas:* Instrumental Music and Vocal Music
Degrees Offered: AA   *Financial Assistance:* Scholarships
Performing Groups: Vocal and Instrumental Groups

MARY HOLMES JUNIOR COLLEGE
West Point   Mississippi 39773, 601 494-6820

Private and 2 Year   *Arts Areas:* Instrumental Music and Vocal Music

MUSIC

Clarence M Simmons, Chairman
Degrees Offered: AA in MusEd, AA in Instrumental Music
Financial Assistance: Scholarships
Performing Groups: Instrumental and Vocal Ensembles

MERIDIAN JUNIOR COLLEGE
Meridian   Mississippi 39301, 601 483-8241 Ext 226

County and 2 Year
Arts Areas: Instrumental Music, Vocal Music, Theatre and Visual Arts
Performance Facilities: MJC Theatre

MUSIC

Dr Robert Hermetz, Chairman   *Number Of Faculty:* 4   *Number Of Students:* 35
Financial Assistance: Scholarships and Work-Study Grants
Performing Groups: College Mixed Chorus, Community Chorus, Select Vocal Ensemble, Concert Band, Jazz Ensemble
Workshops/Festivals: District Band Festival, State Choral Festival

THEATRE

Ronnie Miller, Chairman   *Number Of Faculty:* 2
Technical Training: Stagecraft   *Financial Assistance:* Work-Study Grants
Performing Groups: MJC Theatre Group

MILLSAPS COLLEGE
Jackson   Mississippi 39210, 601 354-5201

Private and 4 Year
Arts Areas: Instrumental Music, Vocal Music, Theatre and Visual Arts

MUSIC

C Leland Byler, Chairman   *Number Of Faculty:* 6   *Number Of Students:* 60
Degrees Offered: BMus, BMusEd   *Teaching Certification Available*
Financial Assistance: Scholarships and Work-Study Grants
Performing Groups: Recitals, Ensembles, Band , Chorus   *Number Of Faculty:* 2
Number Of Students: 20   *Degrees Offered:* BA
Teaching Certification Available
Financial Assistance: Scholarships and Work-Study Grants
Performing Groups: Milsaps Players

MISSISSIPPI COLLEGE
Clinton   Mississippi 39058, 601 924-5131 Ext 202

Private and 4 Year
Arts Areas: Instrumental Music, Vocal Music, Theatre and Visual Arts
Performance Facilities: Aven Hall - Little Theatre; Nelso Hall - Auditorium

(continued on next page)

MUSIC

Dr Jack Lyall, Chairman   **Number Of Faculty:** 17   **Number Of Students:** 115
Degrees Offered: BA; BMus; BMusEd; MMus; MMusEd
Courses Offered: Instrumental Music; Vocal Music; Visual Arts
Teaching Certification Available
Financial Assistance: Assistantships, Scholarships and Work-Study Grants
Performing Groups: Various Ensembles; Choir; Singing Groups; Recitals
Workshops/Festivals: Music Education Workshop each summer

THEATRE

Dr Hollis Todd, Head   **Number Of Faculty:** 4   **Number Of Students:** 38
Degrees Offered: BA; BSEd; MEd (Speech)
Courses Offered: Interpretation; Drama; Mass Media Communications
Teaching Certification Available
Financial Assistance: Assistantships, Scholarships and Work-Study Grants
Performing Groups: Tribal Players

MISSISSIPPI GULF COAST JUNIOR COLLEGE, PERKINSTON CAMPUS
Perkinston   Mississippi 39523, 601 928-7211
State and 2 Year
Arts Areas: Instrumental Music, Vocal Music and Visual Arts
Degrees Offered: AA   **Financial Assistance:** Scholarships
Performing Groups: Vocal and Instrumental Groups

MISSISSIPPI INDUSTRIAL COLLEGE
Memphis St, Holly Springs   Mississippi 38901
601 252-4112
Private and 4 Year   **Arts Areas:** Vocal Music

MUSIC

Harry Winfield, Choir Director   **Number Of Faculty:** 1
Number Of Students: 100
Courses Offered: Music Appreciation; Music for Children
Financial Assistance: Scholarships and Work-Study Grants

MISSISSIPPI STATE UNIVERSITY
State College   Mississippi 39762, 601 325-2644
State and 4 Year
Arts Areas: Dance, Instrumental Music, Vocal Music, Theatre, Film Arts, Television and Visual Arts
Performing Series: Lyceum Program Council, Lecturn Series
Performance Facilities: Lee Hall Auditorium

MUSIC

Tom West, Chairman   **Number Of Faculty:** 21   **Number Of Students:** 200
Degrees Offered: BMusEd, BA, MMusEd, EdD   **Teaching Certification Available**
Financial Assistance: Assistantships, Scholarships and Work-Study Grants
Performing Groups: Marching Band, Symphony Band, Concert Band, Stage Band, Clarinet Choir, Trombone Ensemble, Brass Choir, University Choir, University Chorale, Madrigal Singers, Woodwind Quintet
Workshops/Festivals: District IV Choral Festival, Annual New Band Materials Clinic, Piano Workshop, Piano Master Class, Marching Band Clinic, Mississippi State Stage Band Festival, Mississippi State Junior High Band Festival

THEATRE

Dr Dominic J Cunetto, Chairman   **Number Of Faculty:** 2
Number Of Students: 50   **Degrees Offered:** BA Communication Theatre

(continued on next page)

Teaching Certification Available   Financial Assistance: Scholarships
Performing Groups: Blackfriars Drama Society, Children's Theatre
Workshops/Festivals: State High School Drama Festival

MISSISSIPPI UNIVERSITY FOR WOMEN
Columbus   Mississippi 39701, 601 328-6841
State and 4 Year
Arts Areas: Dance, Instrumental Music, Vocal Music, Theatre, Film Arts, Television and Visual Arts
Performance Facilities: University Auditorium; University Theatre; Music Theatre

DANCE

Dr Dorothy Burdeshaw, Head, Department of Health, PE & Recreation
Degrees Offered: BA   **Teaching Certification Available**
Financial Assistance: Assistantships, Scholarships and Work-Study Grants

MUSIC

Dr Sigfred C Matson, Head   **Degrees Offered:** BA; BMus; BMusEd; MA; MMusEd
Teaching Certification Available
Financial Assistance: Internships, Assistantships, Scholarships and Work-Study Grants
Performing Groups: Chorus, Chapel Choir; Symphonette

THEATRE

Dr Michael Minchew, Head   **Degrees Offered:** BA; MA

MISSISSIPPI VALLEY STATE COLLEGE
Itta Bera   Mississippi 38941, 601 254-2321
State and 4 Year
Arts Areas: Instrumental Music, Vocal Music and Visual Arts

MUSIC

Russell Boone, Chairman   **Degrees Offered:** BMusEd
Teaching Certification Available   Financial Assistance: Scholarships
Performing Groups: Instrumental Ensembles, Choir

UNIVERSITY OF MISSISSIPPI
University   Mississippi 38677, 601 232-7268
Private and 4 Year
Arts Areas: Dance, Instrumental Music, Vocal Music, Theatre, Film Arts, Television and Visual Arts
Performing Series: Artists Series
Performance Facilities: Univeristy of Mississippi Auditorium

DANCE

Nelson Neal, Chairman   **Number Of Faculty:** 2   **Number Of Students:** 30
Financial Assistance: Internships, Assistantships, Scholarships and Work-Study Grants
Performing Groups: University Dancers

MUSIC

Dr James Coleman, Chairman   **Number Of Faculty:** 21
Number Of Students: 200
Degrees Offered: BA, BMus, BMusEd, MMus, MFA, EdD, PhD, D Arts
Teaching Certification Available
Financial Assistance: Internships, Assistantships, Scholarships and Work-Study Grants
Performing Groups: University Symphony, University Chorus, University Singers, University Consort, University Opera Theatre, University Jazz Ensemble
Workshops/Festivals: Orff & Kodaly Workshop, Jazz Workshop, Artists Series, Opera Workshop

(continued on next page)

THEATRE

Dr Donald M McBryde, Chairman   **Number Of Faculty:** 16
Number Of Students: 122
Degrees Offered: BA Speech, Theatre, Radio, Television; MA, MFA
Teaching Certification Available
Financial Assistance: Internships, Assistantships and Work-Study Grants
Performing Groups: University Theatre, Experimental Theatre
Workshops/Festivals: Debate and Platform Speakers Workshop, Community Theater Workshop, Summer Showcase, Junior College Workshop

NORTHEAST MISSISSIPPI JUNIOR COLLEGE
Booneville   Mississippi 38829, 602 728-6208
State and 2 Year
Arts Areas: Instrumental Music, Vocal Music, Theatre and Visual Arts

MUSIC

W T Rutledge, Chairman   **Degrees Offered:** AA Music, A in Applied Music
Financial Assistance: Scholarships
Performing Groups: Instrumental and Vocal Ensembles

THEATRE

Mrs William H Preston, Chairman   **Degrees Offered:** AA Drama & Speech
Financial Assistance: Scholarships

NORTHWEST MISSISSIPPI JUNIOR COLLEGE
Senatobia   Mississippi 38668, 601 562-5262
State and 2 Year
Arts Areas: Dance, Instrumental Music, Vocal Music, Theatre, Television and Visual Arts
Performing Series: Instrumental & Vocal Series
Performance Facilities: Coliseum; Auditorium; Recital Hall

MUSIC

Glenn Triplett, Director   **Number Of Faculty:** 5
Degrees Offered: Associate
Financial Assistance: Scholarships and Work-Study Grants
Performing Groups: Entertainers; Rangerettes
Workshops/Festivals: Sycamore Fair

THEATRE

Sam Christ, Chairman   **Number Of Faculty:** 1   **Degrees Offered:** Associate
Financial Assistance: Scholarships and Work-Study Grants

PEARL RIVER JUNIOR COLLEGE
Poplarville   Mississippi 39470, 601 795-4571
Private and 2 Year   **Arts Areas:** Instrumental Music and Vocal Music
Degrees Offered: AA   **Financial Assistance:** Scholarships
Performing Groups: Instrumental and Vocal Groups

RUST COLLEGE
Rust Ave, Holly Springs   Mississippi 38635
601 252-3555
Private and 4 Year
Arts Areas: Instrumental Music, Vocal Music, Theatre and Visual Arts

MUSIC

Dr Norman Chapman, Chairman   **Number Of Faculty:** 5   **Number Of Students:** 30
Degrees Offered: BMusEd; BA

(continued on next page)

Courses Offered: All traditional & several non-traditional courses
Technical Training: Recording Studio; Musical Theatre; Instrumentation
Teaching Certification Available
Financial Assistance: Internships, Work-Study Grants and Cooperative Educational Program
Performing Groups: Choral & Instrumental Groups; Large & Small Ensemble

THEATRE

John Johnson, Director   **Number Of Faculty:** 1   **Number Of Students:** 6
Technical Training: Introduction to Set Designing & Stage Lighting; Practical Work on Productions
Performing Groups: Theatre Guild   **Workshops/Festivals:** Fine Arts Festival

---

SOUTHEASTERN BAPTIST COLLEGE
Laurel   Mississippi 39440, 601 428-5641
Private and 2 Year   **Arts Areas:** Instrumental Music and Vocal Music
Degrees Offered: AA   **Financial Assistance:** Scholarships
Performing Groups: Vocal and Instrumental Ensembles

SOUTHWEST MISSISSIPPI JUNIOR COLLEGE
Summit   Mississippi 39666, 601 276-7531
Private and 2 Year   **Arts Areas:** Vocal Music and Theatre
Degrees Offered: AA   **Financial Assistance:** Scholarships
Performing Groups: Vocal and Instrumental Groups

TOUGALOO COLLEGE
Tougaloo   Mississippi 39174, 601 982-4242
Private and 4 Year
Arts Areas: Instrumental Music, Vocal Music, Theatre and Visual Arts

MUSIC

Ben Bailey, Chairman   **Number Of Faculty:** 5   **Degrees Offered:** BMus
Teaching Certification Available   **Performing Groups:** Singing Groups

THEATRE

Hollis W Huston Jr, Chairman   **Teaching Certification Available**
Performing Groups: Tougaloo Players

UNIVERSITY OF SOUTHERN MISSISSIPPI
Box 31, Southern Station, Hattiesburg   Mississippi 39401
601 266-7271
State and 4 Year
Arts Areas: Dance, Instrumental Music, Vocal Music, Theatre and Visual Arts
Performing Series: Art Center Series
Performance Facilities: Marsh Auditorium; Performing Arts Center Auditorium; Claude Bennett
Auditorium

DANCE

Dr I Blaine Quarnstrom, Chairman   **Number Of Faculty:** 3
Number Of Students: 150   **Degrees Offered:** BA
Teaching Certification Available
Financial Assistance: Assistantships and Work-Study Grants
Performing Groups: Dance Company

MUSIC

Dr A Norbert Carnovale, Chairman   **Number Of Faculty:** 64
Number Of Students: 450   **Degrees Offered:** BMus; BMusEd; MEd; MMus; PhD; DMA
Teaching Certification Available
Financial Assistance: Assistantships, Scholarships and Work-Study Grants

(continued on next page)

Performing Groups: Band; Chorus; Orchestra; Jazz Lab Band
Workshops/Festivals: Opera; Musical; Southern Fine Arts Festival; Instrumental Conductors; Choral Conductors Conference

THEATRE

Dr I Blaine Quarnstrom, Chairman   **Number Of Faculty:** 7
Number Of Students: 100   **Degrees Offered:** BA; BFA; MFA
Teaching Certification Available

WHITWORTH COLLEGE
Brookhaven   Mississippi 37601, 601 833-4311
Private and 4 Year
Arts Areas: Instrumental Music, Vocal Music and Visual Arts
Degrees Offered: BMus   **Teaching Certification Available**
Performing Groups: Band, Ensembles, Chorus

WILLIAM CAREY COLLEGE
Hattiesburg   Mississippi 39401, 601 582-5051
Private and 4 Year
Arts Areas: Instrumental Music, Vocal Music and Theatre

MUSIC

Dr Donald Winters, Dean   **Number Of Faculty:** 12   **Number Of Students:** 150
Degrees Offered: BMus; BA; MMus   **Teaching Certification Available**
Financial Assistance: Scholarships and Work-Study Grants
Performing Groups: Carey College Chorale; Chapel Choir; Madrigal Singers; Carpenter's Wood
Workshops/Festivals: Church Music Workshops

THEATRE

Obra Quave, Head   **Number Of Faculty:** 2   **Number Of Students:** 30
Degrees Offered: BA; BS   **Teaching Certification Available**
Financial Assistance: Scholarships and Work-Study Grants
Performing Groups: Carey Summer Showcase (dinner theatre)
Workshops/Festivals: Showcase is a student workshop in that students write, produce, direct & act in two summer musical theatre productions

---

WOOD JUNIOR COLLEGE
Mathiston   Mississippi 39752, 601 263-9851
Private and 2 Year
Arts Areas: Instrumental Music, Vocal Music and Theatre
Performing Series: Artist Series   **Performance Facilities:** Bennett Auditorium

MUSIC

Barbara Lott, Head   **Number Of Faculty:** 2   **Number Of Students:** 15
Degrees Offered: AA
Courses Offered: Basic/Advanced Theory, Piano, Voice, Choir
Financial Assistance: Scholarships and Work-Study Grants
Performing Groups: Wood Singers

THEATRE

Wayne Webster, Head   **Number Of Faculty:** 1   **Number Of Students:** 20
Degrees Offered: AA
Courses Offered: Oral Communication; Oral Interpretation; Drama Production; Fundamentals of Theatre
Financial Assistance: Scholarships and Work-Study Grants
Performing Groups: Wood Players

AVILA COLLEGE
11901 Wornall Rd, Kansas City   Missouri 64145
816 942-8400 Ext 289

> Private and 4 Year
> *Arts Areas:* Dance, Instrumental Music, Vocal Music, Theatre, Television and Visual Arts
> *Performance Facilities:* Geppert Theatre; Actors Laborary Theatre

DANCE

William J Louis, Coordinator   *Number Of Faculty:* 2
Number Of Students: 75
Courses Offered: Creative Movement; Ballet, Modern Dance, and Modern Jazz Technique and Theory;
Ballet, Modern Dance, and Modern Jazz Ensemble; Composition
Financial Assistance: Scholarships, Work-Study Grants and Deans Theatre Grants
Performing Groups: Avila Dance Theatre
Workshops/Festivals: KC Ballet annual program

MUSIC

Sister de La Salle McKeen, PhD, Coordinator   *Number Of Faculty:* 10
Number Of Students: 65   *Degrees Offered:* BA
Teaching Certification Available
Performing Groups: Women's Chorus; Mixed Vocal Ensemble; Faculty Soloists; Student Soloists
Workshops/Festivals: Avila Diocesan Music Festival; Vocal, Piano & Church Music Workshop each
summer

THEATRE

Dr Wm J Louis, Coordinator   *Number Of Faculty:* 10   *Number Of Students:* 45
Degrees Offered: BA, BFA concentration in Acting, Directing, Design & Dramatic Literature
Teaching Certification Available
Performing Groups: Actors Laboratory Theatre
Workshops/Festivals: Annual summer Missouri Shakespeare Festival; Annual Fine Arts Festival for
orientation

CENTRAL BIBLE COLLEGE
3000 N Grant, Springfield   Missouri 65802
417 833-2551 Ext 29

> Private and 4 Year   *Arts Areas:* Instrumental Music and Vocal Music
> *Performance Facilities:* College Auditorium; College Chapel

MUSIC

Merlin Mitchell, Assistant Professor, Coordinator
Number Of Faculty: 6 Full-time, 6 Part-time   *Number Of Students:* 100
Degrees Offered: BA in Sacred Music, Applied & Church Music, Theory, Conducting, Hymnology,
Counterpoint, Form & Analysis
Courses Offered: Music History & Literature, Church Music Administration & Applied Lessons;
Composition & Arranging; Keyboard Harmony
Financial Assistance: Scholarships   *Performing Groups:* Choir; Band; Ensembles

---

CENTRAL METHODIST COLLEGE
Fayette   Missouri 65248, 816 248-3391

> Private and 4 Year
> *Arts Areas:* Dance, Instrumental Music, Vocal Music, Theatre and Visual Arts
> *Performance Facilities:* Assembly Hall; Little Theater; Linn United Methodist Church

DANCE

Mrs Phillys Richardson, Physical Education Instructor   *Number Of Faculty:* 1

(continued on next page)

MUSIC

Dr Don Pyle, Acting Dean   **Number Of Faculty:** 9
Degrees Offered: BMus; BMusEd   **Teaching Certification Available**
Financial Assistance: Assistantships, Scholarships and Work-Study Grants
Performing Groups: Marching Band; Concert Band; Jazz Band; Brass Ensemble; A Cappela Choir;
Chamber Choir; Orchestra

THEATRE

Dr Don Eidson, Chairman; Nat Goodwin, Director   **Number Of Faculty:** 6
Teaching Certification Available

CENTRAL MISSOURI STATE UNIVERSITY

Warrensburg   Missouri 64093, 816 429-4111
State and 4 Year
Arts Areas: Dance, Instrumental Music, Vocal Music, Theatre, Television and Visual Arts
Performing Series: Entertainment Series; Convocation Series
Performance Facilities: Hart Recital Hall; Hendrick Hall; Martin Theater

MUSIC

Dr Russell Coleman, Head   **Number Of Faculty:** 26   **Number Of Students:** 300
Degrees Offered: BA; BM; BME; MA; MSE   **Teaching Certification Available**
Financial Assistance: Assistantships and Scholarships
Performing Groups: Three Concert Bands; Marching Band; Four Choirs; Orchestra; Two Jazz Bands;
Brass, Percussion, Woodwind, String, Choral Ensembles
Workshops/Festivals: Missouri State High School Activities Association Music Festival; Jazz Festival;
Summer Music Camp; Marching Contest; Vocal & Instrumental Workshops

THEATRE

James L Highlander, Professor of Theatre   **Number Of Faculty:** 5
Number Of Students: 75   **Degrees Offered:** BA; BFA; BS; BS Ed
Teaching Certification Available
Financial Assistance: Assistantships and Scholarships
Performing Groups: CMSU Players; Theta Alpha Phi
Workshops/Festivals: District Speech & Dramatic Arts Festivals; Directors' Workshop
Artists-In-Residence/Guest Artists: Saint Louis Symphony; Woody Herman Jazz Band; Francis McBeth,
Conductor/Composer; Fisher/Bossart, Pianists; Ossie Davis & Ruby Dee; Danceworks; Pickwick Puppet
Theatre

COLUMBIA COLLEGE

10th & Rogers Sts, Columbia   Missouri 65201
314 449-0531
Private and 4 Year
Arts Areas: Dance, Instrumental Music, Vocal Music and Theatre
Performance Facilities: Launer Auditorium; Dulany Hall

DANCE

Richard Marriott, Chairman   **Number Of Faculty:** 2   **Number Of Students:** 120
Financial Assistance: Assistantships and Scholarships
Performing Groups: Forward Motion - Modern Jazz Precision Performing Group

MUSIC

Richard Marriott, Chairman   **Number Of Faculty:** 4   **Number Of Students:** 50
Degrees Offered: BA   **Teaching Certification Available**
Financial Assistance: Scholarships and Work-Study Grants
Performing Groups: Concert Choir; Camerata Choir; Double Sextet

(continued on next page)

THEATRE

Richard Marriott, Chairman   **Number Of Faculty:** 2   **Number Of Students:** 80
Financial Assistance: Scholarships and Work-Study Grants
Performing Groups: Theatre Workshop

COTTEY COLLEGE
Austin Blvd, Nevada   Missouri 64772
417 667-8181

Private and 2 Year
Arts Areas: Dance, Instrumental Music, Vocal Music and Theatre
Performing Series: Kansas City Philharmonic Orchestra
Performance Facilities: Rosemary Auditorium

DANCE

Donna Needham, Chairman   **Number Of Faculty:** 2   **Degrees Offered:** AA
Financial Assistance: Scholarships and Work-Study Grants
Performing Groups: Modern Dance Club

MUSIC

Forster Day, Chairman   **Number Of Faculty:** 5   **Degrees Offered:** AA
Financial Assistance: Scholarships and Work-Study Grants
Performing Groups: Cottey Choir

THEATRE

Alfred Fenske, Chairman   **Number Of Faculty:** 2   **Degrees Offered:** AA
Financial Assistance: Scholarships and Work-Study Grants
Performing Groups: Children's Theatre Production

CROWDER COLLEGE
Neosho   Missouri 64850, 417 451-3223

2 Year and Community
Arts Areas: Instrumental Music, Vocal Music and Theatre
Performing Series: Crowder College Performing Series
Performance Facilities: Gymnasium Auditorium; Two Multi-purpose Rooms

MUSIC

Edward N Oathour, Chairman   **Number Of Faculty:** 4   **Number Of Students:** 37
Degrees Offered: AA
Courses Offered: Theory I, II, III, IV; Sight Singing; Ear Training; Music History & Appreciation;
Applied Instrumental; Vocal; Keyboard; Piano Lab
Financial Assistance: Scholarships and Work-Study Grants
Workshops/Festivals: Ozark 8 Music Festival; Piano & Voice Workshops

THEATRE

Edward N Oathout, Chairman   **Number Of Faculty:** 1   **Number Of Students:** 9
Degrees Offered: AA
Courses Offered: Intro to Theatre; Theatre Participation; Music - Theatre Participation
Financial Assistance: Scholarships and Work-Study Grants

CULVER-STOCKTON COLLEGE
Canton   Missouri 63425, 314 288-5221 Ext 73

Private and 4 Year
Arts Areas: Instrumental Music, Vocal Music, Theatre, Film Arts and Visual Arts
Performance Facilities: Canton Theatre; Alexander Campbell Auditorium

MUSIC

A Wesley Tower, Chairman   **Number Of Faculty:** 5   **Number Of Students:** 75
Degrees Offered: BA; BS   **Teaching Certification Available**

(continued on next page)

Financial Assistance: Internships, Assistantships, Scholarships and Work-Study Grants
Performing Groups: Chamber Choir; Concert Choir; Symphonic Wind Ensemble; Jazz Lab; Culver-Stockton Singers
Workshops/Festivals: Piano Workshop; Opera Workshop; Woodwind Workshop

THEATRE

Sighard Krueger, Chairman   *Number Of Faculty:* 3   *Number Of Students:* 50
Degrees Offered: BA; BS
Technical Training: Theatre Management; Theatre Lighting; Scene Design
Teaching Certification Available
Financial Assistance: Internships, Assistantships, Scholarships and Work-Study Grants
Performing Groups: Culver-Stockton Players

DRURY COLLEGE
Springfield   Missouri 65802, 417 865-8731
   Private and 4 Year
   Arts Areas: Instrumental Music, Vocal Music, Theatre and Visual Arts

MUSIC

D Wayne Johnson, Chairman   *Number Of Faculty:* 6   *Number Of Students:* 62
Degrees Offered: BA Mus, Mus Ed   *Teaching Certification Available*
Financial Assistance: Scholarships and Work-Study Grants

THEATRE

Robert L Wilhoit, Chairman   *Number Of Faculty:* 3   *Number Of Students:* 46
Degrees Offered: BA Drama   *Teaching Certification Available*
Financial Assistance: Scholarships and Work-Study Grants
Performing Groups: Drury Lane Players

EAST CENTRAL MISSOURI DISTRICT JUNIOR COLLEGE
Union   Missouri 63084, 314 583-5193
   County and 2 Year
   Arts Areas: Instrumental Music, Vocal Music and Visual Arts
   Performing Series: Cultural Events Series
   Performance Facilities: College Auditorium

MUSIC

Carl Walker, Coordinator   *Degrees Offered:* AA
Performing Groups: Vocal and Instrumental Ensembles

EVANGEL COLLEGE
1111 N Glenstone, Springfield   Missouri 65802
417 865-2811
   Private and 4 Year
   Arts Areas: Instrumental Music, Vocal Music, Theatre and Visual Arts

MUSIC

Dr J M Nicholson, Chairman   *Number Of Faculty:* 16   *Number Of Students:* 80
Degrees Offered: BA Mus Ed   *Teaching Certification Available*
Financial Assistance: Scholarships
Performing Groups: Vocal & Instrumental Ensembles

THEATRE

Degrees Offered: BA Drama-Speech   *Teaching Certification Available*
Financial Assistance: Scholarships

FONTBONNE COLLEGE
6800 Wydown, Saint Louis   Missouri 63105
314 862-3456 Ext 201
Private and 4 Year
Arts Areas: Instrumental Music, Vocal Music, Theatre and Visual Arts
Performing Series: Fine Arts Series
Performance Facilities: Fontbonne Theatre

MUSIC

Number Of Faculty: 10   *Number Of Students:* 46
Degrees Offered: BMus; MusEd; Applied Music; Piano Pedagogy
Technical Training: Voice; Organ; Orchestral Instrument; Guitar
Teaching Certification Available
Financial Assistance: Scholarships and Work-Study Grants
Performing Groups: Choir; Jazz Ensemble; String Ensemble
Workshops/Festivals: Various Music Education Workshops; Spring Evaluation Festival

THEATRE

Number Of Faculty: 6   *Number Of Students:* 52   *Degrees Offered:* BA Theatre
Financial Assistance: Scholarships and Work-Study Grants

HANNIBAL LA GRANGE COLLEGE
Hannibal   Missouri 63401, 314 221-3675
Private and 2 Year
Arts Areas: Instrumental Music, Vocal Music and Church Music
Performance Facilities: General Auditorium

MUSIC

Dr Floyd D McCoy, Chairman   *Degrees Offered:* AA; B Church Music
Financial Assistance: Scholarships, Work-Study Grants and Church Vocational Scholarship
Performing Groups: Concert Choir; Concert Band; Campus Choir
Workshops/Festivals: Christmas Festival; Easter Festival; Concert of Art & Music

LINCOLN UNIVERSITY
Jefferson City   Missouri 65101, 314 751-2325
State and 4 Year
Arts Areas: Dance, Instrumental Music, Vocal Music, Theatre, Visual Arts and Radio
Performing Series: Saint Louis Symphony
Performance Facilities: C C Richardson Auditorium; Langston Hughes Theatre

DANCE

Teresa Hunt, Instructor
Dance program under auspices of Physical Education Department
Number Of Faculty: 1
Courses Offered: Modern Dance; Folk, Square & Social Dance; Dance Composition
Financial Assistance: Work-Study Grants   *Performing Groups:* Lincoln University Dance Troupe

MUSIC

Dr F Nathaniel Gatlin, Interim Head of Fine Arts   *Number Of Faculty:* 11
Number Of Students: 75   *Degrees Offered:* BMus; BMusEd
Teaching Certification Available
Financial Assistance: Scholarships and Work-Study Grants
Performing Groups: University Choir; Concert Choir; University Band; University Orchestra; University
Jazz Band
Workshops/Festivals: Festival of the Arts

THEATRE

Dr Thomas Pawley, Head, Department of Communications   *Number Of Faculty:* 4
Number Of Students: 20   *Degrees Offered:* BA; BS Ed   *Teaching Certification Available*

(continued on next page)

Financial Assistance: Scholarships and Work-Study Grants
Performing Groups: Stagecrafters; Readers' Theatre
Workshops/Festivals: Festival of the Arts

LINDENWOOD COLLEGE
Kings Highway, Saint Charles   Missouri 63301
314 723-7152 Ext 219
Private and 4 Year
Arts Areas: Dance, Instrumental Music, Vocal Music, Theatre, Film Arts, Television, Visual Arts and Radio
Performance Facilities: Jelkyl Center for Performing Arts

DANCE

Grazina Amonas, Chairman   **Number Of Faculty:** 1   **Number Of Students:** 48
Degrees Offered: BS
Financial Assistance: Internships, Assistantships, Scholarships and Work-Study Grants
Workshops/Festivals: Gerda Zimmerman In-Residence and Concert; San Francisco Dance Workshop

MUSIC

Dr Ken Greenlaw, Chairman   **Number Of Faculty:** 14   **Number Of Students:** 26
Degrees Offered: BMus; BA; BS; BMusEd   **Teaching Certification Available**
Financial Assistance: Internships, Scholarships and Work-Study Grants
Performing Groups: Lindenwood Choral Society
Workshops/Festivals: Regional Choral Festival for High School Students

THEATRE

Lou Florimonte, Chairman   **Number Of Faculty:** 5   **Number Of Students:** 88
Degrees Offered: BS Communication Arts; BA Communication Arts
Teaching Certification Available
Financial Assistance: Internships, Assistantships and Work-Study Grants
Performing Groups: Theatre Group; Experimental Theatre Projects
Workshops/Festivals: Mime Workshop

LONGVIEW COMMUNITY COLLEGE
500 Longview Rd, Lee's Summit   Missouri 64063
816 763-7777
2 Year and Community College District
Arts Areas: Instrumental Music and Vocal Music

MUSIC

Garland B Reckart, Jr, Instructor   **Number Of Faculty:** 2
Degrees Offered: AA

MAPLE WOODS COMMUNITY COLLEGE
2601 N E Barry Rd, Kansas City   Missouri 64156
816 436-6500
County and 2 Year
Arts Areas: Instrumental Music, Vocal Music and Theatre

MUSIC

Desmond Daniels, Instructor   **Number Of Faculty:** 1   **Degrees Offered:** AA
Courses Offered: Mixed Chorus; Fundamentals of Music; Music Appreciation; Musical Activities; Music Theory I, II; Functional Piano
Financial Assistance: Work-Study Grants   **Performing Groups:** Mixed Chorus

THEATRE

Ronald Brink, Instructor   **Number Of Faculty:** 1   **Degrees Offered:** AA
Courses Offered: Theatre and the Western World; Acting; Elements of Play Production; Theater

(continued on next page)

Practicum; Directed Study in Speech & Drama
Financial Assistance: Work-Study Grants

MINERAL AREA JUNIOR COLLEGE
Flat River   Missouri 63601, 314 431-4593
State and 2 Year
Arts Areas: Instrumental Music, Vocal Music and Visual Arts
Performing Series: Cultural Events Series
Performance Facilities: College Auditorium   *Degrees Offered:* AA
Performing Groups: Vocal and Instrumental Ensembles

MISSOURI SOUTHERN STATE COLLEGE
Newman & Duquesne Rds, Joplin   Missouri 64801
417 624-8100
State and 4 Year
Arts Areas: Instrumental Music, Vocal Music, Theatre and Visual Arts
Performing Series: Performing Arts Series
Performance Facilities: Thomas E Taylor Performing Arts Center; Edward S Phinney Recital Hall; Barn Theatre

MUSIC

Dr F Joe Sims, Associate Professor   *Number Of Faculty:* 7
Number Of Students: 52   *Degrees Offered:* BA & BS in Education
Courses Offered: Music Appreciation; Music Theory; Conducting; History of Music; Music for the Elementary School; Marching Band Techniques; Form & Analysis; Orchestration; Music in the Public School; Instrumental Techniques
Teaching Certification Available
Financial Assistance: Scholarships, Work-Study Grants and Performance Awards
Performing Groups: Choir; Chamber Choir; Brass Choir; Marching Band; Concert Band; Lab Band; Orchestra
Workshops/Festivals: District Piano, Vocal & Instrumental for the High School Activities Association

THEATRE

Milton W Brietzke, Director   *Number Of Faculty:* 4 Full-time, 1 Part-time
Number Of Students: 40
Degrees Offered: BS in Education, Theatre & Speech Emphasis; BA in Theatre & Speech
Courses Offered: Dramatic Literature; Play Production; Acting; Directing; Stage Design; Creative Dramatics; Theatre Appreciation
Teaching Certification Available
Financial Assistance: Scholarships and Performing Aids
Workshops/Festivals: Creative Dramatics; Student Directing

MISSOURI VALLEY COLLEGE
500 E College St, Marshall   Missouri 65340
816 886-6924
Private and 4 Year
Arts Areas: Instrumental Music, Vocal Music, Theatre, Television, Visual Arts and Radio
Performing Series: Concert & Lecture Series

MUSIC

Lyle B King, Assistant Professor   *Number Of Faculty:* 1
Technical Training: Music Appreciation; History; Choir; Band
Financial Assistance: Scholarships and Work-Study Grants
Performing Groups: Choir; Marching Band

THEATRE

Jack Sutton, Chairman   *Number Of Faculty:* 2   *Number Of Students:* 20
Degrees Offered: BA & BS Speech & Drama

(continued on next page)

Courses Offered: Oral Interpretation; Speech Science; Fundamentals of Speech; Voice & Diction
Teaching Certification Available
Financial Assistance: Scholarships and Work-Study Grants
Performing Groups: Valley Players

MISSOURI WESTERN STATE COLLEGE
4525 Downs Dr, Saint Joseph   Missouri 64507
816 233-7192 Ext 272
State and 4 Year
Arts Areas: Instrumental Music, Vocal Music, Theatre and Visual Arts
Performance Facilities: Theater; Art Gallery

MUSIC

Dr Matt Gilmour, Chairman   **Number Of Faculty:** 9   **Degrees Offered:** BS Ed
Teaching Certification Available   **Financial Assistance:** Scholarships
Performing Groups: Vocal Ensemble; Choir; Chorus; Symphony Orchestra; Symphonic Winds; Marching Band; Stage Band; String Ensemble; Swing Choir
Workshops/Festivals: Solo & Ensemble Music Clinic; Vocal Workshop; Band Day; Music Ed Workshop; Mini Jazz Festival

THEATRE

Dr James Mehl, Chairman   **Number Of Faculty:** 4   **Number Of Students:** 24
Degrees Offered: BA, BS Ed   **Teaching Certification Available**
Financial Assistance: Scholarships
Performing Groups: Main Stage Theatre; Projects Productions
Workshops/Festivals: Acting Workshops; Scene Painting Workshops; Mime Workshop; Creative Dramatics Workshops

---

UNIVERSITY OF MISSOURI
140 Fine Arts Bldg, Columbia   Missouri 65201
314 882-3650
State and 4 Year
Arts Areas: Dance, Instrumental Music, Vocal Music, Theatre, Film Arts, Television and Visual Arts
Performance Facilities: Jesse Auditorium   **Number Of Faculty:** 3
Number Of Students: 250
Dance program under auspices of Women's Physical Education Department
Performing Groups: UMC Dancers
Workshops/Festivals: Ballet Workshop; Jazz - Modern Dance Workshop

MUSIC

Charles L Emmons, Chairman   **Number Of Faculty:** 30
Number Of Students: 235   **Degrees Offered:** BMus; BS; MMus; MMusEd; MA
Teaching Certification Available
Financial Assistance: Assistantships, Scholarships and Work-Study Grants
Performing Groups: Band; Orchestra; Chorus; University Singers; Men's Glee Club; Women's Glee Club; Vocal Jazz Ensemble; Stage Band; Chamber Music; Collegium Musicum; Opera Production
Workshops/Festivals: State Music Festival Summer Music Camp; Music Workshops

THEATRE

Stephen M Archer, Chairman   **Number Of Faculty:** 7   **Number Of Students:** 175
Degrees Offered: BA; BS; MA; PhD   **Teaching Certification Available**
Financial Assistance: Assistantships, Scholarships and Work-Study Grants
Performing Groups: University Theatre
Workshops/Festivals: Summer Repertory Theatre; One Act Play Contest

UNIVERSITY OF MISSOURI, KANSAS CITY
51st & Rockhill Rd, Kansas City   Missouri 64110
816 276-2701

State and 4 Year   **Arts Areas:** Theatre, Television and Visual Arts
Performing Series: Cultural Events Series

DANCE

Dance offered at University of Missouri-Kansas City Conservatory of Music

THEATRE

Dr Patricia McIllrath, Chairman   **Number Of Faculty:** 15
Number Of Students: 100   **Degrees Offered:** BA; MA
Technical Training: Professional Training   **Teaching Certification Available**
Financial Assistance: Internships, Assistantships, Scholarships and Work-Study Grants
Performing Groups: Missouri Repertory Theatre (Summer); Missouri Vanguard Theatre (Touring); Missouri Vanguard Children's Theatre

UNIVERSITY OF MISSOURI - KANSAS CITY CONSERVATORY OF MUSIC
4420 Warwick Blvd, Kansas City   Missouri 64111
816 276-2731

State and 4 Year   **Arts Areas:** Dance, Instrumental Music and Vocal Music
Performing Series: Chamber Music Series
Performance Facilities: Stover Auditorium; Pierson Hall

DANCE

Thomas G Owen, Associate Dean   **Number Of Faculty:** 5
Number Of Students: 45   **Degrees Offered:** BA Dance
Courses Offered: Ballet; Modern
Financial Assistance: Scholarships and Work-Study Grants
Performing Groups: Contemporary Dance Ensemble; University Dance Workshop
Workshops/Festivals: Numerous workshops utilizing guest artists and cooperative public performances with the Kansas City Ballet

MUSIC

Dr Lindsey Merrill, Dean   **Number Of Faculty:** 80   **Number Of Students:** 550
Degrees Offered: BA Mus; BMus Performance, Theory, Composition; BME Choral Instruction, Music Theory; MAA; MME; DMA
Technical Training: Piano Tuning; Electronic Music
Teaching Certification Available
Financial Assistance: Internships, Assistantships, Scholarships and Work-Study Grants
Workshops/Festivals: Jazz Festival; Music Ed Workshops; Music Therapy Workshops; Dance, Choral Invitational

UNIVERSITY OF MISSOURI, SAINT LOUIS
8001 Natural Bridge Rd, Saint Louis   Missouri 63121
314 453-0111

State and 4 Year   **Arts Areas:** Instrumental Music and Vocal Music
Performing Series: Concert Series

MUSIC

Leonard W Ott, Chairman   **Number Of Faculty:** 37   **Number Of Students:** 130
Degrees Offered: BA Mus; BMusEd & Performance
Teaching Certification Available
Financial Assistance: Scholarships and Work-Study Grants
Performing Groups: Band; Wind Ensemble; Orchestra; Jazz Ensemble; Chorus; University Singers

NORTHEAST MISSOURI STATE UNIVERSITY
Kirksville   Missouri 63501, 816 665-5121
State and 4 Year
Arts Areas: Dance, Instrumental Music, Vocal Music, Theatre, Visual Arts and Communications
Performing Series: Lyceum Series
Performance Facilities: Auditorium; Little Theater; Activities Room, Student Union

DANCE

Dr William Richerson, Head, Division of Health & Physical Education
Number Of Faculty: 1   **Courses Offered:** Basic courses in Modern Dance
Financial Assistance: Work-Study Grants

MUSIC

Dale Jorgenson, Chairman   **Number Of Faculty:** 24   **Number Of Students:** 160
Degrees Offered: BA; BMus; BME; MA
Courses Offered: Performance; Theory; Literature - History; Music Education
Technical Training: Preparation for performing discipline
Teaching Certification Available
Financial Assistance: Assistantships, Scholarships and Work-Study Grants
Performing Groups: University Symphony Orchestra; University Bands; NEMO Singers; University Chorus; The Jazz Ensembles; Brass Choir; Madrigal Singers; Opera Workshop; String Orchestra; Clarinet Choir
Workshops/Festivals: Workshops in Choral Conducting, Instrumental Conducting, High School Music Camps; Instrument Repair Workshop; Piano Workshop; Jazz Workshop

THEATRE

Edwin Carpenter, Head, Language & Literature Division   **Number Of Faculty:** 3
Number Of Students: 36   **Degrees Offered:** BA & BS in Ed
Courses Offered: Performance; Theory; Literature - History; Theatre Education
Technical Training: Teaching; Preparation for Performance
Teaching Certification Available
Financial Assistance: Assistantships, Scholarships and Work-Study Grants
Performing Groups: University Players; Ice House Players

NORTHWEST MISSOURI STATE UNIVERSITY
Maryville   Missouri 64468, 816 582-7141
State and 4 Year
Arts Areas: Dance, Instrumental Music, Vocal Music, Theatre, Film Arts, Television and Visual Arts
Performing Series: Performing Arts & Lecture Series
Performance Facilities: Charles Johnson Theatre; Administration Building Auditorium

DANCE

Barbara Bernard, Chairman, Women's Physical Education   **Number Of Faculty:** 2
Number Of Students: 10 - 15   **Degrees Offered:** BS
Courses Offered: Beginning, Intermediate & Advanced Modern Dance; Folk & Square Dance; Advanced Folk & Square Dance; Social Dance; Advanced Social Dance
Teaching Certification Available   **Financial Assistance:** Scholarships
Workshops/Festivals: Visiting Dance Groups conduct Workshops annually

MUSIC

Dr Harold Jackson, Chairman   **Number Of Faculty:** 12
Number Of Students: 250 - 300   **Degrees Offered:** BA, BS in Ed; MS in Ed
Teaching Certification Available
Financial Assistance: Assistantships and Scholarships
Performing Groups: Tower Choir; University Chorale; Madralier Singers; Jazz Band; Symphonic Band; Marching Band
Workshops/Festivals: Swing Choir Workshop; Summer Band Camps & Vocal Camps for Junior High & Senior High; Opera Workshop

(continued on next page)

THEATRE

Dr Robert Bohlken, Chairman   **Number Of Faculty:** 13
Number Of Students: 250
Degrees Offered: BS in Ed; BA, BS, MS in Speech Pathology
Teaching Certification Available   Financial Assistance: Scholarships
Performing Groups: Alpha Psi Omega; University Theatre
Workshops/Festivals: Communicative Arts Festival for High School Students

PARK COLLEGE
Kansas City   Missouri 64152, 816 741-2000 Ext 151
Private and 4 Year
Arts Areas: Instrumental Music, Vocal Music, Theatre, Film Arts, Television and Music Theatre
Performing Series: Student Union Board
Performance Facilities: Chapel Music Hall; Alumni Theatre

MUSIC

Robert C Anderson, Professor   **Number Of Faculty:** 7
Number Of Students: 30   **Degrees Offered:** BA Mus; BA MusEd
Courses Offered: Instrumental; Theory; History/Literature; Professional Ed Sequences
Technical Training: Internships; Student Teaching; Orchestra
Financial Assistance: Scholarships and Work-Study Grants
Performing Groups: Northland Symphony; Concert Choir; Park Singers
Workshops/Festivals: KRCHE - Philharmonic Workshops

THEATRE

Robert C Anderson, Professor   **Number Of Faculty:** 4
Number Of Students: 23
Degrees Offered: BA Acting/Directing; Technical Theatre; Music Theatre
Courses Offered: Acting; Directing; All Technical Courses; Make-up; History
Technical Training: Acting/Directing (Experimental Theatre)
Financial Assistance: Scholarships and Work-Study Grants
Performing Groups: Actors Prologue Company; Experimental Theatre
Workshops/Festivals: Mime Festival; Black Contemporary Players; Original Script Repertory Theatre

PENN VALLEY COMMUNITY COLLEGE
3201 SW Trafficway, Kansas City   Missouri 64114
816 756-2800
State and 2 Year
Arts Areas: Instrumental Music, Vocal Music and Theatre
Performing Series: Penn Valley Community College Performing Series
Performance Facilities: Little Theatre/Auditorium

MUSIC

Carder Manning, Chairman   **Number Of Faculty:** 12   **Degrees Offered:** AA
Financial Assistance: BEOG; SEOG

SAINT LOUIS COMMUNITY COLLEGE AT MERAMEC
11333 Big Bend Blvd, Saint Louis   Missouri 63122
314 966-7500
County and 2 Year
Arts Areas: Instrumental Music, Vocal Music, Theatre and Visual Arts
Performing Series: Cultural Events Series & Exhibits; Theatre Productions
Performance Facilities: College Theatre/Auditorium; College Rehearsal Hall; College Gallery

MUSIC

Harold Gamble, Associate Professor   **Number Of Faculty:** 4
Degrees Offered: AA

(continued on next page)

Financial Assistance: Scholarships and Work-Study Grants
Performing Groups: Symphonic Band; Jazz Lab Band; College Choir; College Orchestra

THEATRE

Robert Dixon, Associate Professor   **Number Of Faculty:** 6
Degrees Offered: AA
Financial Assistance: Scholarships and Work-Study Grants
Performing Groups: Meramec Students
Workshops/Festivals: American College Theatre Festival

SAINT LOUIS UNIVERSITY
221 N Grand Blvd, Saint Louis   Missouri 63103
314 535-3300

Private and 4 Year
Arts Areas: Instrumental Music, Vocal Music, Theatre, Film Arts, Television and Visual Arts
Performing Series: University Theatre Series; Dinner Theatre Series
Performance Facilities: University Theatre; Laclede Theatre; Concert Hall; College Church

MUSIC

Dr Robert Neidlinger, Chairman   **Number Of Faculty:** 5
Number Of Students: 25   **Degrees Offered:** BA
Courses Offered: Introduction to Music; Applied Music; Theory; History of Music; Composition; Music in American History & Culture; Counterpoint
Teaching Certification Available
Financial Assistance: Scholarships and Work-Study Grants
Performing Groups: University Chorale; University Chamber Guild; Chamber Singers; Mastersingers; Jazz Band
Workshops/Festivals: Liturgy Institute; Christmas Concert; High School Chorale Festival; Spring Concert

THEATRE

Robert O Butler, Chairman   **Number Of Faculty:** 5   **Number Of Students:** 45
Degrees Offered: MA; BA
Courses Offered: Drama Appreciation; Oral Interpretation; Acting; Movement for the Theatre; Mime; Theatre Practicum; Stagecrafts; History of Theatre; Directing; Theatre Laboratory
Teaching Certification Available
Financial Assistance: Scholarships and Work-Study Grants
Performing Groups: Mime Troup
Workshops/Festivals: Theatre-Go-Round Workshop for High School Students; Copper Mountain, Colorado, Summer Stock Acting Company

---

SCHOOL OF THE OZARKS
Point Lookout   Missouri 65726, 417 334-3101

Private and 4 Year
Arts Areas: Instrumental Music, Vocal Music, Theatre and Visual Arts
Performing Series: Concert Series

MUSIC

W E Hendricks, Chairman   **Number Of Faculty:** 3   **Number Of Students:** 40
Degrees Offered: BA
Financial Assistance: Scholarships and Work-Study Grants
Performing Groups: Band; Chorus

THEATRE

James L Meikle, Chairman   **Number Of Faculty:** 2   **Number Of Students:** 28
Degrees Offered: BA; BS
Financial Assistance: Scholarships and Work-Study Grants
Performing Groups: Thespians; Beacon Hill Theatre
Workshops/Festivals: Summer Theatre

SOUTHEAST MISSOURI STATE UNIVERSITY
900 Normal, Cape Girardeau   Missouri 63701
314 651-2000
   State and 4 Year
   Arts Areas: Instrumental Music, Vocal Music and Theatre

MUSIC

Doyle A Dumas, Chairman   *Number Of Faculty:* 16
Degrees Offered: BME; BA; BS Ed; MAT; MME
Courses Offered: Theory; Applied Music; Music History/Literature
Teaching Certification Available
Financial Assistance: Scholarships and Work-Study Grants
Performing Groups: Choir; Chamber Choir; Male Chorus; Women's Chorus; Marching Band; Concert Band; Wind Ensemble; Symphony Orchestra; Jazz Band; Opera Workshop

THEATRE

M G Lorberg, Jr, Chairman, Department of Speech, Communication & Theatre
Number Of Faculty: 5   *Degrees Offered:* BA; BS Ed
Courses Offered: Acting; Directing; Lighting; Design
Teaching Certification Available
Financial Assistance: Scholarships and Work-Study Grants

SOUTHWEST BAPTIST COLLEGE
623 S Pike, Bolivar   Missouri 65613
417 326-5281
   Private and 4 Year
   Arts Areas: Instrumental Music, Vocal Music and Theatre
   Performance Facilities: SWBC Little Theatre; Grant Davis Theatre; Field House

MUSIC

Dr James Woodward, Chairman   *Number Of Faculty:* 14 Full-time, 7 Part-time
Number Of Students: 300   *Degrees Offered:* BA; BS; BMus; B Church Music
Courses Offered: Church Music Administration & Literature; Ensembles; Conducting; Theory; History; Methods & Techniques; Orchestration
Teaching Certification Available
Financial Assistance: Scholarships and Work-Study Grants
Performing Groups: Collegiate Choral; Contempos; Concert Choir; Campus Singers; Chamber Singers; Lab Band; Symphonic Band; Ensembles; Recitals
Workshops/Festivals: Masterworks Concert; Symphony Orchestra

THEATRE

Number Of Faculty: 1   *Number Of Students:* 150   *Degrees Offered:* BA; BS
Courses Offered: Intro to Theatre; Modern Drama; Acting; Children's Theatre; Directing; Stagecraft; Make-up
Teaching Certification Available   *Financial Assistance:* Scholarships and Work-Study Grants
Performing Groups: Delta Psi Omega
Workshops/Festivals: Summer Community Theatre - co-sponsored

SOUTHWEST MISSOURI STATE UNIVERSITY
901 S National, Springfield   Missouri 65802
417 836-5000
   State and 4 Year
   Arts Areas: Dance, Instrumental Music, Vocal Music, Theatre, Film Arts and Visual Arts
   Performance Facilities: Hammons Student Center; Craig Hall Theatre; Carrington Hall Auditorium
   Ellis Recital Hall; Campus Union

DANCE

Kay Brown, Chairperson   *Number Of Faculty:* 4   *Number Of Students:* 26

(continued on next page)

Courses Offered: Emphasis on Modern Dance, Ballet
Technical Training: Emphasis on Performance & Original Choreography
Teaching Certification Available
Financial Assistance: Scholarships and Work-Study Grants
Performing Groups: Repertory Dance Company

MUSIC

Dr Lloyd J Blakely, Chairman   *Number Of Faculty:* 20 Full-time, 5 Part-time
Number Of Students: 200   *Degrees Offered:* BA; BMus; BS Ed
Teaching Certification Available
Financial Assistance: Assistantships, Scholarships and Work-Study Grants
Performing Groups: Chamber Singers; Collegiate Choral; Concert Chorale; Lyric Singers; University Singers; Opera Workshop; University Symphony Orchestra; Chamber Orchestra; Small String Ensembles; Marching Band; Concert Band; Jazz Ensembles; Chamber Ensembles

THEATRE

Dr Robert H Bradley, Chairman   *Number Of Faculty:* 31
Number Of Students: 275
Degrees Offered: BA; BS Ed; BS Ed (Comprehensive); BS; BS (Comprehensive); BA Theatre & Interpretation; BS Speech Correction; MA Speech & Theatre; MS in Secondary Education with emphasis on Speech & Theatre
Teaching Certification Available
Financial Assistance: Assistantships, Scholarships and Work-Study Grants
Workshops/Festivals: Ozark Spring Interpretation Festival; District Speech Festival

---

ST LOUIS COMMUNITY COLLEGE AT FLORISSANT VALLEY
3400 Pershall Rd, Saint Louis   Missouri 63135
314 595-4366

County and 2 Year
Arts Areas: Instrumental Music, Vocal Music, Theatre, Television and Visual Arts
Performance Facilities: Theatre

MUSIC

Dr Henry Orland, Chairperson   *Number Of Faculty:* 6
Number Of Students: 200
Degrees Offered: AA Arts, Science, Music, Music Therapy, Music Education
Financial Assistance: Internships, Assistantships, Scholarships and Work-Study Grants
Performing Groups: Orchestra; Band; Stage Band; Chorus

STEPHENS COLLEGE
East Broadway, Columbia   Missouri 65201
314 442-2211 Ext 303

Private and 4 Year
Arts Areas: Dance, Instrumental Music, Vocal Music, Theatre, Film Arts, Television and Visual Arts
Performing Series: Faculty Chamber Music Recital Series; Fine Arts Series; Lively Arts Series
Performance Facilities: Assembly Hall; South Campus Auditorium; Windsor Auditorium
Chapel; Playhouse; Warehouse Theatre (Stephens College Performing Arts Center)

DANCE

Harriette Ann Gray, Head   *Number Of Faculty:* 6   *Number Of Students:* 338
Degrees Offered: BFA; BA
Courses Offered: Dance Techniques I, II, III; Choreography I, II; Music Theory for Dance; Dance History
Technical Training: Ballet; Modern; Ethnic; Jazz; Tap; Physical Education with Dance Emphasis
Teaching Certification Available   *Financial Assistance:* Assistantships
Performing Groups: Harriette Ann Gray Dance Company, Inc
Workshops/Festivals: Choreography Workshops; Annual Dance Concert; English Country Dance Festival; Christmas Nutcracker performance; Perry - Mansfield Summer Workshop & Concerts

(continued on next page)

MUSIC

Val Patacchi, Head **Number Of Faculty:** 13 **Number Of Students:** 200
Degrees Offered: BFA; BA; BME
Courses Offered: Fundamentals of Musicianship; Music Theory; Form & Analysis; Music Appreciation; Music History & Literature; Contemporary Music; Orchestration; Conducting; Opera Workshop; Song Literature; Piano Literature; Teaching of Piano; Chamber Music; Concert Chorus; Chapel Choir; Symphony Orchestra; Accompanying; Applied Music: Piano, Voice, Strings, Woodwinds, Brass, Harp
Technical Training: Private Lessons: Music Theory
Teaching Certification Available **Financial Assistance:** Scholarships
Performing Groups: Stephens Symphony Orchestra; Concert Chorus; Faculty Chamber Music; Opera Workshop; Faculty & Student Recitals
Workshops/Festivals: Weekly Student Workshops

THEATRE

Eberle Thomas, Head **Number Of Faculty:** 11 Full-time, 1 Part-time
Degrees Offered: BFA; BA
Courses Offered: Acting; Costuming; Stagecraft Design; Lighting; Directing
Teaching Certification Available **Financial Assistance:** Scholarships
Performing Groups: Playhouse Company; Warehouse Company
Artists-In-Residence/Guest Artists: Luis Rojas; R D T Dance Company, Minnesota Dance Theatre - Karen Kristin; Lilliana Morales; Yannis Nikitakis

---

STEPHENS COLLEGE
Columbia Missouri 65201, 314 442-2211 Ext 303
Private and 4 Year
Arts Areas: Dance, Instrumental Music, Vocal Music, Theatre, Film Arts, Television and Visual Arts
Performing Series: Fine Arts Series; Popular Series
Performance Facilities: Stephens College Performing Arts Center

DANCE

Harriet Ann Gray, Chairman **Number Of Faculty:** 5 **Number Of Students:** 425
Degrees Offered: BA; BFA **Technical Training:** Expressive Arts Therapy
Teaching Certification Available
Financial Assistance: Assistantships, Scholarships and Work-Study Grants
Performing Groups: Stephens Dance Company

MUSIC

Richard Johnson, Chairman **Number Of Faculty:** 11 **Number Of Students:** 242
Degrees Offered: BFA; BA
Technical Training: Expressive Arts Therapy; Music Education
Teaching Certification Available
Financial Assistance: Assistantships, Scholarships and Work-Study Grants
Performing Groups: Symphony Orchestra; Chamber Music Quartet; Campus Chorus; Campus Choir

THEATRE

William West, Chairman **Number Of Faculty:** 9 **Number Of Students:** 294
Degrees Offered: BFA; BA
Technical Training: Technical Theatre; Teacher Education; Expressive Arts Therapy
Teaching Certification Available
Financial Assistance: Internships, Assistantships, Scholarships and Work-Study Grants
Performing Groups: Stephens Summer Theatre Institute; Lake Aokaboji Summer Stock Theatre

---

TARKIO COLLEGE
Tarkio Missouri 64491, 816 736-4131
Private and 4 Year
Arts Areas: Instrumental Music, Vocal Music and Theatre
Performance Facilities: Leitch Chapel; Mule Barn Theatre of Tarkio College

(continued on next page)

MUSIC

Leland D Crapson, Professor   **Number Of Faculty:** 3   **Number Of Students:** 60
Degrees Offered: BA MusEd; BA Mus Performance
Courses Offered: Music Theory; Counterpoint; Music History; Music Ed; Choral Conducting & Arranging; Instrumental Conducting; Applied Music
Teaching Certification Available
Financial Assistance: Scholarships and Work-Study Grants
Performing Groups: Concert Choir; College Singers; Wind Ensemble; Orchestra; Jazz Ensemble
Workshops/Festivals: Kansas City Council for Higher Education & Kansas City Philharmonic Orchestra Workshops; Tarkio College Jazz Festival; Tarkio College Music Camps; Casavant Cavalcade Workshop

THEATRE

John R Dubinski, Chairman, Language & Literature   **Number Of Faculty:** 2
Number Of Students: 50   **Degrees Offered:** BA
Courses Offered: Acting; Stage Movement; Production Lab; Dramatic Literature; Scene Design; Lighting Design; Introduction to Theatre
Teaching Certification Available
Financial Assistance: Scholarships and Work-Study Grants
Workshops/Festivals: Tri - State Area Artist Series; Touring Children's Theatre; Shakespeare-in-the-Barn; Mule Barn Theatre Series; Mule Barn Studio Season

---

THREE RIVERS COMMUNITY COLLEGE
507 Vine St, Poplar Bluff   Missouri 63901
314 785-7794 Ext 26
County and 2 Year   **Arts Areas:** Vocal Music, Theatre and Visual Arts
Performance Facilities: Auditorium

MUSIC

Samuel Coryell, Chairman   **Number Of Faculty:** 3   **Number Of Students:** 40
Degrees Offered: AA   **Courses Offered:** Choral; Applied; Theory
Financial Assistance: Scholarships and Work-Study Grants
Performing Groups: TRCC Chorus; TRCC Singers

THEATRE

Michael Bouland, Chairman   **Number Of Faculty:** 1   **Number Of Students:** 20
Courses Offered: Theatre Production
Financial Assistance: Scholarships and Work-Study Grants

WASHINGTON UNIVERSITY
Saint Louis   Missouri 63130, 314 863-0100
Private and 4 Year
Ralph E MorrowDean, Graduate School of Arts & Sciences
Arts Areas: Dance, Instrumental Music, Vocal Music, Theatre and Visual Arts
Performing Series: Edison Theatre Drama Series; Edison Theatre Dance Series; Edison Theatre Music Series
Performance Facilities: Edison Theatre

DANCE

Annelise Mertz, Chairman   **Number Of Faculty:** 7   **Number Of Students:** 400
Degrees Offered: BA in Dance; BA in Dance & Drama (interdisciplinary major)
Courses Offered: Technique; Theory; History; Composition; Improvisation
Technical Training: Modern Dance (emphasis); Classical Ballet Minor
Teaching Certification Available
Financial Assistance: Scholarships, Work-Study Grants and Loans
Performing Groups: Washington University Dance Theatre
Workshops/Festivals: Summer Dance Institute in cooperation with the Mississippi River Festival

(continued on next page)

MUSIC

Tilford Brooks, Chairman   *Number Of Faculty:* 16 Full-time, 12 Part-time
Number Of Students: 128
Degrees Offered: BA; MA; MAEd; MA in Teaching; MMus; PhD; DEd
Courses Offered: History of Jazz; Theory; Composition; Introduction to Music History; Musicianship;
Collegium Musicum; Choral Rehearsal Techniques; Counterpoint
Teaching Certification Available
Financial Assistance: Assistantships, Scholarships, Work-Study Grants and The Anna May Nussbaum Merit
Scholarship
Performing Groups: Wind Ensemble; University Band; Galant Ensemble; Civic Chorus; University Choir;
Madrigal Singers
Workshops/Festivals: Summer workshops are offered in special areas of music education and choral
techniques

THEATRE

Sidney J Friedman, Area Chairman; Herbert E Metz, Division Chairman
Number Of Faculty: 7   *Number Of Students:* 350
Degrees Offered: BA Drama; BA in Performing Arts (interdisciplinary dance & drama Major); MA in
Literature & Drama
Courses Offered: Stage Performance; Literature; History; Theory; Criticism; Theatre Management
Teaching Certification Available
Financial Assistance: Scholarships, Work-Study Grants and Loans; Mary Wickes Drama Prize
Performing Groups: Thyrsus
Workshops/Festivals: The touring companies offer many master classes & workshops for students, and utilize
student technical crews which contributes to the excellence in technical training
Artists-In-Residence/Guest Artists: Irene Gubrud; Etsuko Tazaki; Trevor Pinnock; Michael Schneider;
James Tyler

WEBSTER COLLEGE
470 E Lockwood, Saint Louis   Missouri 63119
314 968-0500 Ext 376
Private and 4 Year
Arts Areas: Dance, Instrumental Music, Vocal Music, Theatre, Film Arts, Television and Visual Arts
Performance Facilities: Loretto Hilton Center for the Performing Arts

DANCE

Michael Simms, Head   *Number Of Faculty:* 6   *Number Of Students:* 25
Dance program under auspices of Theatre Arts Conservatory
Degrees Offered: BA
Technical Training: Jazz; Primative; Classical; Movement; Choreography; Pointe
Financial Assistance: Scholarships and Work-Study Grants
Performing Groups: Dance Theatre

MUSIC

Eloise Jarvis, Chairman   *Number Of Faculty:* 35   *Number Of Students:* 250
Degrees Offered: BA; BFA   *Teaching Certification Available*
Financial Assistance: Scholarships and Work-Study Grants
Performing Groups: Choir; Choral Union; Chamber Ensemble
Workshops/Festivals: Madrigal Festival

THEATRE

Peter Sargent, Chairman   *Number Of Faculty:* 14   *Number Of Students:* 175
Degrees Offered: BA
Technical Training: Opportunity to work with professional repertory company
Financial Assistance: Scholarships and Work-Study Grants
Performing Groups: Theatre Arts Conservatory; Repertory Company
Workshops/Festivals: Jr Directing Workshops; Sr Workshops

WESTERN NEW MEXICO UNIVERSITY
College Ave, Silver City   Missouri 88061
505 538-6011
    State and 4 Year
    Arts Areas: Instrumental Music, Vocal Music and Theatre
    Performance Facilities: Fine Arts Auditorium; McCray Gallery

MUSIC

Dr William Tietze, Chairman   *Number Of Faculty:* 3   *Degrees Offered:* BA
Courses Offered: Voice; Conducting; Orchestration; Instrumental Technique; University Choir; Harmony;
Elementary Music Methods; History of Music; Counterpoint
Teaching Certification Available
Financial Assistance: Scholarships and Work-Study Grants
Performing Groups: University Choir; Chamber Singers; Marching Caravan; Swing Choir; Orchestras; Jazz
Ensemble; Wind Ensemble
Workshops/Festivals: Gilda Summer Band Camp

THEATRE

James Donohue, Lecturer   *Number Of Faculty:* 1
Courses Offered: Acting; Costume & Stage; Introduction to Bilingual Theatre; The Development of
Theatre & Drama; Playwriting; Children's Theatre & Creative Dramatics; Play Direction
Financial Assistance: Scholarships and Work-Study Grants
Performing Groups: Playmakers

WESTMINISTER COLLEGE
Seventh & Westminister, Fulton   Missouri 65251
314 642-3361
    Private and 4 Year
    Arts Areas: Instrumental Music, Vocal Music, Theatre and Visual Arts

MUSIC

Degrees Offered: BFA; BA
Courses Offered: History; Theory; Analysis; Laboratory
Teaching Certification Available
Financial Assistance: Scholarships and Work-Study Grants
Performing Groups: Mixed Chorus; Chamber Singers; Brass Ensemble; Band

THEATRE

Degrees Offered: BFA; BA   *Teaching Certification Available*
Financial Assistance: Scholarships and Work-Study Grants
Performing Groups: College Theatre; Open Space Theatre
Workshops/Festivals: American College Theatre Competition

WILLIAM JEWELL COLLEGE
Liberty   Missouri 64068, 816 781-3806 Ext 297
    Private and 4 Year
    Arts Areas: Dance, Instrumental Music, Vocal Music, Theatre, Film Arts, Television and Visual Arts
    Performing Series: Fine Arts Program

MUSIC

Dr Wesley L Forbis, Chairman   *Number Of Faculty:* 6
Number Of Students: 68   *Degrees Offered:* BA
Teaching Certification Available
Financial Assistance: Scholarships and Work-Study Grants
Performing Groups: Band; Orchestra; Choirs

(continued on next page)

THEATRE

Dr Georgia Bowman, Chairman   **Number Of Faculty:** 5   **Number Of Students:** 75
Degrees Offered: BA   **Teaching Certification Available**
Financial Assistance: Scholarships and Work-Study Grants
Performing Groups: Players
Artists-In-Residence/Guest Artists: Kurt Meisenbach; Carmen Meisenbach; Veronica Tapsonyi; Nancy Jones

---

WILLIAM WOODS - WESTMINISTER COLLEGE
Fulton   Missouri 65251, 314 642-2251 Ext 241

Private and 4 Year
Arts Areas: Dance, Vocal Music, Theatre and Television
Performing Series: Concert and Lecture Series
Performance Facilities: Campus Center Auditorium; Open Space Theatre; Dulany Auditorium

DANCE

Number Of Faculty: 1   **Number Of Students:** 25

MUSIC

Eugene R Addams, Chairman   **Number Of Faculty:** 5   **Number Of Students:** 25
Degrees Offered: BA; BS; BFA   **Teaching Certification Available**
Financial Assistance: Assistantships and Scholarships
Performing Groups: Brass Ensemble; Swing Choir; Chamber Singers

THEATRE

Christian West, Chairman   **Number Of Faculty:** 5   **Number Of Students:** 40
Degrees Offered: BS; BA; BFA
Technical Training: Scene Design; Technical Direction; Costume Design; Lighting Design; Make-up Design; Summer Stock
Teaching Certification Available
Financial Assistance: Assistantships, Scholarships and Work-Study Grants
Performing Groups: Jesters; Alpha Psi Omega

CARROLL COLLEGE
Capitol Hill, Helena   Montana 59601
406 442-3450

Private and 4 Year
Arts Areas: Instrumental Music, Vocal Music, Theatre and Visual Arts
Performance Facilities: Little Theatre; Fine Arts Center

MUSIC

Joseph Munzenrider, Chairman   *Number Of Faculty:* 2
Teaching Certification Available
Performing Groups: Carrolleers; Carroll College Choir
Workshops/Festivals: Music in the 20th Century; Creative Movement; Music of India

THEATRE

David Haney, Director   *Number Of Faculty:* 2   *Degrees Offered:* BA
Teaching Certification Available   *Financial Assistance:* Scholarships
Performing Groups: Carroll Players

COLLEGE OF GREAT FALLS
1301 20th St S, Great Falls   Montana 59405
406 761-8210 Ext 273

Private and 4 Year
Arts Areas: Dance, Instrumental Music, Vocal Music, Theatre and Visual Arts
Performing Series: Department Concert Series; Montana Arts In Recital

DANCE

Miriam Wolf, Instructor   *Number Of Faculty:* 1   *Number Of Students:* 15
Workshops/Festivals: Two Dance Recitals; Workshop

MUSIC

Lee R Mathews, Chairman   *Number Of Faculty:* 4   *Number Of Students:* 50
Degrees Offered: BA Ed; BA Performance   *Teaching Certification Available*
Financial Assistance: Scholarships and Work-Study Grants
Performing Groups: Concert Choir; Orchestra; Vocal, Brass, Woodwind Ensembles; Jazz, Concert Bands
Workshops/Festivals: Department Recital Series   *Number Of Faculty:* 1
Number Of Students: 15   *Degrees Offered:* Drama Minor
Teaching Certification Available

DAWSON COMMUNITY COLLEGE
PO Box 421, 300 College Dr, Glendive   Montana 59330
406 365-3396

State and 2 Year   *Arts Areas:* Theatre
Performance Facilities: Student Center   *Number Of Faculty:* 1
Degrees Offered: AA
Courses Offered: Acting Lab; Dramatic Activity; Stagecraft; Intro to Theatre; History
Technical Training: Interpretation; Beginning Acting; Historical Costuming; Creative Dramatics; Children's Theatre; Theatre Production

EASTERN MONTANA COLLEGE
1500 N 30th, Billings   Montana 59101
406 657-2011

State and 4 Year
Arts Areas: Instrumental Music, Vocal Music, Theatre and Visual Arts
Performance Facilities: Petro Theatre; Readers Theatre; Little Theatre

(continued on next page)

MUSIC

Rex Sutherland, Associate Professor   **Number Of Faculty:** 8
Number Of Students: 40   **Degrees Offered:** BS; BA
Courses Offered: Vocal; Instrumental   **Teaching Certification Available**
Financial Assistance: Scholarships and Work-Study Grants
Performing Groups: Choir; Stage Band; Concert Band; Madrigals

THEATRE

Vicki Tait, Assistant Professor Speech/Theatre   **Number Of Faculty:** 3
Number Of Students: 20   **Degrees Offered:** BS; BA
Courses Offered: Acting; Stagecraft   **Teaching Certification Available**
Financial Assistance: Scholarships and Work-Study Grants
Performing Groups: Katoya Players; Alpha Psi Omega

FLATHEAD VALLEY COMMUNITY COLLEGE
PO Box 1174, Kalispell   Montana 59901
406 752-3411
State and 2 Year
Arts Areas: Instrumental Music, Vocal Music, Theatre and Visual Arts
Degrees Offered: AA   **Financial Assistance:** Scholarships
Performing Groups: Chorus; Orchestra   **Degrees Offered:** AA
Financial Assistance: Scholarships   **Performing Groups:** Drama Players

MILES COMMUNITY COLLEGE
2600 Dickinson, Miles City   Montana 59301
406 232-3031
County and 2 Year   **Arts Areas:** Vocal Music and Theatre
Performing Series: Miles Community College Arts Series

MUSIC

Jan Wiberg, Instructor   **Number Of Faculty:** 1
Courses Offered: Voice; Piano; Chorus; Music Theory; Introduction to Music
Financial Assistance: Scholarships   **Performing Groups:** Chorus; Pep Band

THEATRE

LeRayne DeJulius, Instructor   **Number Of Faculty:** 1
Courses Offered: Introduction to Theatre; Theatre Workshop
Financial Assistance: Scholarships

MONTANA STATE UNIVERSITY
Bozeman   Montana 59717, 406 994-4405
State and 4 Year
Arts Areas: Dance, Instrumental Music, Vocal Music, Theatre, Film Arts, Television and Visual Arts
Performance Facilities: Student Union Building Theatre; Music Building Recital Hall

DANCE

Rozan Pitcher, Instructor   **Number Of Faculty:** 2   **Number Of Students:** 30
Degrees Offered: BS in Physical Education with Dance Emphasis
Courses Offered: Modern; Ballet; Jazz; Tap   **Technical Training:** Modern
Teaching Certification Available
Financial Assistance: Scholarships and Work-Study Grants
Performing Groups: MSU Repertory Dance Company
Workshops/Festivals: Two workshops a year

MUSIC

Dr H Creech Reynolds, Chairman   **Number Of Faculty:** 18
Number Of Students: 180

(continued on next page)

Degrees Offered: BMusEd (with 4 options); MEd with concentration on Music
Courses Offered: Music Teacher Training; Performance Course; Service Courses for non-majors
Technical Training: Music Teacher Training; Music Industry; Sound Engineering
Teaching Certification Available
Financial Assistance: Scholarships and Work-Study Grants
Performing Groups: Symphonic, Camp, Jazz, Marching & Pep Bands; Symphony Orchestra; University Chorus; Chamber Choir; Chorale; Montanans; Symphonic Choir; Recorder Ensemble; Chamber Ensembles; Opera Workshop
Workshops/Festivals: Adult & High School Chamber Music Festival; Band Workshop; Jazz Festival; Contemporary Music Festival; Summer Workshops

THEATRE

Dr Bruce C Jacobsen, Department Head   *Number Of Faculty:* 4
Number Of Students: 121
Degrees Offered: BA with options in Theatre Arts, Theatre Teaching, Theatre Administration
Teaching Certification Available
Financial Assistance: Scholarships and Work-Study Grants
Performing Groups: Shakespeare in the Parks

UNIVERSITY OF MONTANA, SCHOOL OF FINE ARTS
Missoula   Montana 59812, 406 243-4970
State and 4 Year
Arts Areas: Dance, Instrumental Music, Vocal Music, Theatre and Visual Arts
Performing Series: Program Council of the Associated Students of the University
Performance Facilities: Music Recital Hall; Masquer Theater; University Theater

DANCE

Juliette T Crump, Chairman   *Number Of Faculty:* 2   *Number Of Students:* 25
Degrees Offered: BFA Drama with Dance Emphasis
Financial Assistance: Scholarships and Work-Study Grants
Performing Groups: Montana Dance Company
Workshops/Festivals: Summer Dance Workshop

MUSIC

Dr Donald W Simmons, Chairman   *Number Of Faculty:* 28
Number Of Students: 190
Degrees Offered: BMus; BA; BMusEd; MMusEd; MMus; MA; EdD
Teaching Certification Available
Financial Assistance: Assistantships, Scholarships and Work-Study Grants
Performing Groups: Band; Orchestra; Chorus; Swing Choir; Student & Faculty String Quartets; Woodwind Quintets
Workshops/Festivals: Jazz Workshop; Opera Workshop

THEATRE

James D Kriley, Chairman   *Number Of Faculty:* 8   *Number Of Students:* 80
Degrees Offered: BA; BFA; MA; MFA   *Teaching Certification Available*
Financial Assistance: Assistantships, Scholarships and Work-Study Grants
Performing Groups: Montana Masquers; Touring Montana Repertory Theatre
Workshops/Festivals: Drama Workshop
Artists-In-Residence/Guest Artists: Douglas Dunn; Frank Guerrera; Vohn Biggs Consort

---

NORTHERN MONTANA COLLEGE
Harve   Montana 59501, 406 265-7821
State and 4 Year
Arts Areas: Instrumental Music, Vocal Music and Visual Arts

MUSIC

John P Varnum, Chairman   *Number Of Faculty:* 3   *Number Of Students:* 50
Teaching Certification Available

(*continued on next page*)

Financial Assistance: Scholarships and Work-Study Grants
Workshops/Festivals: Festival of Arts

THEATRE

Mary Clearman, Chairman   *Teaching Certification Available*
Performing Groups: Footlights Club

ROCKY MOUNTAIN COLLEGE
Billings   Montana 59102, 406 245-6151
Private and 4 Year
Arts Areas: Instrumental Music, Vocal Music, Theatre and Visual Arts
Performance Facilities: Losekamp Auditorium; Billings Studio Theatre

MUSIC

Donald F Pihlaja, Chairman   *Number Of Faculty:* 10
Number Of Students: 150   *Degrees Offered:* BA, BS in MusEd
Courses Offered: Vocal; Instrumental; Music Education
Technical Training: Opera   *Teaching Certification Available*
Financial Assistance: Scholarships, Work-Study Grants and Performance Grants; Loans
Performing Groups: Concert Choir; Concert Band; Marching Band; Small Ensembles
Workshops/Festivals: Band Day in October - High School Bands are guests

THEATRE

Neil O'Leary, Chairman   *Number Of Faculty:* 2   *Number Of Students:* 30
Degrees Offered: BA Major in Drama/English
Courses Offered: Acting; Directing; Stagecraft; Shakespeare; Modern Drama; Introduction
Technical Training: Learn all phases of play production
Teaching Certification Available
Financial Assistance: Scholarships, Work-Study Grants and Performance Grants; Loans
Performing Groups: Rocky Mountain Players

WESTERN MONTANA COLLEGE
710 S Atlantic St, Dillon   Montana 59725
406 683-7151
State and 4 Year
Arts Areas: Instrumental Music, Vocal Music and Visual Arts
Performing Series: Performing Artist Series

MUSIC

Samuel E Davis, Chairman   *Number Of Faculty:* 2   *Number Of Students:* 40
Degrees Offered: BS; MS Ed   *Technical Training:* Adult Education Program
Teaching Certification Available   *Financial Assistance:* Scholarships
Performing Groups: Choir; Orchestra; Band; String Ensembles

CHADRON STATE COLLEGE
Chadron Nebraska 69337, 308 432-4451 Ext 317
State and 4 Year
Arts Areas: Instrumental Music, Vocal Music, Theatre and Visual Arts
Performing Series: Mid-America Arts Alliance
Performance Facilities: Memorial Hall: Main Auditorium, Little Theatre

MUSIC

Number Of Faculty: 7   *Number Of Students:* 60
Degrees Offered: BA; BS Ed; MS in Supervision
Teaching Certification Available
Financial Assistance: Internships, Assistantships, Scholarships and Work-Study Grants
Workshops/Festivals: Band/Choral Select Groups; Swing Choir/Stage Band Festival; Solo, Ensemble & Large Group Contests

THEATRE

Number Of Faculty: 3   *Number Of Students:* 40
Degrees Offered: BA; BS Ed; AA
Teaching Certification Available   *Technical Training:* Theatre Technician AA Program
Financial Assistance: Internships, Assistantships, Scholarships and Work-Study Grants
Workshops/Festivals: Mime; Technical Theatre; High School Forensic; One - Act Contests

COLLEGE OF SAINT MARY
1901 S 72nd St, Omaha Nebraska 68124
402 393-8800
Private, 4 Year and Woman's College
Arts Areas: Instrumental Music, Vocal Music and Visual Arts
Performing Series: College Concert Series
Performance Facilities: Gross Center; Marian Hall; Formal Lounge, Student Center

MUSIC

Number Of Faculty: 6   *Number Of Students:* 15
Degrees Offered: BA in Music Education, Piano, or Voice
Technical Training: Piano; Voice; Organ; Guitar; Woodwinds; Brass; Percussion; Strings
Teaching Certification Available
Financial Assistance: Scholarships and Work-Study Grants

THEATRE

Sister Mary Jean, Chairman   *Number Of Faculty:* 5   *Number Of Students:* 50
Degrees Offered: BA   *Teaching Certification Available*
Financial Assistance: Scholarships and Work-Study Grants
Performing Groups: Marian Players

CONCORDIA TEACHERS COLLEGE
800 N Columbia, Seward Nebraska 68434
402 643-3651
Private and 4 Year
Arts Areas: Instrumental Music, Vocal Music, Theatre and Visual Arts
Performance Facilities: Weller Chapel; Heine Hall; St John Church

MUSIC

Theo Beck, Chairman   *Number Of Faculty:* 13   *Number Of Students:* 165
Degrees Offered: BS Ed; BA Mus

(continued on next page)

Courses Offered: Elementary: Primary, Music Ed, Church Music; Secondary: Music Ed
Technical Training: Keyboard; Orchestra Instruments
Teaching Certification Available
Financial Assistance: Scholarships and Work-Study Grants
Performing Groups: A Cappella Choir; Concordia Singers; Nebraska Ensemble; Concordia Chorale; College Band; Orchestra; Collegium Musicum; Brass Choir
Workshops/Festivals: Two workshops annually, one directed toward Music Ed, one toward Church Music

THEATRE

Robert Baden, Chairman, Humanities Division   *Number Of Faculty:* 2
Number Of Students: 31   *Degrees Offered:* BS Ed; BA Communications
Courses Offered: Elementary: Speech/Drama major & minor; Secondary: Speech/Drama minor
Technical Training: Theatre Forms; Play Direction
Teaching Certification Available
Financial Assistance: Scholarships and Work-Study Grants
Performing Groups: Curtain Club; Readers' Theatre

CREIGHTON UNIVERSITY
2500 California St, Omaha   Nebraska 68178
402 449-3035
Private and 4 Year
Arts Areas: Dance, Instrumental Music, Vocal Music, Theatre and Visual Arts
Performance Facilities: Little Theatre

DANCE

Valerie Roche, Chairman   *Number Of Faculty:* 2   *Degrees Offered:* BFA; BA
Courses Offered: Modern & Classical Ballet; Teaching Dance to Children; History; Composition
Teaching Certification Available   *Financial Assistance:* Work-Study Grants
Performing Groups: Creighton University Dance Company

MUSIC

Carole Bean, Assistant Professor   *Number Of Faculty:* 3
Courses Offered: Music Appreciation; Music Literature & Style; Chorus; Brass & Wind Ensemble
Teaching Certification Available   *Financial Assistance:* Work-Study Grants
Performing Groups: Wind & Brass Ensembles; Chorus

THEATRE

Dr Suzanne Dieckman, Professor   *Number Of Faculty:* 3   *Degrees Offered:* BA
Technical Training: Performance   *Teaching Certification Available*

DANA COLLEGE
Blair   Nebraska 68008, 402 426-4101
Private and 4 Year
Arts Areas: Instrumental Music, Vocal Music, Theatre and Visual Arts
Performing Series: Concert Series

MUSIC

Paul Neve, Chairman   *Number Of Faculty:* 7   *Number Of Students:* 89
Degrees Offered: BMus; BMusEd   *Teaching Certification Available*
Financial Assistance: Scholarships and Work-Study Grants
Performing Groups: Orchestra; Band; Woodwind Ensemble; Choral Ensemble; Choir

THEATRE

John Northwall, Chairman   *Number Of Faculty:* 3   *Number Of Students:* 42
Degrees Offered: BA   *Teaching Certification Available*
Financial Assistance: Scholarships and Work-Study Grants
Performing Groups: Alpha Psi Omega

DOANE COLLEGE
Crete   Nebraska 68333, 402 826-2161 Ext 233
> Private and 4 Year
> *Arts Areas:* Instrumental Music, Vocal Music, Theatre and Visual Arts
> *Performance Facilities:* Communications Center Auditorium

MUSIC

> Hubert Brown, Jr, Chairman   *Number Of Faculty:* 5   *Number Of Students:* 40
> *Degrees Offered:* BA   *Teaching Certification Available*
> *Financial Assistance:* Scholarships and Work-Study Grants
> *Performing Groups:* Concert Choir; Concert Band; Marching Band; Stage Band; Varsity Vagabonds; Small Groups
> *Workshops/Festivals:* District Music Contests; Jazz Festival & Workshop

THEATRE

> Walter J Barry, Chairman   *Number Of Faculty:* 1   *Number Of Students:* 20
> *Degrees Offered:* BA   *Teaching Certification Available*
> *Financial Assistance:* Scholarships and Work-Study Grants
> *Performing Groups:* Doane Players
> *Workshops/Festivals:* One-Act Play Festival & Workshop; District One-Act Play Contest

GRACE COLLEGE OF THE BIBLE
1515 S 10th St, Omaha   Nebraska 68108
402 342-3377
> Private and 4 Year   *Arts Areas:* Instrumental Music and Vocal Music

MUSIC

> Henry D Wiebe, Director   *Number Of Faculty:* 6   *Number Of Students:* 67
> *Degrees Offered:* BCM (Bachelor of Church Music, 5 yr): BS
> *Courses Offered:* Theory; Conducting; History; Church Music; Music Ensembles
> *Financial Assistance:* Scholarships and Work-Study Grants
> *Performing Groups:* Two Choirs; Concert Band; Vocal Ensembles; Instrumental Ensembles
> *Workshops/Festivals:* Ban - Collegians - Chorale Retreat; Christian Academy Choir Festival

HASTING COLLEGE
7th & Turner, Hastings   Nebraska 68901
402 463-2402
> Private and 4 Year
> *Arts Areas:* Dance, Instrumental Music, Vocal Music and Theatre
> *Performing Series:* Artist - Lecture Series
> *Performance Facilities:* French Memorial Chapel - Theatre; Perkins Auditorium; Eppley Studio Theatre; Kiewit Gymnasium

MUSIC

> Millard H Cates, Chairman   *Number Of Faculty:* 9   *Number Of Students:* 170
> *Degrees Offered:* BMus; BA
> *Courses Offered:* Performance; Theory; History - Music Methods
> *Teaching Certification Available*
> *Financial Assistance:* Scholarships and Work-Study Grants
> *Performing Groups:* Choir; Band; Symphony; Collegium; Chamber Choir; Jazz Lab Band
> *Workshops/Festivals:* Nebraska High School Honor Band & Honor Choir; Evergreen Pines Summer Music Camp

THEATRE

> Dr Harrold C Shiffler, Chairman, Department of Speech & Theatre Arts
> *Number Of Faculty:* 3   *Number Of Students:* 100   *Degrees Offered:* BA
> *Courses Offered:* Performance; Technical; History; Voice & Articulation
> *Teaching Certification Available*

(continued on next page)

Financial Assistance: Scholarships and Work-Study Grants
Performing Groups: Hastings College Players
Workshops/Festivals: Broken Heart Forensics Tournament

HIRAM SCOTT COLLEGE
Scottsbluff   Nebraska 69361, 308 635-3761
Private and 4 Year
Arts Areas: Instrumental Music, Vocal Music, Theatre and Visual Arts

MUSIC

Degrees Offered: BMus; BMusEd   *Teaching Certification Available*
Financial Assistance: Scholarships and Work-Study Grants

THEATRE

Degrees Offered: BA   *Teaching Certification Available*
Financial Assistance: Scholarships and Work-Study Grants
Performing Groups: HSC Theatre

JOHN F KENNEDY COLLEGE
Wahoo   Nebraska 68066, 402 443-4171
Private and 4 Year
Arts Areas: Instrumental Music, Vocal Music, Theatre and Visual Arts

MUSIC

Degrees Offered: BMus; BMusEd   *Teaching Certification Available*
Financial Assistance: Scholarships and Work-Study Grants

THEATRE

Degrees Offered: BA   *Teaching Certification Available*
Financial Assistance: Scholarships and Work-Study Grants   **Performing Groups:** Theatre Series

KEARNEY STATE COLLEGE
900 W 25th St, Kearney   Nebraska 68847
308 236-4449
State and 4 Year
Arts Areas: Instrumental Music, Vocal Music, Theatre, Television and Visual Arts
Performance Facilities: Fine Arts Building

MUSIC

Dr Gary Thomas, Head   **Number Of Faculty:** 11   **Number Of Students:** 130
Degrees Offered: BA; BA Ed; MSEd   *Teaching Certification Available*
Financial Assistance: Scholarships and Work-Study Grants
Workshops/Festivals: High School Band/Choral Clinic; High School Summer Fine Arts Festival; Piano Workshop

THEATRE

Fred Kootnz, Director   **Number Of Faculty:** 3   **Number Of Students:** 35
Degrees Offered: MA Theatre Arts   *Teaching Certification Available*
Financial Assistance: Scholarships and Work-Study Grants
Performing Groups: College Theatre; Touring Children's Theatre

MC COOK COLLEGE
McCook   Nebraska 69001, 308 345-6303
State and 2 Year
Arts Areas: Instrumental Music, Vocal Music and Visual Arts
Degrees Offered: AA   **Financial Assistance:** Scholarships

MIDLAND LUTHERAN COLLEGE
720 E Ninth St, Fremont   Nebraska 68025
402 721-5480
>Private and 4 Year
>*Arts Areas:* Instrumental Music, Vocal Music, Theatre, Television and Visual Arts
>*Performance Facilities:* Musbach Art Center; Eppley Auditorium; Old Gym; Griffith Chapel in Clemmons Hall

MUSIC

Dr Charles Wilhite, Professor   *Number Of Faculty:* 4
Number Of Students: 110   *Degrees Offered:* BA Mus
Courses Offered: Music Vocabulary; Literature; Conducting; Instrumental Music; Vocal Music
Technical Training: Ensemble   *Teaching Certification Available*
Financial Assistance: Scholarships and Work-Study Grants
Performing Groups: Midland College Choir; Midland College Band; Clef Dwellers; Midland Chamber Singers; Instrumental Ensembles
Workshops/Festivals: Opera Workshop; Midlands Jazz Festival

THEATRE

Dr William Deahl, Jr, Assistant Professor   *Number Of Faculty:* 2
Number Of Students: 50   *Degrees Offered:* BA Speech, Theatre
Courses Offered: Theatre Appreciation; Theatre Interpretation; Shakespeare, Theatre of the Absurd; Role of the Director; Development of Theatre
Technical Training: Internships   *Teaching Certification Available*
Financial Assistance: Scholarships and Work-Study Grants   *Workshops/Festivals:* Hosts Forensic Meets

NEBRASKA CHRISTIAN COLLEGE
Norfolk   Nebraska 68701, 402 371-5960
>Private and 4 Year   *Arts Areas:* Instrumental Music and Vocal Music

MUSIC

Degrees Offered: BA, Sacred Music   *Performing Groups:* Choir; Vocal & Instrumental Ensembles

NEBRASKA WESLEYAN UNIVERSITY
50th & Saint Paul, Lincoln   Nebraska 68504
402 466-2371 Ext 240
>Private and 4 Year
>*Arts Areas:* Instrumental Music, Vocal Music, Theatre and Visual Arts
>*Performance Facilities:* O'Donnell Auditorium; Emerson Recital Hall; Elder Gallery; Enid Miller Theatre; Lucas Loft Theatre; Brownville Village Theatre

MUSIC

Dr Paul R Swanson, Head   *Number Of Faculty:* 13   *Number Of Students:* 150
Degrees Offered: BA; BMus
Courses Offered: Applied Music (Instrumental or Vocal); Sacred Music; Music Education; Music - Theatre
Technical Training: Composition; Conducting; Church Music; Strings; Woodwinds; Brass; Vocal; Organ; Piano
Teaching Certification Available
Financial Assistance: Scholarships and Work-Study Grants
Performing Groups: University Band; University Orchestra; University Choir; Swing Choir; Treble Chorus; Wesleyan Glee; Chamber Singers; Brass Choir; Opera Theatre; Jazz Ensemble
Workshops/Festivals: Plainsman Honors Music Festival

THEATRE

Dr Philip Kaye, Head, Department of Speech, Communication, Theatre Arts
Number Of Faculty: 6   *Number Of Students:* 200   *Degrees Offered:* BA; BS
Courses Offered: Speech Communication; Theatre Arts; Speech Education; Interpersonal Communication

(continued on next page)

Technical Training: Technical Theatre; Debate; Forensics
Teaching Certification Available
Financial Assistance: Scholarships and Work-Study Grants
Performing Groups: Brownville Village Theatre Repertory Company
Workshops/Festivals: Brownville Village Theatre Summer Repertory Company

---

NEBRASKA WESTERN COLLEGE
1601 E 27th St, Scottsbluff   Nebraska 69361
308 635-3606 Ext 62
County and 2 Year
Arts Areas: Instrumental Music, Vocal Music, Theatre, Television and Visual Arts
Performance Facilities: Theater

MUSIC

William French, Instructor   **Number Of Faculty:** 2
Number Of Students: 50 - 75   **Degrees Offered:** AA
Courses Offered: Intro to Music; Music History; Chorus; Band; Theory I, II; Elementary Music
Technical Training: Woodwind; Brass; String; Keyboard
Financial Assistance: Scholarships, Work-Study Grants and Tuition Waivers
Performing Groups: X X T; Stage Band

THEATRE

Dr Dan Steadman, Instructor   **Number Of Faculty:** 1
Number Of Students: 35 - 50   **Degrees Offered:** AA
Courses Offered: Intro to Theater; All College Play; Stage Make-up
Technical Training: Stagecraft I, II
Financial Assistance: Scholarships, Work-Study Grants and Tuition Waivers
Performing Groups: Casts
Workshops/Festivals: One Act Play Festival - District VI

UNIVERSITY OF NEBRASKA, LINCOLN
Lincoln   Nebraska 68588, 402 472-7211
State and 4 Year
Arts Areas: Dance, Instrumental Music, Vocal Music, Theatre and Visual Arts

DANCE

Jim O'Hanlon, Interim Director   **Number Of Faculty:** 4
Number Of Students: 525   **Degrees Offered:** BA; BFA; BA Ed; BS Ed
Courses Offered: Modern & Folk Dance; Modern Jazz; Tap; Social & Square Dance; Ballet; Ethnic Dance; Rhythm Fundamentals/Individual Activity; Dance Workshop; Dance Performance; Practicum in Dance; Dance Composition; Movement Accompaniment; Anatomy; Kinesiology; Rhythmic Motor Movement
Technical Training: Ballet; Jazz; Folk; Ethnic; Social; Square; Tap
Teaching Certification Available   **Financial Assistance:** Scholarships
Performing Groups: The Dance Company; Orchesis; Lecture/Demonstration Group
Workshops/Festivals: Lincoln Community Arts Festival

MUSIC

Raymond Haggh, Director   **Number Of Faculty:** 46   **Number Of Students:** 391
Degrees Offered: BMus; BMusEd; BA; BS Ed; MM
Courses Offered: Music Theory; History; Literature; Musicology; Pedagogy; Ensembles; Applied Music; Music Education
Technical Training: Opera, Piano Design and Mechanics
Teaching Certification Available
Financial Assistance: Assistantships, Scholarships, Work-Study Grants and Hourly Wage
Performing Groups: Faculty Woodwind Quintet; Faculty Trio; Duo Faculty Recitals; Opera Performance; Madrigal Singers; Oratorio Choir; Varsity Glee Club; University Singers; University Chorale; University Orchestra; University Band; Chamber Ensembles

(continued on next page)

Workshops/Festivals: Ten - Twelve Music Ed Workshops Yearly; Performing Arts Series; Individual Touring Events; Czech Music Festival

THEATRE

Rex McGraw, Chairman   ***Number Of Faculty:*** 8   ***Number Of Students:*** 150
Degrees Offered: BA; BFA; MA; MFA; PhD
Teaching Certification Available   ***Financial Assistance:*** Scholarships and Work-Study Grants
Performing Groups: University Theatre; Studio Theatre; Laboratory & Experimental Theatres; Nebraska Repertory Theatre (summers); On The Spot (local touring musical group)
Workshops/Festivals: Nebraska Repertory Theatre; Workshops in all areas of theatre

---

THE UNIVERSITY OF NEBRASKA, OMAHA
60th & Dodge Sts (Box 688), Omaha   Nebraska 68101
402 554-2200
    State and 4 Year
    Arts Areas: Instrumental Music, Vocal Music, Theatre, Television and Visual Arts
    Performance Facilities: UNO Performing Arts Center; University Theatre

MUSIC

Jon J Polifrome, DMA, Chairperson   ***Number Of Faculty:*** 15
Number Of Students: 150   ***Degrees Offered:*** BMus; BMusEd; BS Mus Merchandising
Technical Training: Opera   ***Teaching Certification Available***
Financial Assistance: Assistantships, Scholarships, Work-Study Grants and Fellowships; Tuition Waivers
Performing Groups: The Band; Concert Choir; Choral Union; Town & Gown Orchestra; Brass Ensemble

THEATRE

Robert W Welk, Chairman   ***Number Of Faculty:*** 7   ***Number Of Students:*** 65
Degrees Offered: BA; BFA; MA   ***Teaching Certification Available***
Financial Assistance: Assistantships, Scholarships, Work-Study Grants and Fellowships, Tuition Waivers
Workshops/Festivals: American College Theatre

NORTH PLATTE COLLEGE
5th & Jeffers St, N Platte   Nebraska 69101
308 532-6888
    County and 2 Year
    Arts Areas: Instrumental Music, Theatre and Visual Arts

MUSIC
Robert M Rouch, Chairman   ***Degrees Offered:*** AA
Financial Assistance: Scholarships   ***Performing Groups:*** Instrumental Groups

THEATRE

Degrees Offered: AA   ***Financial Assistance:*** Scholarships
Performing Groups: College Theatre Company

NORTHEASTERN NEBRASKA COLLEGE
Norfolk   Nebraska 68701, 402 371-2020
    State and 2 Year
    Arts Areas: Instrumental Music, Vocal Music and Theatre
    Performing Series: Cultural Events Series   ***Performance Facilities:*** College Auditorium

MUSIC

Degrees Offered: AA   ***Financial Assistance:*** Scholarships and Work-Study Grants
Performing Groups: Instrumental & Vocal Ensembles

THEATRE

Degrees Offered: AA, Speech & Theatre

PERU STATE COLLEGE
Peru   Nebraska 68421, 402 872-3815
  State and 4 Year
  Arts Areas: Instrumental Music, Vocal Music, Theatre and Visual Arts
  Performance Facilities: Fine Arts Auditorium; Main Auditorium

MUSIC

Dr Gilbert Wilson, Chairman   **Number Of Faculty:** 4   **Number Of Students:** 60
Degrees Offered: BFA Ed
Technical Training: Marching Band Techniques; Arranging, Conducting, Woodwind Techniques; Form &
Composition; Music Therapy; Recreation Music
Teaching Certification Available
Financial Assistance: Special Ability Scholarships
Performing Groups: Concert Choir; Concert Band; Marching Band; Woodwind Choir; Clarinet Choir;
Stage Band; Swing Choir; Brass Ensemble
Workshops/Festivals: Band Clinic; Stage Band Clinic; Choir Clinic; Swing Choir Clinic; Homecoming
Parade & Band-O-Rama; Band, Choir, Swing Choir, Stage Band Tours of schools in area

THEATRE

Dr Royal Eckert, Chairman   **Number Of Faculty:** 2   **Number Of Students:** 25
Degrees Offered: BA
Technical Training: Stagecraft; Design (Students design most productions)
Teaching Certification Available
Financial Assistance: Special Ability Scholarships
Performing Groups: Peru Players Drama Club; Windwagon Touring Group
Workshops/Festivals: Summer Theatre Workshop; One - Act Play Festival
Artists-In-Residence/Guest Artists: Frank Erickson; Dr Kenneth Drake; Stewart Newbold; Tim Timmons

PLATTE TECHNICAL COMMUNITY COLLEGE
Box 1027, Columbus   Nebraska 68601
402 564-7132 Ext 267
  State and 2 Year
  Arts Areas: Instrumental Music, Vocal Music, Theatre and Visual Arts
  Performing Series: Fine Arts Festival
  Performance Facilities: College Auditorium

MUSIC

Number Of Faculty: 2   **Number Of Students:** 70   **Degrees Offered:** AA
Technical Training: Minor repair of instruments
Financial Assistance: Scholarships and Work-Study Grants
Performing Groups: Vocal & Instrumental Ensembles
Workshops/Festivals: Jazz Festival; Choral Festival; Choral Workshops; Musical Production Workshop

THEATRE

Number Of Faculty: 1   **Number Of Students:** 40   **Degrees Offered:** AA
Technical Training: Stage Technology   **Financial Assistance:** Scholarships and Work-Study Grants
Performing Groups: Repertory Theatre; Play Production
Workshops/Festivals: Stage Technology Workshop; Summer Theatre Workshop

PLATTE VALLEY BIBLE COLLEGE
305 E 16th St, Scottsbluff   Nebraska 69361
308 632-6933
  Private and 4 Year   **Arts Areas:** Instrumental Music and Vocal Music

MUSIC

Larry Cripe, Music Department Chairman   **Degrees Offered:** BA, Church Music
Performing Groups: Choir; Vocal & Instrumental Ensembles

SOUTHEAST COMMUNITY COLLEGE - FAIRBURY CAMPUS
924 K St, Fairbury   Nebraska 68352
402 729-6148

County and 2 Year
Arts Areas: Instrumental Music, Vocal Music and Theatre

MUSIC

Lewis P Bowling, Director   *Number Of Faculty:* 1½   *Number Of Students:* 24
Degrees Offered: AA
Financial Assistance: Scholarships and Work-Study Grants
Performing Groups: College Chorus; College Band; Vocal & Instrumental Ensemble

THEATRE

Terri Harris, Chairman   *Number Of Faculty:* 1½   *Number Of Students:* 18
Degrees Offered: AA
Financial Assistance: Scholarships and Work-Study Grants
Performing Groups: Drama Club; Traveling Playmakers

UNION COLLEGE
3800 S 48th, Lincoln   Nebraska 68506
402 488-2331 Ext 331

Private and 4 Year
Arts Areas: Instrumental Music, Vocal Music and Visual Arts
Performing Series: Concert & Recital Series
Performance Facilities: Recital Hall; Auditorium; Church

MUSIC

Number Of Faculty: 17   *Number Of Students:* 45
Degrees Offered: BMus; BMusEd   *Teaching Certification Available*
Financial Assistance: Scholarships and Work-Study Grants
Performing Groups: Two Concert Bands; Two Choirs; Brass Ensemble; Two Orchestras
Workshops/Festivals: Music Festival for High School Students

WAYNE STATE COLLEGE
Wayne   Nebraska 68787, 402 375-2200

State and 4 Year
Arts Areas: Instrumental Music, Vocal Music, Theatre, Television, Visual Arts and Radio
Performing Series: Special Program Series (concerts, theatre, lectures)
Performance Facilities: Val Peterson Fine Arts Center

MUSIC

Cornell Runestad, Head   *Number Of Faculty:* 7   *Number Of Students:* 75
Degrees Offered: BA; BA Ed; BFA Ed   *Teaching Certification Available*
Financial Assistance: Scholarships, Work-Study Grants and Federal Loans; Grants
Performing Groups: Concert Band; Concert Choir; Madrigal Singers; Jazz-Rock Ensemble; Concert
Orchestra; String Orchestra; Woodwind Ensemble; String Ensemble; Brass Ensemble
Workshops/Festivals: Summer Music Camp (high school); Festival/Clinics for High School Bands, Stage
Bands, Orchestras, Choirs

THEATRE

Helen J Russell, Professor   *Number Of Faculty:* 2   *Number Of Students:* 30
Degrees Offered: BA; BA Ed   *Teaching Certification Available*
Financial Assistance: Scholarships, Work-Study Grants and Federal Loans; Grants
Performing Groups: Improvisational Troupe
Workshops/Festivals: Make-up Workshop

YORK COLLEGE
9th & Kiplinger St, York   Nebraska 68467
402 362-4441
Private and 2 Year
Arts Areas: Instrumental Music, Vocal Music and Theatre
Performance Facilities: College Auditorium
Degrees Offered: AA, Mus; Certificate of Diploma (Instrumental, Vocal, Theory, Composition)
Performing Groups: Instrumental & Vocal Groups
Degrees Offered: Cert of Diploma; AA, Drama & Speech

UNIVERSITY OF NEVADA, LAS VEGAS
4505 Maryland Pkwy, Las Vegas   Nevada 89154
702 739-3011
State and 4 Year
Arts Areas: Dance, Instrumental Music, Vocal Music, Theatre, Film Arts, Television and Visual Arts
Performing Series: Concert Series
Performance Facilities: Judy Bayley Theatre; Artemus W Ham Concert Hall

DANCE

Carole Ray, Assistant Professor of Physical Education   *Number Of Faculty:* 1
Number Of Students: 250   *Degrees Offered:* BA
Courses Offered: Ballet; Jazz; Modern; Tap; Survey of Dance; Techniques of Recreational Dance;
Improvisation & Basic Stage Movement; Compositional Forms in Dance; Dance for Children; Dance in
Elementary Ed; Dance in Secondary Ed; Choreography; Accompaniment for Dance; Dance Notation
Financial Assistance: Assistantships and Work-Study Grants

MUSIC

Kenneth M Hanlon, Chairman   *Number Of Faculty:* 8   *Number Of Students:* 250
Degrees Offered: BA; BS   *Technical Training:* Opera; Jazz Internship Program
Teaching Certification Available
Financial Assistance: Scholarships, Work-Study Grants and Grants-in-aid
Performing Groups: Choral Group; Opera Theatre; Orchestra; Choir; Chamber Ensembles; Recitals
Workshops/Festivals: Elementary Music Workshop; Contemporary Music Festival

THEATRE

Robert Burgan, Chairman   *Number Of Faculty:* 7   *Number Of Students:* 200
Degrees Offered: BA Drama/Speech   *Teaching Certification Available*
Financial Assistance: Assistantships, Scholarships and Work-Study Grants
Performing Groups: University of Nevada Theatre; Youth - Children's Theatre; Summer Reperatory
Theatre

UNIVERSITY OF NEVADA, RENO
Reno   Nevada 89557, 702 784-6155
State and 4 Year
Arts Areas: Dance, Instrumental Music, Vocal Music, Theatre, Film Arts and Visual Arts
Performing Series: Performing Artist Series
Performance Facilities: Church Fine Arts Theatre

DANCE

Kristen A Avansino, Chairman   *Number Of Faculty:* 1
Number Of Students: 100
Degrees Offered: BA Physical Ed with emphasis in dance
Teaching Certification Available
Financial Assistance: Assistantships and Work-Study Grants
Performing Groups: University Dancers
Workshops/Festivals: Dance Workshop in summer; Spring Dance Review; Master Classes with Guest Artists
in fall & spring

MUSIC

Dr Roscoe Booth, Chairman   *Number Of Faculty:* 9   *Number Of Students:* 130
Degrees Offered: BMusEd; MA; MMus   *Teaching Certification Available*
Financial Assistance: Assistantships, Scholarships and Work-Study Grants
Performing Groups: Opera Workshop; University Symphony Orchestra; Brass Choir; Brass Quintet;
Concert Band; Jazz Band; Faculty Trio; Symphonic Choir; University Singers; Trombone Choir
Workshops/Festivals: Reno International Jazz Festival; Lake Tahoe Music Camp; UNR Arts Festival;
Opera Guild Performance

(continued on next page)

THEATRE

Dr Bob Dillard, Director   **Number Of Faculty:** 6   **Number Of Students:** 75
Degrees Offered: BA Arts & Sciences; BS Ed; MA
Teaching Certification Available
Financial Assistance: Assistantships, Scholarships and Work-Study Grants
Performing Groups: Nevada Repertory Company; Mime Repertory; Merry Miming Minstrals; Summer Festival
Workshops/Festivals: Summer Theatre; High School Drama Day

COLBY COLLEGE
New London   New Hampshire 03257, 603 526-2010
  Private and 4 Year
  Arts Areas: Dance, Instrumental Music, Vocal Music, Theatre, Film Arts and Visual Arts
  Performing Series: Performing Arts Series
  Performance Facilities: Sawyer Fine Arts Center

DANCE

Joel Conrad, Chairman   *Number Of Faculty:* 2   *Number Of Students:* 50
Degrees Offered: BFA   *Financial Assistance:* Assistantships

MUSIC

Nancy Draper, Chairman   *Number Of Faculty:* 5   *Number Of Students:* 50
Degrees Offered: BA

THEATRE

Eugene W Youngken, Chairman   *Number Of Faculty:* 5   *Number Of Students:* 50
Degrees Offered: BFA   *Financial Assistance:* Assistantships

DARTMOUTH COLLEGE
Hanover   New Hampshire 93755, 603 646-1110
  Private and 4 Year
  Arts Areas: Dance, Instrumental Music, Vocal Music, Theatre, Film Arts and Visual Arts
  Performing Series: Concert Series; Dartmouth Players
  Performance Facilities: Hopkins Center for the Creative & Performing Arts: Concert Hall, Two Theatres,
  Recital Hall

MUSIC

Charles E Hamm, Chairman   *Number Of Faculty:* 18   *Number Of Students:* 265
Degrees Offered: BA   *Courses Offered:* History; Theory; Performance
Financial Assistance: Scholarships, Work-Study Grants and Loans
Performing Groups: Collegium Musicum; Dartmouth Glee Clubs; Dartmouth Symphony Orchestra; Handel
Society Chorus; Dartmouth College Marching Band; Wind Ensemble; New Music Ensemble

THEATRE

Errol G Hill, Chairman   *Number Of Faculty:* 16   *Number Of Students:* 197
Degrees Offered: BA
Financial Assistance: Scholarships, Work-Study Grants and Loans
Performing Groups: Dartmouth Players
Artists-In-Residence/Guest Artists: Gyorgy Kepes

DOWLING COLLEGE
Idle Hour Blvd, Oakdale   New Hampshire 11769
516 589-6100
  Private and 4 Year
  Arts Areas: Instrumental Music, Vocal Music and Visual Arts

MUSIC

Carlo Lombardi, Coordinator   *Degrees Offered:* BA

FRANCONIA COLLEGE
Franconia   New Hampshire 03580, 603 823-5545
  Private and 4 Year
  Arts Areas: Dance, Instrumental Music, Vocal Music, Theatre, Film Arts and Visual Arts

(continued on next page)

Performing Series: Concert Series
Performance Facilities: Dow Theatre; Main Bldg Auditorium

DANCE

Marilyn Collins, Chairman   **Number Of Faculty:** 1   **Number Of Students:** 30
Degrees Offered: AA; BA   **Courses Offered:** Ballet; Modern
Financial Assistance: Scholarships and Work-Study Grants

MUSIC

Number Of Faculty: 1   **Number Of Students:** 30   **Degrees Offered:** AA; BA
Courses Offered: Piano; Voice; Composition; Theory; Ethnic Musicology
Financial Assistance: Scholarships and Work-Study Grants
Performing Groups: Chorus; Instrumental Ensembles
Workshops/Festivals: Jazz Workshops

THEATRE

Ken Grantham, Chairman   **Number Of Faculty:** 2   **Number Of Students:** 30
Degrees Offered: AA; BA
Financial Assistance: Scholarships and Work-Study Grants
Performing Groups: Shoestring Theatre

KEENE STATE COLLEGE
229 Main St, Keene   New Hampshire 03431
603 352-1909
State and 4 Year
Arts Areas: Dance, Instrumental Music, Vocal Music, Theatre and Visual Arts
Performing Series: Concert & Lecture Series

DANCE

Alta Lu Townes, Instructor   **Number Of Faculty:** 1   **Number Of Students:** 45
Courses Offered: Beginning & Intermediate Modern Dance

MUSIC

Miriam Goder, Chairman   **Number Of Faculty:** 25   **Number Of Students:** 120
Degrees Offered: BA; BMus   **Teaching Certification Available**
Financial Assistance: Scholarships and Work-Study Grants
Performing Groups: Concert Choir; Concert Band; Collegium Musicum; Vocal Consort; Jazz Ensemble;
Percussion Ensemble; Guitar Ensemble; Recitals
Workshops/Festivals: Jazz Ensemble often gives workshops while on tour in New England

THEATRE

Edith Notman, Chairman   **Performing Groups:** Keene State Theatre
theatre minor offered

NATHANIEL HAWTHORNE COLLEGE
Antrim   New Hampshire 03440, 603 588-6341
Private and 4 Year   **Arts Areas:** Theatre and Visual Arts
Performance Facilities: Fine Arts Studios; Theatre   **Number Of Faculty:** 1
Courses Offered: Modern Dance   **Technical Training:** Theatre Training
Teaching Certification Available
Financial Assistance: Scholarships and Work-Study Grants

NEW ENGLAND COLLEGE
Henniker   New Hampshire 03242, 603 428-2211
Private and 4 Year   **Arts Areas:** Instrumental Music and Theatre

(continued on next page)

MUSIC

Edward F Ulman, Coordinator   **Number Of Faculty:** 3
Performing Groups: Concerts   **Number Of Faculty:** 1   **Degrees Offered:** BA
Technical Training: Honors Program; Independent Study

UNIVERSITY OF NEW HAMPSHIRE
Durham   New Hampshire 03824, 603 862-2600
State and 4 Year
Arts Areas: Dance, Instrumental Music, Vocal Music, Theatre, Film Arts, Television and Visual Arts
Performing Series: UNH Celebrity Series
Performance Facilities: Johnson Theater; Hennessy Theater; Bratton Recital Hall

DANCE

David J Magidson, Chairman; Jean Brown, Director
Dance program under auspices of Theater & Communication Department
Number Of Faculty: 3   **Number Of Students:** 35
Degrees Offered: BA Theater & Communication
Courses Offered: Ballet; Modern; Jazz
Financial Assistance: Scholarships and Work-Study Grants
Performing Groups: UNH Dance Theatre Company
Workshops/Festivals: Lecture Demonstrations; Local & Regional Workshops

MUSIC

Paul F Verrette, Chairman   **Number Of Faculty:** 24   **Number Of Students:** 180
Degrees Offered: BA; BS; BMus; MA; MS   **Teaching Certification Available**
Financial Assistance: Assistantships, Scholarships and Work-Study Grants
Performing Groups: Concert Choir; Chamber Chorus; NH Women's Chorus; Symphony Group; Wind
Ensemble; Concert & Marching Bands; Jazz Ensemble; Chamber Groups
Workshops/Festivals: UNH Summer Youth Music School; Opera Workshops; NE Instrumental Music
Conference

THEATRE

David J Magidson, Chairman   **Number Of Faculty:** 17
Number Of Students: 100   **Degrees Offered:** BA Theatre
Technical Training: Directing; Scene & Light Design; Technical Theatre; Costume; Management;
Television; Film; Puppetry
Teaching Certification Available
Financial Assistance: Assistantships, Scholarships and Work-Study Grants
Performing Groups: University Theater; Durham Summer Theater; UNH Children's Theater; TRY &
Caravan; UNH Dance Theater Company
Workshops/Festivals: ACTF Regional Festivals; NETC Conventions; Durham Summer Theater workshops
Artists-In-Residence/Guest Artists: Arnold Stang

NOTRE DAME COLLEGE
2321 Elm St, Manchester   New Hampshire 03104
603 669-4298
Private and 4 Year
Arts Areas: Instrumental Music, Vocal Music and Visual Arts
Performance Facilities: Auditorium

MUSIC

Sister Anita Marchesseault, Coordinator
Degrees Offered: BA Mus Performance; BA MusEd; AAMus
Courses Offered: Music Theory; Music Education; History & Literature of Music; Studio Courses
Technical Training: Voice; Instrumental   **Teaching Certification Available**
Financial Assistance: Scholarships and Work-Study Grants

(continued on next page)

Performing Groups: Concert Choir; Stage Band; Chamber Singers; Recorder Consort; Opera Workshop
Workshops/Festivals: Organ Workshops annually each summer; Five-day organ & piano pedagogy workshop & three-day organ holiday; Annual Christmas Concert; Spring Opera

PETERBOROUGH PLAYERS
PO Box 1, Peterborough   New Hampshire 03458
603 924-3601

Private and Special   **Arts Areas:** Theatre
Performance Facilities: Peterborough Players Theatre   **Number Of Faculty:** 4
Number Of Students: 20
Technical Training: Concentrated Technical Training for Technical Apprentices
Performing Groups: Peterborough Players Professional Summer Theatre

PLYMOUTH STATE COLLEGE
Plymouth   New Hampshire 93264, 603 536-1550 ext 276
State and 4 Year
Arts Areas: Dance, Instrumental Music, Vocal Music, Theatre and Visual Arts
Performing Series: College Union Programing Board
Performance Facilities: Ernest L Siwer Hall

DANCE

Dr Douglas Wiseman, Chairman, Physical Education Department
Number Of Faculty: 3
Courses Offered: Social Dance; Modern Dance; Classical Ballet

MUSIC

Dr Walter P Smith, Chairman   **Degrees Offered:** BA MusEd; BA Mus
Technical Training: Applied Music   **Teaching Certification Available**
Financial Assistance: Scholarships
Performing Groups: Woodwind Ensemble; Pep & Symphonic Bands; Brass Choir; Jazz Band; Plymouth Singers; Women's Glee Club; Chamber Orchestra; Concerts; Recitals
Workshops/Festivals: PSC Jazz Festival; PSC Band Directors Clinic; PSC Music Education Conference; Rotary - Sponsored Musical Programs; Workshops

THEATRE

Dr Roi White, Director of Plymouth Players   **Number Of Faculty:** 1
Courses Offered: Speech; Intro to Theater; American Drama; World Drama; Oral Interpretation
Technical Training: Stagecraft; Scenery; Lighting; Make-up; Design; Costume Design; Acting
Teaching Certification Available   Financial Assistance: Scholarships
Performing Groups: Plymouth Players
Workshops/Festivals: High School Drama Festivals in the past

RIVIER COLLEGE
S Main St, Nashua   New Hampshire 03060
603 888-1311

Private and 4 Year
Arts Areas: Instrumental Music, Vocal Music and Visual Arts
Performing Series: Rivier College Humanities Series
Performance Facilities: Rivier College Auditorium; Rivier College Center Reception Room; Louis Pasteur Hall Auditorium

MUSIC

Sister Lilly Bergerson, Chairman   **Number Of Faculty:** 3
Number Of Students: 20   **Degrees Offered:** AMus; BMus; BA
Financial Assistance: Assistantships, Scholarships and Work-Study Grants
Performing Groups: Rivier College Glee Club
Workshops/Festivals: Christmas Program; Spring Festival

ALMA WHITE COLLEGE
Zarephath   New Jersey 08890, 201 356-1080
> Private and 4 Year   *Arts Areas:* Instrumental Music and Vocal Music
> *Performance Facilities:* WAWZ - Campus Radio; Auditorium; Chapel; Band Shell

MUSIC

> Eileen Pearsall, Chairman   *Number Of Faculty:* 2
> *Financial Assistance:* Work-Study Grants   *Performing Groups:* Orchestra; Choir

---

ALPHONSUS COLLEGE
87 Overlook Dr, Woodcliff   New Jersey 07680
201 391-8550
> Private and 2 Year
> *Arts Areas:* Instrumental Music, Vocal Music, Theatre and Visual Arts
> *Degrees Offered:* AA   *Performing Groups:* Singing Group

BERGEN COMMUNITY COLLEGE
Paramus   New Jersey 07652, 201 447-1500
> County and 2 Year
> *Arts Areas:* Instrumental Music, Vocal Music and Visual Arts
> *Degrees Offered:* AA   *Performing Groups:* Choir, Band

BLOOMFIELD COLLEGE
Bloomfield   New Jersey 07003, 201 748-9000 Ext 353
> Private and 4 Year
> *Arts Areas:* Instrumental Music, Vocal Music, Theatre and Visual Arts
> *Performance Facilities:* Westminister Theatre

MUSIC

> William Simon, Professor   *Number Of Faculty:* 2   *Degrees Offered:* BA
> *Courses Offered:* Vocal & Instrumental - Private Instructions
> *Financial Assistance:* Work-Study Grants
> *Performing Groups:* Bloomfield College Chorus

THEATRE

> *Number Of Faculty:* 22 *Number Of Students:* 35   *Degrees Offered:* BA
> *Courses Offered:* Theatre Studio & History of Theatre
> *Performing Groups:* Actor's Cafe Theatre
> *Artists-In-Residence/Guest Artists:* Actor's Cafe Theatre; Phoenix Quintet

---

BROOKDALE COMMUNITY COLLEGE
765 Newman Springs Rd, Lincroft   New Jersey 07738
201 842-1900 Ext 380
> County and 2 Year
> Robert SalemChairman, Creative Arts Learning Center
> *Arts Areas:* Dance, Instrumental Music, Vocal Music, Theatre, Film Arts, Television, Visual Arts and Radio
> *Performing Series:* Performing Arts Series; Music at Brookdale Series
> *Performance Facilities:* Brookdale Performing Arts Main Auditorium; Experimental Studio; Little Theatre
> *Number Of Faculty:* 3   *Degrees Offered:* AA
> *Courses Offered:* Introduction to Dance; Modern; Ballet; Jazz; Choreography
> *Financial Assistance:* Scholarships, Work-Study Grants and Student Workers
> *Performing Groups:* Brookdale Dance Company
> *Workshops/Festivals:* Two Evenings of Dance

(continued on next page)

MUSIC

Joseph Szostak, Team Leader, Music/Dance   *Number Of Faculty:* 2
Degrees Offered: AA   *Courses Offered:* Appreciation; Theory; Voice; Piano
Financial Assistance: Scholarships, Work-Study Grants and Student Workers

THEATRE

Phil Smith, Team Leader, Speech/Theatre   *Number Of Faculty:* 2
Degrees Offered: AA
Courses Offered: Acting; History; Appreciation; Musical Theatre; Directing; Children's Theatre; Intro to Technical Theatre; Intro to Visual Elements

---

CALDWELL COLLEGE
Caldwell   New Jersey 07006, 201 228-4424 Ext 45A
  Private and 4 Year
  Arts Areas: Instrumental Music, Vocal Music and Theatre
  Performing Series: Theatre-on-the-Hill
  Performance Facilities: Student Union Building

DANCE

Ballet program under the auspices of Physical Education Department

MUSIC

Sister May Ann, Chairman   *Number Of Faculty:* 12   *Number Of Students:* 30
Degrees Offered: BA Mus, BA MusEd   *Teaching Certification Available*
Financial Assistance: Scholarships and Work-Study Grants
Performing Groups: Concert Choir, Vocal Ensemble, Brass Choir, Stage Band, Caldwell College Singer, Wind Ensemble, String Ensemble
Performing Groups: Upstage Players Group, Theatre Workshop

CAMDEN COUNTY COLLEGE
PO Box 200, Blackwood   New Jersey 08012
609 227-7200 Ext 486
  County and 2 Year
  Arts Areas: Instrumental Music, Vocal Music, Theatre, Film Arts and Visual Arts
  Performing Series: Performing Arts Series
  Performance Facilities: Lincoln Hall

MUSIC

William Marlin, Chairman   *Number Of Faculty:* 1   *Number Of Students:* 40
Degrees Offered: AA
Courses Offered: Applied Music; Basic Musicianship; Music Theory; Survey of Music Literature; Music History; College Choir
Technical Training: Applied Music   *Financial Assistance:* Work-Study Grants
Performing Groups: Choir; Wind Ensemble

THEATRE

Dennis Flyer, Associate Professor of English/Drama   *Number Of Faculty:* 1
Number Of Students: 16   *Degrees Offered:* AA
Courses Offered: History of the Theatre; Dance & Movement for Actors; Voice & Diction; Drama Workshop; Acting; Stagecraft; Children's Theatre; Make-up
Technical Training: Acting; Stagecraft, Make-up; Costuming; Dance
Financial Assistance: Work-Study Grants
Performing Groups: Experimental Theatre

CENTENARY COLLEGE FOR WOMEN
Jefferson St, Hackettstown   New Jersey 07840
201 852-1400
Private and 2 Year
Arts Areas: Instrumental Music, Vocal Music and Theatre

MUSIC

Degrees Offered: BMus   *Technical Training:* Opera
Financial Assistance: Scholarships and Work-Study Grants   *Teaching Certification Available*

THEATRE

John D Babington, Chairman   *Number Of Faculty:* 2   *Number Of Students:* 25
Degrees Offered: BA   *Teaching Certification Available*
Financial Assistance: Scholarships and Work-Study Grants

CUMBERLAND COUNTY COLLEGE
College Dr, Vineland   New Jersey 08360
609 691-8600
County and 2 Year
Arts Areas: Instrumental Music, Vocal Music, Theatre and Visual Arts

MUSIC

Degrees Offered: AA   *Performing Groups:* Band, Choir

THEATRE

John Pyros, Chairman   *Degrees Offered:* AA

FAIRLEIGH DICKINSON UNIVERSITY
1000 River Rd, Teaneck   New Jersey 07666
201 836-6300 Ext 300
Private and 4 Year
Arts Areas: Dance, Instrumental Music, Vocal Music, Theatre, Film Arts, Television and Visual Arts
Performing Series: FDU Concert Series

DANCE

Prof Natalie Duffy, Director   *Number Of Faculty:* 1
Number Of Students: 15   *Financial Assistance:* Work-Study Grants

MUSIC

Prof John F Bullough, Chairman   *Number Of Faculty:* 8
Number Of Students: 25   *Degrees Offered:* BA Fine Arts Music Concentration
Financial Assistance: Work-Study Grants

THEATRE

Prof Theodore Chesler, Chairman   *Number Of Faculty:* 5
Number Of Students: 15   *Degrees Offered:* BA   *Financial Assistance:* Work-Study Grants

DOUGLASS COLLEGE
New Brunswick   New Jersey 08903, 201 247-2757
State and 4 Year
Arts Areas: Dance, Instrumental Music, Vocal Music, Theatre and Visual Arts

DANCE

Degrees Offered: BA, MA   *Teaching Certification Available*
Financial Assistance: Scholarships and Work-Study Grants

(continued on next page)

MUSIC

Number Of Faculty: 17
Number Of Students: 250   *Degrees Offered:* BA, MFA, MA Teaching
Teaching Certification Available
Financial Assistance: Scholarships and Work-Study Grants

THEATRE

Annette L Wood, Director   *Number Of Faculty:* 10   *Number Of Students:* 160
Degrees Offered: BA, MA, PhD   *Teaching Certification Available*
Financial Assistance: Scholarships and Work-Study Grants
Performing Groups: Queens Theatre Guild

DREW UNIVERSITY
36 Madison Ave, Madison   New Jersey 07940
201 377-3000
Private and 4 Year
Arts Areas: Dance, Instrumental Music, Vocal Music, Theatre, Film Arts and Visual Arts
Performance Facilities: Bowne Theatre; Cellar Theatre

DANCE

John Reeves, Associate Professor   *Number Of Faculty:* 1
Number Of Students: 41   *Courses Offered:* Intermediate & Advanced Dance
Financial Assistance: Work-Study Grants and Loans; Financial Aid Grants

MUSIC

Lydia Hailparn, Associate Professor   *Number Of Faculty:* 3
Number Of Students: 191   *Degrees Offered:* BA
Financial Assistance: Work-Study Grants and Financial Aid Grants, Loans
Performing Groups: Performing Ensemble; University Chorus; Madrigal Singers

THEATRE

R G McLaughlin, Assistant Professor   *Number Of Faculty:* 2
Number Of Students: 98   *Degrees Offered:* BA

FELICIAN COLLEGE
260 S Main St, Lodi   New Jersey 07095
201 778-1190 Ext 18
Private and 4 Year
Arts Areas: Instrumental Music, Vocal Music, Theatre, Film Arts and Visual Arts
Performing Series: Concert Series
Performance Facilities: Theatre; Auditorium

MUSIC

Joyce E Zakierski, MM, Chairman   *Number Of Faculty:* 2
Number Of Students: 100   *Degrees Offered:* BA
Financial Assistance: Internships, Scholarships and Work-Study Grants
Performing Groups: Felician Community Chorale; Felician Singers; Felician Folksingers
Workshops/Festivals: Christmas Concert; Spring Festival

THEATRE

Performing Groups: The Twinklers, Children's Theatre Group
Workshops/Festivals: Annual Children's Theatre Production

GEORGIAN COURT COLLEGE
Lakewood Ave, Lakewood   New Jersey 08701
201 364-2200
Private and 4 Year
Arts Areas: Instrumental Music, Vocal Music and Visual Arts
Performing Series: Dramatic Performances, Lectures, Film Series

MUSIC

Number Of Faculty: 3   **Number Of Students:** 30   **Degrees Offered:** BA, BS
Teaching Certification Available
Financial Assistance: Scholarships and Work-Study Grants

GLASSBORO STATE COLLEGE
Glassboro   New Jersey 08028, 609 445-7388
State and 4 Year
Arts Areas: Dance, Instrumental Music, Vocal Music, Theatre and Visual Arts
Performing Series: College Performance Series
Performance Facilities: Wilson Concert Hall, Wilson Recital Hall, Tohill Auditorium

DANCE

Tage Wood, Chairman   **Number Of Faculty:** 3   **Number Of Students:** 200
Degrees Offered: BA   **Technical Training:** Modern, Ethnic, Ballet, Jazz Dance
Teaching Certification Available
Performing Groups: Dance Ensemble; Artist-in-Residence, Alexei Yudenich
Workshops/Festivals: Alvin Ailey City Center Dance Company, Jose Greco Dance Company

MUSIC

Dr Clarke Pfleeger, Chairman   **Number Of Faculty:** 29
Number Of Students: 377   **Degrees Offered:** BA
Technical Training: Musicology, Music Therapy, Church Music, Instrumental, Vocal, Teacher Training, Accordion, Jazz Studies, Electronic Music
Teaching Certification Available
Performing Groups: Madrigal Society, Lab Band, Women's Chorus, College Band, Concert Choir, College - Community Orchestra, Avant Gard Jazz Ensemble, Wind Ensemble, Percussion Ensemble, Woodwind Ensemble, Brass Ensemble, Jazz Ensemble, String Ensemble, Trombone Choir
Workshops/Festivals: Contemporary Music Festival, Solo & Ensemble Festival, Opera Workshop, South Jersey Band, American Music Week, New Jersey Orchestra Festival, High School Jazz Festival, Intercollegiate Jazz Festival

THEATRE

Dr Michael Kelly, Chairman   **Number Of Faculty:** 12
Number Of Students: 119   **Degrees Offered:** BA
Technical Training: Children's Theatre, Costume Design, Acting
Teaching Certification Available   **Performing Groups:** Campus Players
Workshops/Festivals: Mainstage Productions, New Playwrights Workshop, Lab Theatre, Glassboro Summer Theatre

JERSEY CITY STATE COLLEGE
2039 Kennedy Memorial Blvd, Jersey City   New Jersey 07305
201 547-6000
State and 4 Year
Arts Areas: Dance, Instrumental Music, Vocal Music, Theatre, Film Arts, Television and Visual Arts
Performance Facilities: Gothic Theatre, Margaret Williams Auditorium, Student Union Building

DANCE

Stefan Rudnicki, Chairperson   **Number Of Faculty:** 4
Number Of Students: 150

(continued on next page)

MUSIC

Dr Stelio Dubbiosi, Chairperson   **Number Of Faculty:** 24
Number Of Students: 250   **Degrees Offered:** MA MusEd; BA Mus & MusEd
Courses Offered: Musical Theatre   **Teaching Certification Available**
Financial Assistance: Assistantships, Scholarships and Work-Study Grants
Performing Groups: College Choir; Concert Vocal Ensemble; Woman's & Men's Choirs; Madrigal Singers; Jazz/Pop Vocal Ensemble; College-Community Orchestra; JCSC Symphonic Band; Flute, Clarinet, Saxophone, Brass, Early Music Instrumental, Early Music Recorder, Guitar, Percussion Ensembles; String, Brass, Woodwind Quintets; Piano, Jazz Ensembles; Jazz Lab Band; Wind Ensemble; Double Bass Ensemble

THEATRE

Stefan Rudnicki, Chairperson   **Number Of Faculty:** 5
Number Of Students: 200

KEAN COLLEGE OF NEW JERSEY
Morris Ave, Union   New Jersey 07083
201 527-2107

State and 4 Year
Arts Areas: Dance, Instrumental Music, Vocal Music, Theatre, Film Arts, Television and Visual Arts
Performing Series: Concert, Lecture, Drama Series
Performance Facilities: Eugene G Wilkins Theatre for the Performing Arts

DANCE

Dr Nettie Smith, Chairman   **Number Of Faculty:** 4
Technical Training: Modern Dance, Folk Dance, Ballet
Financial Assistance: Work-Study Grants   **Performing Groups:** Dance Theatre (Modern)

MUSIC

Herbert Golub, Chairman   **Number Of Faculty:** 18   **Number Of Students:** 180
Degrees Offered: BA   **Teaching Certification Available**   **Financial Assistance:** Scholarships
Performing Groups: Performing Arts Trio, Concert Chorus, Concert Band, Percussion Ensemble, Woodwind Ensemble

THEATRE

Dr Elizabeth Huberman, Chairman   **Number Of Faculty:** 8
Number Of Students: 40
Technical Training: Acting, Creative Drama, Children's Theatre, Scenic Design, Technical Theater
Financial Assistance: Work-Study Grants
Performing Groups: Theatre Guild, Reader's Theatre Group
Workshops/Festivals: Spring Poetry Reading Contest, Forensic Contests

---

MERCER COUNTY COMMUNITY COLLEGE
1200 Old Trenton Rd, Trenton   New Jersey 08690
609 586-4800 Ext 296

County and 2 Year   **Arts Areas:** Television and County
Performing Series: Performing Arts Series
Performance Facilities: Kelsey Theatre, West Windsor Campus

DANCE

Number Of Faculty: 1   **Number Of Students:** 20   **Degrees Offered:** AA
Financial Assistance: Work-Study Grants
Performing Groups: Mercer Dance Theatre

MUSIC

Number Of Faculty: 3   **Number Of Students:** 85   **Degrees Offered:** AA
Financial Assistance: Work-Study Grants

(continued on next page)

Performing Groups: Stage Band; Chorus; Instrumental Ensemble
Number Of Faculty: 2   *Number Of Students:* 60   *Degrees Offered:* AA
Courses Offered: Introduction to Theatre; Stagecraft; Play Production; Fundamentals of Acting; Theatre
Workshop
Financial Assistance: Work-Study Grants   *Performing Groups:* Mercer College Theatre

MONTCLAIR STATE COLLEGE
Upper Montclair   New Jersey 07043, 201 893-5103
State and 4 Year
Arts Areas: Dance, Instrumental Music, Vocal Music, Theatre, Film Arts, Television and Visual Arts
Performance Facilities: Montclair State College Memorial Auditorium

DANCE

Number Of Faculty: 3   *Number Of Students:* 35   *Degrees Offered:* BA
Financial Assistance: Internships, Assistantships and Work-Study Grants
Performing Groups: Impulse Dance Company
Workshops/Festivals: Spring Dance Festival

MUSIC

Dr Benjamin F Wilkes, Chairman   *Number Of Faculty:* 45
Number Of Students: 445
Degrees Offered: BA Music Education, Therapy, Theory/Composition
Technical Training: Equivalency in Music Therapy
Teaching Certification Available
Financial Assistance: Assistantships, Scholarships and Work-Study Grants
Performing Groups: Faculty String Quartet, Concert Choir, College Choir, Orchestra, Lab Orchestra,
Symphonic Band, Concert Band, Marching Band (Lab), Stage Band (Lab)
Workshops/Festivals: Kodaly - Orff Workshop, Robert Page Workshop sponsored by the National Piano
Foundation

THEATRE

Karl R Moll, Chairman   *Number Of Faculty:* 9   *Number Of Students:* 150
Degrees Offered: BA, MA   *Teaching Certification Available*
Financial Assistance: Internships, Assistantships and Work-Study Grants
Performing Groups: Major Theater Series   *Workshops/Festivals:* ACTF

THE NEW SCHOOL FOR MUSIC STUDY
Box 407, Princeton   New Jersey 08540
609 921-2900
Private and Special   *Arts Areas:* Instrumental Music

MUSIC

Frances O Clark, President, Louise L Goss, Director   *Number Of Faculty:* 8
Number Of Students: 120
Courses Offered: Full-year program in post-graduate piano Pedagogy
Teaching Certification Available   Financial Assistance: Internships and Scholarships
Workshops/Festivals: Workshops, Seminars & Study Courses for Piano Teachers

NORTHEASTERN COLLEGIATE BIBLE INSTITUTE
Oak Lane, Essex Fells   New Jersey 07021
201 226-1074
Private and 4 Year   *Arts Areas:* Instrumental Music and Vocal Music

MUSIC

Frank Johnston, Chairman, Department of Sacred Music   *Number Of Faculty:* 5
Number Of Students: 25   *Degrees Offered:* BS Sacred Music
Courses Offered: Theory; Conducting; Composition; Counterpoint; Music in Elementary Schools; Diction;
Hymnology; Music History

(continued on next page)

Technical Training: Private instruction in any instrument, voice, conducting, composition
Financial Assistance: Scholarships and Work-Study Grants
Performing Groups: Quiet Hope   **Workshops/Festivals:** Artist Series Concerts

---

OCEAN COUNTY COLLEGE
College Dr, Toms River   New Jersey 08753
201 255-4000 Ext 275
County and 2 Year
Arts Areas: Dance, Instrumental Music, Vocal Music, Theatre, Film Arts and Visual Arts
Performing Series: Concert Series; Dramatic Series
Performance Facilities: Auditorium

DANCE

Dr James Doran, Chairman   **Number Of Faculty:** 2   **Number Of Students:** 72
Courses Offered: Ballet; Modern Ballet
Financial Assistance: Work-Study Grants

MUSIC

Dr James Doran, Chairman   **Number Of Faculty:** 4   **Number Of Students:** 26
Courses Offered: Appreciation; Theory; Harmony; Chorus; Band
Financial Assistance: Work-Study Grants
Performing Groups: Community Chorus; College Choir

THEATRE

Dr James Doran, Chairman   **Number Of Faculty:** 2   **Number Of Students:** 16
Courses Offered: Acting, Stagecraft, Script to Stage
Financial Assistance: Work-Study Grants
Performing Groups: Ocean County College Theatre Company

PRINCETON UNIVERSITY
Princeton   New Jersey 08540, 609 452-4240
Private and 4 Year
Arts Areas: Dance, Instrumental Music, Vocal Music, Theatre and Visual Arts
Performing Series: Concert Series
Performance Facilities: McCarter Theatre; Alexander Hall; Woolworth Center; 10 McCosh Hall

DANCE

Ms Ze'eva Cohen, Director of Dance Studies   **Number Of Faculty:** 3
Number Of Students: 200
Courses Offered: Technique; Modern Dance; Choreography; Composition
Financial Assistance: Regular University Financial Aid
Workshops/Festivals: A Dance Recital with pieces choreographed by students and by faculty annually

MUSIC

Peter Westergaard, Chairman, Professor   **Number Of Faculty:** 12
Number Of Students: 60   **Degrees Offered:** AB; MFA; PhD
Financial Assistance: Internships, Assistantships and Scholarships
Performing Groups: P U Orchestra; P U Glee Club; Marching Band; Chapel Choir; Concert Band; Glee Club; Jazz Ensembles; Opera Theatre

THEATRE

Daniel Seltzer, Professor of English; Director, Program in Theatre & Dance
Number Of Faculty: 7   **Number Of Students:** 220
Courses Offered: Acting; Mime; Directing; Movement; Stage Design; Voice; Playwriting

PRINCETON UNIVERSITY

Princeton   New Jersey 08540, 609 452-3000

Private and 4 Year
Arts Areas: Dance, Instrumental Music, Vocal Music, Theatre and Visual Arts
Performing Series: Concert Series
Performance Facilities: Student Theatre, McCarter Theatre

DANCE

Ze'eva Cohen, Director of Program   *Number Of Students:* 100
Dance program under auspices of Theatre Department
Technical Training: Modern, Improvisation

MUSIC

Peter Westergaard, Chairman
Degrees Offered: BA Mus; MFA; PhD Music History, Theory, Composition
Technical Training: Electronic Studio, Computer Synthesis of Sound
Financial Assistance: Assistantships and Scholarships
Performing Groups: Chapel Choir, Orchestra, Chorus, Opera Theatre, Freshman Singers, Band

THEATRE

Dan Seltzer, Director   *Number Of Faculty:* 8   *Number Of Students:* 300
Degrees Offered: Individual Independent Major Degrees may be applied
Technical Training: Acting, Directing, Scene Design, Lighting
The emphasis of the Theatre program is to educate the student into the knowledge of the complexity of performing arts through experience and analysis.

RAMAPO COLLEGE

Mahwah   New Jersey 07430, 201 825-2800

Private and 4 Year
Arts Areas: Instrumental Music, Vocal Music and Theatre
Degrees Offered: BA Speech - Theatre   *Teaching Certification Available*
Financial Assistance: Work-Study Grants   *Performing Groups:* Ramapo Players

RIDER COLLEGE

2083 Lawrenceville Rd, Lawrenceville   New Jersey 08648
609 896-0800 Ext 368

Private and 4 Year
Arts Areas: Instrumental Music, Theatre and Visual Arts
Performance Facilities: Two Theatres; One Studio Theatre

MUSIC

Larry Capo, Chairman, Fine Arts   *Number Of Faculty:* 3
Number Of Students: 20   *Degrees Offered:* BA
Courses Offered: Music History; Music Theory
Technical Training: Piano; Instrumental   *Teaching Certification Available*
Financial Assistance: Work-Study Grants
Performing Groups: Rider Chorale; Rider Instrumental Ensemble

THEATRE

Larry Capo, Chairman, Fine Arts   *Number Of Faculty:* 4
Number Of Students: 40   *Degrees Offered:* BA
Courses Offered: History; Survey
Technical Training: Acting; Technical Theatre; Directing; Make-up
Teaching Certification Available   *Financial Assistance:* Work-Study Grants
Workshops/Festivals: High School Drama Festival

RUTGERS UNIVERSITY
The State University of New Jersey, New Brunswick   New Jersey 08903
201 247-1766
    State and 4 Year
    Arts Areas: Dance, Instrumental Music, Vocal Music and Theatre

MUSIC

George J Buelow, Director   *Number Of Faculty:* 18   *Number Of Students:* 60
Degrees Offered: BMus, BMusEd, MFA, MA Teaching
Financial Assistance: Scholarships and Work-Study Grants
Performing Groups: Orchestra, String Ensembles, Wind Ensembles, Choral Group
Degrees Offered: BA
Financial Assistance: Scholarships and Work-Study Grants
Performing Groups: RU Players

RUTGERS UNIVERSITY, CAMDEN COLLEGE OF ARTS & SCIENCES
311 N Fifth St, Camden   New Jersey 08102
609 757-1766
    State and 4 Year
    Arts Areas: Instrumental Music, Vocal Music, Theatre and Visual Arts
    Performance Facilities: Theatre; Rehearsal Hall

MUSIC

Dr Wilbert Davis Jerome, Chairman   *Number Of Faculty:* 4
Number Of Students: 36   *Degrees Offered:* BA
Courses Offered: Theory; Composition; Performance; Music History; Literature
Technical Training: Applied music instruction is by arrangement
Teaching Certification Available
Financial Assistance: Scholarships and Work-Study Grants
Performing Groups: Rutgers Repertory Singers; Chamber Ensemble

THEATRE

Georgia Gresham, Acting Chairperson & Assistant Professor
Number Of Faculty: 7   *Number Of Students:* 61   *Degrees Offered:* BA
Courses Offered: Acting; Directing; Playwriting; Scenic Design
Technical Training: Lighting Design; Sound Creation; Stage Management
Financial Assistance: Scholarships and Work-Study Grants
Performing Groups: Rutgers Livestock
Workshops/Festivals: Three major productions annually; One - Act play contest

RUTGERS UNIVERSITY, DOUGLASS COLLEGE
New Brunswick   New Jersey 08903, 201 932-9721
    State and 4 Year
    Arts Areas: Dance, Instrumental Music, Vocal Music, Theatre, Film Arts, Television and Visual Arts
    Performance Facilities: Experimental Theater, Little Theater, Voorhees Chapel, Rehearsal Hall

DANCE

Nancy Mitchell, Chairman   *Number Of Faculty:* 6   *Number Of Students:* 51
Degrees Offered: BA   *Technical Training:* Stage Lighting, Choreography

MUSIC

Kunrad Kvam, Chairman   *Number Of Faculty:* 23   *Number Of Students:* 76
Degrees Offered: BA, MFA, MA, PhD   *Teaching Certification Available*
Financial Assistance: Assistantships, Scholarships and Work-Study Grants
Performing Groups: Choir, Orchestra
Workshops/Festivals: American String Teachers Workshop

(continued on next page)

THEATRE

John Bettenbender, Chairman   **Number Of Faculty:** 8   **Number Of Students:** 70
Degrees Offered: BA, MA   **Teaching Certification Available**
Financial Assistance: Assistantships, Scholarships and Work-Study Grants
Performing Groups: Paul Robeson Group, Children's Theatre Program, Root (Black Theatre Group)

RUTGERS UNIVERSITY, NEWARK
392 High St, Newark   New Jersey 07102
201 648-5205
State and 4 Year
Arts Areas: Instrumental Music, Vocal Music, Theatre and Visual Arts

MUSIC

Chester Fanning Smith, Chairman   **Number Of Faculty:** 17
Number Of Students: 80   **Degrees Offered:** BMus   **Technical Training:** Opera
Financial Assistance: Scholarships and Work-Study Grants
Performing Groups: University Chorus, Orchestra, Instrumental Ensembles

THEATRE

Lester L Moore, Chairman   **Number Of Faculty:** 4   **Degrees Offered:** BA
Financial Assistance: Scholarships and Work-Study Grants   **Performing Groups:** The Mummers

SALESIAN COLLEGE
North Haledon   New Jersey 07508, 201 427-0452
Private and 2 Year
Arts Areas: Instrumental Music, Vocal Music, Theatre and Visual Arts
Degrees Offered: AA   **Performing Groups:** Chorus, Band   **Degrees Offered:** AA
Performing Groups: Salesian Dramatic Club

STOCKTON STATE COLLEGE
Pomona   New Jersey 08240, 609 652-1776 Ext 505
State and 4 Year
Arts Areas: Dance, Instrumental Music, Vocal Music, Theatre, Film Arts, Television and Visual Arts
Performing Series: Guest Artist Series
Performance Facilities: Dance Studio; Experimental Theatre; Main House Theatre

DANCE

Pat Hecht, Coordinator   **Number Of Faculty:** 1   **Degrees Offered:** BA
Technical Training: Individual Studies
Financial Assistance: Internships, Assistantships, Scholarships and Work-Study Grants

MUSIC

Number Of Faculty: 5   **Degrees Offered:** BA
Technical Training: Individual attention to Opera, Piano, Woodwind, String
Financial Assistance: Internships, Assistantships, Scholarships and Work-Study Grants
Performing Groups: Chorus; Orchestra; Various Ensembles

THEATRE

Number Of Faculty: 2   **Degrees Offered:** BA   **Technical Training:** Individual Studies
Financial Assistance: Internships, Assistantships, Scholarships and Work-Study Grants

TRENTON STATE COLLEGE
Pennington Rd, Trenton   New Jersey 08625
609 771-1855
State and 4 Year
Arts Areas: Instrumental Music, Vocal Music, Theatre and Visual Arts
Performing Series: Cultural Series

(continued on next page)

MUSIC

Robert J Rittenhouse, Chairman   **Number Of Faculty:** 22
Number Of Students: 325   **Degrees Offered:** BMus, BMusEd, MMus, MMusEd
Technical Training: Opera   **Teaching Certification Available**
Performing Groups: Orchestra, Chorale Ensemble, Instrumental Groups
Workshops/Festivals: Opera Workshop

THEATRE

Harold A Hogstrom, Chairman   **Number Of Faculty:** 12
Number Of Students: 250   **Degrees Offered:** BA Speech - Drama
Teaching Certification Available   **Performing Groups:** Trenton State Theatre

---

UNION COLLEGE
1033 Springfield Ave, Cranford   New Jersey 07016
201 276-2600
　　　Private and 2 Year   **Arts Areas:** Theatre and Visual Arts

THEATRE

Donald H Julian, Chairman   **Number Of Faculty:** 1

UPSALA COLLEGE
East Orange   New Jersey 07019, 201 266-7107
　　　Private and 4 Year
　　　Arts Areas: Instrumental Music, Vocal Music and Theatre
　　　Performing Series: Sundays at Upsala
　　　Performance Facilities: Theatre; Gym; Auditorium

MUSIC

Professor Hugo Lutz, Chairman, Department of Fine Arts
Number Of Faculty: 2   **Number Of Students:** 18   **Degrees Offered:** BA
Courses Offered: Theory; Performance; Composition
Financial Assistance: Scholarships
Performing Groups: College Choir; Chamber Singers

THEATRE

Dr Robert Henson, Chairman, Department of English/Theatre
Number Of Faculty: 14   **Number Of Students:** 40   **Degrees Offered:** BA
Courses Offered: Intro Voice & Diction; Fundamentals of Acting, Producting, Playwriting & Directing
Technical Training: Production; Directing   **Financial Assistance:** Scholarships
Performing Groups: Workshop 90
Workshops/Festivals: High School Drama competition

WESTMINISTER CHOIR COLLEGE
Hamilton & Walnut, Princeton   New Jersey 08540
609 921-7100
　　　Private and 4 Year   **Arts Areas:** Instrumental Music and Vocal Music

MUSIC

Peter D Wright, Dean of College   **Number Of Faculty:** 60
Number Of Students: 450
Degrees Offered: BMus Church Music, Organ, Piano, Voice; BMusEd; MMus Choral Conducting, Church Music, Organ; MMusEd
Technical Training: Opera, Organ
Financial Assistance: Scholarships and Work-Study Grants
Performing Groups: Opera Theatre, Chapel Choir, Symphonic Choir, Instrumental Ensembles

WILLIAM PATERSON COLLEGE
300 Pompton Rd, Wayne   New Jersey 07470
201 595-2314
State and 4 Year
Arts Areas: Instrumental Music, Vocal Music, Theatre, Film Arts and Television
Performance Facilities: Shea Auditorium; Theater II; Coach House; Hobart Hall TV & Film Studio

MUSIC

Robert Latherow, Chairperson   *Number Of Faculty:* 18
Number Of Students: 325   *Degrees Offered:* BS MusEd; BA
Courses Offered: Vocal; Instrumental; Jazz   *Teaching Certification Available*
Financial Assistance: Assistantships, Scholarships and Work-Study Grants
Performing Groups: Orchestra; Band; NJ Percussion Ensemble; Jazz Band; College Chorus
Workshops/Festivals: Performing Artist Series

THEATRE

Dr Bruce Gulbranson, Chairman   *Number Of Faculty:* 12
Number Of Students: 80   *Degrees Offered:* BA
Teaching Certification Available
Financial Assistance: Assistantships, Scholarships and Work-Study Grants
Performing Groups: Pioneer Players

COLLEGE OF ARTESIA
Artesia New Mexico 88210, 505 746-9862
Private and 4 Year
Arts Areas: Instrumental Music, Vocal Music, Theatre and Visual Arts

MUSIC

Degrees Offered: BMus, BMusEd   *Teaching Certification Available*
Financial Assistance: Scholarships   *Performing Groups:* Ensembles, Band, Chorus

THEATRE

Degrees Offered: BA Speech - Theatre   *Teaching Certification Available*
Financial Assistance: Scholarships

COLLEGE OF SANTA FE
St Michael's Dr, Santa Fe   New Mexico 87501
505 982-6439
Private and 4 Year
Arts Areas: Dance, Instrumental Music, Vocal Music, Theatre and Visual Arts
Performance Facilities: Greer Garson Theatre; Kinsella Hall

DANCE

John C Weckesser, Chairman   *Number Of Faculty:* 1   *Number Of Students:* 10
Degrees Offered: Minor in Dance
Courses Offered: Basic Movement; Special Studies in Dance; Mime
Financial Assistance: Scholarships, Work-Study Grants and Service Scholarships

MUSIC

Suzanne M Harkins, Director   *Number Of Faculty:* 2
Courses Offered: Voice; Private Instruction; Theory; Ensembles; Enjoyment of Music; Piano; Guitar
Financial Assistance: Scholarships, Work-Study Grants and Service Scholarships; Grants; Student Loans
Performing Groups: Collegium Musicum of CSF (vocal group)
Workshops/Festivals: Student recitals are held on a regular basis to prepare students for performing

THEATRE

John C Weckesser, Chairman   *Number Of Faculty:* 5
Degrees Offered: BA in Theatre (Acting) or Design/technical Theatre; BFA in Acting or Design/Technical Theatre
Courses Offered: Acting; Directing; Stagecraft; Costuming; Audition Training; Speech; Oral Interpretation
Technical Training: Stagecraft; Lighting Design; Practicum in Theatre; Costuming
Financial Assistance: Scholarships, Work-Study Grants and Service Scholarships; Grants; Student Loans
Workshops/Festivals: Studio production - directed and entirely executed by students
Artists-In-Residence/Guest Artists: Five members of the Royal Shakespeare Co; John Reardon

COLLEGE OF SANTA FE
Santa Fe   New Mexico 87501, 505 982-6131
Private and 4 Year   *Arts Areas:* Theatre
Degrees Offered: BA Theatre Arts   *Teaching Certification Available*
Financial Assistance: Scholarships and Work-Study Grants

EASTERN NEW MEXICO UNIVERSITY, PORTALES
Portales   New Mexico 88130, 505 562-1011
State and 4 Year
Arts Areas: Instrumental Music, Vocal Music, Theatre and Visual Arts

MUSIC

Floren Thompson Jr, Chairman   *Number Of Faculty:* 19
Number Of Students: 180   *Degrees Offered:* BMus, BMusEd, MMus, MMusEd

(continued on next page)

Teaching Certification Available   Financial Assistance: Scholarships
Performing Groups: Ensembles, Band, Chorus

THEATRE

R Lyle Hagan, Chairman   **Number Of Faculty:** 3
Degrees Offered: BA Drama - Speech, MA Drama - Speech
Teaching Certification Available   Financial Assistance: Scholarships
Performing Groups: University Theatre

MOORHEAD STATE UNIVERSITY
Moorhead   New Mexico 56560, 218 236-2762
State and 4 Year
Arts Areas: Instrumental Music, Vocal Music, Theatre, Film Arts, Television and Visual Arts
Performing Series: Performing Arts Series
Performance Facilities: Center for the Arts Auditorium; Weld Hall Auditorium
Center for the Arts Recital Hall ; Wooden Nickel Coffeehouse

MUSIC

Dr Donald Key, Chairperson   **Number Of Faculty:** 22
Number Of Students: 180
Degrees Offered: BS; BA; MSEd with concentration in music
Teaching Certification Available
Financial Assistance: Assistantships, Scholarships and Work-Study Grants
Performing Groups: Choirs; Wind Instrument Groups; Orchestra; Stage Band
Workshops/Festivals: Opera Workshop

THEATRE

Dr Delmar Hansen, Chairperson   **Number Of Faculty:** 5
Number Of Students: 95
Degrees Offered: BS; BA; MSEd with concentration in Speech - Theatre
Teaching Certification Available
Financial Assistance: Assistantships, Scholarships and Work-Study Grants
Performing Groups: MSC Theatre; Readers' Theatre; Children's Theatre
Workshops/Festivals: Full summer program of productions

NEW MEXICO HIGHLANDS UNIVERSITY
Las Vegas   New Mexico 87701, 505 425-7511 Ext 359
State and 4 Year
Arts Areas: Instrumental Music, Vocal Music and Theatre
Performing Series: NMHU Drama Series; NMHU Lyceum Series
Performance Facilities: Ilfeld Auditorium; Sala de Madrid

MUSIC

Dr Grady Greene, Chairman, Department of Fine Arts   **Number Of Faculty:** 6
Number Of Students: 80   **Degrees Offered:** BA; MA
Courses Offered: Instrumental; Vocal; Keyboard; Classical Guitar
Teaching Certification Available
Financial Assistance: Assistantships, Scholarships, Work-Study Grants and Activity Award
Performing Groups: Band; Choir; Instrumental Ensembles; Celebration
Workshops/Festivals: Band & Vocal Festivals; Classical Guitar Workshop

THEATRE

Dr Grady Greene, Chairman, Department of Fine Arts   **Number Of Faculty:** 2
Number Of Students: 40   **Degrees Offered:** BA
Courses Offered: Acting; Directing; Stagecraft
Technical Training: Stagecraft   **Teaching Certification Available**
Financial Assistance: Assistantships, Scholarships, Work-Study Grants and Activity Award
Performing Groups: The Walkaways; Standard University Open Casting

(continued on next page)

Workshops/Festivals: Albuquerque Dance Theater; Theater Arts Corp of Santa Fe; State Theater of New Mexico; El Teatro Campesino
Artists-In-Residence/Guest Artists: Dr Loren E Wise, Composer-in-Residence

NEW MEXICO JUNIOR COLLEGE
Hobbs   New Mexico 88240, 505 392-6526
County and 2 Year
Arts Areas: Instrumental Music, Vocal Music, Theatre and Visual Arts

MUSIC

Joe Walker, Dean of Arts, Business & Humanities   **Number Of Faculty:** 2
Number Of Students: 85   **Degrees Offered:** AA
Courses Offered: Piano; Voice; Theory; Choir; Band; Music Appreciation
Financial Assistance: Scholarships   **Performing Groups:** Choir; Band

NEW MEXICO MILITARY INSTITUTE
501 College Ave, Roswell   New Mexico 88201
505 622-6250 Ext 221
State and 2 Year   **Arts Areas:** Instrumental Music and Theatre
Performing Series: Cadet Activities Forum Series
Performance Facilities: Pearson Auditorium

MUSIC

Gary Sparks, Bandmaster   **Number Of Faculty:** 1   **Number Of Students:** 100
Degrees Offered: AA
Financial Assistance: Scholarships and Work-Study Grants

THEATRE

Travis Reames, Public Information Officer   **Number Of Faculty:** 1
Number Of Students: 25   **Courses Offered:** Intro to Theatre; Acting

NEW MEXICO STATE UNIVERSITY
Las Cruces   New Mexico 88003, 505 646-0111
State and 4 Year
Arts Areas: Dance, Instrumental Music, Vocal Music, Theatre, Film Arts, Television and Visual Arts

DANCE

Clark Rogers, Head of Department of Drama   **Number Of Faculty:** 2
Number Of Students: 15

MUSIC

Dr Guy B Webb, Deparment Head   **Number Of Faculty:** 11
Number Of Students: 125   **Degrees Offered:** BME; BM; BA; MM
Courses Offered: An Introduction to Music; Applied Music; Theory; Counterpoint; Composition
Teaching Certification Available
Financial Assistance: Assistantships, Scholarships, Work-Study Grants and Band Grants
Performing Groups: Brass Ensembles; Brass Quintet; Chamber Arts Ensemble; Chamber Orchestra; Choral Union; Collegium Musicum; Concert Band; Jazz Lab Bands; Marching Band; Percussion Ensemble; String Chamber Groups; Symphonic Winds; University - Civic Orchestra; University Singers; Varsity Pep Band; Woodwind Ensembles
Workshops/Festivals: Music Week; President's Concert; Jazz Festival; Contemporary Music Festival

THEATRE

Clark Rogers, Head   **Number Of Faculty:** 4   **Number Of Students:** 30
Degrees Offered: BA; BS Ed
Courses Offered: Acting; Directing; Technical Theatre; Design; History/Literature
Teaching Certification Available

(continued on next page)

Financial Assistance: Assistantships, Scholarships and Work-Study Grants
Performing Groups: The Experimental Group Theatre
Workshops/Festivals: High School Drama Festival; International Theatre Festival

---

UNIVERSITY OF NEW MEXICO

Albuquerque   New Mexico 87131, 505 277-2111
State and 4 Year
Arts Areas: Dance, Instrumental Music, Vocal Music, Theatre and Film Arts
Performing Series: Keller Hall Chamber Music Series; Major Ensemble Series; Opera Studio Rodey
Theatre Series
Performance Facilities: Keller Hall; Rodey Theatre; Experimental Theatre; Popejoy Hall

DANCE

Jennifer Predock, Coordinator   *Number Of Faculty:* 5
Number Of Students: 70   *Degrees Offered:* BFA; BA
Courses Offered: Ballet; Modern Dance; Ethnic Dance; Choreography; Improvisation
Financial Assistance: Scholarships and Work-Study Grants
Performing Groups: Dance Workshop
Workshops/Festivals: Albuquerque Dance Theatre; Mime Experiment Workshop

MUSIC

William E Rhoads, Chairman   *Number Of Faculty:* 32
Number Of Students: 300
Degrees Offered: BMus; BMusEd; BA Fine Arts; MA; MMus; MMusEd
Courses Offered: Applied Music; Music Education; Theory; Composition; History & Literature
Teaching Certification Available
Financial Assistance: Assistantships, Scholarships and Work-Study Grants
Performing Groups: Symphony Orchestra; Chamber Orchestra; Opera Studio; Wind Ensemble; Seraphim
Trio; Jazz Band; Marching Band; Concert Choir; Collegiate Singers; Madrigal Singers
Workshops/Festivals: All - State Music Festival; Albuquerque Youth Symphony with City Public Schools

THEATRE

Peter Prouse, Chairman   *Number Of Faculty:* 12   *Number Of Students:* 150
Degrees Offered: BFA; BA Fine Arts; MA
Courses Offered: Voice & Diction; Acting; Directing; Technical Design; Stage Design; Lighting; Make-up;
TV; Film History
Teaching Certification Available
Financial Assistance: Assistantships, Scholarships and Work-Study Grants
Workshops/Festivals: High School Theatre Festival
Artists-In-Residence/Guest Artists: Eric Hawkins Dance Company; Gunther Schuller

---

UNIVERSITY OF ALBUQUERQUE

Albuquerque   New Mexico 87120, 505 842-8500
Private and 4 Year
Arts Areas: Instrumental Music, Vocal Music, Theatre and Visual Arts
Degrees Offered: BMus, BMusEd   *Teaching Certification Available*
Financial Assistance: Scholarships and Work-Study Grants
Performing Groups: Chorus, Band, Ensembles

THEATRE

Jim Morley, Chairman   *Degrees Offered:* BA Speech - Drama
Teaching Certification Available
Financial Assistance: Scholarships and Work-Study Grants

ADELPHI UNIVERSITY
Garden City   New York 11530, 516 294-8700
   Private and 4 Year
   Arts Areas: Dance, Instrumental Music, Vocal Music, Theatre, Film Arts and Visual Arts
   Performing Series: "Concerts Plus" Series
   Performance Facilities: Robert G Olmsted Theatre

DANCE

Norman Walker, Chairman   *Number Of Faculty:* 24   *Number Of Students:* 60
Degrees Offered: BA
Courses Offered: Modern Dance; Ballet; Ethnic Dance; Theory; History & Composition
Technical Training: Lighting; Costuming; Set Design; Backstage Work
Financial Assistance: Scholarships and Work-Study Grants
Performing Groups: Adelphi Dance Theatre
Workshops/Festivals: Summer Dance Workshop

MUSIC

Lawrence Rasmussen, Chairman   *Number Of Faculty:* 9
Number Of Students: 29   *Degrees Offered:* BA
Courses Offered: Instrumental Music; Music Education; Theory; Music Appreciation; History
Teaching Certification Available
Financial Assistance: Scholarships and Work-Study Grants
Performing Groups: Glee Club   *Workshops/Festivals:* Opera Workshop

THEATRE

Jacques Burdick, Chairman   *Number Of Faculty:* 13   *Number Of Students:* 96
Degrees Offered: BFA
Courses Offered: Acting; Directing; Voice; Movement; Production; Theatre History; Technical Theatre
Technical Training: Scene, Costume & Lighting Design & Technology; Theatre Administration & Management
Financial Assistance: Scholarships and Work-Study Grants
Performing Groups: Theatre Adelphi; Cabaret Theatre; Mime Theatre; Story Players
Workshops/Festivals: Summer Theatre Workshop

ADIRONDACK COMMUNITY COLLEGE
Glens Falls   New York 12801, 518 793-4491
   State and 2 Year
   Arts Areas: Instrumental Music, Vocal Music, Theatre and Visual Arts
   Performance Facilities: Adirondack Community College Auditorium

DANCE

Several non-credit courses have been offered

MUSIC

Douglas Speicher, Chairman, Humanities Division   *Number Of Faculty:* 9
Number Of Students: 20   *Degrees Offered:* AA; AAS
Financial Assistance: Work-Study Grants
Performing Groups: Instrumental Ensemble; Chorus; Pop-band

THEATRE

Shirley G Weiner, Chairman, Division of English   *Number Of Faculty:* 9
Number Of Students: 500   *Degrees Offered:* AA; AS; AAS
Financial Assistance: Work-Study Grants
Performing Groups: Cue and Curtain Club

ALFRED UNIVERSITY
Alfred   New York 14802, 608 871-2111
>Private and 4 Year
>**Arts Areas:** Dance, Instrumental Music, Vocal Music, Theatre, Film Arts, Television and Visual Arts
>**Performing Series:** Cultural Programs Office of Public Affairs
>**Performance Facilities:** Major Holmes Auditorium

DANCE

Paula Cirulli, Chairman   **Number Of Faculty:** 1   **Number Of Students:** 45
Workshops/Festivals: Solomons Company; Ze'eva Cohen Solo Dance Repertory

MUSIC

David Ohara, Chairman, Division of Humanities   **Number Of Faculty:** 12
Number Of Students: 30   **Degrees Offered:** BA
Teaching Certification Available
Financial Assistance: Scholarships and Work-Study Grants
Performing Groups: Choral Groups; Bands; Jazz Ensemble
Workshops/Festivals: Bach Festival; Rochester Philharmonic Orchestra; Jazz Festival; Piano, Vocal, Woodwind Workshops; Opera Workshop

THEATRE

Number Of Faculty: 4   **Number Of Students:** 15   **Degrees Offered:** BA
Financial Assistance: Scholarships and Work-Study Grants
Performing Groups: DIGGIT (Student Drama Organization)
Workshops/Festivals: City Center Acting Company

AMERICAN ACADEMY OF DRAMATIC ARTS
120 Madison Ave, New York   New York 10016
212 686-9244
>Private and 2 Year   **Arts Areas:** Theatre
>**Performing Series:** Theatre Series
>**Performance Facilities:** Mary Mac Arthur Theatre; Mannie Greenfield Theatre; Lester Martin Theatre

THEATRE

George Cuttingham, Director   **Number Of Faculty:** 30
Number Of Students: 700   **Degrees Offered:** AOS
Courses Offered: Acting; Voice & Speech; Movement; Theatre History; Singing; Make-up; Fencing; Rehearsal & Performance
Performing Groups: All second year students form a repertory company

AMERICAN MUSICAL AND DRAMATIC ACADEMY, INC
150 Bleecker St, New York   New York 10012
212 677-5400
>Private and Special   **Arts Areas:** Dance, Vocal Music and Theatre
>**Performance Facilities:** American Musical & Dramatic Academy Theatre

DANCE

Harry Woolever, Chairman   **Number Of Faculty:** 2   **Number Of Students:** 60
Financial Assistance: Work-Study Grants

MUSIC

Maurice Finnell, Chairman   **Number Of Faculty:** 10   **Number Of Students:** 60
Financial Assistance: Work-Study Grants

THEATRE

David Martin, Chairman   **Number Of Faculty:** 2   **Number Of Students:** 60
Financial Assistance: Work-Study Grants

BARD COLLEGE
Annandale - on - Hudson   New York 12504, 914 758-6822 Ext 257
  Private and 4 Year
  Arts Areas: Dance, Instrumental Music, Vocal Music, Theatre, Film Arts and Visual Arts
  Performing Series: Concert Series
  Performance Facilities: Great Hall, Preston; Theater & Dance Studios;
  Bard Hall; Woods Studio; Chapel; Poetry Room; Committee, College & President's Rooms in Kline
  Commons; Sottery Hall; Proctor Lecture Hall; Ward Manor Social Room; Albee Social Room; Tewksbury
  Social Room

DANCE

Aileen Passloff, Chairman   *Number Of Faculty:* 6   *Number Of Students:* 30
Degrees Offered: BA   *Courses Offered:* Dance Composition; Dance History
Financial Assistance: Scholarships, Work-Study Grants and Student Loans
Performing Groups: Bard Theater of Drama & Dance presenting 6 Dance/Theater productions a year
Workshops/Festivals: Ad Hoc Master Classes

MUSIC

Elie Yarden, Chairmann   *Number Of Faculty:* 5   *Number Of Students:* 50
Degrees Offered: BA
Courses Offered: Fundamentals, Workshops in Music at various levels
Technical Training: Performance; Composition; Improvisation
Financial Assistance: Assistantships, Scholarships and Student Loans
Performing Groups: String Orchestra; Chamber Ensembles; Jazz Ensembles; Community Chorus; Chamber
Chorus

THEATRE

William Driver, Director   *Number Of Faculty:* 7   *Number Of Students:* 77
Degrees Offered: BA
Courses Offered: Play Analysis; History of Theatre; Playwriting; Theories & Styles of Theatre
Technical Training: Studio in Directing
Financial Assistance: Scholarships, Work-Study Grants and Student Loans
Performing Groups: Bard Theatre of Drama & Dance
Workshops/Festivals: Ad Hoc Workshops
Artists-In-Residence/Guest Artists: Robert Craft

BENNETT COLLEGE
Millbrook   New York 12545, 914 677-3441
  Private and 2 Year
  Arts Areas: Dance, Instrumental Music, Vocal Music and Theatre

MUSIC

Degrees Offered: AA   *Financial Assistance:* Scholarships
Performing Groups: Dance Group
Degrees Offered: AA Instrument and Vocal
Performance Facilities: George Gershwin Theatre; Walt Whitman Hall; Recital Hall; New York Theatre
Workshop

(continued on next page)

Performing Groups: Glee Club; Orchestra; Hudson Valley Philharmonic Orchestra
Workshops/Festivals: Hudson Valley Opera Workshop

THEATRE

Frank Ford, Chairman   **Degrees Offered:** AA

BRIARCLIFF COLLEGE
Elm Rd, Briarcliff Manor   New York 10510
914 941-6400
Private and 4 Year
Arts Areas: Instrumental Music, Vocal Music and Theatre
Performing Series: Concerts; Plays; Recitals

THEATRE

Mary D Diks, Chairman   **Degrees Offered:** AA

BRONX COMMUNITY COLLEGE
University Ave at West 181 St, Bronx   New York 10453
212 367-7300 Ext 314
State and 2 Year
Arts Areas: Dance, Instrumental Music, Vocal Music, Theatre, Film Arts, Television and Visual Arts
Performing Series: Heights Gala Performance Series
Performance Facilities: Hall of Fame Playhouse; Schwendler Auditorium; Gould Memorial Library
Auditorium

DANCE

Richard Kor, Chairman, Health & Physical Education   **Number Of Faculty:** 2
Number Of Students: 30   **Degrees Offered:** AAS
Courses Offered: Techniques of Modern, African & Puerto Rican Dance
Financial Assistance: Scholarships, Work-Study Grants and TAP; BEOG
Performing Groups: Modern Dance Club
Workshops/Festivals: Modern Dance Concert

MUSIC

Dr Marvin Salzberg, Chairman   **Number Of Faculty:** 8
Number Of Students: 111   **Degrees Offered:** AAS
Courses Offered: Music Survey; Introduction to Music; Twentieth Century Music; Choral & Orchestral
Performance; Fundamentals of Music; Theory; Keyboard; Instrumental Ensembles; Chamber Chorus; Ear
Training
Technical Training: Vocal & Instrumental
Financial Assistance: Scholarships, Work-Study Grants and TAP; BEOG
Performing Groups: BCC Symphony Orchestra; BCC Choir; BCC Chorus
Workshops/Festivals: Symphony Concerts; Choir Concerts; Thursday Afternoon Concert Series

THEATRE

Dr Robert King, Chairman, Communications, Arts & Sciences Department
Number Of Faculty: 2   **Number Of Students:** 210   **Degrees Offered:** AAS
Courses Offered: Play Production; Principles of Directing; Acting; Theory of the Theatre; Seminar &
Independent Study in Dramatic Arts; Movies; TV
Financial Assistance: Scholarships and Work-Study Grants
Performing Groups: Readers' Theatre
Artists-In-Residence/Guest Artists: Chuck Davis Dance Company

---

BROOKLYN COLLEGE SCHOOL OF PERFORMING ARTS
Brooklyn   New York 11210, 212 780-5006
City and 4 Year
Arts Areas: Dance, Instrumental Music, Vocal Music and Theatre
Performing Series: Guest Artists Series

(continued on next page)

DANCE

Betsy M Carden, Chairperson   **Number Of Faculty:** 18
Number Of Students: 100   **Degrees Offered:** BA; BS
Courses Offered: Modern; Ballet; Ethnic; Repertory/Performance; Anatomy; History; Theory; Labanotation
Technical Training: Dance Theatre Production (Lighting, Stage Management)
Teaching Certification Available
Financial Assistance: Scholarships and Work-Study Grants
Performing Groups: Brooklyn Dance Theatre
Workshops/Festivals: Baroque Dance; Dance Performance Workshops in Ballet, Modern, Ethnic

MUSIC

Dorothy Klotzman, Chairman   **Number Of Faculty:** 53
Number Of Students: 300   **Degrees Offered:** BA; BS; MA
Courses Offered: Performance; Composition; Ear Training; Theory; Music History; Piano, Harpsichord; Organ; Strings; Harp; Voice; Woodwinds; Brass Timpani; Percussion
Teaching Certification Available
Financial Assistance: Assistantships, Scholarships and Work-Study Grants
Performing Groups: Percussion Ensemble; Orchestra; Symphonic Ensemble; Contemporary Music Ensemble; Symphonic Band; Brass Ensemble; Chorus; Woodwind Ensemble

THEATRE

Gordon Rogoff, Chairman   **Number Of Faculty:** 18   **Number Of Students:** 350
Degrees Offered: BA; MA
Courses Offered: Acting; Directing; Design & Technical Playwriting; History; Literature; Criticism; Theatre Management
Technical Training: Theatre Production Practice
Teaching Certification Available
Financial Assistance: Assistantships, Scholarships and Work-Study Grants
Workshops/Festivals: Black Theatre Workshop; Directors' Workshop; Clown Workshop; Musical Comedy Workshop; Chamber Theatre Workshop
Artists-In-Residence/Guest Artists: June Lewis & Company; Vivian Perlis

---

CANTOR'S INSTITUTE & SEMINARY COLLEGE OF JEWISH MUSIC
Columbia University, New York   New York 10027
212 280-1754
Private and Special   **Arts Areas:** Vocal Music

MUSIC

Dr Hugo Weisgall, Chairman
Courses Offered: Cantorial Tradition; Cantorial Art; Musical Literature for Synagogue; Chanting Scriptures

---

CAYUGA COUNTY COMMUNITY COLLEGE
Franklin St, Auburn   New York 13021
315 253-7345 Ext 20
County and 2 Year
Arts Areas: Instrumental Music, Vocal Music, Theatre, Film Arts, Television and Visual Arts
Performing Series: Lecture Series; Performing Arts Series; Art Film Series
Performance Facilities: College Theatre; Gym

MUSIC

Harold M Henderson, Professor   **Number Of Faculty:** 1
Number Of Students: 95

(continued on next page)

Courses Offered: Music Appreciation; History I, II; Essentials; Theory I, II; Recorder Workshop; Instrumental Study
Performing Groups: Concert Choir; Stage Band

THEATRE

Daniel C Labeille, Professor   **Number Of Faculty:** 1
Number Of Students: 40
Courses Offered: Theatre Appreciation; History; Drama Workshop; Varieties of Filmic Experience; Basic Acting; Modern Drama
Technical Training: Scene Construction & Lighting
Performing Groups: Harlequin Productions
Artists-In-Residence/Guest Artists: Steina Vasulka; Theatre Laboratoire Vicinal; Alan Schneider

---

THE CITY COLLEGE, CITY UNIVERSITY OF NEW YORK
Convent Ave & 138th St, New York   New York 10031
212 690-6666
City and 4 Year
Arts Areas: Dance, Instrumental Music, Vocal Music, Theatre, Film Arts and Visual Arts
Performing Series: Edward G Robinson Guest Artist Series
Performance Facilities: Aaron Davis Hall (3 theatres); Shepard Great Hall

DANCE

Dance program under auspices of Department of Theatre Arts
Number Of Faculty: 3   **Number Of Students:** 75   **Degrees Offered:** BFA
Technical Training: Modern; Ballet; Choreography
Financial Assistance: Scholarships and Work-Study Grants
Performing Groups: Davis Center Dance Company
Workshops/Festivals: Workshops in all forms of dance techniques

MUSIC

Virginia Red, Chairperson   **Number Of Faculty:** 22   **Number Of Students:** 200
Degrees Offered: BA; BFA; BA MusEd; MA; MAMus Ed
Technical Training: Professional training for performers; Electronic Music
Teaching Certification Available
Financial Assistance: Scholarships and Work-Study Grants
Performing Groups: Choral Ensemble; Jazz Ensemble; Studio Orchestra; CCNY Orchestra; Early Music Collegium; Chamber Ensemble; Latin Ensemble
Workshops/Festivals: Jazz Workshops; Pop Vocal Workshops; Opera Workshops

THEATRE

Earle R Gister, Chairman   **Number Of Faculty:** 13   **Number Of Students:** 190
Degrees Offered: BA; BFA; MA
Technical Training: All areas of performance and production in theatre and film
Financial Assistance: Scholarships and Work-Study Grants
Performing Groups: Davis Center Theatre Company; Picker Film Institute
Workshops/Festivals: Sydney Meyers Film Festival
Artists-In-Residence/Guest Artists: Jacques Chwat; David Geary; Ira Gitler; Fritz Jahoda; Sheila Jordan; John Knapp; Albin McDuffie; Jan Meyerowitz; Timothy Monich; Judy Padow; Donn Pennebaker; Marjorie Perces; Walter Raines; Judith Raskin; Mariko Sanjo; Jill Silverman; Dennis Tate; Beverly Wideman

---

CITY UNIVERSITY OF NEW YORK
HERBERT H LEHMAN COLLEGE
Bedford Park Blvd W, Bronx   New York 10468
212 960-8881
City and 4 Year
Arts Areas: Instrumental Music, Vocal Music, Theatre and Visual Arts

(continued on next page)

DANCE

Dance program under the auspices of Theatre Department
Degrees Offered: BA; BFA Dance THeatre; BS Dance Education
Teaching Certification Available
Financial Assistance: Scholarships and Work-Study Grants

MUSIC

Edward F Kravik, Chairman   *Number Of Faculty:* 8   *Number Of Students:* 130
Degrees Offered: BA; BS; MA; MA MusEd   *Teaching Certification Available*
Financial Assistance: Scholarships and Work-Study Grants

THEATRE

C J Stevens, Chairman   *Number Of Faculty:* 15   *Number Of Students:* 255
Degrees Offered: BS; MA Drama & Speech   *Teaching Certification Available*
Financial Assistance: Scholarships and Work-Study Grants
Performing Groups: Musical Theatre Society

CITY UNIVERSITY OF NEW YORK, QUEENS COLLEGE
67-30 Kissena Blvd, Flushing   New York 11367
212 445-7500
City and 4 Year
Arts Areas: Instrumental Music, Vocal Music, Theatre and Visual Arts
Performing Series: Performing Arts Series
Performance Facilities: Golden Center

MUSIC

Lawrence W Eisman, Chairman   *Number Of Faculty:* 78
Number Of Students: 936   *Degrees Offered:* BA; MA; MMusEd
Teaching Certification Available   *Financial Assistance:* Scholarships
Performing Groups: Symphony Orchestra Group; Choir Ensemble

THEATRE

Betram L Joseph, Chairman   *Number Of Faculty:* 12   *Number Of Students:* 245
Degrees Offered: BA   *Performing Groups:* Theatre Company

CITY UNIVERSITY OF NEW YORK, YORK COLLEGE
158-11 Jewel Ave, Flushing   New York 11365
212 969-4040
State and 4 Year
Arts Areas: Instrumental Music, Vocal Music and Visual Arts
Degrees Offered: BMus; BMusEd   *Teaching Certification Available*
Financial Assistance: Work-Study Grants

COLGATE UNIVERSITY
Hamilton   New York 13346, 315 824-1000
Private and 4 Year
Arts Areas: Dance, Instrumental Music, Vocal Music, Theatre, Film Arts and Visual Arts
Performing Series: Chamber Music Series; Summer Concert Series
Performance Facilities: Brehmer Theater; Memorial Chapel

DANCE

Thomas Leff & Rachel Hoyd, Co-directors   *Number Of Faculty:* 2
Number Of Students: 25
Courses Offered: Dance Technique; Choreography; History & Aesthetics of Dance
Technical Training: Modern   *Financial Assistance:* Work-Study Grants
Performing Groups: Colgate Dance Theater

(continued on next page)

MUSIC

Joscelyn Godwin, Associate Professor   **Number Of Faculty:** 8
Number Of Students: 100   **Degrees Offered:** BA
Courses Offered: Music History; Theory; Appreciation; Performance
Financial Assistance: Scholarships and Work-Study Grants
Performing Groups: Concert Orchestra; University Chorus; Early Music Ensemble
Workshops/Festivals: Medieval & Renaissance Institute, Summer '78

THEATRE

Atlee Sproul, Director   **Number Of Faculty:** 2   **Number Of Students:** 225
Technical Training: Movement; Voice; Scenic Technique
Financial Assistance: Scholarships and Work-Study Grants
Performing Groups: Colgate University Theater; Colgate Student Theater
Workshops/Festivals: Acting & Directing Workshops
Artists-In-Residence/Guest Artists: Oxford & Cambridge Shakespeare Company

---

COLGATE UNIVERSITY
Hamilton   New York 13346, 315 824-1000
Private and 4 Year
Arts Areas: Instrumental Music, Vocal Music, Theatre, Visual Arts and Radio
Performing Series: Concert & Music Department Recital Series; Lecture Series; Music Department Chamber Series

MUSIC

Dexter Morrill, Chairman   **Number Of Faculty:** 7   **Number Of Students:** 85
Degrees Offered: BA
Financial Assistance: Scholarships and Work-Study Grants
Performing Groups: Colgate Glee Club; University Choir; Colgate Jazz Ensemble
Workshops/Festivals: Instrument Workshop

THEATRE

Brooks W Stoddard, Chairman   **Number Of Faculty:** 4   **Number Of Students:** 50
Degrees Offered: BA
Technical Training: Private instruction in Voice & Instruments
Performing Groups: University Theatre Companies; The Celebrant Ensemble; Junior Recitals; Senior Recitals
Workshops/Festivals: Director & Actor Workshops

COLLEGE OF SAINT ROSE
432 Western Ave, Albany   New York 12203
518 471-5178
Private, 4 Year and Graduate
Arts Areas: Dance, Instrumental Music, Vocal Music, Theatre, Film Arts and Visual Arts
Performance Facilities: Activity Center, College Auditorium

MUSIC

J Robert Sheehan, Chairman   **Number Of Faculty:** 20
Number Of Students: 120   **Degrees Offered:** BA; BS MusEd; MS MusEd
Courses Offered: Instrumental; Vocal; Keyboard; Methodology; History; Theory
Teaching Certification Available
Financial Assistance: Assistantships, Scholarships and Work-Study Grants
Performing Groups: Jazz & Wind Ensembles; Chamber Singers; Masterworks Chorale; Orchestra; Chamber Music
Workshops/Festivals: New York State Student School Music Association Workshop; Eastern New York Orff Association

THE COLLEGE OF WHITE PLAINS OF PACE UNIVERSITY
78 N Broadway, White Plains   New York 10603
914 682-7000
>   Private and 4 Year
>   *Arts Areas:* Dance, Instrumental Music, Vocal Music and Theatre

>   *Courses Offered:* Beginnings to Baroque; Classic to Modern; Musical Understanding Modern Music; Music in America; Music of Baroque Period, Classic Period, Romantic Period

THEATRE

Barbara Eberhardt, Chairman
Courses Offered: Acting I & II; Improvisation; Stagecraft & Scene Design; Directing & Play Production; Readers' Theatre
Performing Groups: Preston Players; Children's Theatre; Cabaret Theatre

COLUMBIA UNIVERSITY
116th St, New York   New York 10027
212 280-1754
>   Private and 4 Year
>   *Arts Areas:* Instrumental Music, Vocal Music and Theatre

MUSIC

Chou Wen-chung, Chairman   *Number Of Faculty:* 8   *Number Of Students:* 125
Degrees Offered: BA; MA; PhD; DMA
Technical Training: Electronic Music; Computer Music; Radio Broadcasts
Financial Assistance: Assistantships, Scholarships and Work-Study Grants
Performing Groups: Public Performances; Columbia University Chamber Music Readings; Columbia Composers Concerts

THEATRE

Bernard Beckerman, Chairman   *Number Of Faculty:* 4   *Number Of Students:* 80
Degrees Offered: BA; MA; PhD   *Teaching Certification Available*
Financial Assistance: Assistantships, Scholarships and Work-Study Grants
Performing Groups: Theatre Company   *Workshops/Festivals:* University Theatre Workshop

COLUMBIA UNIVERSITY, BARNARD COLLEGE
606 W 120th St, New York   New York 10027
212 280-1754
>   Private and 4 Year
>   *Arts Areas:* Dance, Instrumental Music, Vocal Music, Theatre and Visual Arts
>   *Performance Facilities:* Minor Lathan Playhouse

DANCE

Edith G Mason, Athletic Department Chairman   *Number Of Faculty:* 9
Number Of Students: 85
Dance program under the auspices of Recreation & Athletic program
Courses Offered: Modern Dance; Ballet; Jazz; Folk Dance
Workshops/Festivals: Body Movement Workshop; Barnard Dance Theatre Workshop; Master Class

MUSIC

Patricia Carpenter, Chairman   *Number Of Faculty:* 5
Number Of Students: 45   *Degrees Offered:* BA
Technical Training: Conducting; Score Reading; Electronic Music
Financial Assistance: Assistantships, Scholarships and Work-Study Grants
Performing Groups: Orchestra; Barnard - Columbia Chorus; Bands; Various Ensembles; Collegium Musicum; Chamber Music; Symphonic Band; Concert Band

(continued on next page)

THEATRE

Kenneth Janes, Director   **Number Of Faculty:** 5   **Number Of Students:** 35
Performing Groups: The Barnard College Theatre Company

COMMUNITY MUSIC SCHOOL OF BUFFALO
415 Elmwood Ave, Buffalo   New York 14222
716 884-4887

Private and Special
Arts Areas: Dance, Instrumental Music and Vocal Music

DANCE

Janet Springer, Director   **Number Of Faculty:** 2   **Number Of Students:** 80
Courses Offered: Pre - Ballet, Beginning, Intermediate & Advanced Ballet
Technical Training: Russian Classical Ballet (Vaganova)
Financial Assistance: Scholarships, Work-Study Grants and Fee Remission
Performing Groups: The Ballet Centre Ensemble

MUSIC

Daniel D Stevens, Jr, Executive Director   **Number Of Faculty:** 40
Number Of Students: 700
Courses Offered: Theory; History; Orff Schulwerk for Children & Teacher Training; Class & Private
Instrumental/Vocal Instruction
Teaching Certification Available
Financial Assistance: Scholarships, Work-Study Grants and Fee Remission
Performing Groups: The Buffalo Guitar Quartet

CONCORDIA COLLEGE
171 White Plains Rd, Bronxville   New York 10708
914 337-9300

Private and 4 Year   **Arts Areas:** Instrumental Music and Vocal Music
Performing Series: Guest Recital Series
Performance Facilities: Schoenfeld Hall; Maier Hall

MUSIC

James L Brauer, Professor   **Number Of Faculty:** 25   **Number Of Students:** 200
Degrees Offered: BA; BS
Courses Offered: Music Education; Church Music; Applied Music; Music
Technical Training: Voice; Organ; Piano; All Orchestral & Band Instruments
Teaching Certification Available
Performing Groups: Concordia Tour Choir; Concordia Festival Orchestra and Chorus; Symphonic Band
and Instrumental Ensemble; Recorder Consort; Woodwind Quintet; Chapel Singers
Workshops/Festivals: Black Composers Piano Festival; Annual Summer Church Musician Workshops
Performing Groups: The Concordia Players; The Concordia Children's Theatre

---

CORNELL UNIVERSITY
Ithaca   New York 14853, 607 256-1000

Private and 4 Year
Arts Areas: Dance, Instrumental Music, Vocal Music, Theatre, Film Arts and Visual Arts
Performing Series: Bailey Hall Concert Series; Statler Hall String Series
Performance Facilities: Bailey Hall; Barnes Hall; Statler Auditorium
Willard Straight Theatre; Sage Chapel; Drummond Theatre

DANCE

Peggy Lawler, Director
Dance program is co-sponsored by the Physical Education Department and the Department of Theatre Arts
Number Of Faculty: 6   **Number Of Students:** 455   **Degrees Offered:** BA Dance
Courses Offered: Dance & Movement for the Theatre; Beginning Dance Composition; Advanced

(continued on next page)

Composition; Dance Technique; Ballet, Modern; History of Dance; Human Biology for the Performing Arts; Period Dance; Seminar in History of Dance
Financial Assistance: Scholarships and Work-Study Grants
Performing Groups: Cornell Dance Concert
Workshops/Festivals: Seminar in History of Dance, Individual problems in Composition

MUSIC

N A Zaslaw, Chairman   *Number Of Faculty:* 16   *Number Of Students:* 845
Degrees Offered: BA, MA Musicology & Music Theory; MFA Music Composition; PhD Musicology; DMA Music Composition
Courses Offered: Music Appreciation; Music Theory; Music History; Composition; Performance
Financial Assistance: Assistantships, Scholarships, Work-Study Grants and Tuition Grants
Performing Groups: Choral & Instrumental Ensembles; Sage Chapel Choir; Cornell Chorus; Cornell University Glee Club; Marching Band; Wind Ensemble; Symphonic Band; Brass Ensemble; Cornell Symphony Orchestra; Cornell Chamber Orchestra; Chamber Music Groups; Indonesian Gamelon; Collegium Musicum
Workshops/Festivals: Summer viola da gamba institute with John Hsu

THEATRE

Marvin Carlson, Professor   *Number Of Faculty:* 17
Number Of Students: 1097   *Degrees Offered:* BA; MA; MFA; PhD
Courses Offered: Dramatic Literature of various periods; Seminars; American Mime; Acting; Directing; Design (Costume, Scenery); Technical Theatre; Playwriting; Theatre Theory & Criticism; Film History; Cinematography
Technical Training: Acting; Directing; Design
Financial Assistance: Assistantships, Scholarships and Work-Study Grants
Performing Groups: Cornell University Theatre; Ithaca Summer Repertory
Artists-In-Residence/Guest Artists: Amade Trio: Malcolm Bilson;, Sonya Monosoff, John Hsu

---

CORNING COMMUNITY COLLEGE
Corning   New York 14830, 607 962-9011 Ext 321
State and 2 Year
Arts Areas: Instrumental Music, Vocal Music and Theatre
Performance Facilities: Science Amphitheater

MUSIC

Dr James W Hudson, Acting Chairman, Humanities   *Number Of Faculty:* 1
Number Of Students: 30 - 40   *Degrees Offered:* AA; AS
Courses Offered: Introduction to Theory; Introduction to Harmony; Reading Vocal Music; Intro to Music Listening; Modular Courses from Medieval to Jazz; Instrumental Performing Ensemble; Class Voice I & II, Class Piano I & II; Private Music Lessons & Individual Study
Financial Assistance: Work-Study Grants and TAP; BEOG
Performing Groups: Chamber Singers

THEATRE

Henry Moonschein, Professor   *Number Of Faculty:* 1   *Number Of Students:* 30
Degrees Offered: AA; AS
Courses Offered: Theatre History; Intro to Theatre; Theatre Independent Study; Make-up; London Theatre Study Tour
Financial Assistance: Work-Study Grants and TAP; BEOG
Performing Groups: Two Bit Players

DAEMEN COLLEGE
4380 Main St, Amherst   New York 14226
716 839-3600 Ext 225
Private and 4 Year
Arts Areas: Dance, Instrumental Music, Vocal Music and Theatre
Performing Series: Guest Artist Series
Performance Facilities: Wick Campus Center Auditorium; Duns Scotus Auditorium

(continued on next page)

MUSIC

Arthur Ness, Chairman   **Number Of Faculty:** 28   **Number Of Students:** 60
Degrees Offered: BA; BS MusEd; BMus   **Teaching Certification Available**
Financial Assistance: Scholarships
Performing Groups: Band; Orchestra; Chorus
Workshops/Festivals: Faculty Recitals; Student Recitals; Concerts

THEATRE

Dr Katherine Sullivan, Chairperson   **Number Of Faculty:** 4
Number Of Students: 12   **Degrees Offered:** BA
Courses Offered: Acting; Directing; Producting
Financial Assistance: Scholarships   **Performing Groups:** Theatre of Youth

---

DALCROZE SCHOOL OF MUSIC
161 E 73 St, New YOrk   New York 10021
212 879-0316

Private and Special   **Arts Areas:** Instrumental Music and Vocal Music
Performing Series: Artist Faculty Concerts
Performance Facilities: Dalcroze Auditorium; Dalcroze Concert Hall

MUSIC

Number Of Faculty: 42   **Number Of Students:** 750
Courses are accepted toward Master's and Doctor's degree by such colleges as Columbia University, New York University, The City College, Hunter College
Courses Offered: Theory; Harmony; Counterpoint; Composition; Conducting; History of Music; Solfege; Improvisation; Dalcroze Eurhythmics; Indian Music; Montessori; Contemporary Music
Technical Training: Only authorized American Dalcroze Teacher's Training Center
Teaching Certification Available
Financial Assistance: Scholarships and Work-Study Grants
Performing Groups: String Ensemble; Wind Ensemble; Instrumental Ensemble; Choral Ensemble
Workshops/Festivals: Dalcroze Workshops

DUTCHESS COMMUNITY COLLEGE
Pendell Rd, Poughkeepsie   New York 12590
914 471-4500

County and 2 Year
Arts Areas: Dance, Instrumental Music, Vocal Music, Theatre, Television and Visual Arts

DANCE

Richard Skimin, Department Head   **Number Of Faculty:** 1
Courses Offered: Modern Dance

MUSIC

Mrs Helen Baldwin, Chairperson   **Number Of Faculty:** 2
Number Of Students: 494   **Degrees Offered:** AA
Courses Offered: Appreciation; Chorus; Jazz; Madigral Singers; Theory; Brass Ensemble; Piano; Performance Applied
Performing Groups: Instrumental Group & Vocal Music; Jazz Ensemble

THEATRE

Stephen Press, Department Head   **Number Of Faculty:** 6
Number Of Students: 121   **Degrees Offered:** AA
Courses Offered: Stagecraft; Acting; Fundamentals of Theatre; Special Study Project
Workshops/Festivals: Wednesday Night Film; Friday Night Film; Saturday Children's Theatre; Spring Festival

D'YOUVILLE COLLEGE
320 Porter Ave, Buffalo   New York 14201
716 886-8100

Private and 4 Year   *Arts Areas:* Dance and Theatre
Performance Facilities: Dance Studio; Dinner Theater

DANCE

Number Of Faculty: 1   *Number Of Students:* 30
Courses Offered: Modern Creative Dance; Dance Workshop

MUSIC

Courses Offered: Appreciation of Music   *Performing Groups:* D'Youville Singers

THEATRE

Number Of Faculty: 1   *Number Of Students:* 30
Courses Offered: Theater Workshop; Theater Production

EASTMAN SCHOOL OF MUSIC OF THE UNIVERSITY OF ROCHESTER
26 Gibbs St, Rochester   New York 14604
716 275-3032

Private and 4 Year   *Arts Areas:* Instrumental Music and Vocal Music
Performing Series: Kilbourn Concerts Series; The Eastman - Ranlet Concerts; The Eastman Series
Performance Facilities: The Eastman Theatre; Kilbourn Hall; Howard Hanson Recital Hall

MUSIC

Jon Engberg, Associate Director for Academic Affairs
Number Of Faculty: 120   *Number Of Students:* 640
Degrees Offered: BM; BA; MMus; MA; DMA   *Teaching Certification Available*
Financial Assistance: Assistantships, Scholarships and Work-Study Grants
Performing Groups: The Cleveland Quartet; The Eastman Trio; Spectrum, a jazz quintet; The Eastman
Philharmonia Orchestra; Symphony Orchestra; Wind Ensemble; Opera Theatre; Jazz Ensemble; The New
Jazz Ensemble; Wind Orchestra; Graduate String Quartet; Musica Nova; The Inter Musica Chamber
Music Ensemble; Jazz/Lab Band; Studio Orchestra; Trombone Choir; Marimba Band; Percussion
Ensemble
Workshops/Festivals: Summer Institutes in Recording Techniques; Guitar & Jazz Summer Programs for
High School Students in Instrumental Music, Vocal Music, and Jazz

ELIZABETH SETON COLLEGE
1061 W Broadway, Yonkers   New York 10701
914 969-4000

Private and 2 Year
Arts Areas: Instrumental Music, Vocal Music and Theatre

MUSIC

Elizabeth I Carr, Chairman   *Degrees Offered:* AA Mus; AA Mus Ed
Degrees Offered: AA Dramatics - Speech

ELMIRA COLLEGE
Elmira   New York 14901, 607 732-6400

Private and 4 Year
Arts Areas: Dance, Instrumental Music, Vocal Music, Theatre and Visual Arts
Performing Series: Concert, Lecture & Film Series   *Performance Facilities:* Emerson Auditorium

DANCE

Caliope Candianides, Assistant Professor   *Number Of Faculty:* 1
Number Of Students: 20   *Degrees Offered:* BA Dance/Theater
Financial Assistance: Scholarships, Work-Study Grants and Loans
Performing Groups: Orchesis Dance Ensemble

(continued on next page)

MUSIC

Forrest Sanders, Professor   **Number Of Faculty:** 2   **Number Of Students:** 20
Degrees Offered: BA Music
Financial Assistance: Scholarships, Work-Study Grants and Loans
Performing Groups: Mirachords; Chorus

THEATRE

Peter Rodney, Instructor   **Number Of Faculty:** 2   **Number Of Students:** 20
Degrees Offered: BA Theatre   **Performing Groups:** Thespis

FINCH COLLEGE
52 E 78th St, New York   New York 10021
212 288-8450
Private and 4 Year
Arts Areas: Instrumental Music, Vocal Music, Theatre and Visual Arts

MUSIC

Number Of Faculty: 1   **Number Of Students:** 15
Financial Assistance: Assistantships, Scholarships and Work-Study Grants

THEATRE

Number Of Faculty: 2   **Number Of Students:** 30   **Degrees Offered:** AA
Technical Training: Costume Design
Financial Assistance: Assistantships, Scholarships and Work-Study Grants
Performing Groups: Drama Club

FORDHAM UNIVERSITY, LINCOLN CENTER
New York   New York 10023, 212 956-4774
Private and 4 Year
Arts Areas: Dance, Instrumental Music, Vocal Music, Theatre and Visual Arts
Performing Series: Concert Series

MUSIC

Mrs James Reyes, Chairman   **Number Of Faculty:** 3   **Number Of Students:** 350
Degrees Offered: BA   **Technical Training:** Vocal Concentration
Teaching Certification Available
Financial Assistance: Scholarships and Work-Study Grants
Performing Groups: Concert Opera   **Workshops/Festivals:** Concert Series

THEATRE

Degrees Offered: BA Theatre (Liberal Arts & Professional Degrees)
Technical Training: Performance Emphasis
Financial Assistance: Scholarships and Work-Study Grants
Performing Groups: Musicals; 4 Major Productions by Theatre Department each semester
Workshops/Festivals: Student Workshops; Touring in Metro area

GENESEE COMMUNITY COLLEGE
College Rd
PO Box 718, Batavia   New York 14020
716 343-0055 Ext 206
County and 2 Year
Arts Areas: Instrumental Music, Vocal Music, Theatre, Film Arts, Television and Visual Arts
Performing Series: Performing Artists Series
Performance Facilities: Genesee Community College Forum

MUSIC

Dr Frank Jackson, Chairman   **Number Of Faculty:** 2   **Number Of Students:** 20
Degrees Offered: AS
Courses Offered: Violin; Suzuki; Guitar; Continuing Education Courses
Performing Groups: Jazz Ensemble; Choir; Chorale

(continued on next page)

THEATRE

Dr Frank Jackson, Chairman   **Number Of Faculty:** 2   **Number Of Students:** 6
Degrees Offered: AS   **Performing Groups:** Forum Players

HAMILTON COLLEGE
Clinton   New York 13323, 315 859-4011
Private and 4 Year
Arts Areas: Instrumental Music, Vocal Music, Theatre and Visual Arts
Performing Series: Concert & Lecture Series

MUSIC

Stephen Bonts, Chairman   **Number Of Faculty:** 3   **Number Of Students:** 35
Degrees Offered: BA   **Teaching Certification Available**
Financial Assistance: Scholarships and Work-Study Grants

THEATRE

Number Of Faculty: 5   **Number Of Students:** 55
Degrees Offered: BA Drama & Speech   **Teaching Certification Available**
Financial Assistance: Scholarships and Work-Study Grants
Performing Groups: Charlatans

HARLEM SCHOOL OF THE ARTS, INC
645 St Nicholas Ave, New York   New York 10030
212 926-4100
Private and Special
Arts Areas: Dance, Instrumental Music, Vocal Music, Theatre and Visual Arts

DANCE

Courses Offered: Ballet; Modern; Ethnic   **Financial Assistance:** Scholarships
Workshops/Festivals: Dance Workshops for advanced students

MUSIC

Courses Offered: Vocal & Instrumental   **Financial Assistance:** Scholarships

THEATRE

Courses Offered: Acting; Directing; Improvisation
Financial Assistance: Scholarships
Workshops/Festivals: Drama Workshops for Children, Teenagers & Adults

HARTWICK COLLEGE
Oneonta   New York 13820, 607 432-4200 Ext 369
Private and 4 Year
Arts Areas: Dance, Instrumental Music, Vocal Music, Theatre and Visual Arts
Performing Series: Hartwick College Concert/Lecture Series
Performance Facilities: Anderson Center for the Arts; Little Theater; Bresee Hall; Slade Auditorium

MUSIC

Jerome W Campbell, Chairman   **Number Of Faculty:** 18
Number Of Students: 50
Degrees Offered: BS MusEd; BA with concentration in Liberal Arts; Orff Certification
Courses Offered: Theory; Literature; Appreciation; History; Applied Methods; Acoustics; Student Teaching
(Orff included) begining freshman year
Technical Training: Private instruction for all instruments & voice; Electronic Music
Teaching Certification Available   **Financial Assistance:** Scholarships and Work-Study Grants
Performing Groups: Wind Ensemble; Jazz Ensemble; Choir; Chorale; Madrigal Group; Male Choir;
Church Choirs; Membership in the Catskill Symphony Orchestra; Renaissance Wind & String Hartwick
College Choir; Community Chorale; Symphony Orchestra
Workshops/Festivals: Performance, "Verdi Requiem", Dr Thruston J Dox, Conducting

(continued on next page)

(Hartwick College — cont'd)

THEATRE

Dr David M Ferrell, Assistant Professor   **Number Of Faculty:** 5
Number Of Students: 8   **Degrees Offered:** BA Theatre Arts
Courses Offered: History; Applied Theatre; Seminar; Acting Courses; Touring groups
Technical Training: Make-up; Technical Theatre
Performing Groups: Cardboard Alley Players; Alpha Psi Omega

HASTINGS TALENT EDUCATION CENTRE, INC
126 Fort Hill Rd, Scarsdale   New York 10583
914 472-9762

Private and Special   **Arts Areas:** Instrumental Music

MUSIC

L Shapiro, Director   **Number Of Faculty:** 8   **Number Of Students:** 70
Degrees Offered: Suzuki Certificates   **Courses Offered:** Suzuki; Violin; Cello
Technical Training: Suzuki Training   **Teaching Certification Available**
Financial Assistance: Scholarships   **Performing Groups:** Kurtis String Ensemble

---

HEBREW ARTS SCHOOL FOR MUSIC AND DANCE
15 W 65th St, New York   New York 10023
212 787-0650

Private and Special
Arts Areas: Dance, Instrumental Music, Vocal Music and Visual Arts

MUSIC

Dr T Jochsberger, Director   **Number Of Faculty:** 45
Number Of Students: 500   **Financial Assistance:** Scholarships
Performing Groups: Hebrew Arts Chamber Players; Zamir Chorale; Hebrew Arts Orchestra

---

HEBREW UNION COLLEGE - JEWISH INSTITUTE OF RELIGION SCHOOL OF SACRED MUSIC
40 W 68th St, New York   New York 10023
212 873-0200

Private and Five Year   **Arts Areas:** Vocal Music   **Performance Facilities:** College Auditorium

MUSIC

Cantor Lawrence Avery, Academic Coordinator   **Number Of Faculty:** 20
Number Of Students: 50   **Degrees Offered:** BA and MA, Sacred Music
Teaching Certification Available
Financial Assistance: Tuition Grants (based on need)

HERKIMER COUNTY COMMUNITY COLLEGE
Reservoir Rd, Herkimer   New York 13350
315 866-0300 Ext 51

County and 2 Year   **Arts Areas:** Theatre, Television and Visual Arts
Performance Facilities: Theater

MUSIC

Number Of Faculty: 1   **Degrees Offered:** AA
Courses Offered: American Music; Music Appreciation; Music Theory; Music and the Child; American Folk Music
Financial Assistance: Scholarships and Work-Study Grants   **Performing Groups:** Lyric Theater

THEATRE

Number Of Faculty: 2   **Degrees Offered:** AA
Courses Offered: Verbal Communication; Oral Interpretation; Acting Technique; Introduction to the Theater
Financial Assistance: Scholarships and Work-Study Grants   **Performing Groups:** Society of Dionysus

HOBART & WILLIAM SMITH COLLEGES
Geneva   New York 14456, 315 789-5500
Private and 4 Year
Arts Areas: Instrumental Music, Vocal Music and Visual Arts
Performing Series: Community Concert Series; Artistic Lecture Series

MUSIC

Nicholas U D'Angelo, Chairman   *Number Of Faculty:* 3
Number Of Students: 50   *Degrees Offered:* BA; BMusEd
Teaching Certification Available
Financial Assistance: Assistantships and Scholarships
Performing Groups: Orchestra; Instrumental Ensembles; Chorale Group; Band; Chamber Music; Jazz Ensemble
Workshops/Festivals: The Creative Workshop

THEATRE

Benjamin P Atkinson, English Department Chairman
Theatre Program under auspices of English Department
Performing Groups: Little Theatre Company
Workshops/Festivals: The Creative Workshop

HOFSTRA UNIVERSITY
Fulton Ave, Hempstead   New York 11550
516 560-3491
Private and 4 Year
Arts Areas: Dance, Instrumental Music, Vocal Music, Theatre, Television and Visual Arts
Performing Series: Concert Series; Performing Art Series
Performance Facilities: John Cranford Adams Playhouse; West End Theater; Little Theater

DANCE

Carl Morris, Chairman   *Number Of Faculty:* 2   *Number Of Students:* 180
Degrees Offered: BA; BFA; BS   *Courses Offered:* Body Movement; Modern Dance
Teaching Certification Available   *Financial Assistance:* Scholarships

MUSIC

Herbert Deutsch, Chairman   *Number Of Faculty:* 18   *Number Of Students:* 290
Degrees Offered: BA; BS   *Teaching Certification Available*
Financial Assistance: Scholarships
Performing Groups: Collegium Musicum; Band; Orchestra; Jazz Ensemble; Mixed Chorus; Chamber Music Series; Hofstra Quartet

THEATRE

James Van Wart, Chairman   *Number Of Faculty:* 8   *Number Of Students:* 180
Degrees Offered: BA; BFA   *Teaching Certification Available*
Financial Assistance: Scholarships
Performing Groups: Hofstra Repertory Theater
Workshops/Festivals: Shakespeare Festival

HOUGHTON COLLEGE
Houghton   New York 14744, 716 567-2211
Private and 4 Year
Arts Areas: Instrumental Music, Vocal Music and Visual Arts
Performing Series: Houghton College Artist Series
Performance Facilities: Wesley Chapel - Auditorium

MUSIC

Dr Donald Bailey, Chairman, Division of Fine Arts   *Number Of Faculty:* 15

(continued on next page)

Number Of Students: 135   **Degrees Offered:** BA; BMus
Teaching Certification Available
Financial Assistance: Scholarships and Work-Study Grants
Performing Groups: Madrigal Chamber Singers; College Choir; Chapel Choir; Woman's Choir; Men's Choir; Orchestra; Wind Ensemble; Concert Band
Workshops/Festivals: Annual Festival; Various Workshops
Artists-In-Residence/Guest Artists: William Allen; Charles H Finney

---

HUDSON VALLEY COMMUNITY COLLEGE
Vandenburgh Ave, Troy   New York 12180
518 283-1100

State and 2 Year   **Arts Areas:** Instrumental Music and Theatre
Performing Series: College Cultural Series; Student Performing Art Series; Student Film Series
Performance Facilities: Campus Center Theatre; Hudson Hall Auditorium; Lang Hall Auditorium

MUSIC

H R Vincent, Coordinator of Instrumental Music   **Number Of Faculty:** 1
Number Of Students: 15 - 25   **Degrees Offered:** AA Liberal Arts
Courses Offered: Band; Music Appreciation
Financial Assistance: Work-Study Grants and Based on PCS (financial need)
Performing Groups: Summer Community Band; Concert & Pep Bands
Workshops/Festivals: Two Concerts during the summer program

THEATRE

Professor Robert Couture, Chairperson   **Number Of Faculty:** 1
Number Of Students: 15- 20   **Degrees Offered:** AA
Courses Offered: Intro to Theatre; Youth Theatre Arts; Elements of Acting; Contemporary Drama
Financial Assistance: Work-Study Grants and Based on PCS (financial need)
Performing Groups: Valley Players
Workshops/Festivals: Two four-performance presentations annually
Artists-In-Residence/Guest Artists: Chuck Mangione, Albany Symphony Orchestra

---

HUNTER COLLEGE,
CITY UNIVERSITY OF NEW YORK
695 Park Ave, New York   New York 10021
212 570-5566

City and 4 Year
Arts Areas: Dance, Instrumental Music, Vocal Music, Theatre, Film Arts, Television and Visual Arts
Performance Facilities: Assembly Hall; Playhouse; Little Theatre

DANCE

Dorothy Vislocky, Chairman
Dance program under auspices of Music Department
Number Of Faculty: 6   **Number Of Students:** 75
Degrees Offered: BA Dance; MA Dance Therapy
Courses Offered: Theory & Practice
Performing Groups: Hunter College Dance Company
Workshops/Festivals: Little Studio Series; Balkan Dance Festival; Workshops

MUSIC

James Harrison, Chairman   **Number Of Faculty:** 41   **Number Of Students:** 200
Degrees Offered: BA; BS; BMus Performance; MA
Courses Offered: Introduction to Music; Literature & History of Music; Theory; Musical Performance
Technical Training: Electronic Music   **Teaching Certification Available**
Financial Assistance: Internships, Assistantships, Scholarships and Work-Study Grants
Performing Groups: Concert & Dance Bands; Orchestra; College Choir; Collegium Musicum; Jazz Workshop

(continued on next page)

THEATRE

Vera Mowry Roberts, Chairman   **Number Of Faculty:** 29
Number Of Students: 340   **Degrees Offered:** BA; MA
Courses Offered: Introduction to Theatre; History of the Theatre; Children's Theatre; Acting; Playwriting; Directing; Stage Lighting; Stagecraft; Make-up; Scene Design
Technical Training: Film Production   **Teaching Certification Available**
Financial Assistance: Internships, Assistantships, Scholarships and Work-Study Grants
Performing Groups: Children's Theatre; Hunter College Undergraduate Productions; Hunter Playwright's Project

---

IONA COLLEGE
715 North Ave, New Rochelle   New York 10801
914 636-2100
    Private and 4 Year   **Arts Areas:** Theatre

THEATRE

Stephanie Schwartz, Director Speech & Dramatic Arts
Extracurricular Activities

ITHACA COLLEGE
Danby Rd, Ithaca   New York 14850
607 274-3401
    Private and 4 Year
    Arts Areas: Dance, Instrumental Music, Vocal Music, Theatre, Film Arts, Television, Visual Arts and Radio
    Performing Series: The College Theatre Season; The College Concert Series
    Performance Facilities: Walter Ford Hall Auditorium; Dillingham Center for the Performing Arts

MUSIC

Dr Joel Stegall, Dean   **Number Of Faculty:** 65   **Number Of Students:** 500
Degrees Offered: BM; MM; MS; BA; BFA
Courses Offered: Applied Music; Music Education; Composition; Music Theory
Technical Training: Piano Technology; Brass & Woodwind Repairs
Teaching Certification Available
Financial Assistance: Scholarships and Work-Study Grants
Performing Groups: Orchestra; Chorus; Band; Opera Workshop; Jazz Workshop; Chamber Groups; Brass Choir; Percussion Ensemble; Madrigal Singers
Workshops/Festivals: The Roberta Peters Annual Concert

THEATRE

Dr Firman H Brown, Chairperson   **Number Of Faculty:** 22
Number Of Students: 200   **Degrees Offered:** BA; BFA; BS
Courses Offered: Speech; Drama; Acting/Directing; Technical Production
Technical Training: Theatrical Design; Theatre Management
Teaching Certification Available
Financial Assistance: Scholarships and Work-Study Grants
Performing Groups: Theta Alpha Pi
Workshops/Festivals: Participation in the Ithaca Repertory Company each summer
Artists-In-Residence/Guest Artists: Alfred Reed; Judith Raskin; John Browning; Leonard Rose; Cleveland Quartet; Phyllis Curtin; Goldovsky Opera Company; New York Brass Quintet; Gary Karr & Harmon Lewis

---

JEWISH THEOLOGICAL SEMINARY OF AMERICA
3080 Broadway, New York   New York 10027
212 479-8000
    Private and 4 Year   **Arts Areas:** Instrumental Music and Vocal Music
    Performing Series: Concert & Lecture Series   **Degrees Offered:** BA Sacred Music
    Financial Assistance: Scholarships and Work-Study Grants

THE JUILLIARD SCHOOL
Lincoln Center, New York   New York 10023
212 799-5000

Private and 4 Year
Arts Areas: Dance, Instrumental Music, Vocal Music and Theatre
Performance Facilities: Alice Tully Hall; The Juilliard Theater; Paul Recital Hall; The Drama Theater

DANCE

Ms Martha Hill, Chairman   *Number Of Faculty:* 25   *Number Of Students:* 75
Degrees Offered: BA   *Courses Offered:* Modern Dance; Composition; Notation
Financial Assistance: Assistantships, Scholarships and Work-Study Grants
Performing Groups: The Juilliard Dance Ensemble
Workshops/Festivals: Spring Dance season of new & repertory works

MUSIC

Peter Mennin, President   *Number Of Faculty:* 135   *Number Of Students:* 700
Degrees Offered: Certified Diploma; BMus; MMus; DMA
Courses Offered: Piano; Organ; Stringed Instruments; Voice; Composition; Orchestral Instruments
Financial Assistance: Assistantships, Scholarships and Work-Study Grants
Performing Groups: The Juilliard Orchestra; Juilliard Philharmonia; Juilliard Symphony; 20th Century
Music Ensemble; Juilliard Conducting Orchestra

THEATRE

Alan Schneider, Chairman   *Number Of Faculty:* 28   *Number Of Students:* 75
Degrees Offered: BFA
Financial Assistance: Assistantships, Scholarships and Work-Study Grants
Performing Groups: Juilliard Theater Center Company

KEUKA COLLEGE
Lodge Rd, Keuka Park   New York 14478
315 536-4411

Private and 4 Year
Arts Areas: Instrumental Music, Vocal Music and Visual Arts
Performing Series: Performing Artist Series

MUSIC

Gerald M Hansen, Chairman   *Number Of Faculty:* 4   *Number Of Students:* 50
Degrees Offered: BA   *Teaching Certification Available*
Financial Assistance: Scholarships and Work-Study Grants
Performing Groups: Recital Concerts; Orchestra; Ensembles; Chorale Group

THE KING'S COLLEGE
Briarcliff Manor   New York 10510, 914 941-7200

Private and 4 Year   *Arts Areas:* Instrumental Music and Vocal Music
Performing Series: College Cultural Affairs Series; Music Department Faculty & Guest Artist Series
Performance Facilities: Chapel/Auditorium; Gymnasium/Auditorium

MUSIC

James W Terry, Chairman   *Number Of Faculty:* 5   *Number Of Students:* 60
Degrees Offered: BS MusEd; BS in Applied
Courses Offered: Theory; History; Applied Music; Music Education
Teaching Certification Available   *Financial Assistance:* Scholarships
Performing Groups: Concert Band; Concert Choir; Oratorio Chorus; Orchestra; Jazz Ensemble; Vocal
Ensemble
Workshops/Festivals: Choral Festival; Church Music Workshop
Artists-In-Residence/Guest Artists: Irene Jordan

KIRKLAND COLLEGE
Clinton   New York 13323, 315 859-7462
>   Private and 4 Year
>   **Arts Areas:** Instrumental Music, Vocal Music and Visual Arts
>   **Degrees Offered:** BMus

LEMOYNE COLLEGE
LeMoyne Heights, Syracuse   New York 13214
315 446-2882 Ext 476
>   Private and 4 Year
>   **Arts Areas:** Theatre, Film Arts, Television and Visual Arts
>   **Performance Facilities:** LeMoyne College Auditorium; TV Center

THEATRE

>   Thomas R Hogan, Chairman   **Number Of Faculty:** 3
>   **Number Of Students:** 50 - 60   **Degrees Offered:** BA
>   **Courses Offered:** Voice; Acting; Directing; Shakespeare Workshop
>   **Performing Groups:** Performing Arts Association
>   **Workshops/Festivals:** Workshop in Shakespeare for High Schools
>   **Artists-In-Residence/Guest Artists:** Kenneth Bowles

MANHATTAN SCHOOL OF MUSIC
120 Claremont Ave, New York   New York 10027
212 749-2802
>   Private and 4 Year   **Arts Areas:** Instrumental Music and Vocal Music
>   **Number Of Faculty:** 179   **Number Of Students:** 800
>   **Degrees Offered:** BMus; MMusEd; MMus; PhD Mus
>   **Teaching Certification Available**
>   **Financial Assistance:** Scholarships and Work-Study Grants
>   **Performing Groups:** Percussion Ensemble; String Ensemble; Brass Ensemble; Woodwind Ensemble; Choral
>   Ensembles; Chamber Music Groups; Symphony Orchestras; Opera Theatre
>   **Workshops/Festivals:** Repetoire Workshops; Composers Forums; Master Class Series
>   **Artists-In-Residence/Guest Artists:** Aaron Rosand

MANHATTANVILLE COLLEGE
Purchase St, Purchase   New York 10577
914 946-9600 Ext 470
>   Private and 4 Year
>   **Arts Areas:** Dance, Instrumental Music, Vocal Music and Theatre
>   **Performing Series:** Faculty Artist Series
>   **Performance Facilities:** Little Theatre of Brownston Hall; Pius X Hall

DANCE

>   Greta Levart, Director   **Number Of Faculty:** 2   **Number Of Students:** 90
>   **Courses Offered:** History of American Dance; Modern Dance Technique, Improvisation & Composition
>   Workshop; Workshop in Music for Dancers & Body Mechanics for Dancers
>   **Teaching Certification Available**
>   **Financial Assistance:** Scholarships and Job Opportunities on Campus; Grant Assistance
>   **Performing Groups:** Dance Club
>   **Workshops/Festivals:** Summer Dance Festival; workshops offered on campus during the academic year by
>   guest artists

MUSIC

>   Anthony LaMagra, Chairman   **Number Of Faculty:** 26   **Number Of Students:** 90
>   **Degrees Offered:** BA; BMus; MA in Teaching   **Teaching Certification Available**
>   **Financial Assistance:** Scholarships and Job Opportunities on campus; Grant Assistance

(continued on next page)

Performing Groups: Chorus; Orchestra; Chamber Choir; Opera Players; Early Music Ensemble; Ensemble for 20th Century Music
Workshops/Festivals: Instrumental workshops; workshops and recitals by guest artists

THEATRE

Jonathan C Huberth, Director   **Number Of Faculty:** 1
Number Of Students: 52
Courses Offered: Acting; Classical Theater & Theater Games; Improvisation & Story Theater
Financial Assistance: Scholarships and Job Opportunities on campus; Grant Assistance
Performing Groups: Drama Club

MANNES COLLEGE OF MUSIC
157 E 74th St, New York   New York 10021
212 737-0700
Private and 4 Year
Arts Areas: Instrumental Music, Vocal Music and Visual Arts

MUSIC

David Tcimpidis, Chairman
Degrees Offered: BS; BMus; Diploma; Past Graduate Diploma
Financial Assistance: Scholarships
Performing Groups: Orchestra; Chamber Ensembles; Symphonic Ensembles; Choral Groups; Woodwind Ensembles; String Ensembles; Bands
Workshops/Festivals: Opera Workshop

MARIA REGINA COLLEGE
1024 Court St, Syracuse   New York 13208
315 474-4891
Private and 2 Year   **Arts Areas:** Instrumental Music and Vocal Music

MUSIC

Sister M Arcadia, Director   **Degrees Offered:** AA Music

MARYMONT MANHATTAN COLLEGE
221 E 71st St, New York   New York 10021
212 472-3800 Ext 506
Private and 4 Year
Arts Areas: Dance, Instrumental Music, Vocal Music, Theatre, Film Arts, Television and Visual Arts
Performance Facilities: Marymount Manhattan College Theatre

DANCE

L Elaine Lewnau, Chairperson   **Number Of Faculty:** 3
Number Of Students: 20   **Degrees Offered:** BA Dance
Technical Training: Stagecraft/Scene Design; Work opportunities for independent study with Phoenix Theatre
Financial Assistance: Assistantships, Scholarships and Work-Study Grants

THEATRE

L Elaine Lewnau, Chairperson   **Number Of Faculty:** 8
Number Of Students: 50   **Degrees Offered:** BA
Technical Training: Performance; Dramatic Theorys Criticism
Teaching Certification Available
Financial Assistance: Assistantships, Scholarships and Work-Study Grants

MARYMOUNT COLLEGE
Tarrytown   New York 10591, 914 631-3200 Ext 202
Private and 4 Year
Arts Areas: Dance, Instrumental Music, Vocal Music, Theatre and Visual Arts
Performance Facilities: Spellman Hall; Rita Concert Hall

DANCE

Margot Lehman, Chairman   **Number Of Faculty:** 1   **Number Of Students:** 120
Degrees Offered: BFA
Technical Training: Technique; Improvisation; Composition; Rhythmic Training, Dance Education
Performing Groups: Dance Club

MUSIC

Prof Wolfgang Schanzer, Chairman   **Number Of Faculty:** 9
Number Of Students: 80-90   **Degrees Offered:** BA; BMus
Technical Training: Music Therapy   **Teaching Certification Available**
Financial Assistance: Scholarships and Work-Study Grants
Performing Groups: Glee Club; Ensemble Groups
Workshops/Festivals: Musical Theatre Workshop

THEATRE

Prof Ron Weyand, Chairman   **Number Of Faculty:** 9   **Number Of Students:** 27
Degrees Offered: BA
Technical Training: Stagecraft; Fundamental Training in Acting and Directing
Teaching Certification Available
Workshops/Festivals: Drama Workshops; Theatre Seminar; Black Drama Workshop

MERCY COLLEGE
555 Broadway, Dobbs Ferry   New York 10522
914 693-4500 Ext 56
Private and 4 Year
Arts Areas: Dance, Instrumental Music, Vocal Music, Theatre and Film Arts
Performing Series: Department of Fine Arts Concert Series; Concert Artists Guild NYC
Performance Facilities: Mercy College Lecture Hall

DANCE

Scott Devroe, Chairman   **Courses Offered:** Introduction to Dance

MUSIC

Dr John Rayburn, Chairman   **Degrees Offered:** BS; BA
Technical Training: Electronic Techniques; All Keyboard & Orchestral Instruments; Theory and Composition
Teaching Certification Available   **Performing Groups:** Chorus; Orchestra

MOHAWK VALLEY COMMUNITY COLLEGE
1101 Sherman Dr, Utica   New York 13501
315 792-5000
County and 2 Year
Arts Areas: Instrumental Music, Vocal Music, Film Arts and Visual Arts

MUSIC

Anthony Millagrand, Director   **Number Of Faculty:** 1
Number Of Students: 60   **Courses Offered:** Music Appreciation; Theory

MOUNT KISCO SCHOOL OF MUSIC
520 Lexington Ave, Mount Kisco   New York 10549
914 666-3529

Private and Special   *Arts Areas:* Instrumental Music and Vocal Music

MUSIC

Alan Gramson, Director   *Number Of Faculty:* 20   *Number Of Students:* 350
Courses Offered: Private Instruction; Yamaha Music Course
Financial Assistance: Scholarships

NAZARETH COLLEGE OF ROCHESTER
4245 East Ave, Rochester   New York 14612
716 586-2525

Private and 4 Year
Arts Areas: Instrumental Music, Vocal Music, Theatre and Visual Arts

MUSIC

Sister Jeanne Troy, Chairman   *Number Of Faculty:* 17
Number Of Students: 91
Degrees Offered: BS in Music, Music Education, Applied Music, Music Theory; BA Mus
Courses Offered: Music Education; Music Theory; Applied Music
Technical Training: Applied Music in individual instruments; Teacher Education Courses
Teaching Certification Available
Financial Assistance: Assistantships, Scholarships and Work-Study Grants
Performing Groups: Mixed Chorus; Chamber Choir; Jazz Lab; Chamber Orchestra

THEATRE

James Kolb, Chairman   *Number Of Faculty:* 7   *Number Of Students:* 28
Degrees Offered: BA   *Courses Offered:* Theatre Arts
Financial Assistance: Assistantships, Scholarships and Work-Study Grants
Performing Groups: Drama Club

COLLEGE OF NEW ROCHELLE
New Rochelle   New York 10801, 914 632-5300

Private and 4 Year   *Arts Areas:* Dance, Film Arts and Visual Arts
Performance Facilities: Little Theatre; Auditorium

DANCE

Dance program under auspices of Physical Education Department

MUSIC

Sister Elizabeth Monaghan, Chairman   *Number Of Faculty:* 1
Number Of Students: 90   *Courses Offered:* Music Theory; History of Music
Financial Assistance: Internships, Assistantships, Scholarships and Work-Study Grants

---

NEW YORK INSTITUTE OF TECHNOLOGY
Old Westbury   New York 11568, 516 686-7616

Private, 4 Year and Graduate
Arts Areas: Theatre, Film Arts, Television, Visual Arts and Communications
Performing Groups: Whitney Players

NEW YORK UNIVERSITY
Washington Sq, New York   New York 10003
212 598-1212

Private and 4 Year
Arts Areas: Dance, Instrumental Music, Vocal Music, Theatre, Film Arts, Television and Visual Arts

(continued on next page)

DANCE

Degrees Offered: BA, MA, PhD Theatre Dance & Dance Education
Financial Assistance: Assistantships, Scholarships and Work-Study Grants

MUSIC

David L Burrows, Chairman
Degrees Offered: BA; MA; PhD Musicology; BA Mus, MusEd   **Teaching Certification Available**
Financial Assistance: Assistantships, Scholarships and Work-Study Grants
Workshops/Festivals: Member MENC

THEATRE

Michael Kirby, Chairman   **Number Of Faculty:** 24   **Number Of Students:** 265
Degrees Offered: BA, BFA, MA Theatre & Theatre Design; PhD
Technical Training: Directing   **Teaching Certification Available**
Financial Assistance: Assistantships, Scholarships and Work-Study Grants
Performing Groups: Children's Theatre; Theatre Program Group; Hall of Fame Players

---

NIAGARA UNIVERSITY
Niagara University   New York 14109, 716 285-1212 Ext 525
  Private and 4 Year
  Arts Areas: Dance, Theatre, Film Arts, Television and Visual Arts
  Performing Series: University Theatre Series
  Performance Facilities: Niagara University Theatre

THEATRE

Brother Augustine Towey, C M, Director   **Number Of Faculty:** 9
Number Of Students: 15   **Degrees Offered:** BA
Courses Offered: Acting; Dance; Mime; History of Theatre; Criticism; Production; Independent Study; Directing; Management; Design
Technical Training: Design; Management   **Teaching Certification Available**
Performing Groups: University Players; Artpark Repertory Theatre Company; AM - Dance in Concert
Workshops/Festivals: General Theatre Workshops

NYACK COLLEGE
Nyack   New York 10960, 914 358-1710
  Private and 4 Year
  Arts Areas: Instrumental Music, Vocal Music and Film Arts
  Performing Series: Artist-Lecture Series

MUSIC

Paul F Liljestrand, Chairman   **Number Of Faculty:** 7
Number Of Students: 100   **Degrees Offered:** BA; BMusEd   **Teaching Certification Available**
Financial Assistance: Assistantships, Scholarships and Work-Study Grants
Performing Groups: Chamber Orchestra; Choir; Ensembles

ONONDAGA COMMUNITY COLLEGE
Hill Campus, Syracuse   New York 13210
315 469-7741
  County and 2 Year   **Arts Areas:** Instrumental Music and Theatre
  Degrees Offered: AA   **Degrees Offered:** AA

PACE UNIVERSITY
861 Bedford Rd, Pleasantville   New York 10570
914 769-3200 Ext 437
  Private and 4 Year   **Arts Areas:** Theatre, Film Arts and Television
  Performing Series: Performing Art Series
  Performance Facilities: Campus Center; Willcox Hall

(continued on next page)

MUSIC

Dr Richard Podgorski, Chairman   *Number Of Faculty:* 4
Number Of Students: 40
Financial Assistance: Scholarships and Work-Study Grants
Performing Groups: Glee Club; Band; Jazz, Dance, Vocal, Orchestra Concerts

THEATRE

Dr Richard Podgorski, Chairman   *Number Of Faculty:* 7
Number Of Students: 150
Financial Assistance: Scholarships and Work-Study Grants
Performing Groups: Parnassus Players; Comedy Series; Experimental Theatre

---

C W POST CENTER OF LONG ISLAND UNIVERSITY

Greenvale   New York 11548, 516 299-2395
Private and 4 Year
Arts Areas: Dance, Instrumental Music, Vocal Music, Theatre, Film Arts, Television and Visual Arts
Performing Series: Weekly Concert Series
Performance Facilities: Little Theatre; Hillwood Commons

MUSIC

Raoul Pleskow, Professor   *Number Of Faculty:* 9   *Number Of Students:* 300
Degrees Offered: BFA; BA; BA MusEd; BFA MusEd; MA Mus; MA MusEd
Courses Offered: Theory; Composition; Music History; Music Literature; Instruments; Music Ed
Teaching Certification Available
Financial Assistance: Assistantships, Scholarships, Work-Study Grants and Performance Scholarship
Performing Groups: Chorus; Chamber Singers; Madrigal Singers; Chamber Orchestra; Band; Collegeum
Musicum
Workshops/Festivals: Pierrot Consort - in - Residence; American Theatre Festival

THEATRE

Lucille Rhodes, Professor   *Number Of Faculty:* 9   *Number Of Students:* 100
Degrees Offered: BA; BFA   *Courses Offered:* Dance; Theatre; Film
Technical Training: Lighting; Stage Management; Design; Lighting; Sound
Financial Assistance: Assistantships, Scholarships and Work-Study Grants
Performing Groups: Post Theatre Company; Post Theatre Film Association
Workshops/Festivals: American Theatre Festival; Film Festival; Dance Workshops; Playwrights Unit

---

PRATT INSTITUTE

215 Ryerson St, Brooklyn   New York 11205
212 636-3600
Private and 4 Year
Arts Areas: Dance, Theatre, Film Arts, Television and Visual Arts
Performing Series: March of Drama Series; Contemporary Playwrights Series

DANCE

Number Of Faculty: 12   *Number Of Students:* 15   *Degrees Offered:* BFA
Courses Offered: Modern Dance; Choreography; Dance History
Financial Assistance: Internships, Scholarships and Work-Study Grants
Performing Groups: Dance Workshop

THEATRE

Dr Nick Manning, Chairman   *Number Of Faculty:* 20   *Number Of Students:* 100
Degrees Offered: BFA
Technical Training: Technical Production; Scene Design; Costume Design; Lighting
Workshops/Festivals: Shakespeare Festival; Isben Festival
Artists-In-Residence/Guest Artists: Lou Bunin; Andre Gregory

QUEENSBOROUGH COMMUNITY COLLEGE,
CITY UNIVERSITY OF NEW YORK
56th Ave & Springfield Blvd, Bayside   New York 11364
212 631-6262

City and 2 Year
Arts Areas: Dance, Instrumental Music, Vocal Music, Theatre, Film Arts, Television and Visual Arts
Performing Series: Performing Arts Series
Performance Facilities: QCC Theatre; Kurzweil Memorial Hall

DANCE

Professor Alfred Kahn, Chairman, Health, Physical Education & Dance
Number Of Faculty: 7   *Degrees Offered:* AA
Courses Offered: Modern; Social; Folk; Square; Ballet; African & Afro - Caribbean; Foundation of Dance Movement; Dance Workshop; Movement Training for the Theatre
Technical Training: Dance Workshop I & II
Financial Assistance: Scholarships, Work-Study Grants and TAP; BEOG; Tuition Waiver Program
Performing Groups: Dance Workshop

MUSIC

Dr Marvin R Schwartz, Chairman   *Number Of Faculty:* 8   *Degrees Offered:* AA
Courses Offered: Introduction to Music; History of Western Music; Twentieth - Century; Opera; Music on the Modern Stage; Fundamentals; Theory; Sight Singing; Keyboard Harmony; Conducting; Music Therapy; Piano; The Synthesizer
Technical Training: Collegium Musicum; Vocal & Instrumental; Chorus; Orchestra; Band
Financial Assistance: Scholarships, Work-Study Grants and TAP; BEOG; Tuition Waiver Program
Performing Groups: Collegium Musicum; Queensborough Chorus, Queensborough Orchestra; Queensborough Symphonic Band

THEATRE

Richard G Heath, Chairman, Department of Speech, Communication & Theatre Arts
Number Of Faculty: 14   *Degrees Offered:* AA
Courses Offered: Acting; Theatre; Contemporary Cinema & Television; Dramatic Writing for Theatre; Film & Television; Theater Production; American Film History
Technical Training: Technical Theater Production
Financial Assistance: Scholarships, Work-Study Grants and TAP; BEOG; Tutition Waiver Program
Performing Groups: QCC Theatre; QCC Professional Theatre-in-Residence

RIVERDALE SCHOOL OF MUSIC
253rd St & Post Rd, Bronx   New York 10471
212 549-8034

Private and Special   *Arts Areas:* Instrumental Music and Vocal Music
Performing Series: Chamber Music Series; Faculty Recitals; Special Concerts
Performance Facilities: Auditorium; Recital Room

MUSIC

Robert Rudie, Director   *Number Of Faculty:* 30   *Number Of Students:* 250
Courses Offered: Individual & Group Instruction in all Instruments; Voice; Theory; Composition; Electronic Music; Music for Young Children
Financial Assistance: Scholarships
Performing Groups: The Riverdale String Quartet

ROBERTS WESLEYAN COLLEGE
2301 Westside Dr, Rochester   New York 14624
716 594-9471

Private and 4 Year
Arts Areas: Instrumental Music, Vocal Music and Visual Arts

(continued on next page)

Performing Series: Cultural Life Series
Performance Facilities: Cox Hall Auditorium; Parmeter Chapel

MUSIC

Robert Shewan, Chairman   *Number Of Faculty:* 11   *Number Of Students:* 70
Degrees Offered: BA Mus; BS MusEd; AS Mus with emphasis in Piano Pedagogy
Teaching Certification Available
Financial Assistance: Scholarships and Work-Study Grants
Performing Groups: Chorale; Band; Mixed Choir; Chamber Singers; Brass Ensemble

---

SAINT JOHN'S UNIVERSITY
Grand Central & Utopia Pkwys, Jamaica   New York 11439
212 969-8000 Ext 249
Private and 4 Year
Arts Areas: Instrumental Music, Vocal Music and Film Arts
Performing Series: Lecture Program

MUSIC

Prof Thomas J Flanagan, Director   *Number Of Faculty:* 7
Performing Groups: Chorus; Orchestra

SAINT LAWRENCE UNIVERSITY
Canton   New York 13617, 315 379-5011
Private and 4 Year
Arts Areas: Dance, Instrumental Music, Vocal Music, Theatre, Visual Arts and Radio
Performing Series: Concert-Lecture Program; Steinman Festival of the Arts
Performance Facilities: Noble Center Auditorium; Gilbert Recital Hall; Black Box Theater

MUSIC

Dr J Kenneth Munson, Chairman
Number Of Faculty: 4
Number Of Students: 50
Degrees Offered: BA; BS
Courses Offered: Composition; Performance; Music History
Performing Groups: Laurentian Singers; Saint Lawrence Chorale; Early Music Ensemble; Brass Quintet;
University Chorus; Chapel Choir; Instrumental Groups
Workshops/Festivals: Helps with Steinman Festival of the Arts

THEATRE

Dr Philip E Larson, Chairman   *Number Of Faculty:* 2
Number Of Students: 20   *Degrees Offered:* BA; BS
Courses Offered: Stagecraft; Acting; Scene Design; Costume Design; Theater History; Drama Study
Performing Groups: Mummers
Workshops/Festivals: Helps with Steinman Festival of the Arts

---

SARAH LAWRENCE COLLEGE
1 Meadway, Bronxville   New York 10708
914 337-0700
> Private and 4 Year
> **Arts Areas:** Dance, Instrumental Music, Vocal Music, Theatre, Film Arts and Visual Arts
> **Performance Facilities:** Reisinger Auditorium; Marshall Field House

DANCE

> Bessie Schonberg, Director   **Number Of Faculty:** 4   **Number Of Students:** 35
> **Degrees Offered:** BA; MA; MFA
> **Technical Training:** Continuing Education Program
> **Teaching Certification Available**
> **Financial Assistance:** Assistantships, Scholarships and Work-Study Grants
> **Performing Groups:** Dance Group

MUSIC

> Stanley Lock, Chairman   **Number Of Faculty:** 13   **Number Of Students:** 105
> **Degrees Offered:** BA; MA Theory & Composition; MFA
> **Technical Training:** Continuing Education Program
> **Financial Assistance:** Assistantships, Scholarships and Work-Study Grants
> **Performing Groups:** Music For Awhile; Collegium Musicum: Chorus; Laurentian Chamber Players;
> Orchestra Contemporary Music Ensembles

THEATRE

> Charles Carshen, Chairman   **Number Of Faculty:** 9   **Number Of Students:** 75
> **Degrees Offered:** DA; MA; MFA
> **Technical Training:** Continuing Education Program
> **Teaching Certification Available**
> **Financial Assistance:** Assistantships, Scholarships and Work-Study Grants
> **Performing Groups:** Sarah Lawrence Theatre; Children's Theatre

SCHOOL OF PERFORMING ARTS
LA GUARDIA HIGH SCHOOL OF MUSIC & THE ARTS
120 W 46th St, New York   New York 10036
212 582-4197
> County and Special   **Arts Areas:** Dance, Instrumental Music and Theatre

DANCE

> Lydia Joel, Coordinator   **Technical Training:** Ballet
> **Workshops/Festivals:** Ballet & Modern Dance Workshop

MUSIC

> Vivian Orzach, Coordinator
> **Performing Groups:** Band; Orchestra; Solo; Ensemble

THEATRE

> Jerome Eskow, Assistant Principal
> **Workshops/Festivals:** Lectures and guests weekly
> The school is geared to provide intensive professional training for students who, through audition,
> demonstrate interest, determination and potential to succeed in dance, drama and music professions

SHUMIATCHER SCHOOL OF MUSIC
2005 Palmer Ave, Larchmont   New York 10538
914 834-8946
> Private and Special
> **Arts Areas:** Instrumental Music, Vocal Music and Theatre
> **Performing Series:** East & West Performances; Faculty Performances

(continued on next page)

Number Of Faculty: 27   **Number Of Students:** 105
Degrees Offered: Certificates   **Teaching Certification Available**
Financial Assistance: Assistantships, Scholarships and Work-Study Grants
Performing Groups: Trio; Quartets; Orchestra Ensembles
Workshops/Festivals: Art and Music Festivals; Opera Workshop

SKIDMORE COLLEGE
Saratoga Springs   New York 12866, 518 584-5000
Private and 4 Year
Arts Areas: Dance, Instrumental Music, Vocal Music, Theatre and Visual Arts
Performing Series: Skidmore Performing Arts Series
Performance Facilities: Skidmore Theatre; Filene Recital Hall

DANCE

Dr Beverly J Becker, Chairman of the Department of Physical Education & Dance
Number Of Faculty: 6   **Number Of Students:** 500   **Degrees Offered:** BS
Courses Offered: Ballet; Modern; History; Methods; Improvosation; Choreography
Technical Training: Ballet; Modern   **Performing Groups:** Skidmore Dancers
Workshops/Festivals: Summer Dance Program

MUSIC

George C Green, Chairman   **Number Of Faculty:** 12   **Number Of Students:** 450
Degrees Offered: BS; BA
Courses Offered: Theory; Music History & Literature; Performance; Music Education
Technical Training: Concentration in Performance
Teaching Certification Available
Financial Assistance: Scholarships and Work-Study Grants
Performing Groups: Chamber Orchestra; Madrigal Singers & Collecium Musicum; Chorus; Sonneteers;
Bandersnatchers
Workshops/Festivals: Annual Guest Composer; Performing Artist Workshops

THEATRE

Alan Brody, Chairman   **Number Of Faculty:** 6   **Number Of Students:** 60
Degrees Offered: BS
Courses Offered: Introductory, Advanced & Intermediate courses in Acting; Directing; Technical Theatre
Financial Assistance: Scholarships and Work-Study Grants
Performing Groups: Skidmore Players; Centerstage
Workshops/Festivals: The Acting Company; The Talking Band; Reality Theatre of Boston

---

SOUTHAMPTON COLLEGE OF LONG ISLAND UNIVERSITY
Southampton   New York 11968, 516 283-4000 Ext 241
Private and 4 Year
Arts Areas: Dance, Instrumental Music, Vocal Music, Theatre and Visual Arts
Number Of Faculty: 1   **Number Of Students:** 25   **Courses Offered:** Modern Dance

MUSIC

Robert Shaughnessy, Chairman   **Number Of Faculty:** 2
Number Of Students: 75
Courses Offered: Piano; Choir; Voice; Orchestra; Music History; Theory; Classical Guitar; Music Criticism
Performing Groups: Madrigal Ensemble; Chorus
Workshops/Festivals: Art Festival   **Number Of Faculty:** 1
Number Of Students: 25

STATE UNIVERSITY AGRICULTURAL & TECHNICAL COLLEGE
Delhi   New York 13753, 607 746-4216
State and 2 Year   **Arts Areas:** Theatre
Performance Facilities: The Little Theatre

(continued on next page)

MUSIC

Donald O Shauer, Chairman   **Number Of Faculty:** 1   **Number Of Students:** 35
Performing Groups: Concert Choir; Fidelitones

THEATRE

William Campbell, Chairman   **Number Of Faculty:** 1   **Number Of Students:** 45
Performing Groups: College Players

STATE UNIVERSITY OF NEW YORK, ALBANY
1400 Washington Ave, Albany New York 12222
518 457-3300
    State and 4 Year
    Arts Areas: Instrumental Music, Vocal Music, Theatre, Film Arts, Television, Visual Arts and Radio

MUSIC

Nathan Gottschalk, Chairman   **Number Of Faculty:** 19
Number Of Students: 270   **Degrees Offered:** BA; MA
Teaching Certification Available
Financial Assistance: Internships, Assistantships, Scholarships and Work-Study Grants
Performing Groups: Instrumental & Vocal Ensembles; Mixed Chorus; University Singers; Orchestra; Band

THEATRE

Jarka Burian, Chairman   **Number Of Faculty:** 12   **Number Of Students:** 165
Degrees Offered: BA; MA
Technical Training: Experimental Production Techniques; Children's Theatre
Teaching Certification Available
Financial Assistance: Internships, Assistantships, Scholarships and Work-Study Grants
Performing Groups: Theatre Group   **Workshops/Festivals:** Theatrical Productions

---

STATE UNIVERSITY OF NEW YORK, BINGHAMTON
Vestal Parkway E, Binghamton New York 13901
607 798-2000
    State and 4 Year
    Arts Areas: Instrumental Music, Vocal Music, Theatre, Film Arts and Visual Arts
    Performing Series: Concert Series; Meet - the - Composer Series; Link Organ Series;
    Thursday Concert Series; Watters Mainstage, Studio Theater Series
    Performance Facilities: Casadesus Hall; Watters Theater; Cider Mill Playhouse; "Black Box" theaters

MUSIC

Alice Mitchell, Chairman   **Number Of Faculty:** 30   **Number Of Students:** 110
Degrees Offered: BA; MA; MM   **Teaching Certification Available**
Financial Assistance: Assistantships and Work-Study Grants
Performing Groups: University Symphony Orchestra; Wind Ensemble; Opera Workshop; Jazz Workshop;
Collegium Musicum; Renaissance Consort; Harpur Chorale; University Chorus; Chamber Groups
Workshops/Festivals: Summer Jazz Workshop; Folk Music/Dance Workshop

THEATRE

John Bielenberg, Chairman   **Number Of Faculty:** 17   **Number Of Students:** 80
Degrees Offered: BA; MA
Technical Training: Scene Design; Lighting; Stagecraft; Sound
Teaching Certification Available
Financial Assistance: Assistantships and Work-Study Grants
Workshops/Festivals: Lessac Workshop in Voice & Body for Actors; Dance Festival; Creative Writing
Festival; Various Symposia through the Center for Modern Theater Research
Artists-In-Residence/Guest Artists: Alan Simpson

STATE UNIVERSITY OF NEW YORK, BUFFALO
Main St, Buffalo   New York 14214
716 831-5306
State and 4 Year
Arts Areas: Dance, Instrumental Music, Vocal Music, Theatre, Film Arts, Television and Visual Arts

DANCE

Linda Swiniuch, Program Director   *Number Of Faculty:* 4
Number Of Students: 300   *Degrees Offered:* BA; MA
Financial Assistance: Assistantships

THEATRE

Dr Saul Elkin, Professor & Chairman   *Number Of Faculty:* 12
Number Of Students: 200   *Degrees Offered:* BA; MA Humanities
Financial Assistance: Assistantships
Performing Groups: Center for Theatre Research

STATE UNIVERSITY OF NEW YORK COLLEGE, BROCKPORT
Brockport   New York 14420, 716 395-2543
State and 4 Year
Arts Areas: Dance, Instrumental Music, Vocal Music and Theatre
Performing Series: Second Season Productions; Nickel Theatre; Dime - A - Dance;
The Rainbow Gallery; Fine Arts Main Gallery Series; Jazz in the "Rat"; Chamber Music Ensemble
Performance Facilities: Hartwell Hall; Fine Arts Theatre; College Union Ballroom; Rathskeller

DANCE

Ms Irma Pylyshenko, Area Spokesperson   *Number Of Faculty:* 14
Number Of Students: 125   *Degrees Offered:* BA; BS
Courses Offered: Improvisation; Composition; Repertory; Workshop; Music; Methods; Folk; Square;
Ethnic; Therapy; Research; Technique; Children's Theatre Dance; Methods of Teaching Dance & Related
Arts
Technical Training: Stage Design; Lighting
Financial Assistance: Work-Study Grants and Awards
Performing Groups: Bottom of the Bucket, But; Gumdrop Dragon Dance Company; The New York
Chamber Dance Group
Workshops/Festivals: S U N Y Dance Festival; Folk Festival

MUSIC·

Ms Susan Edmunds, Spokesperson   *Number Of Faculty:* 14
Number Of Students: 70   *Degrees Offered:* BA Mus Ed; BS Mus
Technical Training: Keyboard Technology
Financial Assistance: Scholarships and Work-Study Grants
Performing Groups: Symphony Orchestra; Band; Early Music Ensemble; Jazz Chorus; Chamber Chorus;
Men's & Women's Glee Club; Jazz Ensemble; Woodwind Ensemble; Brass Ensemble; Gospel Chorus
Workshops/Festivals: Keyboard Symposium; May Festival for Children; Jazz Residency; Arts for Children
Workshop

THEATRE

Sri Ram V Bakshi, Chairman   *Number Of Faculty:* 15
Number Of Students: 140
Degrees Offered: BA & BS Theatre; BS in Arts for Children
Technical Training: Technical Theatre; History & Criticism; Performance; Child Drama
Financial Assistance: Scholarships and Work-Study Grants
Performing Groups: Second Season; Hichel Theatre; Harlequins
Workshops/Festivals: Media Festival; World Theatre Day

STATE UNIVERSITY OF NEW YORK COLLEGE, CORTLAND
Cortland   New York 13045, 607 753-2011

State and 4 Year
Arts Areas: Instrumental Music, Vocal Music, Theatre and Visual Arts
Number Of Faculty: 14   *Number Of Students:* 215   *Degrees Offered:* BA
Teaching Certification Available
Financial Assistance: Assistantships, Scholarships and Work-Study Grants
Performing Groups: Orchestra; Choir; Ensembles; Band

THEATRE

Joseph A Elfenbein, Chairman   *Number Of Faculty:* 12
Number Of Students: 175   *Degrees Offered:* BA in Speech and Theatre
Teaching Certification Available
Financial Assistance: Assistantships, Scholarships and Work-Study Grants
Performing Groups: Hilltop Masquers

STATE UNIVERSITY OF NEW YORK COLLEGE, FREDONIA
Fredonia   New York 14063, 716 673-3111

State and 4 Year
Arts Areas: Instrumental Music, Vocal Music, Theatre and Visual Arts

MUSIC

Thomas Carpenter, Chairman   *Number Of Faculty:* 42
Number Of Students: 715   *Degrees Offered:* BA; BA Mus Ed; BFA; MA; MA MusEd
Teaching Certification Available
Financial Assistance: Assistantships, Scholarships and Work-Study Grants
Performing Groups: Chorus; Woodwinds; Strings; Percussion; Various Ensembles
Workshops/Festivals: Percussion & Timpani Workshop; String Instruments Workshop

THEATRE

Alice E Bartlett, Chairman   *Number Of Faculty:* 5   *Number Of Students:* 90
Degrees Offered: BA; BFA; MA   *Teaching Certification Available*
Financial Assistance: Assistantships, Scholarships and Work-Study Grants
Performing Groups: Theatre Company

STATE UNIVERSITY OF NEW YORK COLLEGE AT GENESEO
Geneseo   New York 14454, 716 245-5211

State and 4 Year
Arts Areas: Dance, Instrumental Music, Vocal Music, Theatre and Visual Arts
Performing Series: Limelight Artists Series
Performance Facilities: Brodie Fine Arts Center; Fallbrook Theatre; Black Box Theatre; Wadsworth Auditorium

DANCE

Scott Ray, Chairman   *Number Of Faculty:* 2   *Number Of Students:* 50
Degrees Offered: BA   *Teaching Certification Available*
Financial Assistance: Work-Study Grants
Workshops/Festivals: Annual Dance Concerts

MUSIC

Robert Isgro, Chairman   *Number Of Faculty:* 12   *Number Of Students:* 350
Degrees Offered: BA   *Teaching Certification Available*
Financial Assistance: Work-Study Grants
Performing Groups: Chamber Singers; Concert Band

THEATRE

Bruce Klee, Chairman   *Number Of Faculty:* 10   *Number Of Students:* 200

(continued on next page)

Degrees Offered: BA   **Teaching Certification Available**
Financial Assistance: Work-Study Grants   **Performing Groups:** Cothurnus
Workshops/Festivals: High School Drama Festival

STATE UNIVERSITY OF NEW YORK COLLEGE, NEW PALTZ
New Paltz   New York 12562, 914 257-2448
State and 4 Year
Arts Areas: Dance, Instrumental Music, Vocal Music, Theatre, Film Arts, Television and Visual Arts
Performance Facilities: McKenna Theatre; Parker Theatre; Main Building Auditorium; Gymnasium;
Student Union Building

DANCE

Gloria Bonali, Coordinator Dance Programs   **Number Of Faculty:** 4
Number Of Students: 248   **Degrees Offered:** Minor in Dance
Courses Offered: Technique; Choreography; History; Production; Children's Dance
Technical Training: Modern Dance; Ballet
Financial Assistance: Work-Study Grants
Performing Groups: New Paltz Dance Ensemble
Workshops/Festivals: Summer Workshop in Dance/Movement Education

MUSIC

Lee H Pritchard, Chairman   **Number Of Faculty:** 17   **Number Of Students:** 250
Technical Training: Applied Music; Music Therapy
Financial Assistance: Assistantships, Work-Study Grants and NYSTAP; BEOG
Performing Groups: Concert Choir; Symphonic Band; College - Community Orchestra; Women's Chorale;
Collegium Musicum; Chamber Singers; Jazz Ensemble; New Paltz Chamber Music Series
Workshops/Festivals: Summer Workshops

THEATRE

Joseph C Paparone, Chairman   **Number Of Faculty:** 7
Number Of Students: 200   **Degrees Offered:** BA
Courses Offered: History; Literature; Acting; Directing; Design
Financial Assistance: Work-Study Grants
Performing Groups: McKenna Productions; Children's Theatre; Summer Repertory Theatre; Players
Workshops/Festivals: State wide Student Directed Play Festivals

STATE UNIVERSITY OF NEW YORK COLLEGE, ONEONTA
Oneonta   New York 13820, 607 431-3500
State and 4 Year
Arts Areas: Instrumental Music, Vocal Music, Theatre and Visual Arts

MUSIC

John P Mazarak, Chairman   **Number Of Faculty:** 11   **Number Of Students:** 520
Degrees Offered: BA   **Courses Offered:** Music History; Theory & Performance
Technical Training: Applied Music
Financial Assistance: Work-Study Grants and Temporary Service Employment
Performing Groups: Chamber Singers; Concert Choir; Swing Choir; Concert Band; Catskill Symphony
Orchestra; Brass Ensemble; String Chamber Music; Woodwind Ensemble; Recorder Consort; Baroque
Ensemble
Workshops/Festivals: Music Festival of the New York State School Music Association; Workshops in Orff,
Ethnic Music, Folk Instrument Construction, Overseas Orchestral & Choral Institutes

THEATRE

Dr Josef A Elfenbein, Chairman   **Number Of Faculty:** 10
Degrees Offered: BA
Courses Offered: Appreciation; Introduction to Theatre as a Performing Art; Acting; Stage, Scenery &
Lighting; Make-up; Directing; Costuming; Creative Dramatics; Children's Theater; History; American
Theater; Greek Theater; Black Theater

(continued on next page)

Teaching Certification Available   *Financial Assistance:* Work-Study Grants
Performing Groups: Mask & Hammer; SUCO Summer Community Theater

---

STATE UNIVERSITY OF NEW YORK COLLEGE, OSWEGO
Oswego   New York 13126, 315 341-2500
State and 4 Year
Arts Areas: Instrumental Music, Vocal Music, Theatre and Visual Arts
Performing Series: Cultural Events Program

MUSIC

James J Soluri, Chairman   *Number Of Faculty:* 15   *Number Of Students:* 255
Degrees Offered: DA   *Teaching Certification Available*
Financial Assistance: Assistantships, Scholarships and Work-Study Grants
Performing Groups: Orchestra; Chamber Ensemble; Jazz Ensemble; Madrigals; Choir

THEATRE

Sanford Sternlight, Chairman   *Number Of Faculty:* 15
Number Of Students: 250   *Degrees Offered:* BA Speech-Theatre
Teaching Certification Available
Financial Assistance: Assistantships, Scholarships and Work-Study Grants
Performing Groups: Blackfriars

STATE UNIVERSITY OF NEW YORK COLLEGE, PLATTSBURGH
Broad St, Plattsburgh   New York 12901
518 564-2000
State and 4 Year
Arts Areas: Dance, Instrumental Music, Vocal Music, Theatre, Film Arts, Television and Visual Arts
Performing Series: Concert Series
Performance Facilities: Hartman Theatre; Hawkins Hall Auditorium; Studio Theatre

MUSIC

Alan Frank, Chairman   *Number Of Faculty:* 8   *Number Of Students:* 700
Degrees Offered: BA   *Teaching Certification Available*
Financial Assistance: Assistantships, Scholarships and Work-Study Grants
Performing Groups: College - Community Orchestra; Collage Chorale; College Symphonic Band; Jazz & Contemporary Ensemble; Faculty Trio

THEATRE

Daniel J Watermeier, Chairman   *Number Of Faculty:* 6
Number Of Students: 50   *Degrees Offered:* BA
Courses Offered: Theatre History; Theory; Acting; Directing; Design; Theatre Technology; Children's Theatre
Financial Assistance: Assistantships, Scholarships and Work-Study Grants
Performing Groups: The New Theatre Association
Workshops/Festivals: Summer Theatre Workshop

STATE UNIVERSITY OF NEW YORK COLLEGE, POTSDAM
Pierrepont Ave, Potsdam   New York 13676
315 268-2973
State and 4 Year
Arts Areas: Dance, Instrumental Music, Vocal Music, Theatre, Film Arts, Television and Visual Arts
Performing Series: Faculty Performance Series; School of Music Convocation Series; Celebrity Artist Series
Performance Facilities: Sara M Snell Music Theater; Helen M Hosmer Concert Hall; College Theater

DANCE

K Wright Dunkley, Coordinator   *Number Of Faculty:* 3
Number Of Students: 260
Courses Offered: Techniques; Composition; Repertory; History; Notation

(continued on next page)

Financial Assistance: Work-Study Grants
Performing Groups: College Dance Ensemble
Workshops/Festivals: Summer Dance Workshop in Technique, Composition & Improvisation

MUSIC

Robert W Thayer, Chairman   *Number Of Faculty:* 55   *Number Of Students:* 600
Degrees Offered: BMus; BA
Courses Offered: Music Education; Composition; History/Literature; Theory; Performance; Church Music; Special Education Music; Piano Pedagogy
Technical Training: Recording Technology; Instrument Repair
Teaching Certification Available
Financial Assistance: Scholarships and Work-Study Grants
Performing Groups: Wind Ensemble; Jazz Ensemble & Jazz Band; Concert Bands; String Quartets, Chamber Wind Groups; Woodwind Quintets; Brass Quintets; Percussion, Live/Electronic, Opera, Chamber Ensembles; Chorus; Symphony Orchestra; Chamber Choir; Collegiate Singers; Concert Choir
Workshops/Festivals: Spring Music Festival; Convocations - Guest Presentors; Crane Youth Music Summer Program; Potsdam/Saratoga Choral Institute (summer); Summer Music Theater; Opera

THEATRE

Dorothy Gmucs, Coordinator   *Number Of Faculty:* 3   *Number Of Students:* 200
Degrees Offered: BA
Courses Offered: Acting; Directing; History Design; Children's Theatre; Reader's Theatre; Technical Theatre
Technical Training: Design & Stagecraft; Stage Make-up
Financial Assistance: Assistantships, Scholarships and Work-Study Grants
Performing Groups: Children's Theatre Tour; Major Productions; Reader's Theatre
Workshops/Festivals: Student directed one - act plays & Workshops

---

STATE UNIVERSITY OF NEW YORK COLLEGE, PURCHASE
PROFESSIONAL SCHOOL OF ARTS
Purchase   New York 10577, 914 253-5000
State and 4 Year
Arts Areas: Dance, Instrumental Music, Vocal Music, Theatre and Visual Arts
Performance Facilities: Theatre D; Humanities Auditorium

DANCE

William Bales, Dean   *Number Of Faculty:* 16   *Number Of Students:* 340
Degrees Offered: BFA, 4 Areas; Certificate, 4 Areas
Technical Training: Modern; Ballet; Professional; Composition; Body Correctives; Ballet & Modern Variations; Lighting for Dance
Performing Groups: Purchase Dance Repertory Company
Workshops/Festivals: Dance Workshop; Repertory Work with Anna Sokolow, Nel Wong

MUSIC

Michael Hammond, Dean   *Number Of Faculty:* 23   *Number Of Students:* 100
Degrees Offered: BFA; Certificate
Technical Training: Professional Training in Performance

THEATRE

Norris Houghton, Chairman   *Number Of Faculty:* 17   *Number Of Students:* 135
Degrees Offered: BFA   *Technical Training:* Professional Program

---

STATE UNIVERSITY OF NEW YORK, OSWEGO
Tyler Hall, Oswego   New York 13126
315 341-2500
State and 4 Year
Arts Areas: Dance, Instrumental Music, Vocal Music, Theatre, Film Arts, Television and Visual Arts
Performing Series: Faculty Concert Series; Student Concerts & Recital Series; Drama Series; Cultural Series

(*continued on next page*)

Performance Facilities: Waterman Theatre; Experimental Theatre; Sheldon Hall Theatre; Hewitt Union Ballroom; Lee Hall Gym

DANCE

Joan Huff, Chairman   *Number Of Faculty:* 2   *Number Of Students:* 50
Financial Assistance: Work-Study Grants

MUSIC

Marilynn J Smiley, Chairman   *Number Of Faculty:* 15 Full-time, 3 Part-time
Number Of Students: 1,200   *Degrees Offered:* BA
Courses Offered: Music Theory; History & Literature; Applied Music; Performance
Financial Assistance: Scholarships and Work-Study Grants
Performing Groups: College Band; College Orchestra; College Choir; Chamber Singers; Choralaires (Women's Chorus); Men's Glee Club; Statesingers (Pop Vocal Group); Solid State (Jazz/Rock Ensemble); Festival Chorus (College/Community Group); Opera Workshop

THEATRE

Sanford Sternlight, Chairperson   *Number Of Faculty:* 10
Degrees Offered: BA Theatre; BS Speech & Theatre, Secondary Education
Courses Offered: Acting; Directing; History, Criticism
Technical Training: Acting; Stagecraft; Lighting; Design; Costuming
Teaching Certification Available
Financial Assistance: Scholarships and Work-Study Grants
Performing Groups: Black Friars; Chamber Readers
Workshops/Festivals: H S Theatre Festival; Children's Theatre Festival

---

STATE UNIVERSITY OF NEW YORK, STONY BROOK
Stony Brook   New York 11794, 516 246-5000
State and 4 Year
Arts Areas: Instrumental Music, Vocal Music and Theatre
Performing Series: University Concert Series; Electronic Music Series
Performance Facilities: Fine Arts Center; Stony Brook Union; Claerone Theatre; Auditorium

MUSIC

Leo Treitler, Chairman   *Number Of Faculty:* 35   *Number Of Students:* 350
Degrees Offered: BA; MA; MMus; PhD; DMA
Courses Offered: History; Theory; Composition; Performance
Financial Assistance: Work-Study Grants and Fellowships; N Y State residents - Tuition Assistance Program
Performing Groups: University Orchestra; Chamber Orchestra; University Band; The Stony Brook University Chorus; Chamber Singers; Ensembles; Opera Workshop
Workshops/Festivals: Electronic Music Workshop; Lecture - Workshop in the Performance of Baroque Music; Opera Workshop

THEATRE

Alfred G Brooks, Chairman   *Number Of Faculty:* 12   *Number Of Students:* 70
Degrees Offered: BA
Courses Offered: Acting; Voice; Directing; Design; Technical Theatre; Film; Movement; Scriptwriting
Technical Training: Scenery Construction; Scenery Painting; Stage Lighting; Costume Design & Construction; Motion Picture Operation; Film Editing
Financial Assistance: Work-Study Grants and Fellowships; N Y State residents - Tuition Assistance Program
Performing Groups: University Theatre; Opera Company; Summer Playhouse

---

STATEN COLLEGE COMMUNITY COLLEGE,
CITY UNIVERSITY OF NEW YORK
130 Stuyvesant Place, Staten Island   New York 10301
212 720-3073
City and 4 Year
Arts Areas: Dance, Instrumental Music, Vocal Music, Theatre, Film Arts, Television and Visual Arts

(continued on next page)

Performing Series: Sunday Concert Series
Performance Facilities: The Theatre; College Hall; Television Studio

DANCE

Professor Carolyn Watson, Coordinator   **Number Of Faculty:** 1
Number Of Students: 200   **Degrees Offered:** AA; BA
Technical Training: Internships; Independent Study; Practicum in Stage Work
Financial Assistance: Work-Study Grants and TAP; BEOG
Performing Groups: SI Ethnic Dance Company; Elizabeth Keene Dance Workshops
Workshops/Festivals: Master Classes with Professionals; Workshops with Professional Groups;
Annual Festival of the Arts at the Snug Harbor Cultural Center

MUSIC

Professor Victor Mattfeld, Coordinator   **Number Of Faculty:** 4
Number Of Students: 50   **Degrees Offered:** AA; BA
Technical Training: Internships; Independent Study; Practicum in Stage Work
Financial Assistance: Work-Study Grants and TAP; BEOG
Performing Groups: The College of State Island Chorus; College of Staten Island Jazz Ensemble
Workshops/Festivals: Annual Festival of the Arts at Snug Harbor Cultural Center

THEATRE

Professor Martin Blank, Chairman   **Number Of Faculty:** 4
Number Of Students: 50   **Degrees Offered:** AA; BA
Technical Training: Internships; Independent Study; Practicum in Stage Work
Financial Assistance: Work-Study Grants and TAP; BEOG
Performing Groups: Black Theatre Workshop
Workshops/Festivals: Annual Festival of the Arts at Snug Harbor Cultural Center

---

STUART OSTROW FOUNDATION, INC
PO Box 188, Pound Ridge   New York 10576
914 764-4412
Private and Special; Graduate School
Arts Areas: Dance, Instrumental Music, Vocal Music and Visual Arts
Performance Facilities: Musical Theatre Lab at the John F Kennedy Center for the Performing Arts

THEATRE

Edward Berkeley, Artistic Director of Musical Theatre Lab
The aim of the Foundation is to advance education and development of musical theatre in the United States
and to integrate the training and education of musical theatre into the colleges and universities at a graduate
level
Performing Groups: Musical Theatre Lab at Kennedy Center - Nine Productions
Workshops/Festivals: Workshops and Readings of original musicals

---

SUFFOLK COMMUNITY COLLEGE
533 College Rd, Selden   New York 11784
516 732-1600
State and 2 Year
Arts Areas: Instrumental Music, Vocal Music and Theatre
Number Of Faculty: 6   **Degrees Offered:** AA
Financial Assistance: Work-Study Grants

THEATRE

Shirley Cox, Director   **Number Of Faculty:** 7   **Degrees Offered:** AA
Financial Assistance: Work-Study Grants

SUFFOLK COUNTY COMMUNITY COLLEGE
533 College Rd, Selden   New York 11784
516 233-5240

County and 2 Year
Arts Areas: Dance, Instrumental Music, Vocal Music, Theatre, Film Arts, Television and Visual Arts
Performance Facilities: Islip Arts Theatre; I - 119 - Mini Theatre
Number Of Faculty: 1   *Number Of Students:* 350
Courses Offered: Folk, Square & Social Dance; Modern Dance & Composition; Dance for Theatre
Financial Assistance: Work-Study Grants
Performing Groups: Student Dance Productions
Workshops/Festivals: Summer Dance Workshop conducted by visiting dancer

MUSIC

Russell A Stevenson, Department Head   *Number Of Faculty:* 6
Number Of Students: 1,371
Courses Offered: Understanding Music; Music in Recreation; Theory; Music History; Sightsinging; Jazz; Folk Music; Piano; 20th Century Music
Financial Assistance: Work-Study Grants
Performing Groups: Chamber Orchestra; Concert Band; Suffolk Singers; Brass Ensemble; Jazz Ensemble; College Choir
Workshops/Festivals: May Arts Festival

THEATRE

Richard D Britton, Department Head   *Number Of Faculty:* 8
Number Of Students: 400
Courses Offered: Understanding Theatre; Stagecraft; Acting I, II; Dance for Theatre; Directing; Classical Theatre; Modern Theatre; Summer Theatre Workshop; Rehearsing & Performing I, II, III, IV
Technical Training: Production Work   *Performing Groups:* Student Drama Groups

SYRACUSE UNIVERSITY
Lowe Art Center, Syracuse   New York 13210
315 423-2611

Private and 4 Year
Arts Areas: Dance, Instrumental Music, Vocal Music, Theatre and Visual Arts
Performance Facilities: Concert Hall; Regent Theatre; Experimental Theatre

DANCE

Peter P Cataldi, Chairman   *Number Of Faculty:* 2   *Number Of Students:* 250
Degrees Offered: BS; MS
Courses Offered: Choreography; History; Appreciation of Dance
Financial Assistance: Internships and Assistantships
Performing Groups: Modern Dance Interest Group
Workshops/Festivals: Modern Dance Workshops

MUSIC

M Douglas Soyars, Assist Dean for Music   *Number Of Faculty:* 40
Number Of Students: 140
Degrees Offered: BMus; BA MusEd, Theory, Composition; BMus Performance Honors; MMus; MA; EdD in Mus Ed
Teaching Certification Available
Financial Assistance: Internships, Assistantships, Scholarships and Work-Study Grants
Performing Groups: Student Faculty Orchestra; Chorus; Schola Cantorum; Wind Ensemble; Stage Band; Symphony Band
Workshops/Festivals: Jazz Workshop

THEATRE

Arthur Storch, Chairman   *Number Of Faculty:* 12   *Number Of Students:* 157
Degrees Offered: BS; MA   *Technical Training:* Design; Technical Theatre

(continued on next page)

Financial Assistance: Internships, Assistantships and Work-Study Grants
Performing Groups: Syracuse Stage
Workshops/Festivals: Guest Speakers for Master Classes

UNION COLLEGE
Schenectady   New York 12308, 518 370-6000
Private and 4 Year
Arts Areas: Dance, Instrumental Music, Vocal Music, Theatre and Visual Arts
Performing Series: Union College - Schenectady Museum Concert Series; Contemporary Composer's Series
(with workshop)
Performance Facilities: Memorial Chapel; Nott Memorial

MUSIC

Number Of Faculty: 3   *Degrees Offered:* BA
Courses Offered: Introduction to Music; Composition; Ear Training & Sight Singing; Composition II, III;
Traditional Harmony; Sixteenth Century Counterpoint; Keyboard Harmony & Sight Reading; Introduction
to Electronic Music; Independent Study; Classic Musicians, 1750 -1825; Musical Romanticism, 1825 -1900;
Origins of Twentieth Century Music; Music in the 20th Century
Technical Training: Instrumental; Vocal; Electronic Music
Financial Assistance: Scholarships and Work-Study Grants

THEATRE

Number Of Faculty: 2   *Degrees Offered:* BA
Technical Training: Stage Design; Lighting; Set & Costume Construction; Make-up; Drafting
Financial Assistance: Scholarships and Work-Study Grants
Performing Groups: Mountebands (Student Theatre Group)
Workshops/Festivals: Costume, Make-up & Student Directing Workshops
Artists-In-Residence/Guest Artists: Elbert Weinberg

VASSAR COLLEGE
Ramond Ave, Poughkeepsie   New York 12601
914 452-7000
Private and 4 Year
Arts Areas: Instrumental Music, Vocal Music, Theatre and Visual Arts

MUSIC

Robert Middleton, Chairman   *Number Of Faculty:* 15
Degrees Offered: BA Music   *Technical Training:* Junior Year Abroad Program
Financial Assistance: Scholarships and Work-Study Grants
Performing Groups: Weekly Concerts Program

THEATRE

Evert Sprinchorn, Chairman   *Number Of Faculty:* 7   *Degrees Offered:* BA
Financial Assistance: Scholarships and Work-Study Grants
Performing Groups: Vassar Experimental Theatre

VILLA MARIA COLLEGE OF BUFFALO
240 Pine Ridge Rd, Buffalo   New York 14225
716 896-0700
Private and 2 Year
Arts Areas: Instrumental Music, Vocal Music and Visual Arts
Degrees Offered: AA   *Teaching Certification Available*
Financial Assistance: Work-Study Grants

WAGNER COLLEGE
631 Howard Ave, Staten Island   New York 10301
212 390-3000
Private and 4 Year
Arts Areas: Dance, Instrumental Music, Vocal Music, Theatre and Visual Arts
Performing Series: Theatre Production Series   *Performance Facilities:* Auditorium; Gymnasium

DANCE

Robert Hicks, Chairman, Physical Education Department   *Number Of Faculty:* 1
Courses Offered: Beginning, Intermediate & Advanced Modern Dance; Dances of India; Tap; Ballet;
Exploring Dance in NY
Financial Assistance: Scholarships
Performing Groups: Staten Island Dance Theatre (resident dance company)

MUSIC

Dr Harald Normann, Chairman   *Number Of Faculty:* 11
Number Of Students: 51   *Degrees Offered:* BA
Courses Offered: Vocal; Instrumental; Conducting; Music Education; Orchestration; Exploring
Opera/Symphony in NY
Financial Assistance: Scholarships
Performing Groups: Band; Choir; Collegium Musicum; College Community Orchestra

THEATRE

Dr Lowell Matson, Chairman   *Number Of Faculty:* 11   *Number Of Students:* 49
Degrees Offered: BA
Courses Offered: Stagecraft; Stage Lighting; Acting Techniques; Stage Directing; Stage Design; Performing
Arts Management; Exploring Theatre in NY; Art of the Cinema
Teaching Certification Available   *Financial Assistance:* Scholarships
Performing Groups: Wagner College Theatre   *Workshops/Festivals:* Wagner College Summer Theatre

WELLS COLLEGE
Aurora   New York 13026, 315 364-3011
Private and 4 Year   *Arts Areas:* Dance, Vocal Music and Theatre
Performing Series: Wells Concert Series; Music Department Series
Performance Facilities: Smith Hall (Dance); Barler Recital Hall (Music); Phipps Auditorium (Theatre,
Music, Dance)

Number Of Faculty: 4   *Number Of Students:* 260   *Degrees Offered:* BA
Teaching Certification Available   *Financial Assistance:* Assistantships and Work-Study Grants
Performing Groups: Early Music Consort; Chamber Singers; Choir

THEATRE

Number Of Faculty: 1   *Number Of Students:* 46   *Degrees Offered:* BA
Financial Assistance: Assistantships and Work-Study Grants   *Performing Groups:* Kastalia

YESHIVA UNIVERSITY
New York   New York 10033, 212 568-8400
Private and 4 Year
Arts Areas: Instrumental Music, Vocal Music, Theatre and Visual Arts

MUSIC

Number Of Faculty: 6   *Number Of Students:* 60   *Degrees Offered:* BA
Financial Assistance: Assistantships, Scholarships and Work-Study Grants

THEATRE

Number Of Faculty: 7   *Number Of Students:* 70   *Degrees Offered:* BA Speech and Drama
Financial Assistance: Assistantships, Scholarships and Work-Study Grants
Performing Groups: Dramatics Society

APPALACHIAN STATE UNIVERSITY
Boone   North Carolina 28607, 704 262-3036
>State, 4 Year and Graduate
>*Arts Areas:* Dance, Instrumental Music, Vocal Music, Theatre, Film Arts, Television and Visual Arts
>*Performing Series:* Artist & Lecture Series
>*Performance Facilities:* I G Gree Auditorium; Farthing Auditorium

DANCE

Lawrence Horine, Chairperson, Health, Physical Education & Recreation
Number Of Faculty: 2   *Number Of Students:* 100

MUSIC

Dr Frank Carroll, Chairman   *Number Of Faculty:* 26
Number Of Students: 300   *Degrees Offered:* BMus; BA; MA
Technical Training: Performance; Musical Education; Church Music; Composition
Teaching Certification Available
Financial Assistance: Assistantships, Scholarships and Work-Study Grants
Performing Groups: Symphony Orchestra; Chamber Orchestra; Wind Ensemble; Band; University Singers; Madrigal Singers; Men's & Women's Choruses; Percussion Ensemble
Workshops/Festivals: Cannon Music Camp; Contemporary Music Festival; Music Education Workshops

THEATRE

Charles Porterfield, Chairman, Communication Arts Department
Number Of Faculty: 10   *Number Of Students:* 120   *Degrees Offered:* BS
Technical Training: Radio; TV; Communication Media
Teaching Certification Available
Financial Assistance: Assistantships, Scholarships and Work-Study Grants
Performing Groups: Theatre Group; Radio Station WASU; Forensics Groups; Debate Team
Workshops/Festivals: Professional Summer Theatre

ATLANTIC CHRISTIAN COLLEGE
Lee St, Wilson   North Carolina 27893
919 237-3161
>Private and 4 Year
>*Arts Areas:* Instrumental Music, Vocal Music, Theatre and Visual Arts
>*Performing Series:* Concert & Lecture Series; AAUP Faculty Forum

MUSIC

Ross Albert, Chairman   *Number Of Faculty:* 16   *Number Of Students:* 75
Degrees Offered: BS MusEd; BA Mus   *Teaching Certification Available*
Financial Assistance: Scholarships, Work-Study Grants and College Work Grants
Performing Groups: Choir; Band; Ensembles: Brass, Percussion, Vocal, Recorder, String, New Music
Workshops/Festivals: Concert & Lecture Committee; Contemporary Music Festival

THEATRE

Paul Crouch, Director   *Number Of Faculty:* 1   *Number Of Students:* 20
Technical Training: Directing
Financial Assistance: Scholarships, Work-Study Grants and College Work Grants
Performing Groups: Stage & Script Club

BENNETT COLLEGE
Greensboro   North Carolina 27420, 919 273-4431
>Private and 4 Year
>*Arts Areas:* Dance, Instrumental Music, Vocal Music, Theatre, Film Arts, Television and Visual Arts
>*Performance Facilities:* Little Theatre; Annie Merner Pfeiffer Chapel

(continued on next page)

MUSIC

Dr Charlotte Alston, Chairman   **Number Of Faculty:** 4
Number Of Students: 80   **Degrees Offered:** BA MusEd
Courses Offered: Musicianship; Music Literature & Appreciation
Technical Training: Voice; Piano; Private Instruction
Teaching Certification Available
Financial Assistance: Scholarships and Work-Study Grants
Performing Groups: Choir; Choral Ensemble; Gospel Choir; Band Quartet; Octet; Jazz/Rock Group

THEATRE

Denise Troutman, Instructor of Speech & Drama   **Number Of Faculty:** 1
Number Of Students: 60   **Degrees Offered:** BA
Courses Offered: Play Production; Stage Acting; Stage Lighting; Film Making
Technical Training: Little Theatre Guild Workshop
Financial Assistance: Scholarships and Work-Study Grants
Performing Groups: Little Theatre Guild

BREVARD COLLEGE
Brevard   North Carolina 28712, 704 883-8292
Private and 2 Year
Arts Areas: Instrumental Music, Vocal Music and Theatre
Performing Series: Lyceum Concert Series
Performance Facilities: Dunham Music Center

MUSIC

Dr John D Upchurch, Chairman   **Number Of Faculty:** 12
Number Of Students: 63   **Degrees Offered:** AFA
Courses Offered: Theory; Composition; History & Literature; Electronic Music
Financial Assistance: Scholarships and Work-Study Grants
Performing Groups: Collegiate Singers; Oratorio Chorus; Chamber Singers; Wind Ensemble; Stage & Concert Bands

THEATRE

Sam Cope, Chairman   **Number Of Faculty:** 1
Courses Offered: Introduction to Theatre Arts; Theatre Arts Workshop
Financial Assistance: Scholarships and Work-Study Grants

CAMPBELL COLLEGE
Buies Creek   North Carolina 27406, 919 893-4111
Private and 4 Year
Arts Areas: Instrumental Music, Vocal Music and Theatre
Performing Series: Campbell College Concert Series
Performance Facilities: Turner Auditorium

MUSIC

Dr Paul M Yoder, Chairman   **Number Of Faculty:** 11   **Number Of Students:** 80
Degrees Offered: BA; BMusEd   **Teaching Certification Available**
Financial Assistance: Scholarships and Work-Study Grants
Performing Groups: Concert Choir; Campbell Singers (chamber); Chorale; Girls' Ensemble; Men's Ensemble; Concert Band; Stage Band; Woodwind Ensemble

THEATRE

Daniel Linney, Director   **Number Of Faculty:** 2   **Number Of Students:** 20
Financial Assistance: Scholarships and Work-Study Grants
Performing Groups: Campbell Players

CATAWBA COLLEGE
West Innes St Ext, Salisbury   North Carolina 28144
704 637-4111
Private and 4 Year
Arts Areas: Instrumental Music, Vocal Music, Theatre, Film Arts and Visual Arts
Performing Series: Catawba - Community Artist Series; College Union Board Series
Performance Facilities: Hedrick Little Theatre; Goodman Gymnasium; Keffel Auditorium

MUSIC

Lawrence Bond, Chairman   **Number Of Faculty:** 5   **Number Of Students:** 30
Degrees Offered: BA
Courses Offered: Theory; Literature; Applied Music; Ensemble; Music Education
Teaching Certification Available
Financial Assistance: Scholarships and Work-Study Grants

THEATRE

Hoyt McCachren, Chairman   **Number Of Faculty:** 8   **Number Of Students:** 68
Degrees Offered: BA
Courses Offered: Acting; Directing; Design; Technique; History & Literature
Technical Training: Lighting; Costuming; Construction; Design
Teaching Certification Available
Financial Assistance: Assistantships and Grant - In - Aid Scholarships
Performing Groups: Blue Masque; Piedmont Players; Experimental Theatre
Workshops/Festivals: High School Workshop; Teacher Certification Workshop; Creative Dramatics
Workshop

CHOWAN COLLEGE
Murfreesboro   North Carolina 27855, 919 398-4101 Ext 236
Private and 2 Year
Arts Areas: Dance, Instrumental Music and Vocal Music
Performing Series: Community Concerts Series
Performance Facilities: McDowell Columns Auditorium; Daniel Recital Hall

DANCE

Stacey Williams, Director   **Number Of Faculty:** 1   **Number Of Students:** 40
Degrees Offered: AA; AS
Courses Offered: Ballet; Modern; Folk; Contemporary; Dance History
Performing Groups: Dance Theater   **Workshops/Festivals:** Summer Dance Camp

MUSIC

James M Chamblee, Director, Daniel School of Music   **Number Of Faculty:** 5
Number Of Students: 25   **Degrees Offered:** AA; AS; AM
Courses Offered: Music Theory; Music Literature; Methods; Applied (all areas); Music Appreciation;
Choir; Stage Band; Concert Band
Technical Training: Voice; Piano & Organ; Brass; Woodwind; Percussion
Financial Assistance: Scholarships and Work-Study Grants
Performing Groups: College Choir; Touring Choir; Stage Band; Concert Band; Chamber Singers; Brass
Quintet
Workshops/Festivals: Summer String Camp; High School Stage Band Festival; Area Piano Teacher's
Workshop; Piano Guild Auditions

COLLEGE OF THE ALBEMARLE
Elizabeth City   North Carolina 27909, 919 335-0821 266
State and 2 Year
Arts Areas: Instrumental Music, Vocal Music, Theatre and Visual Arts
Performance Facilities: College Auditorium

(continued on next page)

MUSIC

Anna W Bair, Chairman   *Number Of Faculty:* 3   *Number Of Students:* 27
Degrees Offered: AA   *Financial Assistance:* Scholarships
Performing Groups: College of Albermarle Chorale, Albemarle Choral Society

THEATRE

Lucy Vaughan, Chairman   *Number Of Faculty:* 1   *Number Of Students:* 22
Degrees Offered: AA
Financial Assistance: Scholarships and Work-Study Grants
Performing Groups: College of the Albemarle Satyrs

DAVIDSON COLLEGE
Davidson   North Carolina 28036, 704 892-2000
Private and 4 Year
Arts Areas: Instrumental Music, Vocal Music, Theatre, Film Arts and Visual Arts
Performing Series: Artists Series; Chamber Music Series; Public Lectures
Performance Facilities: Love Auditorium; Hodson Hall; 900 Room

MUSIC

Donald B Plott, Chairman   *Number Of Faculty:* 3 Full-time, 5 Part-time
Number Of Students: 200   *Degrees Offered:* BA; BS
Courses Offered: Applied Music   *Technical Training:* Individual Instruction
Financial Assistance: Scholarships and Work-Study Grants
Performing Groups: The Male Chorus; Women's Chorus; Madrigal Singers; Chamber Chorus; Chamber Music Ensemble; Pep Band; Stage Band; Student Guild of Organists
Workshops/Festivals: Sacred Music Convocation; Alumni Organ Recital

THEATRE

Rupert T Barber, Jr, Chairman   *Number Of Faculty:* 4
Number Of Students: 210
Financial Assistance: Scholarships and Work-Study Grants
Performing Groups: Drama Department; Studio Theatre; Readers' Theatre
Workshops/Festivals: Studio Productions

DUKE UNIVERSITY
Durham   North Carolina 27706, 919 684-8111
Private and 4 Year
Arts Areas: Dance, Instrumental Music, Vocal Music and Theatre
Performing Series: Duke University Artist Series
Performance Facilities: Page Auditorium; Duke Chapel; Baldwin Auditorium; East Duke Music Room; Small Chamber Music Halls

DANCE

Julia Wray, Director
Dance program under auspieces of Physical Education Department
Number Of Faculty: 3   *Number Of Students:* 300
Courses Offered: Modern Dance; Ballet; Folk; Improvisation; Tap; History of Dance
Technical Training: Contemporary Dance Composition; Creative Movement for Children
Financial Assistance: Work-Study Grants   *Performing Groups:* Duke Dance Group
Workshops/Festivals: Workshops for students working in local public schools

MUSIC

Dr Frank Tirro, Chairman   *Number Of Faculty:* 38   *Number Of Students:* 1200
Degrees Offered: BA
Courses Offered: Theory; Composition; History of Music; Literature; Music Education; Pedagogy
Technical Training: Applied Music; All Strings; Brass; Woodwinds; Piano; Percussion; Voice; Organ; Ensembles; Electronic Recording Studio
Financial Assistance: Assistantships, Scholarships and Work-Study Grants

(continued on next page)

Performing Groups: Chorale; Chapel Choir; Symphony Orchester; Wind Symphony; Marching Band; Pep Band; Chamber Orchestra; Collegium Musicum
Workshops/Festivals: Annual performances of Messiah at Christmas; Outdoor fall & spring garden concerts by band & chamber groups

THEATRE

Dr John Clum, Director   **Number Of Faculty:** 3   **Number Of Students:** 200
Courses Offered: History of Theatre; Stagecraft; Play Production; Broadcasting; Speaking Voice Acting; Set Design; Directing
Technical Training: Practical Theatre Training; Work in Production Techniques
Financial Assistance: Assistantships, Scholarships and Work-Study Grants
Performing Groups: Duke Players
Workshops/Festivals: Annual Summer Theater Program
Artists-In-Residence/Guest Artists: Mary Lou Williams

EAST CAROLINA UNIVERSITY
Greenville   North Carolina 27834, 919 757-6390
State and 4 Year
Arts Areas: Dance, Instrumental Music, Vocal Music, Theatre, Television and Visual Arts
Number Of Faculty: 5   **Number Of Students:** 300   **Degrees Offered:** BFA
Courses Offered: Ballet; Jazz; Modern; Dance History; Choreography
Financial Assistance: Assistantships, Scholarships and Work-Study Grants

MUSIC

Everett Pittman, Dean   **Number Of Faculty:** 46   **Number Of Students:** 380
Degrees Offered: BMus; MMus
Courses Offered: Performance; Music Education; Theory/Composition; Music Therapy
Teaching Certification Available
Financial Assistance: Assistantships, Scholarships and Work-Study Grants
Performing Groups: Symphony Orchestra; Wind Ensemble; Marching Band; Two Bands; Five Choruses; Two Lab Bands; Collegium Musicum; Woodwind Quintet
Workshops/Festivals: Piano; Choral; Band; Various Instruments; Fine Arts Festival

THEATRE

Edgar R Loessin, Chairman   **Number Of Faculty:** 18
Number Of Students: 300 - 400   **Degrees Offered:** BA; BS; BFA
Courses Offered: Acting; Directing; Design; Dance

ELON COLLEGE
Elon College   North Carolina 27244, 919 584-9711
Private and 4 Year
Arts Areas: Dance, Instrumental Music, Vocal Music, Theatre and Visual Arts
Performing Series: Lyceum Series
Performance Facilities: Whitley Auditorium; Mooney Theatre

DANCE

Number Of Faculty: 1   **Number Of Students:** 20
Courses Offered: Folk, Square, Social & Creative; Modern Dance; Methods & Materials of Rhythms

MUSIC

Walter Westafer, Chairman, Department of Fine Arts   **Number Of Faculty:** 9
Number Of Students: 92   **Degrees Offered:** BA; BS
Courses Offered: Applied Music; Theory; History of Music; Form; Counterpoint; Music Education; Arranging; Conducting
Financial Assistance: Scholarships and Work-Study Grants
Performing Groups: Band; Choir; Orchestra; "The Emanons" (a stage band)
Workshops/Festivals: Annual Brass Clinic

(continued on next page)

THEATRE

Number Of Faculty: 1   **Number Of Students:** 15
Courses Offered: Introduction to Theater; Theater Workshop
Financial Assistance: Scholarships and Work-Study Grants

FAYETTEVILLE STATE UNIVERSITY
Murchinson Rd, Fayetteville   North Carolina 28301
919 483-6144 Ext 219
State and 4 Year
Arts Areas: Dance, Instrumental Music, Vocal Music, Theatre and Television
Performing Series: Lyceum Series   **Performance Facilities:** Seabrook Auditorium

MUSIC

Number Of Faculty: 7   **Number Of Students:** 49   **Degrees Offered:** BS MusEd
Teaching Certification Available
Performing Groups: Choir, Band, Vocal Octet, Brass Ensemble, Woodwind Ensemble, Jazz Band
Workshops/Festivals: Clinics, Guest Artists   **Financial Assistance:** Scholarships and Work-Study Grants

---

GARDNER - WEBB COLLEGE
Boiling Springs   North Carolina 28017, 704 434-2361 Ext 333
Private and 4 Year   **Arts Areas:** Instrumental Music and Vocal Music
Performing Series: Distinguished Artist Series
Performance Facilities: Hamrick Auditorium; O Max Gardner Fine Arts Center; Boiling Springs Baptist Church; Bost Gymnasium

MUSIC

Dr George R Cribb, Chairman, Department of Fine Arts   **Number Of Faculty:** 15
Number Of Students: 94   **Degrees Offered:** BA
Courses Offered: Applied (voice, piano, organ, instrumental); Theory; Music History & Literature; Sacred Music; Music Education; Performance Organizations
Teaching Certification Available   **Financial Assistance:** Work-Study Grants
Performing Groups: Choral Ensemble; Chamber Chorus; College Chorus; Band; Orchestra; Opera Workshop
Workshops/Festivals: Choral Clinic/Workshop; Piano Workshop

THEATRE

David W Smith, Chairman   **Number Of Faculty:** 1
Courses Offered: Applied Theatre; Intro to the Drama
Financial Assistance: Work-Study Grants   **Performing Groups:** Applied Theatre

---

GREENSBORO COLLEGE
815 W Market St, Greensboro   North Carolina 27420
919 272-7102 Ext 272
Private and 4 Year
Arts Areas: Instrumental Music, Vocal Music and Theatre
Performance Facilities: Greenboro College Auditorium

MUSIC

Mr Don Hansen, Chairman   **Number Of Faculty:** 11   **Number Of Students:** 48
Degrees Offered: BA, BMus, BMusEd   **Teaching Certification Available**
Financial Assistance: Scholarships and Work-Study Grants
Performing Groups: Chorale, Glee Club, Chamber Orchestra
Workshops/Festivals: Music Performance Workshop

THEATRE

Mr Leonard Hart, Chairman   **Number Of Faculty:** 1   **Number Of Students:** 57
Degrees Offered: BA; BS   **Teaching Certification Available**
Financial Assistance: Scholarships and Work-Study Grants   **Performing Groups:** Players

HIGH POINT COLLEGE
933 Montlieu Ave, High Point   North Carolina 27262
919 885-5101

Private and 4 Year
Arts Areas: Vocal Music, Theatre, Film Arts, Television and Visual Arts
Performing Series: Performing Artists Series
Performance Facilities: Memorial Auditorium; "The Empty Space Theatre"

MUSIC

Dr James M Elson, Professor of Music   *Number Of Faculty:* 2
Number Of Students: 15   *Degrees Offered:* BA
Courses Offered: Applied music in Voice & Piano, Organ & Theory
Teaching Certification Available
Performing Groups: High Point College Choir; High Point College Singers; College - Community Band

THEATRE

David Christovich, Associate Professor   *Number Of Faculty:* 2
Number Of Students: 15
Courses Offered: Performing; Technical; Theory; History
Teaching Certification Available   *Performing Groups:* Tower Players

JOHNSON C SMITH UNIVERSITY
100 - 152 Beatties Ford Rd, Charlotte   North Carolina 28216
704 372-2370 Ext 255

Private and 4 Year
Arts Areas: Instrumental Music, Vocal Music, Theatre, Visual Arts and Radio

MUSIC

Christopher W Kemp, Professor & Head of Department   *Number Of Faculty:* 5
Number Of Students: 60   *Degrees Offered:* BA; BMus
Courses Offered: Instrumental; Vocal   *Teaching Certification Available*
Financial Assistance: Scholarships and Work-Study Grants
Performing Groups: Marching Band; Choir; Glee Club; Ensembles
Workshops/Festivals: Christmas Cantata; Spring Concert

THEATRE

Theatre Department under auspices of Communication Arts Department
Number Of Faculty: 3   *Number Of Students:* 40
Degrees Offered: BA Communication Arts
Technical Training: Stage & Lighting; Radio
Financial Assistance: Work-Study Grants and Word Aid
Performing Groups: Ira Aldridge Drama Guild
Workshops/Festivals: Dramatic Productions; Reading

LEES MCRAE COLLEGE
Banner Elk   North Carolina 28604, 704 898-6625

Private and 2 Year
Arts Areas: Instrumental Music, Vocal Music and Visual Arts
Performing Series: Lees McRae Concert Series
Performance Facilities: College Auditorium   *Degrees Offered:* AA
Financial Assistance: Scholarships and Work-Study Grants
Performing Groups: Vocal and Instrumental Ensembles; Cast 139

LENOIR - RHYNE COLLEGE
Hickory   North Carolina 28601, 704 328-1741 Ext 272
Private and 4 Year
Arts Areas: Instrumental Music, Vocal Music, Theatre and Visual Arts
Performance Facilities: P E Monroe Auditorium; Mauney Music Building

MUSIC

E Ray McNeely, Jr, Assistant Professor   *Number Of Faculty:* 9
Number Of Students: 60   *Degrees Offered:* BA; BM
Courses Offered: Harmony; Sight Singing; Intro to Music; Music Appreciation; Fundamentals of Music for Classroom Teachers; Keyboard Harmony; Music Literature Survey for Teachers; Fundamentals & Methods for Intermediate Teachers; Counterpoint; Orchestration; Music History & Literature; Intro to Church Music; Composition; Form & Analytical Technique
Technical Training: Applied Music in Piano, Organ, Strings, Woodwinds, Brass; Voice Class; Piano Class; Brass/Percussion Class; String Class; Instrumental Conducting; Public School Music Methods; Piano Pedagogy; Voice Pedagogy; Field Experience in Music Education; Choral Conducting & Literature; Woodwind Class; High School Music Methods; Instrumental Methods
Teaching Certification Available
Financial Assistance: Scholarships and Work-Study Grants
Performing Groups: Marching Band; Wind Ensemble; Stage Band; A Cappella; Choir; College Singers

THEATRE

Dr Marion H Love, Chairman   *Number Of Faculty:* 4   *Number Of Students:* 22
Degrees Offered: BA
Courses Offered: Acting; Directing; Stagecraft; Scene Design; Lighting; Costuming - Make-up; Theatre History; Dramatic Literature
Technical Training: Acting; Directing; Stage Design; Properties; Light Design
Teaching Certification Available
Financial Assistance: Scholarships and Work-Study Grants
Performing Groups: Playmakers; Summer Theatre
Workshops/Festivals: Regular Production Season; Laboratory Productions
Artists-In-Residence/Guest Artists: Ronald Aulgar

LIVINGSTONE COLLEGE
701 W Monroe, Salisbury   North Carolina 28144
704 633-7960
Private and 4 Year
Arts Areas: Instrumental Music, Vocal Music, Theatre and Visual Arts

MUSIC

Number Of Faculty: 7   *Number Of Students:* 35   *Degrees Offered:* BA
Teaching Certification Available
Financial Assistance: Scholarships and Work-Study Grants
Performing Groups: Band, Concert Choir, Mens Glee Club

THEATRE

Clyde Williams, Chairman   *Number Of Faculty:* 2   *Number Of Students:* 28
Teaching Certification Available
Financial Assistance: Scholarships and Work-Study Grants
Performing Groups: Julia B Duncan Players

MARS HILL COLLEGE
Mars Hill   North Carolina 28754, 704 689-1203
Private and 4 Year
Arts Areas: Dance, Instrumental Music, Vocal Music, Theatre and Visual Arts
Performing Series: Visiting Lecturers & Artists Series
Performance Facilities: Owen Theatre, Robert More Fine Arts Auditorium

(continued on next page)

MUSIC

Joel Stegal, Chairman   **Number Of Faculty:** 17   **Number Of Students:** 185
Degrees Offered: BMus, BMusEd   **Teaching Certification Available**
Financial Assistance: Internships, Scholarships and Work-Study Grants
Performing Groups: Touring Choir, Chorus, Marching Band, Concert Band, Stage Band, Brass Ensemble
Workshops/Festivals: Regular Workshops for High School Choruses and Band

THEATRE

James W Thomas, Chairman   **Number Of Faculty:** 3   **Number Of Students:** 35
Degrees Offered: BA, B Theatre Arts Education, B Arts & MusEd, BA Musical Theatre Performance
Teaching Certification Available
Financial Assistance: Internships, Assistantships, Scholarships and Work-Study Grants
Performing Groups: College Theatre, Lab Theatre, Southern Appalacian Repertory Theatre (Summer)
Workshops/Festivals: Summer Theatre Workshop for College, High School Students and High School
Teachers

MAYLAND TECHNICAL INSTITUTE
Spruce Pine   North Carolina 28777, 704 765-7351 Ext 60
  State and 2 Year   **Arts Areas:** Instrumental Music and Vocal Music
  Number Of Faculty: 2 Part-time
  Courses Offered: Chorus; Music Appreciation; Instrumental Ensemble; Recorder
  Artists-In-Residence/Guest Artists: Patrick Cauble; Shayna Hollander

MEREDITH COLLEGE
Hillsborough St, Raleigh   North Carolina 27611
919 833-6461
  Private and 4 Year
  Arts Areas: Dance, Instrumental Music, Vocal Music, Theatre and Visual Arts
  Performance Facilities: Jones Auditorium; Cate Center Auditorium; Studio Theatre; Carswell Concert Hall

MUSIC

Dr David Lynch, Chairman   **Number Of Faculty:** 36   **Number Of Students:** 130
Degrees Offered: BMus; BA
Courses Offered: Theory; Literature; History; Education; Composition; Applied Music
Teaching Certification Available
Financial Assistance: Scholarships and Loans; Student Employment
Performing Groups: Meredith Chorale; Renaissance Singers; Ensemble; Orchestra; Handbell Choir
Workshops/Festivals: Spring Choral Festival; Orff Workshop; Master Classes in Piano, Organ & Voice

THEATRE

Nancy Truesdale, Instructor   **Number Of Faculty:** 2
Courses Offered: Play Production; Intro to the Theater
Technical Training: Play Production; Independent Studies
Performing Groups: Meredith Playhouse; Children's Theatre Company; Oral Interpretation Class

METHODIST COLLEGE
Raleigh Rd, Fayetteville   North Carolina 28301
919 488-7110
  Private and 4 Year
  Arts Areas: Instrumental Music, Vocal Music, Theatre and Visual Arts
  Performing Series: College Convocation Series
  Performance Facilities: Reeves Auditorium; Science Building Auditorium; Hensdale Chapel
  Student Union Building; Michael Terrence O'Hanlon Memorial Amphitheater

MUSIC

Dr Willis Gates, Chairman   **Number Of Faculty:** 4   **Degrees Offered:** BA
Teaching Certification Available

(continued on next page)

North Caroli

Financial Assistance: Scholarships and Work-Study Grants
Performing Groups: College Chorus; Wind Ensemble; Vocal Ensemble; Stage Band; English Handbell Ensemble; Orchestra

THEATRE

Dr Jack Peyrouse, Associate Professor of Speech & Theater
Number Of Faculty: 1
Financial Assistance: Scholarships and Work-Study Grants
Performing Groups: Green and Gold Masque Keys

MITCHELL COMMUNITY COLLEGE

West Broad St, Statesville   North Carolina 28677
704 873-2201 Ext 233
State and 2 Year
Arts Areas: Dance, Instrumental Music, Vocal Music, Theatre and Visual Arts
Performance Facilities: Shearer Hall

MUSIC

Jane Heyman, Division Chairman   **Number Of Faculty:** 3
Number Of Students: 30   **Degrees Offered:** AFA
Courses Offered: Vocal; Strings; Keyboard; Choir
Financial Assistance: Scholarships and Work-Study Grants
Performing Groups: Choir

MONTREAT ANDERSON COLLEGE

Montreat   North Carolina 28757, 704 669-8425
Private and 2 Year   **Arts Areas:** Instrumental Music and Vocal Music
Performance Facilities: College Auditorium

MUSIC

Degrees Offered: AA Mus, AA MusEd
Financial Assistance: Scholarships
Performing Groups: Vocal and Instrumental Ensembles

MOUNT OLIVE COLLEGE

Mount Olive   North Carolina 28365, 919 658-2502
Private and 2 Year
Arts Areas: Instrumental Music, Vocal Music and Visual Arts
Performance Facilities: College Auditorium

MUSIC

Irene S Patten, Chairman   **Number Of Faculty:** 3   **Degrees Offered:** AA
Financial Assistance: Scholarships and Work-Study Grants
Performing Groups: Instrumental and Vocal Ensembles

NORTH CAROLINA AGRICULTURE AND TECHNICAL STATE UNIVERSITY

327 N Dudley St, Greensboro   North Carolina 27411
919 379-7500
Private and 4 Year
Arts Areas: Instrumental Music, Vocal Music and Visual Arts
Performing Series: A&T State University Lyceum Series
Performance Facilities: Harrison Auditorium

(continued on next page)

MUSIC

Jimmy J Williams, Chairman   **Number Of Faculty:** 6   **Number Of Students:** 60
Degrees Offered: BA   **Teaching Certification Available**
Financial Assistance: Scholarships and Work-Study Grants

NORTH CAROLINA CENTRAL UNIVERSITY
Durham   North Carolina 27707, 919 682-2172
State and 4 Year
Arts Areas: Dance, Instrumental Music, Vocal Music, Theatre and Visual Arts
Performing Series: NCCU Lyceum Program
Performance Facilities: B N Duke Auditorium

DANCE

Nancy Pinckney, Chairman   **Number Of Faculty:** 1   **Number Of Students:** 72
Performing Groups: NCCU Dance Club

MUSIC

Dr Gene Strassler, Chairman   **Number Of Faculty:** 11
Number Of Students: 350   **Degrees Offered:** BA, MA
Teaching Certification Available   **Financial Assistance:** Work-Study Grants
Performing Groups: NC String Trio, Concert and Touring Choirs, Concert and Marching Bands

THEATRE

Dr Randolph Unberger, Chairman   **Number Of Faculty:** 6
Number Of Students: 360   **Degrees Offered:** BA
Technical Training: Standard Technical Courses
Teaching Certification Available   **Financial Assistance:** Work-Study Grants
Performing Groups: Reader's Theatre, Children's Theatre, Ivan Dixon Players

---

NORTH CAROLINA SCHOOL OF THE ARTS
PO Box 12189, Winston - Salem   North Carolina 27107
919 784-7170
State, 4 Year and Includes high school and college
Arts Areas: Dance, Instrumental Music, Vocal Music, Theatre, Visual Arts and Design & Production
Performance Facilities: Crawford Hall; Agnes de Mille Theatre; Recital Hall; Sound Studio

DANCE

Robert Lindgren, Dean   **Number Of Faculty:** 10   **Number Of Students:** 150
Degrees Offered: BFA
Courses Offered: Modern & Ballet Technique; Pointe; Character; Adagio; Acting; Dance History;
Composition & Notation; Stage Presence
Technical Training: Modern & Ballet Technique
Financial Assistance: Scholarships, Work-Study Grants and Tuition Reductions; Loans
Performing Groups: North Carolina Dance Theatre (professional company affiliated with school)
Workshops/Festivals: "The Nutcracker"; One other Major Ballet; Two Workshops; Touring Modules

MUSIC

Robert Hickok, Dean   **Number Of Faculty:** 37   **Number Of Students:** 235
Degrees Offered: BMus
Courses Offered: Literature & Materials; Solfege; Music History; Orchestration; Composition Techniques;
Keyboard Studies; Score Reading - Conducting; Chamber Music; Accompanying; Vocal Repertoire;
Diction; Secondary Piano; Orchestra
Financial Assistance: Scholarships, Work-Study Grants and Tuition Reductions; Loans
Performing Groups: Clarion Wind Quintet; Piedmont Chamber Orchestra; NCSA Orchestra; NCSA
Chamber Choir
Workshops/Festivals: One Opera Workshop; One Fully Staged Opera; Eight Orchestra Concerts; Various
Recitals; Touring Modules

(continued on next page)

THEATRE

Malcolm Morrison, Dean   **Number Of Faculty:** 13   **Number Of Students:** 90
Degrees Offered: BFA
Courses Offered: Acting; Voice & Speech; Singing; Movement; Stage Fighting; Mime; Mask Work; Clowning
Financial Assistance: Scholarships, Work-Study Grants and Tuition Reductions; Loans
Performing Groups: Senior Students' Company
Workshops/Festivals: Three Major Productions; Five Workshops; Touring Modules
Artists-In-Residence/Guest Artists: Charles Czarny; Alexandra Danilova; James Dodding; Barnet Kellman; Max Rudolf; Robert Israel; John Gosling

---

NORTH CAROLINA WESLEYAN COLLEGE
Hwy 301 North, Rocky Mount   North Carolina 27801
919 442-7121
Private and 4 Year
Arts Areas: Instrumental Music, Vocal Music and Theatre
Performing Series: Rocky Mount - Wesleyan Performing Arts Series
Performance Facilities: Everett Gymnasium; Garber Chapel

MUSIC

Dr William Sasser, Chairman   **Number Of Faculty:** 3   **Number Of Students:** 25
Degrees Offered: BA
Courses Offered: Music Appreciation; Survey of Music Literature; Basic Music; Form & Analysis; Music Fundamentals for Classroom Teachers; Orchestration; History & Composition; Music in Public Schools; Keyboard Pedagogy; Vocal Pedagogy; Conducting; Piano; Organ; Voice; Woodwinds; Brasses; Percussion; Performing Ensembles; Class Instrumental & Vocal
Teaching Certification Available
Financial Assistance: Scholarships and Work-Study Grants
Performing Groups: Wesleyan Singers; Pro Arte; Wesleyan Concert Band; Wesleyan Jazz Band

THEATRE

John Tobinski, Chairman   **Number Of Faculty:** 2   **Number Of Students:** 40
Degrees Offered: BA
Courses Offered: Theatre Lab; Acting; Introduction to Technical Theatre; Make-up; Introduction to Theatre; Video-tape Production; Directing; Scenic Design
Technical Training: Lighting Design; Costume Design; History of Theatre; Oriental; Theatre; Film Appreciation; Advanced Studies; Methods in Creative Drama
Teaching Certification Available
Financial Assistance: Scholarships and Work-Study Grants
Performing Groups: Wesleyan Players
Workshops/Festivals: Several workshops are scheduled throughout the year for high school and junior college students

---

UNIVERSITY OF NORTH CAROLINA, ASHEVILLE
University Heights, Asheville   North Carolina 28804
704 258-0200
State and 4 Year
Arts Areas: Instrumental Music, Vocal Music, Theatre and Speech
Performing Series: Asheville Chamber Music Series
Performance Facilities: Belk Theatre; Lipinsky Auditorium; Carmichael Humanities Lecture Hall

MUSIC

Dr E Frank Edwinn, Associate Professor   **Number Of Faculty:** 1
Number Of Students: 10   **Teaching Certification Available**
Financial Assistance: Scholarships and Work-Study Grants

THEATRE

Arnold K Wengrow, Associate Professor   **Number Of Faculty:** 3

(continued on next page)

Number Of Students: 20   **Degrees Offered:** BA in Drama or Drama/Literature
Teaching Certification Available
Financial Assistance: Scholarships and Work-Study Grants
Performing Groups: Theatre UNC- Asheville; Forum Theatre; Readers' Theatre
Workshops/Festivals: Summer workshop in conjunction with Asheville Community Theatre for Youth

---

UNIVERSITY OF NORTH CAROLINA, CHARLOTTE
Charlotte   North Carolina 28223, 704 597-2387
State and 4 Year
Arts Areas: Dance, Instrumental Music, Vocal Music, Theatre, Visual Arts and Creative Writing
Performance Facilities: Rowe Theatre; Rowe Studio Theatre; Rowe Recital Hall

DANCE

Gerda Zimmermann, Department Coordinator   **Number Of Faculty:** 2
Number Of Students: 50   **Degrees Offered:** BCA
Courses Offered: Dance Skills; Related Theoretical Studies (Anatomy, Kinesiology, Dance History); Mime; Jazz; Ethnic; Choreography; Performance
Teaching Certification Available   **Financial Assistance:** Work-Study Grants
Performing Groups: UNCC Creative Dance Ensemble

MUSIC

Robert Gehner, Coordinator   **Number Of Faculty:** 10
Number Of Students: 120   **Degrees Offered:** BCA
Courses Offered: Independent Projects & Seminars
Teaching Certification Available   **Financial Assistance:** Work-Study Grants
Performing Groups: UNCC Sinfonietta; UNCC Chorale; UNCC Symphony; UNCC Oratorio Chorus

THEATRE

William Rackley, Coordinator   **Number Of Faculty:** 6
Number Of Students: 70   **Degrees Offered:** BCA
Courses Offered: Acting; Directing; Designing; Writing; A Colloquium on Selected Periods; Seminars & Workshops
Teaching Certification Available   **Financial Assistance:** Work-Study Grants
Performing Groups: UNCC Theatre Ensemble

UNIVERSITY OF NORTH CAROLINA, GREENSBORO
1000 Spring Garden St, Greensboro   North Carolina 27412
919 379-5494
State and 4 Year
Arts Areas: Dance, Instrumental Music, Vocal Music, Theatre, Television and Visual Arts
Performing Series: Concert - Lecture Series
Performance Facilities: Aycock Auditorium; Taylor Theatre; Curry Auditorium; Parkway Playhouse

DANCE

Lois Andreasen, Chairman   **Number Of Faculty:** 9   **Number Of Students:** 120
Degrees Offered: BFA; BS; MFA; MS; EdD   **Courses Offered:** Performance; Dance
Technical Training: Ballet; Modern; Ethnic; Dance History; Literature; Labonation; Artist - in - Residence Program
Teaching Certification Available
Financial Assistance: Scholarships and Work-Study Grants
Performing Groups: Concert Company; Touring Company; Ensemble
Workshops/Festivals: Summer Workshops with Guest Artists

MUSIC

Lawrence Hart, Dean   **Number Of Faculty:** 41   **Number Of Students:** 800
Degrees Offered: BM; BA; MM; MFA; EdD
Courses Offered: Applied Music; Music Education; Composition/Theory
Teaching Certification Available

(continued on next page)

Financial Assistance: Assistantships, Scholarships and Work-Study Grants
Performing Groups: Concert Band; Wind & Jazz Ensembles; Symphony & Chamber Orchestra; Glee Club; Choir; Chorale; Symphonic Chorus; Madrigal Singers; Opera & Musical Comedy

THEATRE

John Lee Jellicorse, Head, Department of Communication & Theatre
Number Of Faculty: 11   **Number Of Students:** 500
Degrees Offered: BA; BFA; MA; MEd; MFA
Courses Offered: Acting/Directing; Design/Technical Theatre; Child Drama; Broadcasting/Cinema
Teaching Certification Available
Financial Assistance: Assistantships, Scholarships and Work-Study Grants
Performing Groups: UNCG Theatre; UNCG Summer Repertory Theatre; Studio Theatre; Parkway Playhouse; Theatre for Young People; Theatre for Young People Touring Professional Repertory Company; Kaleidoscope; Mime Troupe
Workshops/Festivals: Carolina Drama Association Southeastern Theatre Conference (home institution); Two Dance Concerts; Opera; Cinema Workshop & Cinema House Production Unit

UNIVERSITY OF NORTH CAROLINA, WILMINGTON

PO Box 3725, Wilmington   North Carolina 28401
919 791-4330 Ext 225
State and 4 Year
Arts Areas: Instrumental Music, Vocal Music, Theatre and Visual Arts
Performing Series: UNCW Fine Arts Series; University Music Series
Performance Facilities: S R O Theatre; Sarah Graham Kenan Memorial Auditorium

MUSIC

Richard Deas, Chairman   **Number Of Faculty:** 9 Full-time, 2 Part-time
Number Of Students: 37   **Degrees Offered:** BA MusEd; BA in Creative Arts
Teaching Certification Available
Financial Assistance: Scholarships and Work-Study Grants
Performing Groups: Concert Choir; Chamber Singers; Wind Ensemble; Jazz Ensemble; The Wilmington Pro Musica and the UNCW Community Orchestra

THEATRE

W Terry Rogers, Chairman   **Number Of Faculty:** 6   **Number Of Students:** 25
Degrees Offered: BA in Creative Arts
Financial Assistance: Scholarships and Work-Study Grants
Performing Groups: University Theatre; University Readers' Theatre; S R O Straw - Hat Summer Theatre
Workshops/Festivals: Blockade Runner Invitational Debate Tournament

PEACE COLLEGE

15 E Peace St, Raleigh   North Carolina 27604
919 832-2881
Private and 2 Year
Arts Areas: Dance, Instrumental Music, Vocal Music and Theatre
Performing Series: Mary Howard Clark Arts & Lecture Series
Performance Facilities: Recital Hall; Brown - McPherson Music Bldg

DANCE

Margaret Westcott, Instructor   **Number Of Faculty:** 1
Number Of Students: 22
Courses Offered: Beginning & Intermediate Modern Dance
Performing Groups: Dance Club
Workshops/Festivals: Annual May Day Performance

MUSIC

Dr Joan Duyk, Instructor   **Number Of Faculty:** 3   **Number Of Students:** 117
Courses Offered: Voice; Piano; Organ; Strings; Woodwinds; Brass; Music Appreciation; Theory; Music

(continued on next page)

History; Piano Ensemble; Instrumental Ensemble
Financial Assistance: Scholarships
Performing Groups: Peace College Choir; Chamber Singers
Workshops/Festivals: Spring Concert Tour

THEATRE

Terry McGovern, Drama Instructor   *Number Of Faculty:* 1
Number Of Students: 28
Courses Offered: Acting; Theatre Participation; Play Production
Financial Assistance: Scholarships   *Performing Groups:* Theatre Arts Group

---

PEMBROKE STATE UNIVERSITY
Pembroke   North Carolina 28372, 919 521-4214 Ext 230
State and 4 Year
Arts Areas: Dance, Instrumental Music, Vocal Music and Theatre
Performing Series: Lyceum Series
Performance Facilities: Moore Hall Recital Auditorium; Performing Arts Center

DANCE

Gloria Canonizedo, Instructor   *Number Of Faculty:* 1
Financial Assistance: Scholarships

MUSIC

Harold C Slagle, Chairman   *Number Of Faculty:* 8   *Number Of Students:* 50
Degrees Offered: BS in Instrument and/or Vocal; BA
Teaching Certification Available
Financial Assistance: Scholarships and Work-Study Grants
Performing Groups: Concert Choir; Concert Band; Singers & Swingers; Small Ensembles
Workshops/Festivals: Instrument Festival; Jazz Festival; Summer Band Camps

THEATRE

Al Dunovan, Senior Member   *Number Of Faculty:* 3
Financial Assistance: Scholarships and Work-Study Grants
Performing Groups: Pembroke Players

PFEIFFER COLLEGE
Misenheimer   North Carolina 28109, 704 463-7343
Private and 4 Year
Arts Areas: Instrumental Music, Vocal Music, Theatre and Visual Arts
Performing Series: Pfeiffer College Concert Series
Performance Facilities: Henry Pfeiffer Chapel; Pfeiffer Theatre

MUSIC

Stanley R Scheer, Head   *Number Of Faculty:* 6   *Number Of Students:* 50
Degrees Offered: BA   *Courses Offered:* Church Music; Music Education
Teaching Certification Available
Financial Assistance: Scholarships and Work-Study Grants
Performing Groups: Chapel Choir; Concert Choir; Symphonic Choir; Chamber Singers; Wind Ensemble;
Stage Band

THEATRE

James B Wood, Head   *Number Of Faculty:* 1   *Number Of Students:* 10
Degrees Offered: BA   *Courses Offered:* Drama; English - Drama
Financial Assistance: Scholarships and Work-Study Grants
Performing Groups: Pfeiffer Playmakers

QUEENS COLLEGE
1900 Selwyn Ave, Charlotte   North Carolina 28274
704 332-7121 Ext 213
Private and 4 Year
Arts Areas: Instrumental Music, Vocal Music, Theatre and Visual Arts
Performance Facilities: Dana Auditorium; Suzanne Little Recital Hall

MUSIC

Dr George A Stegner, Chairman   **Number Of Faculty:** 15
Number Of Students: 50   **Degrees Offered:** BMus; BMusEd; BA
Courses Offered: Theory; History; Applied; Therapy; Music Ed
Teaching Certification Available
Financial Assistance: Scholarships and Work-Study Grants

THEATRE

Dr Charles O Hadley, Professor, English & Drama   **Number Of Faculty:** 3
Number Of Students: 15   **Degrees Offered:** BA
Courses Offered: Technical; Dramatic; Literature; Speech
Teaching Certification Available
Financial Assistance: Scholarships and Work-Study Grants
Performing Groups: Queens Players   **Workshops/Festivals:** Showcase of the Arts

SACRED HEART COLLEGE
Belmont   North Carolina 28012, 704 825-5146
Private and 4 Year   **Arts Areas:** Instrumental Music and Vocal Music

MUSIC

Sister M Cecelia Lewis, RSM, Chairperson   **Number Of Faculty:** 4
Degrees Offered: AA Church Music
Financial Assistance: Assistantships, Scholarships and Work-Study Grants

SAINT ANDREWS PRESBYTERIAN COLLEGE
McCall Hwy, Laurinburg   North Carolina 28352
919 276-3652
Private and 4 Year
Arts Areas: Instrumental Music, Vocal Music, Theatre and Visual Arts
Performing Series: Concert & Artist Series
Performance Facilities: Avinger Auditorium; Vardell Hall

DANCE

Anne Woodson Art, Chairperson   **Number Of Faculty:** 2
Number Of Students: 18   **Degrees Offered:** BA
Teaching Certification Available
Financial Assistance: Internships, Assistantships, Scholarships and Work-Study Grants

MUSIC

David Wilkins, Chaiperson   **Number Of Faculty:** 8   **Number Of Students:** 33
Teaching Certification Available
Financial Assistance: Internships, Assistantships, Scholarships and Work-Study Grants
Performing Groups: Chamber Singers; Concert Choir; Opera Theater; Stage Band; Dixieland Band; Jazz Band; Chamber Ensembles; Concert Band

THEATRE

Arthur McDonald, Chairperson   **Number Of Faculty:** 3
Number Of Students: 44   **Degrees Offered:** BA
Financial Assistance: Internships, Assistantships, Scholarships and Work-Study Grants
Performing Groups: Highland Players; Instant Theater

SAINT AUGUSTINE'S COLLEGE
Oakwood Ave, Raleigh   North Carolina 27611
919 828-4451 Ext 213
> Private and 4 Year
> *Arts Areas:* Dance, Instrumental Music, Vocal Music and Visual Arts

MUSIC

Dr Addison Reed, Chairman   *Number Of Faculty:* 5   *Degrees Offered:* BA
Teaching Certification Available
Financial Assistance: Scholarships and Work-Study Grants
Performing Groups: College Band; College Choir

SALEM COLLEGE
Winston - Salem   North Carolina 27108, 919 723-7961
> Private and 4 Year
> *Arts Areas:* Dance, Instrumental Music, Vocal Music and Visual Arts
> *Performance Facilities:* Hanes Auditorium; Shirley Recital Hall; Drama Workshop

DANCE

Nan Rufty, Assistant Professor of Physical Education   *Number Of Faculty:* 1
Number Of Students: 20   *Performing Groups:* Dansalems

MUSIC

Clemens Sandresky, Dean, School of Music   *Number Of Faculty:* 22
Number Of Students: 220   *Degrees Offered:* BA; BMus
Teaching Certification Available   *Financial Assistance:* Scholarships
Performing Groups: Chorus; Madrigal Singers
Workshops/Festivals: Organ Academy; Piano Workshops

THEATRE

Dr Mary Homrighous, Professor of Drama   *Number Of Faculty:* 1
Number Of Students: 30   *Financial Assistance:* Scholarships
Performing Groups: Pierrette Players

SHAW UNIVERSITY
118 E South St, Raleigh   North Carolina 27602
919 833-3812
> Private and 4 Year
> *Arts Areas:* Instrumental Music, Vocal Music and Visual Arts
> *Number Of Faculty:* 3   *Number Of Students:* 42   *Degrees Offered:* BA
> *Teaching Certification Available*
> *Financial Assistance:* Scholarships and Work-Study Grants
> *Performing Groups:* Band, Choir, Ensembles

UNIVERSITY OF NORTH CAROLINA
Chapel Hill   North Carolina 27514, 919 933-1132
> State and 4 Year
> *Arts Areas:* Dance, Instrumental Music, Vocal Music, Theatre and Television
> *Performance Facilities:* The Playmaker Theatre, The Forest Theatre, The Lounge Theatre, The Laboratory Theatre

DANCE

Dance program under auspices of Department of Dramatic Arts - Theatre

MUSIC

Edgar Alden, Chairman   *Number Of Faculty:* 26   *Number Of Students:* 175

(continued on next page)

Degrees Offered: BA, BMus, BEd, MA, MMus, PhD
Teaching Certification Available
Financial Assistance: Assistantships, Scholarships and Work-Study Grants
Performing Groups: University Symphony Orchestra, Chamber Orchestra, Wind Ensemble, Jazz Lab Band, NC String Quartet
Workshops/Festivals: Piano Clinic, Choral Workshop, Choral Institutes, Band Clinic, Elementary School Music Educators

THEATRE

Arthur L Housman, Chairman   **Number Of Faculty:** 15
Number Of Students: 135
Degrees Offered: BA, BFA, MA, MFA, LDA, PhD (with Comparative Literature)
Financial Assistance: Assistantships, Scholarships and Work-Study Grants
Performing Groups: The Carolina Playmakers, The Laboratory Theatre
Workshops/Festivals: The Carolina Dramatic Association State Festival

---

WAKE FOREST UNIVERSITY
Winston - Salem   North Carolina 27109, 919 761-5000
Private and 4 Year
Arts Areas: Dance, Instrumental Music, Vocal Music, Theatre, Film Arts, Television, Visual Arts and Composition
Performing Series: WF Artist Series (International Artists); WF Chamber Music Series

MUSIC

Dr Annette LeSiege, Chairman   **Number Of Faculty:** 11
Number Of Students: 60   **Degrees Offered:** BA Mus
Courses Offered: Performance (private & ensemble); Theory; History; Composition
Teaching Certification Available
Financial Assistance: Internships, Scholarships and Work-Study Grants
Performing Groups: Orchestra; Wind & Jazz Ensembles; Marching Band; Concert & Touring Choir; Madrigals
Workshops/Festivals: Jazz Festival; Marching Band Festival; Special Workshops & Lectures

---

WARREN WILSON COLLEGE
Swannanoa   North Carolina 28778, 704 298-3325
Private and 4 Year
Arts Areas: Instrumental Music, Vocal Music, Theatre, Visual Arts and Appalachian Music, Dance, Crafts
Performing Series: NC Music in the Mountains
Performance Facilities: Kittredge Community Arts Center; Gladfelter Student Center; Bannerman Hall; College Chapel

MUSIC

Dr Schuyler Robinson, Chairman   **Number Of Faculty:** 6   **Degrees Offered:** BA
Teaching Certification Available
Financial Assistance: Scholarships and Work-Study Grants
Performing Groups: College Choir; Community Choir; Band; Wind Ensemble; Appalachian String Band; Chamber Choir

THEATRE

Dr Richard Homan, Chairman   **Number Of Faculty:** 2   **Degrees Offered:** BA
Teaching Certification Available
Financial Assistance: Scholarships and Work-Study Grants
Workshops/Festivals: High School Drama Workshops

WESTERN CAROLINA UNIVERSITY
Cullowhee   North Carolina 28723, 704 293-7337
> State and 4 Year
> *Arts Areas:* Instrumental Music, Vocal Music, Theatre, Film Arts, Television and Visual Arts
> *Performing Series:* Lecture, Concerts & Exhibition Series; Thursday Evening Music Series
> *Performance Facilities:* Hoey Auditorium; Forsyth Auditorium; Reid Gymnasium

MUSIC

Dr Thomas Tyra, Head   *Number Of Faculty:* 18   *Number Of Students:* 125
Degrees Offered: BA & BS in Music Education
Teaching Certification Available
Financial Assistance: Assistantships, Scholarships and Work-Study Grants
Performing Groups: Symphonic Band; Stage Band; Woodwind Quintet; Brass Choir; Percussion Ensemble:
Concert Choir; University Chorus; Madrigal Singers
Workshops/Festivals: Cullowhee Music Festival; Summer Music Camp

THEATRE

Dr Donald Loeffler, Head   *Number Of Faculty:* 9   *Number Of Students:* 55
Degrees Offered: BA; BFA; BS Ed   *Teaching Certification Available*
Financial Assistance: Assistantships, Scholarships and Work-Study Grants
Performing Groups: University Theatre; Reader's Theatre
Workshops/Festivals: The Summer Repertory Company (Fontana Village); Children's Theatre Tour
Artists-In-Residence/Guest Artists: David Nichols

WINSTON - SALEM STATE UNIVERSITY
Winston - Salem   North Carolina 27103, 919 725-3563
> State and 4 Year   *Arts Areas:* Instrumental Music and Vocal Music
> *Performing Series:* Concert - Lecture Series
> *Performance Facilities:* University Auditorium

MUSIC

P F Dunston, Chairman   *Degrees Offered:* BA
Teaching Certification Available
Financial Assistance: Scholarships and Work-Study Grants
Performing Groups: Vocal and Instrumental Ensembles

BISMARK JUNIOR COLLEGE
Shafer Heights, Bismark   North Dakota 58501
701 223-4500
  2 Year   *Arts Areas:* Instrumental Music and Vocal Music
  Degrees Offered: AA
  Courses Offered: Individual Instruction; Transfer Programs
  Financial Assistance: Scholarships
  Performing Groups: Vocal & Instrumental Ensembles

LAKE REGION JUNIOR COLLEGE
Devils Lake   North Dakota 58301, 701 662-4951
  County and 2 Year   *Arts Areas:* Theatre   *Degrees Offered:* AA
  Financial Assistance: Work-Study Grants

MAYVILLE STATE COLLEGE
Mayville   North Dakota 58257, 701 786-2301 Ext 284
  State and 4 Year
  Arts Areas: Instrumental Music, Vocal Music, Theatre, Television and Visual Arts

MUSIC

  Merwyn A Green, Chairman   *Number Of Faculty:* 4   *Number Of Students:* 75
  Degrees Offered: BA; BS   *Teaching Certification Available*
  Financial Assistance: Scholarships and Work-Study Grants
  Performing Groups: Concert Band; Concert Choir; Stage Band; Pop Singers; Choral; Instrumental

THEATRE

  Dr Christopher Jones, Chairman   *Number Of Faculty:* 2
  Number Of Students: 20   *Degrees Offered:* BS; BA
  Teaching Certification Available   *Financial Assistance:* Work-Study Grants

MINOT STATE COLLEGE
Minot   North Dakota 58701, 701 838-6101
  State and 4 Year
  Arts Areas: Instrumental Music, Vocal Music, Theatre and Visual Arts

MUSIC

  John A Strohm, Chairman   *Number Of Faculty:* 9   *Number Of Students:* 89
  Degrees Offered: BA   *Teaching Certification Available*
  Financial Assistance: Scholarships
  Performing Groups: Instrumental Ensembles; Chorus; Singing Ensembles; Band

THEATRE

  Kenneth R Robbins, Chairman   *Number Of Faculty:* 2   *Number Of Students:* 34
  Degrees Offered: BA   *Teaching Certification Available*
  Financial Assistance: Scholarships   *Performing Groups:* Campus Players

NORTH DAKOTA STATE UNIVERSITY
Fargo   North Dakota 58102, 701 237-7131
  State and 4 Year
  Arts Areas: Dance, Instrumental Music, Vocal Music, Theatre and Visual Arts

DANCE

  Ms M Naas, Associate Professor of Physical Education   *Number Of Faculty:* 2
  Courses Offered: American Dance; Ballroom; Folk; Beginning Modern Dance; Intermediate Modern
  Dance; Advanced Modern Dance; Teaching Dance & Gymnastics; History of Dance in Art & Ed

(continued on next page)

MUSIC

Edwin R Fissinger, Chairman   **Number Of Faculty:** 9
Number Of Students: 125   **Degrees Offered:** BSMusEd; A in Performance
Courses Offered: Fundamentals of Music; Theory; Arranging; Contemporary Harmonic Techniques; Counterpoint; Music History & Literature; Music Education; Applied Music
Teaching Certification Available
Financial Assistance: Scholarships and Work-Study Grants
Performing Groups: Concert Band; Varsity Band; State Band; Marching Band; Wind Ensemble; Brass Chorus; Madrigal Singers; Opera Workshop
Workshops/Festivals: Choral - Vocal Workshops; Instrumental Workshops

THEATRE

E James Ubbelohde, Chairman, Speech & Drama   **Number Of Faculty:** 5
Number Of Students: 12   **Degrees Offered:** BA; BS; BFA; MA
Courses Offered: Introduction to Theatre; Make-up; Stage Production; Acting; Design for Stage; Summer Theatre Practicum; Playwriting; History of the Theatre; Directing; Theory of Drama; Drama Criticism
Teaching Certification Available
Financial Assistance: Scholarships and Work-Study Grants

NORTH DAKOTA STATE UNIVERSITY OF AGRICULTURE & APPLIED SCIENCE
Fargo   North Dakota 58203, 701 237-8011
State and 4 Year
Arts Areas: Instrumental Music, Vocal Music, Theatre and Visual Arts

MUSIC

Dr Edwin R Fissinger, Chairman   **Number Of Faculty:** 9
Number Of Students: 20   **Degrees Offered:** BA Mus, MusEd
Teaching Certification Available   **Financial Assistance:** Scholarships
Performing Groups: Choir; Band; Instrumental Ensembles

THEATRE

Frederick G Walsh, Chairman   **Number Of Faculty:** 7
Degrees Offered: BA, MA Speech   **Teaching Certification Available**
Financial Assistance: Scholarships   **Performing Groups:** Little County Theatre

---

VALLEY CITY STATE COLLEGE
College St, Valley City   North Dakota 58072
701 845-4321
State and 4 Year
Arts Areas: Instrumental Music, Vocal Music and Visual Arts

MUSIC

Ronald Q Johnson, Chairman   **Number Of Faculty:** 6   **Number Of Students:** 75
Degrees Offered: BA
Financial Assistance: Scholarships and Work-Study Grants
Performing Groups: Band; Chorus; Glee Club

UNIVERSITY OF AKRON
COLLEGE OF FINE AND APPLIED ARTS
302 E Buchtel Ave, Akron   Ohio 44325
216 375-7564

> State and 4 Year
> **Arts Areas:** Dance, Instrumental Music, Vocal Music, Theatre, Film Arts, Television and Visual Arts
> **Performance Facilities:** Nola Guzzetta Recital Hall; Experimental Theatre; E J Thomas Performing Arts Hall

DANCE

Marc Ozanick, Department Head   **Number Of Faculty:** 3
Number Of Students: 125   **Degrees Offered:** BA Ballet
Financial Assistance: Scholarships and Work-Study Grants
Performing Groups: Experimental Dance Company

MUSIC

Frank Bradshaw, Department Head   **Number Of Faculty:** 25
Number Of Students: 200   **Degrees Offered:** BA; BM; MM
Courses Offered: Applied   **Teaching Certification Available**
Financial Assistance: Assistantships, Scholarships and Work-Study Grants
Performing Groups: Faculty Brass Quintet; Akron Jazz Ensemble; UA Orchestra; UA Trombone Ensemble; UA Concert Band; Cambini Wind Quintet; UA Glee Clubs; UA Symphony Band; UA Brass Choir; UA Singers; UA Tuba Ensemble; Chamber Chorale; Choral Ensemble; Piano Trio; Marching Band; Faculty Vocal Ensemble; Evening Chorus; Pops Chorale; Opera Workshop

THEATRE

Dr James F Dunlap, Head, Theatre Arts and Dance Department
Number Of Faculty: 9   **Number Of Students:** 200   **Degrees Offered:** BA
Teaching Certification Available
Financial Assistance: Assistantships, Scholarships and Work-Study Grants
Performing Groups: University Theatre; Experimental Dance Company
Artists-In-Residence/Guest Artists: The Ohio Ballet (in residence)

ANTIOCH COLLEGE
Yellow Springs   Ohio 45387, 513 767-7331

> Private and 4 Year
> **Arts Areas:** Instrumental Music, Vocal Music, Theatre, Film Arts, Television and Visual Arts
> **Performing Series:** Antioch College Concert Series; Artists Series

MUSIC

Walter F Anderson, Chairman   **Number Of Faculty:** 6   **Degrees Offered:** BA
Technical Training: Antioch Experimental Program; Advanced Theory Courses; Advanced Composition
Teaching Certification Available
Financial Assistance: Assistantships, Scholarships and Work-Study Grants
Performing Groups: Antioch Orchestra; Antioch Chorus; Black Ensemble
Workshops/Festivals: Music-At-Antioch Series

THEATRE

Meredith Dallas, Chairman   **Number Of Faculty:** 5
Degrees Offered: BA; MA Teaching   **Teaching Certification Available**
Financial Assistance: Internships, Assistantships, Scholarships and Work-Study Grants
Performing Groups: Antioch Dance Theatre; Antioch Area Theatre
Workshops/Festivals: Workshop of Student Directed One - Act Plays

ASHLAND COLLEGE
Ashland Ohio 44805, 419 289-4085
> Private and 4 Year
> *Arts Areas:* Instrumental Music, Vocal Music, Theatre, Television and Visual Arts
> *Performing Series:* Ashland College Artists Series
> *Performance Facilities:* Hugo Young Theatre; Convocation Center; Chapel; Small Recital Halls

MUSIC

Dr Joseph E Thomas, Chairman, Music Department *Number Of Faculty:* 6½
Number Of Students: 55 *Degrees Offered:* BM; BA Music
Teaching Certification Available
Financial Assistance: Scholarships and Grants-in-Aid
Performing Groups: Band; College Choir; Chapel Choir; Jazz Ensemble; Chamber Ensembles; The Ashland Orchestra (in association with community)

BALDWIN - WALLACE COLLEGE
275 Eastland Rd, Berea Ohio 44017
216 826-2900
> Private and 4 Year
> *Arts Areas:* Instrumental Music, Vocal Music and Theatre
> *Performing Series:* Concerts; Dramas; Art Exhibits; Dance Concerts; Films
> *Performance Facilities:* Art and Drama Center - Proscenium and Studio Theatres
> Kulas Musical Arts Building - Fanny Nast Gamble Auditorium and Chamber Music Hall

MUSIC

Dr Warren A Scharf, Director, Conservatory of Music *Number Of Faculty:* 40
Number Of Students: 250 *Degrees Offered:* BM; BME; BA Music
Courses Offered: Voice and All Instruments *Teaching Certification Available*
Financial Assistance: Scholarships and Work-Study Grants
Performing Groups: Orchestra; Symphonic Wind Ensemble; Concert Wind Ensemble; College Choir; Motet Choir; Festival Chorus; Brass Choir; Woodwind Choir; Percussion Ensemble; Jazz Ensemble; Guitar Ensemble; Collegium Musicum
Workshops/Festivals: Annual Bach Festival (May); Opera Workshop Productions

THEATRE

Dr James A Ross, Head, Department of Speech and Theatre Arts
William A Allman; Director of Drama
Number Of Faculty: 12 *Number Of Students:* 85 *Degrees Offered:* BA
Courses Offered: Full range of Theatre and Speech
Teaching Certification Available *Workshops/Festivals:* Berea Summer Theatre

---

BLUFFTON COLLEGE
Bluffton Ohio 45817, 419 358-8015 Ext 291
> Private and 4 Year
> *Arts Areas:* Instrumental Music, Vocal Music, Theatre and Visual Arts
> *Performing Series:* Forum and Artist Series; Music Department Series
> *Performance Facilities:* Mosiman Hall; Founders Hall

MUSIC

Dr Earl W Lehman, Chairman, Music Department *Number Of Faculty:* 8
Number Of Students: 40 *Degrees Offered:* BA
Courses Offered: Music Theory, Education, History; Conducting; Applied Music; Church Music
Teaching Certification Available
Financial Assistance: Scholarships and Work-Study Grants
Performing Groups: Chorale; Concert Band; Orchestra; Choral Society; Small Vocal and Instrumental Ensembles
Workshops/Festivals: Junior High School Music Enrichment Workshop; Piano Workshop

BOWLING GREEN STATE UNIVERSITY
Bowling Green   Ohio 43403, 419 372-2531
   State and 4 Year
   Arts Areas: Dance, Instrumental Music, Vocal Music, Theatre, Television and Visual Arts
   Degrees Offered: BA; BFA; MA   *Teaching Certification Available*
   Financial Assistance: Assistantships, Scholarships and Work-Study Grants
   Performing Groups: Modern Dance Group

MUSIC

Robert Glidden, Dean, Department of Music   *Number Of Faculty:* 53
Number Of Students: 700   *Degrees Offered:* BM; MM
Courses Offered: Full complement of undergraduate and graduate courses in music education, music
performance, composition-theory, and history-literature
Teaching Certification Available
Financial Assistance: Assistantships and Scholarships
Performing Groups: Brass Quintet; String Trio; Woodwind Quintet; Marching Band; Symphonic Band;
Concert Bands I, II, III; Symphony Orchestra; Chamber Orchestra; Collegiate Chorale; A Cappella Choir;
Men's Chorus; Women's Chorus; Lab Bands I and II; New Music Ensemble; Percussion Ensemble; Brass
Choirs I, II
Workshops/Festivals: New Band Reading Clinic; Orchestral Clinic; Choral Reading Clinic; Jazz Festival;
Kodaly Workshop; Orf Workshop; Marching Band Workshop; Conducting Workshop

THEATRE

Mildred Theatre Area Program Director   *Number Of Faculty:* 14
Number Of Students: 210   *Degrees Offered:* BA; BS Ed; BAC; MA; PhD
Courses Offered: Theatre History; Criticism; Literature; Directing; Acting; Design; Lighting; Costuming;
Musical Theatre
Teaching Certification Available
Financial Assistance: Assistantships and Scholarships
Performing Groups: University Players; Second Season Players; Third World Theatre; Huron Playhouse;
Cabaret Theatre
Workshops/Festivals: Summer Musical Theatre Workshop; The Huron Playhouse (at Huron, OH)

BOWLING GREEN STATE UNIVERSITY - FIRELANDS CAMPUS
901 Rye Beach Rd, Huron   Ohio 44839
419 433-5560
   State and Regional Branch Campus   *Arts Areas:* Theatre
   Performing Series: Foreign Film Festival; Opera Performance; Winter and Spring Theatre Performances
   Performance Facilities: Theatre

THEATRE

Dr Ronald Ruble, Chair, Humanities Department   *Number Of Faculty:* 2
Number Of Students: 20   *Degrees Offered:* AA
Courses Offered: Speech; Theatre-Acting; Design
Technical Training: Set Design; Makeup   *Performing Groups:* Huron Playhouse

CAPITAL UNIVERSITY
Columbus   Ohio 43209, 614 236-6101
   Private and 4 Year
   Arts Areas: Instrumental Music, Vocal Music and Visual Arts
   Performing Series: Capitol Music Series; Capitol Music Programs

MUSIC

Dr Marceau C Myers, Dean of Music   *Number Of Faculty:* 31
Number Of Students: 215   *Degrees Offered:* BMus
Teaching Certification Available

(continued on next page)

Financial Assistance: Assistantships, Scholarships and Work-Study Grants
Performing Groups: Orchestra; Instrumental Ensembles; Chorus

THEATRE

Armin Langholz, Chairman   *Number Of Faculty:* 4   *Degrees Offered:* BA
Teaching Certification Available
Financial Assistance: Assistantships, Scholarships and Work-Study Grants
Performing Groups: Masquers

CASE WESTERN RESERVE UNIVERSITY
2040 Adelbert Rd, Cleveland   Ohio 44106
216 368-2000
Private and 4 Year
Arts Areas: Dance, Instrumental Music, Vocal Music, Theatre and Visual Arts
Performing Series: Symphonic Band Concerts; Glee Club Concerts; Theatre Performances; Dance Performances
Performance Facilities: Strosacker Auditorium; Eldred Hall; Harkness Chapel; Amasa Stone Chapel

DANCE

Kathryn Karipides, Associate Professor
Dance program under auspices of Theatre Department
Performing Groups: Kathryn Karipides/Henry Kurth Dance Theatre

MUSIC

John G Suess, Chairman   *Number Of Faculty:* 7   *Number Of Students:* 55
Degrees Offered: BA; BS Music Ed; BH; MA; MA-MLS
Courses Offered: Music; Music Education; Applied Music; Music Librarianship; Music Therapy
Teaching Certification Available
Financial Assistance: Scholarships and Work-Study Grants
Performing Groups: Instrumental Ensembles; Choir

THEATRE

Kenneth Albers, Chairman   *Number Of Faculty:* 8   *Number Of Students:* 60
Degrees Offered: BA; BFA; MA; MFA   *Courses Offered:* Theatre (Dance and Drama)
Technical Training: Technical Theatre; Design
Financial Assistance: Scholarships and Work-Study Grants
Performing Groups: University Theatre
Artists-In-Residence/Guest Artists: Doris Ornstein, Artist-in-Residence (Harpsichord)

CEDARVILLE COLLEGE
Box 601, Cedarville   Ohio 45314
513 766-2211 Ext 370
Private and 4 Year   *Performing Series:* Artist Series
Performance Facilities: Alford Auditorium; Chapel/Convocation Center

MUSIC

David L Matson, Chairman, Department of Music   *Number Of Faculty:* 13
Number Of Students: 75   *Degrees Offered:* BA; BME
Courses Offered: Music Theory; Form & Analysis; Music History; Music Education; Church Music; Applied Music; Instrumental and Vocal Ensembles
Teaching Certification Available
Financial Assistance: Scholarships and Work-Study Grants
Performing Groups: Concert Choir; Choralaires; Brass Choir; Wind Ensemble

CENTRAL STATE UNIVERSITY
Wilburforce   Ohio 45384, 513 376-6001
State and 4 Year
Arts Areas: Instrumental Music, Vocal Music, Film Arts, Television and Visual Arts

MUSIC

Stanley D Kirton, Chairman   *Number Of Faculty:* 8   *Number Of Students:* 60
Degrees Offered: BA   *Teaching Certification Available*
Financial Assistance: Scholarships and Work-Study Grants
Performing Groups: Various Ensembles; Chorus; Band

THEATRE

Essie K Payne, Chairman   *Degrees Offered:* BA
Financial Assistance: Scholarships and Work-Study Grants
Performing Groups: Univ Players

THE CINCINNATI BIBLE SEMINARY
2700 Glenway Ave, Cincinnati   Ohio 45204
513 471-4800
Private and 4 Year
Arts Areas: Instrumental Music, Vocal Music and Church Music

MUSIC

Earl W Sims, Vice President and Dean   *Number Of Faculty:* 4
Degrees Offered: AS and BS in Church Music
Courses Offered: Theory; History and Literature; Conducting; Ministry of Music
Financial Assistance: Scholarships and Work-Study Grants
Performing Groups: Watchmen; Women's Chorus; Concert Choir; Madrigal Singers

UNIVERSITY OF CINCINNATI
COLLEGE - CONSERVATORY OF MUSIC
Cincinnati   Ohio 45221, 513 475-6338
State
Arts Areas: Dance, Instrumental Music, Vocal Music, Theatre, Film Arts, Television and Visual Arts
Performing Series: Faculty Artist Series; New Music Series
Cincinnati Chamber Music Series; Orchestral Series; Opera/Music Theater; Wind Ensemble Series; Choral Series
Performance Facilities: Patricia Corbett Pavilion Theater; Watson Recital Hall; Corbett Auditorium

DANCE

David McLain, Division Head   *Number Of Faculty:* 7   *Number Of Students:* 40
Degrees Offered: BFA; MA in Ballet
Courses Offered: Ballet; Modern Dance; Ballet History; Techniques; Choreography; Ensembles
Financial Assistance: Assistantships and Scholarships
Performing Groups: Ballet Ensemble; Modern Dance Ensemble; Preparatory Dance Ensemble; Cincinnati Ballet Company

MUSIC

Eugene Bonelli, Dean   *Number Of Faculty:* 140   *Number Of Students:* 1,050
Degrees Offered: BM in Performance, Composition, Theory, Music History, Music Education, and Jazz Studies; BA; BFA in Ballet, Musical Theater, Opera/Musical Theater Production, and Broadcasting; MM in Performance, Composition, Theory, Music History, Music Education, Conducting, and Accompanying; MA in Arts Administration, Ballet, and Broadcasting; DMA in Performance, Composition, and Conducting; D Music Ed; PhD in Music
Teaching Certification Available
Financial Assistance: Assistantships, Scholarships and Work-Study Grants
Performing Groups: Black Earth Percussion Group; Vocal Ensembles (8); Instrumental Ensembles; Orchestras (2); Chamber Ensembles

(continued on next page)

Workshops/Festivals: Opera/Musical Theater Workshop and Productions; Summer Workshops in Opera, Composition, Music Education, Jazz Studies, Applied Music, and Conducting

THEATRE

Helen Laird, Curriculum Coordinator   ***Number Of Faculty:*** 15
Number Of Students: 80
Degrees Offered: BFA in Musical Theater; Artist Certificate in Opera
Courses Offered: Acting; Dance; Make-Up; Stage-Craft; Costuming; Characterization; Directing
Technical Training: Applied Music Instruction; Coaching; Studio; Workshop; Production
Financial Assistance: Assistantships, Scholarships and Work-Study Grants
Performing Groups: Opera and Musical Theatre groups

CLEVELAND INSTITUTE OF MUSIC
11021 E Boulevard, Cleveland   Ohio 44106
216 791-5165

Private and 4 Year
Arts Areas: Dance, Instrumental Music and Vocal Music
Performing Series: Weekly faculty recital series; Special guest concerts; Student recitals; Alumni recitals
Performance Facilities: CIM Concert Hall

DANCE

Joy Kane, Chairman
Degrees Offered: BMus; Diploma; Artist Diploma; MMus; MusD
Financial Assistance: Assistantships, Scholarships and Work-Study Grants
Workshops/Festivals: Area Dalcroze Workshops

MUSIC

Grant Johannesen, Director   ***Number Of Faculty:*** 152
Number Of Students: 250
Degrees Offered: BMus; Diploma; Artist Diploma; MMus; MusD
Financial Assistance: Assistantships, Scholarships and Work-Study Grants
Performing Groups: CIM Orchestra; Wind Ensemble; Brass Ensemble; String Ensemble

THEATRE

Anthony Addison, Opera Theatre Department Chairman
Degrees Offered: BMus; Diploma; Artist Diploma; MMus; MusD
Financial Assistance: Assistantships, Scholarships and Work-Study Grants
Performing Groups: CIM Opera Theater

CLEVELAND MUSIC SCHOOL SETTLEMENT
11125 Magnolia Dr, Cleveland   Ohio 44106
216 421-5806

Private and Special
Arts Areas: Dance, Instrumental Music and Vocal Music
Performing Series: Faculty Recital Series; Community Enrichment Recitals
Performance Facilities: Cleveland Music School Settlement Hall

DANCE

Nancy Sample, Chairman   ***Number Of Faculty:*** 4

MUSIC

Howard Whittake, Exectuive Director   ***Number Of Faculty:*** 200
Number Of Students: 5,000
Numerous grade levels must be passed to receive Certificate of Performance and Certificate of Accomplishment
Financial Assistance: Scholarships
Performing Groups: String Ensemble; Wind Ensemble; Choral Group Ensemble

CLEVELAND STATE UNIVERSITY
1983 E 24th St, Cleveland   Ohio 44115
216 687-2000
State and 4 Year
Arts Areas: Dance, Instrumental Music, Vocal Music, Theatre and Visual Arts
Performing Series: Concert Series; Lecture Series; Theatre Season
Performance Facilities: Main Classroom Building Auditorium; University Center Auditorium; Theatre Arts Building

DANCE

Gretchan Moran, Associate Professor   *Number Of Faculty:* 1
Financial Assistance: Scholarships   *Performing Groups:* Modern Dance Company

MUSIC

Julius Drossin, Professor   *Number Of Faculty:* 14   *Number Of Students:* 225
Degrees Offered: BA; MM
Courses Offered: History; Theory; Composition; Music Education; Music Therapy; Performance
Technical Training: Applied Music - all instruments
Teaching Certification Available
Financial Assistance: Assistantships and Scholarships
Performing Groups: CSU Chorus, Chorale, Orchestra, and Band; Collegium Musicum; Jazz Ensemble
Workshops/Festivals: Orff Workshops

THEATRE

Reuben Silver, Area Head and Professor of Theatre Arts
Number Of Faculty: 5   *Number Of Students:* 35   *Degrees Offered:* BA
Courses Offered: Full range in Theatre Arts
Financial Assistance: Assistantships and Scholarships
Performing Groups: CSU Players

THE COLLEGE OF STEUBENVILLE
Franciscan Way, Steubenville   Ohio 43952
614 283-3771 Ext 285
Private and 4 Year   *Arts Areas:* Theatre, Film Arts and Television
Performance Facilities: Anathan Theatre

MUSIC

Courses Offered: Chorus; Band; Music Education; Elementary Music Methods
Music Program under auspices of Education Department
Performing Groups: College Chorus

THEATRE

Donald Rowe, Chairman, English Department   *Number Of Faculty:* 2
Degrees Offered: BA in English-Drama   *Performing Groups:* College Players

CONNORS STATE COLLEGE
Warner   Ohio 74469, 918 463-2931
State and 2 Year
Arts Areas: Instrumental Music, Vocal Music and Visual Arts
Thomas O Webb, Chairman   *Degrees Offered:* AA   *Technical Training:* Opera
Financial Assistance: Scholarships and Work-Study Grants

CUYAHOGA COMMUNITY COLLEGE
7300 York Rd, Parma   Ohio 44130
216 845-4000
County and 2 Year
Arts Areas: Dance, Instrumental Music, Theatre and Visual Arts
Performance Facilities: Campus Theatre

(continued on next page)

DANCE

Jerry Burr, Chairman   **Number Of Faculty:** 1   **Number Of Students:** 55
Financial Assistance: Work-Study Grants
Performing Groups: W Campus Dance Theatre

MUSIC

Joseph Howard, Chairman   **Number Of Faculty:** 3   **Number Of Students:** 120
Degrees Offered: AA   **Financial Assistance:** Work-Study Grants

THEATRE

Lawrence C Vincent, Chairman   **Number Of Faculty:** 2
Number Of Students: 80   **Degrees Offered:** AA
Financial Assistance: Work-Study Grants   **Performing Groups:** W Campus Theatre

---

UNIVERSITY OF DAYTON
300 College Park, Dayton   Ohio 45469
513 229-2539
Private and 4 Year
Arts Areas: Instrumental Music, Vocal Music, Theatre and Visual Arts
Performing Series: University Art Series; Dayton Bach Society; Dayton Philharmonic String Quartet
Performance Facilities: Boll Theatre; UD Arena; Kennedy Union Ballroom

MUSIC

Dr Patrick S Gilvary, Acting Chairman   **Number Of Faculty:** 10
Number Of Students: 100
Degrees Offered: BA in Music; BM in Performance, Theory, Composition, Music Therapy, and Music Education
Courses Offered: Theory; History; Composition; Pedagogy; Performance Ensembles; Therapy
Teaching Certification Available
Financial Assistance: Scholarships and Work-Study Grants
Performing Groups: UD Marching Band; Concert Band; Jazz Lab Band; Wind Ensemble; Brass Quintet; Woodwind Quintet; Brass Choir; Clarinet Choir; Pep Bands (2); University Choir

THEATRE

Dr Patrick S Gilvary, Acting Chairman   **Number Of Faculty:** 3
Number Of Students: 15   **Degrees Offered:** BA in Theatre
Courses Offered: Theory; History; Criticism; Directing; Design; Acting
Technical Training: Lighting; Set Design; Costumes
Teaching Certification Available
Financial Assistance: Scholarships and Work-Study Grants
Performing Groups: Spotlight Theatre

DEFIANCE COLLEGE
701 N Clinton St, Defiance   Ohio 43512
419 784-4010
Private and 4 Year
Arts Areas: Instrumental Music, Vocal Music and Visual Arts
Performing Series: Schomburg Concert Series
Performance Facilities: Schomburg Auditorium

MUSIC

Richard Stroede, Chairman, Music Department   **Number Of Faculty:** 4
Number Of Students: 20   **Degrees Offered:** BA; BS
Courses Offered: Music Ed and Liberal Arts Music Courses
Teaching Certification Available
Financial Assistance: Internships, Assistantships, Scholarships and Work-Study Grants
Performing Groups: Concert Choir; Chamber Choir; Concert Band; Dance Band; Chamber Ensembles

DENISON UNIVERSITY

Granville   Ohio 43023, 614 587-0810

Private and 4 Year
Arts Areas: Dance, Instrumental Music, Vocal Music, Theatre, Film Arts and Visual Arts
Performing Series: University Theatre; Music Recitals; Dance Performances
Performance Facilities: Burke Hall of Music and Art; Ace Morgan Theatre; Doane Dance Center; Swasey Chapel

DANCE

Anne Andersen, Chairman   *Number Of Faculty:* 2   *Degrees Offered:* BA; BFA
Courses Offered: Composition; Movement; Forms; History; Applied Anatomy and Kinesiology; Directed Study; Workshop; Notation
Teaching Certification Available
Financial Assistance: Scholarships and Work-Study Grants
Performing Groups: Dance Performance Workshop

MUSIC

Dr William Osborne, Chairman   *Number Of Faculty:* 8
Degrees Offered: BA; BFA
Courses Offered: Vocal Music; Applied Music; Theory; History and Literature; Conducting; Analysis; Composition
Teaching Certification Available
Financial Assistance: Scholarships and Work-Study Grants
Performing Groups: Concert Choir; Licking County Symphony Orchestra; Women's Chorale; Concert Band; Denison Singers

THEATRE

Dr Bruce Halverson, Chairman, Department of Theatre and Cinema
Number Of Faculty: 7   *Degrees Offered:* BA; BFA
Courses Offered: Theatre Courses: Acting; Production Management; Makeup; History; Development; Design; Drafting; Lighting; Costume History and Design; Theory; Directed Study. Cinema Courses: World Cinema; Production; History; Theory; Workshop
Teaching Certification Available
Financial Assistance: Scholarships and Work-Study Grants
Performing Groups: University Theatre; Theatre II
Workshops/Festivals: Film Festival
Artists-In-Residence/Guest Artists: William Feuer and Richard Kimble (Artists-in-Residence, Dance)

EDGECLIFF COLLEGE

2220 Victory Pkwy, Cincinnati   Ohio 45206
513 961-3770

Private and 4 Year
Arts Areas: Instrumental Music, Vocal Music, Theatre and Visual Arts
Performance Facilities: Indoor Theater in the Round; Outdoor Theater on the Green; Gothic Music Room

MUSIC

Helmut J Roehrig, Department Chairman   *Number Of Faculty:* 6
Number Of Students: 25   *Degrees Offered:* BA; BS; BFA
Courses Offered: Full degree music curriculum
Teaching Certification Available
Financial Assistance: Scholarships and Work-Study Grants
Performing Groups: Edgecliff Singers; Edgecliff Chorus; Vocal and Instrumental Ensembles

THEATRE

Barbara Kay, Department Chairperson   *Number Of Faculty:* 4
Number Of Students: 37   *Degrees Offered:* BA; BFA
Courses Offered: Full degree theatre curriculum
Technical Training: Set Design; Costume Design
Teaching Certification Available

(continued on next page)

Financial Assistance: Scholarships and Work-Study Grants
Performing Groups: Edgecliff Players; Senior Thesis Group
Workshops/Festivals: Shakespeare Festival; Summer Theater Festival; High School Workshop
Artists-In-Residence/Guest Artists: Paul Chidlaw, Artist-in-Residence

---

FAIRMOUNT CENTER FOR CREATIVE & PERFORMING ARTS
1925 Coventry Rd, Cleveland Heights   Ohio 44118
216 932-2000
OR:
8400 Fairmount Rd, Novelty, OH 44072
Telephone: 216 338-3171
Private   **Arts Areas:** Dance, Vocal Music, Theatre and Visual Arts
Performance Facilities: Fairmount Center

DANCE

John Begg, Director of Dance at Coventry
Libby Lubingers, Director of Dance at Novelty
Financial Assistance: Internships, Scholarships and Work-Study Grants
Performing Groups: Fairmount Spanish Dancers; Fairmount Dance Theatre
Workshops/Festivals: Teacher Training Workshops

THEATRE

Kenneth Long, Director
Financial Assistance: Internships, Scholarships and Work-Study Grants
Performing Groups: Fairmount Theatre; Fairmount Theatre of the Deaf

---

FINDLAY COLLEGE
1000 N Main St, Findlay   Ohio 45840
419 422-8313
Private and 4 Year
Arts Areas: Instrumental Music, Vocal Music, Theatre, Television and Visual Arts
Performing Series: Theatre Season; Concerts and Recitals
Performance Facilities: Egner Theatre; Egner Gallery

MUSIC

Number Of Faculty: 4   **Number Of Students:** 30
Degrees Offered: BA; BS in Music and Music Ed   **Teaching Certification Available**
Financial Assistance: Internships, Assistantships, Scholarships and Work-Study Grants
Performing Groups: Band; Choir; Chamber Ensemble

Number Of Faculty: 2   **Number Of Students:** 30
Degrees Offered: BA; BS in Speech - English Education, Communications, Speech - Theatre
Teaching Certification Available
Financial Assistance: Internships, Assistantships, Scholarships and Work-Study Grants
Workshops/Festivals: Summer Stock Season

HAWKEN SCHOOL
Box 249, Gate Mills   Ohio 44040
216 423-4446
Private Prep School
Arts Areas: Dance, Instrumental Music, Vocal Music, Theatre and Visual Arts
Performing Series: "Overture" Series   **Performance Facilities:** Theatre

MUSIC

David Rosenzweig, Chairman   **Number Of Faculty:** 4

HEIDELBURG COLLEGE
Tiffin   Ohio 44883, 419 447-2310
> Private and 4 Year
> *Arts Areas:* Instrumental Music, Vocal Music, Theatre and Visual Arts

MUSIC

Dr Ferris Ohl, Chairman   *Number Of Faculty:* 23   *Number Of Students:* 140
Degrees Offered: BMus   *Teaching Certification Available*
Financial Assistance: Scholarships and Work-Study Grants
Performing Groups: Orchestra; Various Ensembles

THEATRE

James Lee Austin, Chairman   *Number Of Faculty:* 6   *Number Of Students:* 78
Degrees Offered: BA   *Teaching Certification Available*
Financial Assistance: Scholarships and Work-Study Grants
Performing Groups: Heidelburg College Theatre

HIRAM COLLEGE
Hiram   Ohio 44234, 216 569-3211
> Private and 4 Year
> *Arts Areas:* Instrumental Music, Vocal Music, Theatre and Visual Arts
> *Performing Series:* Hiram College Concert & Artist Series

MUSIC

Benn Gibson, Chairman   *Number Of Faculty:* 9   *Number Of Students:* 40
Degrees Offered: BMus   *Teaching Certification Available*
Financial Assistance: Scholarships and Work-Study Grants
Performing Groups: Orchestra; Band; Various Ensembles; Choir

THEATRE

Richard Beachman, Chairman   *Number Of Faculty:* 5   *Number Of Students:* 45
Degrees Offered: BA   *Teaching Certification Available*
Financial Assistance: Scholarships and Work-Study Grants
Performing Groups: Hirman College Theatre

JOHN CARROLL UNIVERSITY
Cleveland   Ohio 44118, 216 491-4911
> Private and 4 Year
> *Arts Areas:* Instrumental Music, Television and Visual Arts
> *Performance Facilities:* Kulas Auditorium   *Number Of Faculty:* 3
> *Degrees Offered:* BA   *Teaching Certification Available*

KENT STATE UNIVERSITY
Kent   Ohio 44242, 216 672-2760
> State and 4 Year
> *Arts Areas:* Dance, Instrumental Music, Vocal Music, Theatre, Film Arts, Television and Visual Arts
> *Performing Series:* Performing Arts Series
> *Performance Facilities:* E Turner Stump Theatre; Experimental Theatre; Porthouse Theatre; Recital Hall

DANCE

Eugenia Schoettler, Coordinator   *Number Of Faculty:* 3 - 4
Number Of Students: 40   *Teaching Certification Available*
Performing Groups: Kent Dance Theatre; KSU Performing Dancers
Workshops/Festivals: Dance Masters of America (Summer Workshop)

(continued on next page)

MUSIC

Ralph E Verrastro, Director   *Number Of Faculty:* 54
Number Of Students: 400   *Degrees Offered:* BMus; BSEd; BA; MMus; MA; MEd; PhD
Teaching Certification Available
Financial Assistance: Assistantships and Scholarships
Performing Groups: Orchestra; Sinfonia; Choir; Kent Chorus; University Chorus; Chorale; Concert
Band; Wind Ensemble; Woodwind Quintet; Brass Quintet; University Madrigal Singers; Brass Ensemble;
Marching Band; Repertory Light Opera Company; Opera Workshop
Workshops/Festivals: Blossom Festival School

THEATRE

Dr William H Zucchero, Coordinator   *Number Of Faculty:* 7
Number Of Students: 195   *Degrees Offered:* BA; BFA; MA; PhD
Courses Offered: Acting; Directing; Theatre History & Criticism; Oral Playwriting; Design & Technical
Theatre; Costuming; Theatre Management
Technical Training: Stage Design; Costuming; Technical Lighting
Teaching Certification Available   *Financial Assistance:* Scholarships
Performing Groups: University Theatre; Children's Theatre Touring Company; Repertory Theatre Touring
Company; Summer Repertory Theatre Company
Workshops/Festivals: High School Drama Clinic; Blossom Festival School of Theatre

---

KENT STATE UNIVERSITY
Kent   Ohio 44242, 216 672-2760
State and 2 Year
Arts Areas: Dance, Instrumental Music, Vocal Music, Theatre, Film Arts, Television and Visual Arts
Performing Series: KSU Artist Lecture Series
Performance Facilities: Turner Stump Theater; Music Recital Hall

DANCE

Eugenia V Schoettler, Dance Coordinator   *Number Of Faculty:* 2
Number Of Students: 40
Degrees Offered: BS in Physical Education with concentration in Dance
Performing Groups: KSU Performing Dancers; Porthouse Theater Dance Company
Workshops/Festivals: Theater - Dance Workshop offered through The Blossom Festival School

MUSIC

Lindsey Merrill, Chairman   *Number Of Faculty:* 53   *Number Of Students:* 400
Degrees Offered: BMus; BMusEd; BS; BSEd; BA; MMus; MA; MEd; PhD in Education
Teaching Certification Available
Financial Assistance: Assistantships, Scholarships and Work-Study Grants
Performing Groups: Orchestra; Sinfonia; Choir; Chorale; Oratorio Guild; Symphony Band; Concert Band;
Wind Ensemble; New Kent Singers; Brass Choir; Percussion Ensemble; Lab Band; String Quartet;
Woodwind Quintet; Brass Quintet; Repertory Light Opera Company
Workshops/Festivals: The Blossom Festival; The Cleveland Orchestra; Opera Workshop

THEATRE

Dr William Zucchero, Chairman   *Number Of Faculty:* 9
Number Of Students: 145   *Degrees Offered:* BA; BFA; MA; PhD
Teaching Certification Available
Financial Assistance: Internships, Assistantships, Scholarships and Work-Study Grants
Performing Groups: University Theatre; Children's Theater Touring Company; Repertory Theater Touring
Company; Summer Repertory Theater Company
Workshops/Festivals: High School Drama Clinic; Blossom Festival School of Theater

KENT STATE UNIVERSITY, TUSCARAWAS CAMPUS
University Drive NE, New Philadelphia   Ohio 44663
216 364-5561
State and 2 Year   *Arts Areas:* Vocal Music, Theatre and Visual Arts
Performance Facilities: Tuscarawas Campus Auditorium

MUSIC

Dorothy Lutsch, Chairman   *Number Of Faculty:* 1   *Number Of Students:* 20   *Degrees Offered:* AA

THEATRE

Robert C Liberatore, Chairman   *Number Of Faculty:* 1
Number Of Students: 20   *Degrees Offered:* AA   *Performing Groups:* Tuscarawas Campus Theatre

KENYON COLLEGE
Gambier   Ohio 43022, 614 427-2244
Arts Areas: Instrumental Music, Vocal Music and Theatre

MUSIC

Number Of Faculty: 4   *Number Of Students:* 52   *Degrees Offered:* BMus
Financial Assistance: Scholarships and Work-Study Grants   *Performing Groups:* Band; Chorus

THEATRE

Number Of Faculty: 2   *Number Of Students:* 26   *Degrees Offered:* BA
Financial Assistance: Scholarships and Work-Study Grants
Performing Groups: Kenyon College Drama Club

LAKE ERIE COLLEGE
Painesville   Ohio 44077, 352-3361 Ext 276
Private and 4 Year
Arts Areas: Dance, Instrumental Music, Vocal Music, Theatre and Television
Performing Series: Guild of the Arts Concert Series
Performance Facilities: Helen Rockwell Morley Music Building

MUSIC

Harold Fink, Chairman   *Number Of Faculty:* 3   *Number Of Students:* 45
Degrees Offered: BMus   *Teaching Certification Available*
Financial Assistance: Scholarships and Work-Study Grants   *Performing Groups:* Orchestra Quartet

THEATRE

Jake L Rufi, Chairman   *Number Of Faculty:* 2   *Number Of Students:* 30
Degrees Offered: BA   *Teaching Certification Available*
Financial Assistance: Scholarships and Work-Study Grants
Performing Groups: Children's Theatre; Community Theatre

LAKELAND COMMUNITY COLLEGE
Mentor   Ohio 44060, 216 951-1000
County and 2 Year
Arts Areas: Dance, Instrumental Music, Vocal Music, Theatre, Film Arts and Television

DANCE

Number Of Faculty: 1   *Number Of Students:* 50   *Performing Groups:* Lakeland Dance Ensemble

MUSIC

Number Of Faculty: 2   *Number Of Students:* 85   *Degrees Offered:* AA with emphasis in Music
Financial Assistance: Scholarships
Performing Groups: Lakeland Band; Lakeland Jazz Ensemble; Lakeland Chorus
Workshops/Festivals: High School Music Contest; Annual Junior College of Ohio Music Festival

THEATRE

Number Of Faculty: 1   *Number Of Students:* 60   *Performing Groups:* Lakeland Theater Company

MALONE COLLEGE
515 25th St NW, Canton   Ohio 44709
216 454-3011 Ext 248
Private and 4 Year
Arts Areas: Instrumental Music, Vocal Music, Theatre and Visual Arts
Performing Series: Faculty - Artist Series
Performance Facilities: Performing Arts Hall; College - Community Room; Osborne Hall

MUSIC

Donald R Murray, Chairman, Division of Fine Arts   *Number Of Faculty:* 6
Number Of Students: 50   *Degrees Offered:* BA; BS in Education
Teaching Certification Available
Financial Assistance: Scholarships and Work-Study Grants
Performing Groups: Vocal and Instrumental Ensembles; College Chorale; College - Community Band

THEATRE

Morris R Pike, Chairman   *Number Of Faculty:* 1   *Number Of Students:* 20
Degrees Offered: BA
Financial Assistance: Scholarships and Work-Study Grants
Performing Groups: Malone Players

MARIETTA COLLEGE
Marietta   Ohio 45750, 614 373-4643
Private and 4 Year
Arts Areas: Instrumental Music, Vocal Music, Theatre, Television and Visual Arts
Performing Series: Thomas Series; Assembly Program Series

MUSIC

Dr Harold Mueller, Chairman   *Number Of Faculty:* 9   *Number Of Students:* 25
Degrees Offered: BA Music   *Teaching Certification Available*
Financial Assistance: Assistantships and Work-Study Grants
Performing Groups: Singers; Band; Oratorio Chorus; Orchestra

THEATRE

Willard J Friederick, Chairman   *Number Of Faculty:* 4   *Degrees Offered:* BA
Teaching Certification Available
Financial Assistance: Assistantships and Work-Study Grants
Performing Groups: Children's Theatre; Readers' Theatre; One-Act Play Series; College Theatre

MARY MANSE COLLEGE
2436 Parkwood, Toledo   Ohio 43620
419 243-9241
Private and 4 Year
Arts Areas: Instrumental Music, Vocal Music, Theatre and Visual Arts

MUSIC

Sister M Gretchen, Chairman   *Number Of Faculty:* 9   *Number Of Students:* 30
Degrees Offered: BMus   *Teaching Certification Available*
Financial Assistance: Scholarships and Work-Study Grants   *Performing Groups:* Choir

THEATRE

Number Of Faculty: 2   *Performing Groups:* The Mary Manse Players

MIAMI UNIVERSITY
Oxford   Ohio 45056, 513 529-6010

State and 4 Year

Arts Areas: Dance, Instrumental Music, Vocal Music, Theatre, Television, Visual Arts
Performing Series: Miami University Artists Series
Performance Facilities: Gates - Abegglen Theatre; Millett Hall

DANCE

Dr Marjorie Price, Chairman Physical Education Department
Number Of Faculty: 2   *Number Of Students:* 25
Technical Training: Performance   *Financial Assistance:* Assistantships
Performing Groups: Dance Theatre; Orchesis; Performing Groups; Dance Repertory

MUSIC

Dr Paul A Aliapoulios, Chairman   *Number Of Faculty:* 29
Number Of Students: 282
Degrees Offered: BMus; BMusEd; MMus; MA; Cooperative PhD and DMA with University of Cincinnati
Teaching Certification Available
Financial Assistance: Assistantships and Scholarships
Performing Groups: Symphony Orchestra; Marching Band; Symphonic Band; A Cappella Singers; Men's Glee Club; Choraliers; Choral Union; Chamber Orchestra

THEATRE

Dr Donald L Rosenberg, Chairman   *Number Of Faculty:* 7
Number Of Students: 100   *Degrees Offered:* BA; MA
Teaching Certification Available
Financial Assistance: Internships, Assistantships, Scholarships and Work-Study Grants
Performing Groups: Miami University Theatre

MOUNT SAINT JOSEPH ON THE OHIO COLLEGE
5700 Delhi Rd, Mount Saint Joseph   Ohio 45051
513 244-4863

Private and 4 Year

Arts Areas: Instrumental Music, Vocal Music, Theatre and Visual Arts
Performing Series: Performing Artists Series

MUSIC

Number Of Faculty: 5   *Number Of Students:* 65   *Degrees Offered:* BA
Teaching Certification Available
Financial Assistance: Scholarships and Work-Study Grants
Performing Groups: Choir; Vocal & Instrumental Ensembles

THEATRE

Number Of Faculty: 3   *Number Of Students:* 40   *Degrees Offered:* BA in Speech
Teaching Certification Available   *Financial Assistance:* Scholarships and Work-Study Grants

MOUNT UNION COLLEGE
219 W State St, Alliance   Ohio 44601
216 821-5320

Private and 4 Year

Arts Areas: Instrumental Music, Vocal Music, Theatre and Visual Arts

MUSIC

Dr Lewis A Philps, Chairman   *Number Of Faculty:* 18
Number Of Students: 85   *Degrees Offered:* BMus; BMusEd
Financial Assistance: Scholarships and Work-Study Grants   *Teaching Certification Available*
Performing Groups: Vocal & Instrumental Ensembles

(continued on next page)

THEATRE

Number Of Faculty: 3   **Number Of Students:** 45   **Degrees Offered:** BA
Financial Assistance: Scholarships and Work-Study Grants   **Performing Groups:** Mount Union Players

---

MOUNT VERNON NAZERENE COLLEGE
Martinsburg Rd, Mount Vernon   Ohio 43050
614 392-1244

Private and 4 Year   **Arts Areas:** Instrumental Music and Vocal Music
Performing Series: Concert & Lecture Series   **Degrees Offered:** BA
Financial Assistance: Scholarships and Work-Study Grants

MUSKINGUM COLLEGE
New Concord   Ohio 42762, 614 826-8211

Private and 4 Year
Arts Areas: Dance, Instrumental Music, Vocal Music, Theatre, Film Arts, Television and Visual Arts
Performing Series: Fine Arts Series
Performance Facilities: Johnson Hall Theatre; E Sue Cook Dance Studio; Brown Chapel;
Muskingum Science Center Auditorium; John Glenn Gymnasium

DANCE

Joyce Krumpe, Instructor
Dance program under auspices of Physical Education Department
Number Of Faculty: 1   **Number Of Students:** 22
Courses Offered: Modern Dance; Methods of Teaching Dance

MUSIC

Woodrow Pickering, Department Chairman   **Number Of Faculty:** 6
Number Of Students: 84
Degrees Offered: BM; BA in Music, Applied Music, Music Ed
Financial Assistance: Scholarships and Work-Study Grants
Performing Groups: College Band; Stage Band; A Cappella Choir; Hi-Liters; Choral Society; Vocal
Ensembles; Southeastern Ohio Symphony Orchestra

THEATRE

Donald Hill, Chairman, Department of Speech, Communication, and Theatre
Number Of Faculty: 5   **Number Of Students:** 85
Degrees Offered: BA in Speech and Drama   **Teaching Certification Available**
Financial Assistance: Scholarships and Work-Study Grants
Performing Groups: Muskingum Players
Workshops/Festivals: High School Communication Workshop

NOTRE DAME COLLEGE OF OHIO
4545 College Rd, Cleveland   Ohio 44121
216 381-1680

Private and 4 Year
Arts Areas: Dance, Instrumental Music, Vocal Music, Theatre, Film Arts and Visual Arts
Performance Facilities: The Little Theatre

MUSIC

Sister Mary Electa, SND, Department Chairman   **Number Of Faculty:** 1
Degrees Offered: BA in Music Ed

OBERLIN COLLEGE
Oberlin   Ohio 44074, 216 775-8121

Private and 4 Year
Arts Areas: Dance, Instrumental Music, Vocal Music, Theatre, Film Arts and Visual Arts

(continued on next page)

Performing Series: Oberlin Artist Recital Series; New Directions Series
Performance Facilities: Conservatory of Music; Hall Auditorium; Warner Center for the Perofrming Arts; Finney Chapel

DANCE

David Newman, Acting Director of Inter-Arts   *Number Of Faculty:* 3
Number Of Students: 200   *Degrees Offered:* BA
Courses Offered: History and Literature; Criticism; Modern Dance; Choreography and Aesthetics; Ballet; Kinesiology; Improvisation
Financial Assistance: Scholarships and Work-Study Grants
Performing Groups: The Oberlin Dance Company
Workshops/Festivals: Workshops by guest dancers

MUSIC

David Boe, Dean, Conservatory of Music   *Number Of Faculty:* 65
Number Of Students: 500
Degrees Offered: BM; BFA; BM/M Music Ed; BM/M Music Teaching; MM in Conducting; MM in Music Theater
Courses Offered: Applied Music; Composition; Ethnomusicology; Music Education; History; Literature; Music Theater; Theory; Music Therapy; Technology in Music
Teaching Certification Available
Financial Assistance: Scholarships and Work-Study Grants
Performing Groups: Musical Union; Oberlin College Choir, Chorus, and Black Ensemble; Oberlin Orchestra, Chamber Orchestra, and Wind Ensemble; Collegium Musicum; Large Jazz Ensemble; Small Jazz Ensemble; Javanese Gamelan; Chamber Music; Chamber Music for Winds; Viola da Gamba Consort; Baroque Ensemble Class; Piano Ensemble; Harp Ensemble; Trombone Ensemble; Oberlin Percussion Group; Ensembles for Harpists; Ensembles for Percussionists
Workshops/Festivals: Summer Institutes: Baroque Performance Institute; Organ Institute; Contemporary Choral Institute

THEATRE

David Newman, Acting Director of Inter-Arts   *Number Of Faculty:* 5
Number Of Students: 175   *Degrees Offered:* BA
Courses Offered: History and Literature; Criticism; Acting; Vocal Training; Analysis
Technical Training: Lighting; Costume Construction; Technical Production; Sound
Artists-In-Residence/Guest Artists: Tom MacIntyre, Playwright-in-Residence

---

OHIO NORTHERN UNIVERSITY
Ada   Ohio 45810, 419 634-9921 Ext 218
Private and 4 Year
Arts Areas: Instrumental Music, Vocal Music, Theatre and Visual Arts
Performing Series: University Artist Series; Music Department Faculty Recitals; Music Department Student Recitals; University Touring Concerts
Performance Facilities: King - Horn Center; Lehr Auditorium; Presser Hall

MUSIC

Dr Alan Drake, Department Chairman
Number Of Faculty: 7 Full-time, 8 Part-time   *Number Of Students:* 42
Degrees Offered: BA; BM
Courses Offered: Music Ed; Sacred Music; Applied Music
Teaching Certification Available
Financial Assistance: Internships, Scholarships and Work-Study Grants
Performing Groups: Symphonic Band; Concert Band; Jazz Lab Band; University Singers; University Chorus; Chapel Choir; Small Ensembles
Workshops/Festivals: Annual Jazz Festival; Summer Music Camp

THEATRE

Ronald Ladwig, Department Chairman
Number Of Faculty: 6 Full-time, 3 Part-time   *Number Of Students:* 21

(continued on next page)

Degrees Offered: BA in Speech - Theatre   **Teaching Certification Available**
Financial Assistance: Internships, Scholarships and Work-Study Grants
Performing Groups: University Theatre; Children's Theatre; Lab Theatre; Reader's Theatre; Polar Bear Puppet Theatre Mobile

OHIO UNIVERSITY
Athens   Ohio 45701, 614 594-5664
State
Arts Areas: Dance, Instrumental Music, Vocal Music, Theatre, Film Arts and Visual Arts
Performance Facilities: Forum Theater; Patio Theater; Memorial Auditorium; Putnam Studio; School of Music

DANCE

Shirley Wimmer, Director   **Number Of Faculty:** 5   **Number Of Students:** 57
Degrees Offered: BFA   **Teaching Certification Available**
Financial Assistance: Assistantships, Scholarships and Work-Study Grants
Performing Groups: The Movement   **Workshops/Festivals:** Summer Dance Workshop

MUSIC

Dr Clyde H Thompson, Director   **Number Of Faculty:** 32
Number Of Students: 309   **Degrees Offered:** BM; MM; M Music Ed
Teaching Certification Available
Financial Assistance: Assistantships, Scholarships and Work-Study Grants
Performing Groups: Marching Band; Center Band; Wind Ensemble; Choir; Jazz Ensembles; Opera Workshop; OU Trio; Baroque Trio; Trombone Choir; Percussion Ensemble; University Orchestra
Workshops/Festivals: Summer Music Workshops

THEATRE

Robert Winters, Acting Director   **Number Of Faculty:** 14
Number Of Students: 201   **Degrees Offered:** BFA; MA; MFA
Teaching Certification Available
Financial Assistance: Assistantships, Scholarships and Work-Study Grants
Performing Groups: Appalachian Green Parks Project; Ohio University Theater; Experimental Theater; Ohio Valley Summer Theater; Monomoy Theater
Workshops/Festivals: Summer Musical Theater Festival

OHIO WESLEYAN UNIVERSITY
50 N Liberty 1, Delaware   Ohio 43015
614 369-4431
Private and 4 Year
Arts Areas: Dance, Instrumental Music, Vocal Music, Theatre, Film Arts, Television and Visual Arts
Performing Series: Ohio Wesleyan University Lecture - Artist Series
Performance Facilities: Chappelear Drama Center, Main and Studio Theatres;
Gray Chapel Auditorium; Sanborn Recital Hall; Branch Rickey Physical Education Center Arena

DANCE

Mary Titus, Associate Professor, Physical Education Department
Number Of Faculty: 1   **Number Of Students:** 30
Financial Assistance: All aid based on financial need
Performing Groups: Orchesis
Workshops/Festivals: Workshops by visiting troupes

MUSIC

Willis Olson, Chairman   **Number Of Faculty:** 10   **Number Of Students:** 50
Degrees Offered: BM; BM in Music Ed; BA; Combined BM/BA
Courses Offered: Performance; Theory and Composition; Church Music
Teaching Certification Available
Financial Assistance: All aid based on financial need

(continued on next page)

Performing Groups: Choral Society; Choral Union; Symphonic Band; Orchestra; Jazz Band; Bishop Band
Workshops/Festivals: High School Music Festival; Spring Festival

THEATRE

Llewellyn Rabby, Chairman   *Number Of Faculty:* 3   *Number Of Students:* 25
Degrees Offered: BA   *Courses Offered:* Acting; Directing; Design; Survey
Teaching Certification Available
Financial Assistance: All aid based on financial need
Performing Groups: Wesleyan Players' Club
Workshops/Festivals: High School Drama Festival

OTTERBEIN COLLEGE
Westerville   Ohio 43081, 614 890-8000
Private and 4 Year
Arts Areas: Dance, Instrumental Music, Vocal Music, Theatre, Television and Visual Arts
Performing Series: Otterbein Artist Series; Otterbein College Theatre; Music Department Concerts and Recitals
Performance Facilities: Cowan Hall; Hall Auditorium, Lambert Hall

MUSIC

Dr Morton Achter, Chairman   *Number Of Faculty:* 21   *Number Of Students:* 75
Degrees Offered: BA; B Music Ed
Courses Offered: Theory/Composition; Applied Music; History/Literature; Musical Theatre
Teaching Certification Available
Financial Assistance: Scholarships and Work-Study Grants
Performing Groups: Opus Zero; Concert Choir; Orchestra; Marching Band; Concert Band; Various Ensembles

THEATRE

Dr Charles Dodrill, Director of Theatre   *Number Of Faculty:* 3
Number Of Students: 65   *Degrees Offered:* BA; BFA
Courses Offered: Performing Theatre; Technical Theatre; Theatre Grad School; Children's Theatre; Management; Theatre Education; Musical Theatre
Teaching Certification Available
Financial Assistance: Scholarships and Work-Study Grants
Performing Groups: College Theatre; Otterbein Summer Theatre; Chancel Drama

RIO GRANDE COLLEGE AND COMMUNITY COLLEGE
Rio Grande   Ohio 45674, 614 245-5353
4 Year and 2 Year
Arts Areas: Instrumental Music, Vocal Music and Theatre

MUSIC

Merlyn Ross, Chairman   *Number Of Faculty:* 2
Degrees Offered: Validation to teach elementary grades 1 - 8
Teaching Certification Available
Financial Assistance: Scholarships and Work-Study Grants
Performing Groups: The Grande Chorale; College Choir; College Band
Number Of Faculty: 1

SCHOOL OF FINE ARTS
38660 Mentor Ave, Willoughby   Ohio 44094
216 951-7500
Private and 2 Year
Arts Areas: Dance, Instrumental Music, Vocal Music, Theatre and Visual Arts
Performing Series: Faculty Performing Arts Series; Community - based Performers
Performance Facilities: Fine Arts Association Auditorium

(continued on next page)

DANCE

Raymond Smith, Chairman **Number Of Faculty:** 2 **Number Of Students:** 140
Dance program under auspices of Lakeland College
Financial Assistance: Scholarships
Performing Groups: Student Performing Group; Lecture - Recitals by Jan and Ray Smith
Workshops/Festivals: Summer Fine Arts Festival

MUSIC

Edith Reed, Chairman **Number Of Faculty:** 40 **Number Of Students:** 800
Financial Assistance: Scholarships
Performing Groups: Touring Opera Company; Musical Ensembles
Workshops/Festivals: Summer Fine Arts Festival

THEATRE

Timothy Ryan, Chairman **Number Of Faculty:** 7 **Number Of Students:** 100
Financial Assistance: Scholarships and Work-Study Grants
Performing Groups: Performing Arts Ensemble; Children's Theatre Group
Workshops/Festivals: Fine Arts Festival

SINCLAIR COMMUNITY COLLEGE
444 W Third St, Dayton Ohio 45402
513 226-2500

County and 2 Year
Arts Areas: Dance, Instrumental Music, Vocal Music, Theatre and Visual Arts
Performance Facilities: Blair Hall Theatre

DANCE

Dr Clarance Walls, Chairman **Number Of Faculty:** 6
Number Of Students: 172

MUSIC

Dr Clarence Walls, Chairman **Number Of Faculty:** 22
Number Of Students: 500 **Degrees Offered:** AA
Performing Groups: Band; Choir; Community Chorus; Sinclair Singers; Jazz Lab Band

THEATRE

Dr Robert Mac Clannan **Number Of Faculty:** 1 **Number Of Students:** 80

UNIVERSITY OF TOLEDO
2801 W Bancroft St, Toledo Ohio 43606
419 537-2675

State and 4 Year
Arts Areas: Dance, Instrumental Music, Vocal Music, Theatre, Film Arts, Television and Visual Arts
Performing Series: University Convocations; Faculty and Student Concert Series; Theatre Season
Performance Facilities: Center for Performing Arts - Recital Hall, Center Theater;
Studio Theatres; University Hall - Doermann Theater; Student Union - Ingman Room and Auditorium;
Centennial Hall

MUSIC

Bernard R Sanchez, Chairman **Number Of Faculty:** 27
Number Of Students: 170 **Degrees Offered:** BA in Music; BM; BE in Music
Courses Offered: History and Literature; Class Instruction; Theory; Applied Music Education
Teaching Certification Available
Financial Assistance: Scholarships and Work-Study Grants
Performing Groups: University Orchestra; University Chorus; Varsity Singers; Brass Ensemble; Jazz Lab
Band; Woodwind Quintet; Chamber Orchestra; Marching Band; Concert Band; Brass Quintet

(continued on next page)

Workshops/Festivals: Choral Music Workshop; Career Day (Toledo Symphony); Music in Elementary Classroom; Junior High Solo and Ensemble Contest

THEATRE

Dr Julian Olf, Chairman   **Number Of Faculty:** 8   **Number Of Students:** 100
Degrees Offered: BA in Theatre
Courses Offered: Acting; History; Stagecraft; Design; Voice; Playwriting; Filmmaking; Makeup; Directing; Drama-in-Education
Financial Assistance: Scholarships and Work-Study Grants
Performing Groups: Theatre-in-the-Streets; Theatre-in-the-Schools

---

URSULINE COLLEGE
2550 Lander Rd, Cleveland   Ohio 44124
216 449-4200
Private and 4 Year
Arts Areas: Instrumental Music, Vocal Music, Theatre and Visual Arts
Performance Facilities: Little Theater

MUSIC

Sister Janet Moore, Chairman   **Number Of Faculty:** 6
Number Of Students: 15   **Degrees Offered:** BA
Teaching Certification Available
Financial Assistance: Scholarships and Work-Study Grants
Performing Groups: Choral; Orchestra; Small Vocal Ensemble

THEATRE

Dr Mary P Daley, Chairman   **Number Of Faculty:** 2   **Number Of Students:** 15
Degrees Offered: BA
Teaching Certification Available
Financial Assistance: Scholarships and Work-Study Grants
Performing Groups: UC Little Theater; UC Reader's Theater; Ursuline Children's Theater; Matinee Theater

---

WESTERN COLLEGE OF MIAMI UNIVERSITY
Oxford   Ohio 45056, 513 529-8131
Private and 4 Year
Arts Areas: Instrumental Music, Vocal Music, Theatre and Visual Arts

MUSIC

Number Of Faculty: 6   **Number Of Students:** 48   **Degrees Offered:** BMus
Teaching Certification Available
Financial Assistance: Scholarships and Work-Study Grants
Performing Groups: Various Ensembles; Choir; Orchestra

THEATRE

Jack V Booch, Chairman   **Number Of Faculty:** 2   **Number Of Students:** 16
Degrees Offered: BA   **Teaching Certification Available**
Financial Assistance: Scholarships and Work-Study Grants

WILMINGTON COLLEGE
Wilmington   Ohio 45177, 513 382-6661
Private and 4 Year
Arts Areas: Instrumental Music, Vocal Music, Theatre and Visual Arts

MUSIC

Number Of Faculty: 2   **Number Of Students:** 26   **Degrees Offered:** BA Mus
Teaching Certification Available
Financial Assistance: Scholarships and Work-Study Grants

(continued on next page)

(*Wilmington College — cont'd*)

THEATRE

Degrees Offered: BA Theatre   **Teaching Certification Available**
Financial Assistance: Scholarships and Work-Study Grants
Performing Groups: Wilmington College Theatre

WITTENBERG UNIVERSITY
Springfield   Ohio 45501, 513 327-6231
Private and 4 Year
Arts Areas: Instrumental Music, Vocal Music and Theatre

MUSIC

Dr L David Miller, Dean, School of Music
Number Of Faculty: 21 Full-time, 13 Part-time   **Number Of Students:** 571
Degrees Offered: BM; MM
Courses Offered: Applied; Theory; History; Conducting; Accompaniment; Literature; Teaching; Church Music; Composition; Scoring
Teaching Certification Available
Financial Assistance: Scholarships and Work-Study Grants
Performing Groups: Bach Chorale; Chapel Choir; Choristers; Collegium Musicum; Schola; Wittenberg Choir; Brass Choir; Chamber Ensemble; Hand Bell Choir; Jazz Ensemble; String Ensemble; Symphonic Band; Opera Workshop
Workshops/Festivals: Festival of Music, Worship, and the Arts; Festival of the Hymn Society of America; Horn Festival; Performing Arts Spring Festival

THEATRE

Dr Dorothy Laming, Director of Theater   **Number Of Faculty:** 4
Number Of Students: 300
Degrees Offered: BA in Theater, Speech and Theater, Speech and Theater Education, and Music Theater
Courses Offered: Acting; Directing; Stagecraft; Scene Design and Stage Lighting; Child Drama
Teaching Certification Available
Financial Assistance: Scholarships and Work-Study Grants
Performing Groups: University Theater; WU Children's Theater

THE COLLEGE OF WOOSTER
Wooster   Ohio 44691, 216 264-1234
Private and 4 Year
Arts Areas: Instrumental Music, Vocal Music, Theatre, Film Arts and Visual Arts
Performance Facilities: Freedlander Theatre; Shoolroy Arena Theatre; McGaw Chapel; Mateer Auditorium; Mackey Hall

MUSIC

Daniel W Winter, Chairman   **Number Of Faculty:** 8 Full-time, 5 Part-time
Number Of Students: 52   **Degrees Offered:** BA; BM; B Music Education
Courses Offered: Theory/Composition; Music History and Literature; Applied Music; Music Education
Teaching Certification Available
Financial Assistance: Scholarships and Work-Study Grants
Performing Groups: Concert Choir; Westminster Choir; Wooster Symphony Orchestra; Wooster Chorus; Scot Band; Jazz Ensemble

THEATRE

Gerald Sanders, Chairman   **Number Of Faculty:** 6   **Number Of Students:** 54
Degrees Offered: BA in Speech
Courses Offered: Performing and Technical Theatre; Radio and Television; Speech Pathology; Theatre History
Teaching Certification Available
Financial Assistance: Scholarships and Work-Study Grants
Performing Groups: The Little Theatre; Black Theatre

WRIGHT STATE UNIVERSITY
Dayton   Ohio 45435, 513 873-3333

    State and 4 Year
    Arts Areas: Dance, Instrumental Music, Vocal Music, Theatre, Film Arts and Visual Arts
    Performing Series: Artist and Lecture Series
    Performance Facilities: Creative Arts Center; Concert Hall; Recital Hall; Festival Playhouse; Celebration
    Theatre

DANCE

Dr Abe J Bassett, Chairman   **Number Of Faculty:** 2   **Degrees Offered:** BFA
Courses Offered: Modern Dance
Financial Assistance: Internships, Scholarships and Work-Study Grants
Performing Groups: Dance Ensemble

MUSIC

Dr William Fenton, Chairman   **Number Of Faculty:** 14
Number Of Students: 170   **Degrees Offered:** BA; BM; MM
Teaching Certification Available   **Financial Assistance:** Scholarships
Performing Groups: Chamber Singers; Brass Choir; Symphony Orchestra; Symphony Band; Concert Band;
Jazz Ensemble; Varsity Band

THEATRE

Dr Abe J Bassett, Chairman   **Number Of Faculty:** 10
Number Of Students: 150 majors   **Degrees Offered:** BA; BFA; B Secondary Ed
Courses Offered: Studio Acting; Design - Technology; Arts Management; Dance; Directing; Motion Picture
Teaching Certification Available   **Financial Assistance:** Scholarships
Performing Groups: University Theatre; Children's Theatre Tour
Workshops/Festivals: American College Theatre Festival (Great Lakes Region); High School Theatre
Workshops; Southwest Ohio Thespian Workshop; WOBC Motion Picture Workshop

XAVIER UNIVERSITY
Victor Pkwy, Cincinnati   Ohio 45207
513 745-3000

    Private and 4 Year   **Arts Areas:** Theatre, Film Arts and Television
    Performing Series: XU Players Theatre Series
    Performance Facilities: Theatre; Television Studios; Radio Studios

MUSIC

Constantine Soriano, Band Director   **Number Of Faculty:** 1
Music Program under auspices of Fine Arts Department
Performing Groups: Band; Clef Club; Dance Band
Workshops/Festivals: Xavier Piano Series

THEATRE

Dr Ernest Fontana, Chairman, English Department
Theatre Program under auspices of English Department
Number Of Faculty: 2   **Number Of Students:** 15
Degrees Offered: BA in English with Theatre major
Courses Offered: History; Acting; Theatre Appreciation; Production; Directing
Teaching Certification Available   **Performing Groups:** XU Players

YOUNGSTOWN STATE UNIVERSITY
410 Wick Ave, Youngstown   Ohio 44555
216 746-1851 Ext 586

    State and 4 Year
    Arts Areas: Instrumental Music, Vocal Music, Theatre, Film Arts, Television and Visual Arts
    Performance Facilities: Ford Auditorium; Bliss Recital Hall; Dana Recital Hall

(continued on next page)

MUSIC

Donald W Byo, Director, Dana School of Music   **Number Of Faculty:** 28
Number Of Students: 350   **Degrees Offered:** BM; MM
Teaching Certification Available
Financial Assistance: Assistantships and Scholarships
Performing Groups: Brass Ensemble; Woodwind Ensemble; Band; Orchestra; Wind Ensemble; Concert Choir; University Chorus
Workshops/Festivals: Music Education Workshops

THEATRE

Donald Elser, Chairman, Speech, Communication, and Theatre Department
Number Of Faculty: 5   **Number Of Students:** 80   **Degrees Offered:** BFA
Teaching Certification Available
Financial Assistance: Assistantships and Scholarships
Performing Groups: Spotlight Theatre

BACONE COLLEGE
Muskogee   Oklahoma 74401, 918 683-4581 Ext 205
   Private and 2 Year   *Arts Areas:* Vocal Music

MUSIC

Jeannine Rainwater, Chairman   *Number Of Faculty:* 2   *Degrees Offered:* AA
Courses Offered: Chorus; Applied Voice; Applied Instruments; Harmony and Sight Singing; Fundamentals
Financial Assistance: Scholarships and·Work-Study Grants
Performing Groups: Bacone Choir

BARTLESVILLE WESLEYAN COLLEGE
Bartlesville   Oklahoma 74003, 918 333-6151
   Private and 4 Year   *Arts Areas:* Instrumental Music and Vocal Music

MUSIC

Dr Robert Hauck, Chairman   *Number Of Faculty:* 5   *Degrees Offered:* BA; BS
Teaching Certification Available   *Financial Assistance:* Work-Study Grants
Performing Groups: Freedom Singers; Wesleyan Singers

BETHANY NAZARENE COLLEGE
39th Expressway, Bethany   Oklahoma 73008
405 789-6400
   Private and 4 Year   *Arts Areas:* Instrumental Music and Vocal Music
   Performing Series: BNC Music Series; BNC Culture Series
   Performance Facilities: Cantrell Recital Hall; Herrick Auditorium

MUSIC

Howard Oliver, Chairman, Division of Fine Arts   *Number Of Faculty:* 10
Number Of Students: 80   *Degrees Offered:* BA; BS; B Music Ed
Teaching Certification Available
Financial Assistance: Assistantships, Scholarships and Work-Study Grants
Performing Groups: Concert Band; Stage Band; Male Chorus; Master Chorale; Chamber Singers; Oratorio;
Community Chorus

CENTRAL STATE UNIVERSITY
100 N University Dr, Edmond   Oklahoma 73034
405 341-2980 Ext 575
   State and 4 Year
   Arts Areas: Dance, Instrumental Music, Vocal Music, Theatre and Visual Arts
   Performing Series: Drama Series; Concert Series
   Performance Facilities: Mitchell Hall; Music Building; Exhibit Hall

DANCE

Dr Virginia Peters, Chairman, Physical Education Department
Dance program under auspices of Physical Education Department
Number Of Faculty: 2   *Number Of Students:* 200   *Degrees Offered:* BA
Courses Offered: Folk; Square Dance; Ballroom; Modern; Dance Forms
Teaching Certification Available
Financial Assistance: Scholarships and Work-Study Grants

MUSIC

Dr Jack Sisson, Chairman, Music Department   *Number Of Faculty:* 22
Number Of Students: 500   *Degrees Offered:* BA; MME
Teaching Certification Available

(continued on next page)

Financial Assistance: Scholarships and Work-Study Grants
Performing Groups: Tunesmiths; Choirs; Stage Band; Marching Band; Orchestra; Woodwind Quintet; String Quartet; Vocal Groups
Workshops/Festivals: State High School Band Festival

THEATRE

Dr Lee Hicks, Chairman   *Number Of Faculty:* 8   *Number Of Students:* 250
Degrees Offered: BA
Courses Offered: Speech; Drama; Broadcasting; Oral Communication
Teaching Certification Available

CLAREMORE JUNIOR COLLEGE
College Hill, Claremore   Oklahoma 74017
918 341-7510 Ext 249
State and 4 Year
Arts Areas: Instrumental Music, Vocal Music, Theatre and Visual Arts
Performance Facilities: Will Rogers Auditorium

MUSIC

Dr James Willis, Chairman   *Number Of Faculty:* 6   *Number Of Students:* 120
Degrees Offered: AA
Technical Training: Country-Western Music; Folk Music; Music Industry; Recording Techniques
Financial Assistance: Internships, Assistantships, Scholarships and Work-Study Grants
Performing Groups: Choral; Stage Band; Jazz Band; Bluegrass; Countrypolitan; Traditional Country; American Traditional
Workshops/Festivals: Country Music Composition Workshop; Country Music Industry Workshop; Stringed Instrument Workshop

THEATRE

Dr James Willis, Chairman   *Number Of Faculty:* 2   *Number Of Students:* 20
Degrees Offered: AA
Financial Assistance: Scholarships and Work-Study Grants
Performing Groups: Claremore Community College Players

EAST CENTRAL OKLAHOMA STATE UNIVERSITY
Ada   Oklahoma 74820, 405 332-8000
State and 4 Year
Arts Areas: Instrumental Music, Vocal Music and Theatre
Performance Facilities: Science Hall Auditorium; Horace Mann Auditorium; Robert S Kerr Activities Center

MUSIC

Dr Douglas Nelson, Chairman   *Number Of Faculty:* 8
Degrees Offered: BA in Education   *Teaching Certification Available*
Financial Assistance: Scholarships and Work-Study Grants
Performing Groups: Oklahomans; Choir; Concert Band; Jazz Ensemble
Workshops/Festivals: Little Dixie Choral Festival; Messiah Festival; National Teachers Piano Workshop; District Band Workshop; District XII Music Contest

THEATRE

Robert Payne, Chairman, Speech Department   *Number Of Faculty:* 4
Degrees Offered: BA in Education; BA, Speech major and Theatre major
Courses Offered: General theatre curriculum
Technical Training: Stagecraft; Makeup; Lighting; Scene Design; Costumes
Teaching Certification Available
Financial Assistance: Scholarships and Work-Study Grants
Performing Groups: Alpha Psi Omega
Workshops/Festivals: Annual Forensic Tournaments (2)

EASTERN OKLAHOMA STATE COLLEGE
Wilburton Oklahoma 74578, 918 465-2361 Ext 222
State and 2 Year
Arts Areas: Instrumental Music, Vocal Music and Theatre
Performance Facilities: Pratt Hall; Mitchell Auditorium

MUSIC

Edwin Ashmore, Chairman **Number Of Faculty:** 3 **Number Of Students:** 20
Degrees Offered: AA **Courses Offered:** Instrumental; Vocal; Theory
Financial Assistance: Scholarships and Work-Study Grants
Performing Groups: Many Sounds
Workshops/Festivals: High School Marching Band Contest; Instrumental Music Regional Workshop

THEATRE

Johnny Wray, Chairman **Number Of Faculty:** 2 **Number Of Students:** 15
Degrees Offered: AA **Courses Offered:** BA in Speech/Drama
Financial Assistance: Scholarships and Work-Study Grants
Workshops/Festivals: District Speech Contest; Regional Speech Contest; Carl Albert Oratorial High School Speech Contest

LANGSTON UNIVERSITY
PO Box 907, Langston Oklahoma 73050
405 466-2281
State and 4 Year
Arts Areas: Instrumental Music, Vocal Music and Visual Arts

MUSIC

John Smith, Chairman
Number Of Faculty: 6 **Number Of Students:** 63
Degrees Offered: BA **Teaching Certification Available**
Financial Assistance: Scholarships and Work-Study Grants

MOUNT HOOD COMMUNITY COLLEGE
26000 SE Stark, Gresham Oklahoma 97030
503 666-1306
County
Arts Areas: Instrumental Music, Vocal Music, Television, Visual Arts and Radio

MUSIC

Degrees Offered: AA **Financial Assistance:** Scholarships
Performing Groups: Chorus; Orchestra; Instrumental Ensembles

THEATRE

Degrees Offered: AA Speech-Theatre **Financial Assistance:** Scholarships

MURRAY STATE COLLEGE
Tishomingo   Oklahoma 73460, 405 371-2371 Ext 30
   State and 2 Year
   Arts Areas: Instrumental Music, Vocal Music and Television

MUSIC

Larry Metcalf, Chairman   *Number Of Faculty:* 3   *Degrees Offered:* AS
Financial Assistance: Scholarships and Work-Study Grants
Performing Groups: MSC "Entertainers"

THEATRE

Fred Poe, Chairman   *Number Of Faculty:* 3   *Degrees Offered:* AS

NORTHEAST OKLAHOMA STATE UNIVERSITY
Tahlequah   Oklahoma 74464, 918 456-5511
   State and 4 Year
   Arts Areas: Dance, Instrumental Music, Vocal Music, Theatre, Television and Visual Arts
   Performing Series: Allied Arts Series
   Performance Facilities: Fine Arts Auditorium

MUSIC

Dr Ralph Whitworth, Chairman   *Number Of Students:* 80   *Degrees Offered:* BA
Teaching Certification Available   Financial Assistance: Work-Study Grants
Performing Groups: Band; Stage Band; Brass Choir; Woodwind Ensemble; German Band; Chorus; Vocal Ensemble
Workshops/Festivals: Choral Festival; Green Country Jazz Festival
Number Of Faculty: 2   *Number Of Students:* 50
Financial Assistance: Work-Study Grants

NORTHEASTERN OKLAHOMA A & M COLLEGE
2nd & I, NE, Miami   Oklahoma 74354
918 542-8441 Ext 249
   State and 2 Year
   Arts Areas: Instrumental Music, Vocal Music, Theatre and Visual Arts
   Performance Facilities: Auditorium

MUSIC

Kenneth Richards, Chairman of Fine Arts   *Number Of Faculty:* 6
Number Of Students: 55   *Degrees Offered:* AA
Courses Offered: Applied Music; Voice; Music Literature
Financial Assistance: Scholarships and Work-Study Grants
Performing Groups: Chorus; Meistersingers; Band; Stage Band
Workshops/Festivals: High School Choral Festival; High School Band Festival

THEATRE

Shirl White, Chairman   *Number Of Faculty:* 5   *Number Of Students:* 30
Degrees Offered: AA
Courses Offered: Introduction to Theatre; Speech; Makeup; Technical Courses; History of Costumes
Performing Groups: Speech - Drama Club

NORTHEASTERN STATE COLLEGE
Tahlequah   Oklahoma 74464, 918 456-5511
   State
   Arts Areas: Instrumental Music, Vocal Music, Theatre and Visual Arts
   Performing Series: Northeastern State College Allied Arts Series
   Performance Facilities: College Auditorium

(continued on next page)

MUSIC

Dr Theo M Mix, Chairman   **Number Of Faculty:** 10   **Number Of Students:** 50
Degrees Offered: BA   **Teaching Certification Available**
Financial Assistance: Scholarships   **Performing Groups:** College Choir

THEATRE

Dr Frank Vesley, Chairman, Communications Div   **Number Of Faculty:** 2
Number Of Students: 55   **Degrees Offered:** BA Speech
Teaching Certification Available   **Financial Assistance:** Scholarships
Performing Groups: Au-Ger-Du-Ho Players

NORTHERN OKLAHOMA COLLEGE
1220 E Grand, Tonkawa   Oklahoma 74653
405 628-2581

State and 2 Year
Arts Areas: Instrumental Music, Vocal Music, Theatre, Visual Arts and Radio
Performance Facilities: Wilkin Auditorium

MUSIC

Bill Heilmann, Chairman   **Number Of Faculty:** 4   **Number Of Students:** 40
Degrees Offered: AA   **Financial Assistance:** Scholarships
Performing Groups: Roustabouts; Nocquints; Nocturnes

THEATRE

James Morgan, Chairman   **Number Of Faculty:** 1   **Number Of Students:** 40
Degrees Offered: AA   **Financial Assistance:** Scholarships
Performing Groups: Thespians

NORTHWESTERN OKLAHOMA STATE UNIVERSITY
Alva   Oklahoma 73717, 405 327-1700

State and 4 Year
Arts Areas: Instrumental Music, Vocal Music and Theatre

MUSIC

Ed Huckeby, Chairman   **Number Of Faculty:** 3   **Number Of Students:** 100
Degrees Offered: BA; BAEd   **Teaching Certification Available**
Financial Assistance: Scholarships, Work-Study Grants and Participation Awards
Performing Groups: Northwest Soundsation (pop rock group); Rangerettes (women's vocal ensemble); Jazz Band; Marching Band

THEATRE

John Barton, Chairman, Speech Department   **Number Of Faculty:** 3
Number Of Students: 100   **Degrees Offered:** BA; BAEd
Teaching Certification Available

NORTHWESTERN OKLAHOMA STATE UNIVERSITY
Alva   Oklahoma 73717, 405 327-1700

State and 4 Year
Arts Areas: Instrumental Music, Vocal Music and Theatre
Performance Facilities: Auditorium

MUSIC

Ed Huckeby, Chairman   **Number Of Faculty:** 4   . **Number Of Students:** 100
Degrees Offered: BA Education; MMus Ed   **Teaching Certification Available**

THEATRE

John Barton, Chairman   **Number Of Faculty:** 3   **Number Of Students:** 100
Degrees Offered: BA; MEd   **Teaching Certification Available**

OKLAHOMA BAPTIST UNIVERSITY
Shawnee   Oklahoma 74801, 405 273-2300

Private and 4 Year
Arts Areas: Instrumental Music, Vocal Music, Theatre and Visual Arts
Performing Series: Cultural Events Series
Performance Facilities: University Auditorium   *Number Of Faculty:* 28

MUSIC

Number Of Students: 285   *Degrees Offered:* BA; BA Mus Ed
Technical Training: Opera   *Teaching Certification Available*
Financial Assistance: Scholarships and Work-Study Grants
Performing Groups: Choir; Orchestra; Vocal and Instrumental Ensembles
Workshops/Festivals: Opera Workshop

THEATRE

Mrs O Craig, Chairman   *Number Of Faculty:* 3   *Number Of Students:* 44
Teaching Certification Available
Financial Assistance: Scholarships and Work-Study Grants

OKLAHOMA CITY SOUTHWESTERN COLLEGE
4700 NW 10th St, Oklahoma City   Oklahoma 73127
403 947-2331

Private and 2 Year   *Arts Areas:* Vocal Music and Theatre

MUSIC

Ray Ballen, Chairman   *Degrees Offered:* AA
Financial Assistance: Scholarships
Performing Groups: Choir; Great Life Singers

OKLAHOMA CITY UNIVERSITY
SCHOOL OF MUSIC AND PERFORMING ARTS
23rd & Blackwelder, Oklahoma City   Oklahoma 73106
405 521-5315

Private and 4 Year
Arts Areas: Dance, Instrumental Music, Vocal Music and Theatre
Performance Facilities: Fine Arts Auditorium; Small Auditorium; Smith Chapel

DANCE

Conrad Ludlow, Chairman   *Number Of Faculty:* 3   *Degrees Offered:* BA
Courses Offered: Ballet; Theater Dance; Modern Dance
Performing Groups: Metropolitan Ballet Company

MUSIC

Dr Fred C Mayer, Dean   *Number Of Faculty:* 37   *Number Of Students:* 260
Degrees Offered: BM; BA in Music; MM; M in Performing Arts
Courses Offered: Applied (Music and Voice); Music Education
Teaching Certification Available
Financial Assistance: Scholarships and Work-Study Grants
Performing Groups: Band; Symphony Orchestra; Stage Band; University Singers; Madrigal Singers; Surrey Singers; Opera Theater

THEATRE

Bob Varga, Chairman   *Number Of Faculty:* 6   *Number Of Students:* 60
Degrees Offered: BA; M Performing Arts   *Teaching Certification Available*
Financial Assistance: Scholarships and Work-Study Grants
Performing Groups: University Theatre; Let's Pretend Players; Puppet People Studio

OKLAHOMA STATE UNIVERSITY
Stillwater   Oklahoma 74074, 405 372-6211 Ext 224
State and 4 Year
Arts Areas: Dance, Instrumental Music, Vocal Music, Theatre, Television and Visual Arts
Performing Series: Allied Arts   *Performance Facilities:* Concert Hall; Theatre

DANCE

Myr-Lou Rollins, Director   *Number Of Faculty:* 3   *Number Of Students:* 100
Degrees Offered: BA
Technical Training: Modern Dance; Some Folk Dance and Social Dance
Teaching Certification Available   *Financial Assistance:* Work-Study Grants
Performing Groups: OSU Modern Dance Group

MUSIC

Dr Max A Mitchell, Department Head   *Number Of Faculty:* 18
Number Of Students: 975   *Degrees Offered:* BA; BMus; BMus Ed
Technical Training: Individual Lesson in Piano, Organ, Woodwinds, Brass
Teaching Certification Available
Financial Assistance: Scholarships and Work-Study Grants
Performing Groups: Univ. Symphony; OSU Marching Band; Univ Choir; OSU Glee Club; OSU Concert Band

THEATRE

Viva Locke, Director   *Number Of Faculty:* 5   *Number Of Students:* 1,250
Degrees Offered: BA; BS; MA; MS   *Teaching Certification Available*
Financial Assistance: Assistantships, Scholarships and Work-Study Grants
Performing Groups: Theatre Guild

UNIVERSITY OF OKLAHOMA
540 Parrington Oval, Norman   Oklahoma 73019
405 325-2771
State and 4 Year
Arts Areas: Dance, Instrumental Music, Vocal Music, Theatre, Film Arts, Visual Arts and Opera/Music Theatre
Performance Facilities: Rupel J Jones Theatre; Holmberg Hall Auditorium

DANCE

Miguel Terekhov, Chairman and Artist-in-Residence   *Number Of Faculty:* 5
Number Of Students: 94   *Degrees Offered:* BFA and MFA in Dance
Courses Offered: Ballet Performance and Pedagogy; Modern Dance Performance and Pedagogy
Financial Assistance: Assistantships, Scholarships and Work-Study Grants

MUSIC

Dr Jerry Neil Smith, Director   *Number Of Faculty:* 46
Number Of Students: 374
Degrees Offered: BM; B Music Ed; MM; M Music Ed; D Music Ed; DMA
Courses Offered: History; Theory; Composition; Applied; Conducting; Music Ed
Teaching Certification Available
Financial Assistance: Assistantships, Scholarships and Work-Study Grants
Performing Groups: Symphony Orchestra; Chamber Orchestra; Concert Band; Symphonic Band; Marching Band; Concert Choirs I & II; Trombone Choir; Trumpet Choir; Opera/Music Theatre Company; Flute Ensemble; OU Percussion Ensemble; Collegium Musicum; OU Jazz Ensemble
Workshops/Festivals: Women in Music Festival; Woodwind Workshop; Trumpet Symposium; Contemporary Music Festival; Percussion Workshop & Festival

THEATRE

Dr Theodore Herstand, Director   *Number Of Faculty:* 11
Number Of Students: 157   *Degrees Offered:* BFA; MA; MFA

(continued on next page)

Courses Offered: Acting; Directing; Design and Technical Production; Drama/Speech Education
Teaching Certification Available
Financial Assistance: Assistantships, Scholarships and Work-Study Grants
Performing Groups: University Theatre Company; Graduate Production Company; Southwest Repertory Theatre Company
Workshops/Festivals: High School Drama Workshops
Artists-In-Residence/Guest Artists: Yvonne Chouteau and Miguel Terekhov, Artists-in-Residence

---

UNIVERSITY OF SCIENCE AND ARTS OF OKLAHOMA
2000 S 17th St, Chickasha   Oklahoma 73018
405 224-3140
State and 4 Year
Arts Areas: Instrumental Music, Vocal Music, Theatre, Film Arts and Music Theatre
Performing Series: Chickasha Community Concerts; Exchange Artist Program
Performance Facilities: Administration Auditorium; Frances D Davis Little Theatre; Davis Hall Amphitheatre

MUSIC

Dr Elaine Minton, Chairman   *Number Of Faculty:* 6   *Number Of Students:* 40
Degrees Offered: BA in Music and Theory
Courses Offered: Fundamentals; Materials; Literature; Performance; Technique; Pedagogy; Conducting; Teaching Methods; Musical Theatre
Teaching Certification Available
Financial Assistance: Scholarships and Work-Study Grants
Performing Groups: USAO Pep Band; Chorale

THEATRE

Dr Charles DeShong, Chairman   *Number Of Faculty:* 4
Number Of Students: 20
Degrees Offered: BA in Drama; BA in Drama with Technical Theatre Emphasis
Courses Offered: Acting; Oral Interpretation and Reader's Theatre; Design; Directing; Dramatic Literature; Teaching Methods
Teaching Certification Available

ORAL ROBERTS UNIVERSITY
7777 S Lewis Ave, Tulsa   Oklahoma 74171
918 492-6161 Ext 2514
Private and 4 Year
Arts Areas: Instrumental Music, Vocal Music, Theatre, Television and Visual Arts
Performance Facilities: Howard Auditorium; Mabee Center; Zoppelt Auditorium; Christ's Chapel

MUSIC

Dr Paul Wohlgemuth, Chairman, Fine Arts Department   *Number Of Faculty:* 19
Number Of Students: 500   *Degrees Offered:* BA in Music; BM; B Music Ed
Teaching Certification Available   *Financial Assistance:* Scholarships
Performing Groups: Concert Band; Chamber Singers; Wind Ensemble; Jazz Ensembles; Concert Choir; Souls A'Fire Choir; University Chorale; University Orchestra
Workshops/Festivals: Opera Workshops; Summer Music Camps

THEATRE

Dr Robert Primrose, Chairman of Communication Arts
Dr Raymond Lewandowski Director of Theatre
Number Of Faculty: 2   *Number Of Students:* 100
Degrees Offered: BA in Communication Arts, Drama Concentration
Teaching Certification Available   *Financial Assistance:* Scholarships
Performing Groups: World Action Drama; Children's Theatre
Workshops/Festivals: High School Drama Day; Forensic Tournaments

OSCAR ROSE JUNIOR COLLEGE
6420 SE 15th St, Midwest City   Oklahoma 73110
405 737-6611 Ext 211
State and 2 Year   *Arts Areas:* Vocal Music and Theatre
Performance Facilities: Oscar Rose Junior College Theater

THEATRE

Jean Miller, Chairman   *Number Of Faculty:* 2   *Number Of Students:* 30
Degrees Offered: AA   *Financial Assistance:* Internships
Performing Groups: Theatre Guild
Workshops/Festivals: Oklahoma College Theatre Festival

PANHANDLE STATE UNIVERSITY
Goodwell   Oklahoma 73939, 405 349-2611 Ext 255
State and 4 Year
Arts Areas: Instrumental Music, Vocal Music, Theatre and Television
Performance Facilities: McKee Auditorium; Hughes - Strong Auditorium

MUSIC

Milton Bradley, Chairman   *Number Of Faculty:* 3   *Number Of Students:* 40
Degrees Offered: BA in Music and Music Ed
Courses Offered: Applied; Theory and History; Music Education
Teaching Certification Available
Financial Assistance: Scholarships, Work-Study Grants and BEOG
Performing Groups: Band; Choir

THEATRE

Jim Roach   *Number Of Faculty:* 3   *Number Of Students:* 40
Degrees Offered: BA in Speech
Courses Offered: Speech - Communication; Radio - Television; Drama
Teaching Certification Available
Financial Assistance: Scholarships, Work-Study Grants and BEOG
Workshops/Festivals: Drama Workshops; Radio Workshops; Television Workshops
Artists-In-Residence/Guest Artists: Oklahoma City Symphony

PHILLIPS UNIVERSITY
University Station, Enid   Oklahoma 73701
405 237-4433 Ext 200
Private and 4 Year
Arts Areas: Instrumental Music, Vocal Music and Theatre
Performing Series: Enid/Phillips Symphony Series
Performance Facilities: Briggs Auditorium

MUSIC

Dr Max Tromblee, Acting Chairman   *Number Of Faculty:* 17
Number Of Students: 110   *Degrees Offered:* BM; B Music Ed; M Music Ed
Teaching Certification Available
Financial Assistance: Scholarships and Work-Study Grants
Performing Groups: Band; Chorus; Orchestra; Stage Band; Chamber Groups
Workshops/Festivals: Tri-State Music Festival

THEATRE

Jerry Turpin, Chairman   *Number Of Faculty:* 2   *Number Of Students:* 35
Degrees Offered: BA; BS; MA in Education   *Teaching Certification Available*

SOUTHEASTERN OKLAHOMA STATE UNIVERSITY
Durant   Oklahoma 74701, 405 924-0121 Ext 244
State and 4 Year   *Arts Areas:* Instrumental Music and Vocal Music
Performing Series: Musical Arts Series
Performance Facilities: Little Theatre; Montgomery Auditorium

MUSIC

Paul M Mansur, Chairman   *Number Of Faculty:* 10   *Number Of Students:* 100
Degrees Offered: BA in Music and Music Ed; MA in Music Ed
Teaching Certification Available
Financial Assistance: Scholarships and Work-Study Grants
Performing Groups: Stage Band; Concert Band; Marching Band; Chorale; Chorvettes; Madrigals; Opera Workshop; Brass Ensembles; Woodwind Ensembles; Percussion Ensembles
Workshops/Festivals: All-District Band and Choral Festival; Musical Arts Series; Elementary Music Ed Workshop

SOUTHWESTERN OKLAHOMA STATE UNIVERSITY
Weatherford   Oklahoma 73096, 405 772-6611 Ext 44305
State and 4 Year   *Arts Areas:* Instrumental Music and Vocal Music
Performance Facilities: University Auditorium; Student Center Ballroom

MUSIC

Dr James W Jurrens, Chairman   *Number Of Faculty:* 21
Number Of Students: 250   *Degrees Offered:* BMusEd; BA; MMusEd
Teaching Certification Available
Financial Assistance: Assistantships, Scholarships and Work-Study Grants
Performing Groups: Women's Glee Club; Men's Glee Club; Southwestern Singers; Choraliers; Wind Symphony; Concert Band; Jazz Ensembles; Woodwind Choir; Percussion Ensemble; Brass Choir; Orchestra
Workshops/Festivals: Senior High Choral Festival; Junior High Choral Festival; Day of Jazz Festival & Contest; Band Camp; Choral Camp; Double Reed Camp; Flag/Rifle Camp; Cheerleading Camp; Piano Workshop; Bach Festival

UNIVERSITY OF TULSA
600 S College, Tulsa   Oklahoma 74104
918 939-6351 Ext 261
Private and 4 Year
Arts Areas: Instrumental Music, Vocal Music, Theatre, Film Arts, Television and Visual Arts
Performance Facilities: Kendall Hall; Tyrrell Hall

MUSIC

Ronald E Predl   *Number Of Faculty:* 14   *Number Of Students:* 175
Degrees Offered: BMus; BMus Ed; MMus; MMus Ed
Teaching Certification Available
Financial Assistance: Assistantships, Scholarships and Work-Study Grants
Performing Groups: Wind Ensemble; Jazz Ensemble; Orchestra; Chamber Choir; Concert Chorus; Marching Band; Chamber Ensemble; Opera Workshop

THEATRE

Dr Nancy Vunovich, Chairman   *Number Of Faculty:* 4 plus 1 part-time
Number Of Students: 32   *Degrees Offered:* BA; MFA
Teaching Certification Available
Financial Assistance: Scholarships and Work-Study Grants

BLUE MOUNTAIN COMMUNITY COLLEGE
PO Box 100, Pendleton   Oregon 97801
503 276-1260
> State and 2 Year
> ***Arts Areas:*** Instrumental Music, Vocal Music, Theatre, Television and Visual Arts
> ***Performance Facilities:*** College Auditorium; College Theatre

MUSIC

William Hughes, Chairman   ***Number Of Faculty:*** 2   ***Number Of Students:*** 150
Degrees Offered: AA   ***Courses Offered:*** Applied; Theory; History and Literature
Financial Assistance: Scholarships and Work-Study Grants

THEATRE

Number Of Faculty: 1   ***Number Of Students:*** 15   ***Degrees Offered:*** AA
Courses Offered: Principles; Workshop

CENTRAL OREGON COMMUNITY COLLEGE
Bend   Oregon 97701, 503 382-6112
> State and 2 Year
> ***Arts Areas:*** Instrumental Music, Vocal Music and Visual Arts
> ***Degrees Offered:*** AA in Music   ***Performing Groups:*** Instrumental & Vocal Ensembles

---

CLATSOP COMMUNITY COLLEGE
16th & Jerome, Astoria   Oregon 97103
503 325-0910
> State and 2 Year
> ***Arts Areas:*** Dance, Instrumental Music, Vocal Music, Theatre, Television and Visual Arts
> ***Performance Facilities:*** Performing Arts Auditorium

DANCE

Jack Brown, Coordinator
Dance program under auspices of Physical Education Department
Number Of Faculty: 3   ***Number Of Students:*** 50   ***Courses Offered:*** Modern; Jazz; Square
Financial Assistance: Work-Study Grants

MUSIC

Arthur Vaughn, Coordinator   ***Number Of Faculty:*** 6   ***Number Of Students:*** 75
Degrees Offered: AA   ***Financial Assistance:*** Work-Study Grants
Workshops/Festivals: Annual North Coast High School Honor Band Festival

THEATRE

Edwin Collier, Director   ***Number Of Faculty:*** 1   ***Number Of Students:*** 40
Degrees Offered: AA   ***Financial Assistance:*** Work-Study Grants
Performing Groups: Clatsop College Players

COLEGIO CESAR CHEVEZ
Mount Angel   Oregon 97362, 503 843-2234
> Private and 4 Year
> ***Arts Areas:*** Instrumental Music, Vocal Music, Theatre and Visual Arts
> ***Performing Series:*** Fine Arts & Lecture Series

MUSIC

Number Of Faculty: 4   ***Number Of Students:*** 20   ***Degrees Offered:*** BMus
Teaching Certification Available

(continued on next page)

(Colegio Cesar Chevez — cont'd)

Financial Assistance: Internships, Assistantships, Scholarships and Work-Study Grants
Performing Groups: Chorus; Orchestra

THEATRE

Carl Ritchie, Chairman   *Number Of Faculty:* 3   *Number Of Students:* 15
Degrees Offered: BA   *Teaching Certification Available*
Financial Assistance: Internships, Assistantships, Scholarships and Work-Study Grants
Performing Groups: Mt Angel Players

COMMUNITY MUSIC CENTER
3350 SE Francis, Portland   Oregon 97202
503 235-8222

City and Special   *Arts Areas:* Instrumental Music
Performance Facilities: David Campbell Recital Hall

MUSIC

Phillip K Murthe, Director   *Number Of Faculty:* 15
Number Of Students: 240   *Technical Training:* Ear Training; Theory
Financial Assistance: Scholarships

CONCORDIA COLLEGE
2811 NE Holman, Portland   Oregon 97211
503 284-1148

Private and 4 Year   *Arts Areas:* Theatre
Performance Facilities: College Auditorium

THEATRE

Hans Spalteholz, Chairman   *Performing Groups:* The Concordia Players

EASTERN OREGON STATE COLLEGE
9th & K Ave, La Grande   Oregon 97850
503 963-2171

State and 4 Year
Arts Areas: Instrumental Music, Vocal Music, Theatre and Visual Arts
Performance Facilities: EOSC Theatre; Arena Theatre

MUSIC

Dr John L Cobb, Chairman   *Number Of Faculty:* 5   *Number Of Students:* 100
Degrees Offered: BA in Music
Courses Offered: Applied (Vocal and Instrumental); History; Theory; Composition; Conducting
Teaching Certification Available
Financial Assistance: Scholarships and Work-Study Grants
Performing Groups: Grande Ronde Symphony Orchestra; Blue and Gold Singers; EOSC Choir; EOSC Band
Workshops/Festivals: Summer Music Camp

THEATRE

Richard G Hiatt, Chairmant   *Number Of Faculty:* 2   *Number Of Students:* 30
Courses Offered: Acting; Directing; Technical Theatre; History and Literature
Teaching Certification Available
Financial Assistance: Scholarships and Work-Study Grants
Performing Groups: EOSC Theatre

GEORGE FOX COLLEGE
Newberg   Oregon 97132, 503 538-2101

Private and 4 Year
Arts Areas: Instrumental Music, Vocal Music and Theatre   *Performing Series:* Concert & Lecture Series

(continued on next page)

MUSIC

Number Of Faculty: 10   **Number Of Students:** 150   **Degrees Offered:** BA; BMus; BMus Ed
Technical Training: Opera   **Teaching Certification Available**
Financial Assistance: Scholarships and Work-Study Grants
Performing Groups: Chorale Ensemble; Orchestra; Band; Instrumental Ensembles

THEATRE

Geraldine H Mitsch, Chairman   **Number Of Faculty:** 6
Number Of Students: 90   **Degrees Offered:** BA
Teaching Certification Available
Performing Groups: Delta Psi Players

JUDSON BAPTIST COLLEGE
9201 NE Fremont, Portland   Oregon 97220
503 252-5563

Private and 2 Year
Arts Areas: Instrumental Music, Vocal Music, Theatre and Visual Arts

MUSIC

Per O Walthinsen, Chairman   **Number Of Faculty:** 3   **Number Of Students:** 125
Degrees Offered: AA; AS
Courses Offered: Fundamentals; Theory I & II; Literature; Applied; Conducting; Performance; Appreciation
Financial Assistance: Scholarships and Work-Study Grants
Performing Groups: Concert Choir; Women's Chorale; Stage Band; Madrigal Singers
Workshops/Festivals: Fine Arts Festival

THEATRE

Rhonda A Miller, Chairman   **Number Of Faculty:** 1   **Number Of Students:** 30
Degrees Offered: AA; AS
Courses Offered: Acting Techniques; Appreciation; Production
Financial Assistance: Scholarships and Work-Study Grants
Performing Groups: Reader's Theatre; Department Theatre Company

---

LANE COMMUNITY COLLEGE
4000 E 30th Ave, Eugene   Oregon 97405
503 747-4501

State and 2 Year   **Arts Areas:** Theatre, Television and Visual Arts

THEATRE

Edward W Ragozzine, Chairman   **Degrees Offered:** AA
Financial Assistance: Scholarships and Work-Study Grants

LEWIS AND CLARK COLLEGE
Portland   Oregon 97219, 503 244-6161

Private and 4 Year
Arts Areas: Instrumental Music, Vocal Music, Theatre and Visual Arts
Performing Series: Cultural Arts Series
Performance Facilities: Evans Auditorium

MUSIC

Jerry D Luedders   **Number Of Faculty:** 47   **Number Of Students:** 190
Degrees Offered: BA in Music; BM in Performance, Theory/Composition, and Music Ed; MM; MMEd
Courses Offered: Survey; Specialized Theory/History; Applied
Teaching Certification Available
Financial Assistance: Scholarships, Work-Study Grants and BEOG, SEOG, NDSL, and State Grants
Performing Groups: Orchestra; Wind Ensemble; Choir; Community Chorale; Opera Workshop; Stage

(continued on next page)

Band; Collegium Musicum; Pioneer Band; Instrumental Ensembles
Workshops/Festivals: Opera Workshop; Summer Workshops and Master Classes

THEATRE

James Ostolthoff, Chairman   *Number Of Faculty:* 5   *Number Of Students:* 50
Degrees Offered: BA; BS
Courses Offered: History and Theory; Acting; Directing; Design
Teaching Certification Available
Financial Assistance: Scholarships, Work-Study Grants and BEOG, SEOG, NDSL, and State Grants

---

LINFIELD COLLEGE
McMinnville   Oregon 97128, 503 472-4121
Private and 4 Year   *Arts Areas:* Theatre, Television and Radio
Performance Facilities: Linfield Little Theatre; Pioneer Hall Auditorium; Melrose Hall

DANCE

Warren L Baker, Chairman, Music and Ballet Department   *Number Of Faculty:* 1
Number Of Students: 50
Courses Offered: Ballet Theory and Technique; Choreography
Financial Assistance: Scholarships and Work-Study Grants
Workshops/Festivals: Summer School Ballet Camps

MUSIC

Warren L Baker, Chairman, Music and Ballet Department
Number Of Faculty: 18   *Number Of Students:* 30   *Degrees Offered:* BA
Courses Offered: Applied; History and Literature; Education; Conducting
Teaching Certification Available
Financial Assistance: Scholarships and Work-Study Grants
Performing Groups: A Cappella Choir; Band; String Orchestra; Swing Choir; Stage Band; Choral Union; Brass Choir; Trombone Choir
Workshops/Festivals: Summer Vocal Music Camp; Summer Brass Workshop

THEATRE

Ted Desel, Director   *Number Of Faculty:* 2   *Number Of Students:* 30
Degrees Offered: BA   *Teaching Certification Available*

MARYLHURST EDUCATION CENTER
Marylhurst   Oregon 97036, 503 636-8141
Private and 4 Year
Arts Areas: Instrumental Music, Vocal Music and Visual Arts
Performance Facilities: St Anne's Chapel

MUSIC

Sister Lucie Hutchinson, Director   *Number Of Faculty:* 20
Number Of Students: 100   *Degrees Offered:* BM; BA in Music
Courses Offered: Performance; Jazz Studies; Pedagogy; Composition; History and Literature; Accompanying
Financial Assistance: Scholarships
Performing Groups: Marylhurst Philharmonic Orchestra; Jazz Studies Ensemble

---

MOUNT HOOD COMMUNITY COLLEGE
26000 SE Stark St, Gresham   Oregon 97030
503 667-1561
2 Year
Arts Areas: Dance, Instrumental Music, Vocal Music, Theatre, Film Arts, Television and Visual Arts
Performance Facilities: Theatres (3)

(continued on next page)

DANCE

Gael Tower, Division Chairperson   *Number Of Faculty:* 4 Part-time
Number Of Students: 200   *Degrees Offered:* AA
Courses Offered: Modern; Ballet; Jazz; Tap; Theater
Financial Assistance: Work-Study Grants

MUSIC

Gael Tower, Division Chairperson   *Number Of Faculty:* 12
Number Of Students: 350   *Degrees Offered:* AA
Courses Offered: Voice; Instrumental
Financial Assistance: Scholarships and Work-Study Grants
Performing Groups: Vocal Jazz Groups I & II; Stage Bands I & II; String Ensemble; Wind Ensemble; Dixieland Group; Repertoire Singers; Madrigals I & II
Workshops/Festivals: Northwest Vocal Jazz Festival; Northwest Orchestra Festival; Northwest Stage Band Festival; Northwest Small Groups Festival

THEATRE

Gael Tower, Division Chairperson   *Number Of Faculty:* 2
Degrees Offered: AA   *Courses Offered:* Acting; Technical Courses

---

NORTHWEST CHRISTIAN COLLEGE
Eugene   Oregon 97401, 503 343-1641
Private and 4 Year   *Arts Areas:* Instrumental Music and Vocal Music

MUSIC

Guy E Aydelott, Chairman   *Number Of Faculty:* 4
Degrees Offered: BA or BS, in Biblical Major with Music Concentration
Courses Offered: Theory; History; Applied; Church Music; Conducting

---

OREGON COLLEGE OF EDUCATION
345 N Monmouth Ave, Monmouth   Oregon 97361
503 838-1220 Ext 281
State and 4 Year
Arts Areas: Dance, Instrumental Music, Vocal Music, Theatre and Visual Arts
Performing Series: Fine Arts Series
Performance Facilities: Fine Arts Auditorium; Music Recital Hall

MUSIC

Edgar H Smith, Chairman   *Number Of Faculty:* 22   *Number Of Students:* 220
Degrees Offered: BA/BS in Education; BA/BS in Music; BA/BS in the Arts; M Music Ed
Courses Offered: Theory and Analysis; History and Literature; Music Education; Performance (Voice and Instrumental)
Teaching Certification Available
Financial Assistance: Scholarships and Work-Study Grants
Performing Groups: Orchestra; Concert Band; Jazz Ensemble; Wind, String, Percussion, and Brass Ensembles; Concert Choir; Women's Chorale; Select Singers; Chamber Ensemble; Opera Workshop
Workshops/Festivals: Summer Arts Festival; High School Stage Band Festival; Fine Arts Series; Public Schools Voice and Ensemble Contest; State Solo Voice and Instrumental Contest

THEATRE

Allen J Adams, Chairman   *Number Of Faculty:* 5   *Number Of Students:* 65
Degrees Offered: BA/BS in Education; BA/BS in Humanities; BA/BS in the Arts
Courses Offered: Acting; Direction; Production; Technical Theater
Technical Training: Scenecraft; Lighting; Costuming; Makeup; Scene Design
Teaching Certification Available
Financial Assistance: Internships, Scholarships and Work-Study Grants
Performing Groups: Alpha Psi Omega Studio Theatre; Humanities Night; Lunchbox Theatre; Children's Theatre
Workshops/Festivals: Summer Arts Festival; Mainstage Theater

OREGON STATE UNIVERSITY
Corvallis   Oregon 97330, 503 754-1061
State and 4 Year
Arts Areas: Dance, Instrumental Music, Vocal Music, Theatre, Film Arts, Television and Visual Arts
Performing Series: ATA International Liaison Committee speakers and performers
Civic Concert Series; University Service Group "Encore"
Performance Facilities: Oregon State Univ Performing Arts Center

DANCE

Georgia Brock, Coordinator   **Number Of Faculty:** 3   **Number Of Students:** 500
Degrees Offered: BA or BS in Physical Education with Dance Option; MA; MS; MEd
Financial Assistance: Assistantships
Performing Groups: Promenaders (Folk Dance); Orchesis (Modern Dance)
Workshops/Festivals: Folk Dance Festivals; Modern Dance Workshops

MUSIC

William A Campbell, Chairman   **Number Of Faculty:** 14
Number Of Students: 80 majors
Degrees Offered: BA or BS in Music; Music Education; MA in Interdisciplinary Studies
Teaching Certification Available   *Financial Assistance:* Work-Study Grants
Performing Groups: Symphony Orchestra; Chamber Orchestra; University Choir; Civic University Chorus;
Madrigal Singers; Chamber Choir; Baroque Ensemble; Marching Band; Symphonic Band; Concert Band;
Jazz Band
Workshops/Festivals: Summer Music Camps

THEATRE

Dr C V Bennett, Coordinator   **Number Of Faculty:** 4
Number Of Students: 75 majors; 250 non-majors   **Degrees Offered:** BA; BS; BSEd
Teaching Certification Available
Financial Assistance: Assistantships, Scholarships and Work-Study Grants
Performing Groups: Faculty and student directed productions
Workshops/Festivals: Mime; Summer Theatre

UNIVERSITY OF OREGON
Eugene   Oregon 97403, 503 686-3111
State and 4 Year
Arts Areas: Dance, Instrumental Music, Vocal Music, Theatre, Film Arts, Television, Visual Arts and Radio
Performing Series: Chamber University Music Series
Performance Facilities: McArthur Court; Robinson Theatre; Beall Concert Hall; Dougherty Dance Theatre

DANCE

Linda Hearn, Chairman   **Number Of Faculty:** 7   **Number Of Students:** 140
Degrees Offered: BA; BS; MA; MS
Courses Offered: Notation; Production; History; Music in Dance
Financial Assistance: Assistantships
Performing Groups: Modern, Ballet, and Folk Repertory Groups

MUSIC

Morrette Rider, Dean   **Number Of Faculty:** 38   **Number Of Students:** 450
Degrees Offered: BS; BA; BM; MA; MM; DMA; PhD; DED
Courses Offered: Performance; Music Ed; Composition; Theory; History; Conducting
Technical Training: Piano Technician   *Teaching Certification Available*
Financial Assistance: Internships, Assistantships, Scholarships, Work-Study Grants and Competitive
Fellowships
Performing Groups: Choirs; Orchestras; Bands; Collegium; Opera Workshop; Vocal Jazz Ensemble;
Instrumental Jazz Ensembles; Brass Choir; Percussion Ensemble
Workshops/Festivals: International Festival, International Center for Music, England (year-round)

(continued on next page)

THEATRE

Marya Bednerik, Chairman   **Number Of Faculty:** 7   **Number Of Students:** 200
Degrees Offered: BA; MA; MS; MFA; PhD   **Teaching Certification Available**
Financial Assistance: Internships, Assistantships, Scholarships and Work-Study Grants
Performing Groups: University Theatre; Action Theatre

PACIFIC UNIVERSITY
Forest Grove   Oregon 97116, 503 357-6151 Ext 251
Private and 4 Year
Arts Areas: Dance, Instrumental Music, Vocal Music, Theatre, Television and Visual Arts
Performing Series: Pacific University Artist Series
Performance Facilities: Brighton Auditorium; Miles Theatre; Washburn Hall

DANCE

Mr John Neff, Chairman   **Number Of Faculty:** 1   **Number Of Students:** 10
Degrees Offered: BA   **Teaching Certification Available**
Financial Assistance: Internships, Scholarships and Work-Study Grants
Performing Groups: Pacific Univ Dancers

MUSIC

Dr Albert C Shaw, Dean   **Number Of Faculty:** 11   **Number Of Students:** 45
Degrees Offered: BMus; BMus Ed; BA; MA Teaching
Teaching Certification Available
Financial Assistance: Internships, Scholarships and Work-Study Grants
Performing Groups: Pacific Community Orchestra; Pacific Univ Band; Pacific Singers; Pacific Univ
Chamber Singers; Stage Band; Pep Band
Workshops/Festivals: Music in May Festival, Suzuki Institute

THEATRE

Mr Theodore Sizer, Chairman   **Number Of Faculty:** 2   **Number Of Students:** 14
Degrees Offered: BA   **Teaching Certification Available**
Financial Assistance: Internships, Scholarships and Work-Study Grants
Performing Groups: Pacific Univ Theatre

PORTLAND STATE UNIVERSITY
PO Box 751, Portland   Oregon 97207
503 229-3514
State and 4 Year
Arts Areas: Dance, Instrumental Music, Vocal Music, Theatre, Film Arts and Visual Arts
Performance Facilities: Lincoln Hall Auditorium; Studio Theater

DANCE

Nancy R Matschek, Director   **Number Of Faculty:** 4   **Number Of Students:** 175
Degrees Offered: Certificate in Dance
Courses Offered: Choreography; Composition; Production; History; Aesthetics
Financial Assistance: Scholarships and Work-Study Grants
Performing Groups: Portland Ballet Company; Repertory Dancers
Workshops/Festivals: Spring Festival of Dance

MUSIC

Wilma Sheridan, Acting Head   **Number Of Faculty:** 11
Number Of Students: 260   **Degrees Offered:** BM; B Music Ed; M Music Ed
Teaching Certification Available
Financial Assistance: Internships, Assistantships, Scholarships and Work-Study Grants
Performing Groups: Opera Theatre; Orchestra; Chorus; Instrumental Ensembles

(continued on next page)

THEATRE

Jack L Featheringill, Head   **Number Of Faculty:** 6   **Number Of Students:** 135
Degrees Offered: BA; BS; MA; MAT; MST   **Teaching Certification Available**
Financial Assistance: Internships, Assistantships, Scholarships and Work-Study Grants
Performing Groups: PSU Players
Workshops/Festivals: Coaster Theater Summer Stock

UNIVERSITY OF PORTLAND
5000 N Willamette Blvd, Portland   Oregon 97203
503 283-7228
Private and 4 Year
Arts Areas: Instrumental Music, Vocal Music, Theatre and Television
Performance Facilities: Mago Hunt Center for the Performing Arts

MUSIC

Paul S Melhuish, Chairman   **Number Of Faculty:** 4   **Number Of Students:** 35
Degrees Offered: BM; B Music Ed; MM; M Music Ed
Teaching Certification Available
Financial Assistance: Assistantships, Scholarships and Work-Study Grants
Performing Groups: Band; Choir; Ensemble; Orchestra; Symphony
Workshops/Festivals: Festival of Jazz; Choral Clinic; Summer Jazz Clinic

THEATRE

Paul S Melhuish, Chairman   **Number Of Faculty:** 4
Number Of Students: 10 - 15   **Degrees Offered:** BA; MFA; MA
Courses Offered: Acting; Production; Directing; Reader's Theatre; Lighting; Makeup; Stage Design;
Costume Design; History
Teaching Certification Available
Financial Assistance: Assistantships, Scholarships and Work-Study Grants
Performing Groups: Shakespearean Company; Classical Company; Comedy Company; Musical Theatre;
Children's Theatre
Artists-In-Residence/Guest Artists: Cliff Smith, Artist-in-Residence; Rev Harry C Cronin,
Playwright-in-Residence

REED COLLEGE
Portland   Oregon 97202, 503 771-1112 Ext 381
Private and 4 Year
Arts Areas: Dance, Instrumental Music, Theatre and Visual Arts
Performing Series: Reed Music Associates; Cultural Affairs Board
Performance Facilities: The Theatre

DANCE

Judy Massee, Chairman   **Number Of Faculty:** 1   **Number Of Students:** 50
Degrees Offered: BA Dance-Theatre   **Teaching Certification Available**
Financial Assistance: Scholarships and Work-Study Grants
Performing Groups: Reed Dance Ensemble

MUSIC

Leila Birnbaum, Chairman   **Number Of Faculty:** 4   **Number Of Students:** 30
Degrees Offered: BA   **Technical Training:** Instrumental Music
Teaching Certification Available

THEATRE

Larry Oliver, Chairman   **Number Of Faculty:** 2   **Number Of Students:** 50
Degrees Offered: BA   **Teaching Certification Available**
Financial Assistance: Scholarships and Work-Study Grants

SOUTHERN OREGON COLLEGE
1250 Siskiyou Blvd, Ashland   Oregon 97520
503 482-3311
State and 4 Year
Arts Areas: Instrumental Music, Vocal Music, Theatre and Visual Arts
Performing Series: Performing Artist Series; Oregon Shakespeare Festival

MUSIC

William C Bushnell, Chairman   **Number Of Faculty:** 12
Number Of Students: 220   **Degrees Offered:** BA; BMus; BMus Ed; MMus
Technical Training: Opera   **Teaching Certification Available**
Financial Assistance: Assistantships, Scholarships and Work-Study Grants
Performing Groups: Opera Theatre; Orchestra; String Ensembles; Wind Ensembles; Chorus
Workshops/Festivals: Britt Music Festival; Opera Workshop; Fine Arts Workshop

THEATRE

Dorothy E Stolp, Chairman   **Number Of Faculty:** 11   **Number Of Students:** 200
Degrees Offered: AS; BA; BFA; MA; MFA   **Teaching Certification Available**
Financial Assistance: Assistantships, Scholarships and Work-Study Grants
Performing Groups: Soc Players
Workshops/Festivals: Oregon Shakespeare Festival; Fine Arts Week

SOUTHWESTERN STATE COLLEGE
Weatherford   Oregon 73096, 405 772-5511
State and 4 Year
Arts Areas: Instrumental Music, Vocal Music, Theatre and Visual Arts

MUSIC

Dr James W Junens, Chairman   **Number Of Faculty:** 18
Number Of Students: 225   **Degrees Offered:** BA; BA Mus Ed
Teaching Certification Available
Financial Assistance: Scholarships and Work-Study Grants
Performing Groups: Christmas Oratorio

THEATRE

Dr G Bellamy, Chairman, English Department   **Number Of Faculty:** 1
Degrees Offered: BA Drama; MA Drama   **Teaching Certification Available**
Financial Assistance: Scholarships and Work-Study Grants
Performing Groups: Alpha Psi Omega

TREASURE VALLEY COMMUNITY COLLEGE
650 College Blvd, Ontario   Oregon 97914
503 889-6493
State and 2 Year
Arts Areas: Instrumental Music, Vocal Music and Visual Arts
Performance Facilities: College Auditorium   **Degrees Offered:** AA in Music
Financial Assistance: Scholarships and Work-Study Grants
Performing Groups: Instrumental & Vocal Ensembles

WARNER PACIFIC COLLEGE
2219 SE 68th St, Portland   Oregon 97215
503 775-4368
Private and 4 Year
Arts Areas: Instrumental Music, Vocal Music, Theatre and Visual Arts
Performing Series: Concert and Lecture Series
Performance Facilities: Speech Arts Bldg

(continued on next page)

MUSIC

Dr Denon Helbling, Chairman   **Number Of Faculty:** 8
Number Of Students: 150   **Degrees Offered:** AA; BA; BMus; BMus Ed
Technical Training: Electronic Music   **Teaching Certification Available**
Financial Assistance: Internships, Scholarships and Work-Study Grants
Performing Groups: Chorus; Instrumental Ensembles; Orchestra; Wind Ensembles (Touring); Lab Band; Music Stage Productions

THEATRE

Mary Boyce, Chairman   **Number Of Faculty:** 6   **Number Of Students:** 70
Degrees Offered: BA   **Teaching Certification Available**
Financial Assistance: Scholarships and Work-Study Grants
Performing Groups: University Theatre

WESTERN BAPTIST BIBLE COLLEGE
5000 Deer Park Dr SE, Salem   Oregon 97302
508 581-8600
Private and 4 Year   **Arts Areas:** Instrumental Music and Vocal Music

MUSIC

Dr Robert Whittaker, Chairman   **Number Of Faculty:** 8
Number Of Students: 36   **Degrees Offered:** BS with Music Major or Minor
Courses Offered: Performance; Theory/Composition; History; Conducting
Financial Assistance: Scholarships and Work-Study Grants
Performing Groups: Orchestra; Chorus; Vocal Ensembles; Instrumental Ensembles
Workshops/Festivals: Spring Music Festival

WILLAMETTE UNIVERSITY
Salem   Oregon 97301, 503 370-6300
Private and 4 Year
Arts Areas: Instrumental Music, Vocal Music, Theatre and Visual Arts
Performing Series: Concert Series

MUSIC

Richard H Stewart, Acting Dean   **Number Of Faculty:** 12
Number Of Students: 170   **Degrees Offered:** BA; BMus; BMus Ed; MMus Ed
Technical Training: Overseas Study; Music Therapy; Opera
Teaching Certification Available
Financial Assistance: Assistantships, Scholarships and Work-Study Grants
Performing Groups: Symphony Concerts; Chamber Music Ensembles; Chorale Ensemble; Band; Orchestra
Workshops/Festivals: Opera Workshop

THEATRE

Robert M Putnam, Chairman   **Number Of Faculty:** 2   **Number Of Students:** 30
Degrees Offered: BFA   **Teaching Certification Available**
Financial Assistance: Assistantships, Scholarships and Work-Study Grants
Performing Groups: Willamette Univ Players

ALBRIGHT COLLEGE
13th & Exeter Sts, Reading   Pennsylvania 19604
215 921-2381

Private and 4 Year
Arts Areas: Instrumental Music, Vocal Music, Theatre, Film Arts, Television and Visual Arts
Performing Series: Arts and Lecture Series
Performance Facilities: Campus Center Theater; Memorial Chapel; Bollman Physical Education Center

MUSIC

Dr Francis H Williamson, Chairman   *Number Of Faculty:* 2
Degrees Offered: BA
Courses Offered: Survey; Theory; History and Organization; Vocal and Instrumental Literature
Financial Assistance: Scholarships, Work-Study Grants and Loans
Performing Groups: Concert Band; Marching Band; Instrumental Ensembles; Concert Choir; Chapel Choir

THEATRE

Dr Lynn S Morrow, Director of Theatre and Asst Professor of English
Number Of Faculty: 1   *Degrees Offered:* BA
Courses Offered: Introduction; Survey; Literature
Technical Training: Set Design; Lighting Design
Financial Assistance: Scholarships, Work-Study Grants and Loans
Performing Groups: Domino Players; Summer Dinner Theatre
Workshops/Festivals: Interim Semester Workshop

ALLEGHENY COLLEGE
Meadville   Pennsylvania 16335, 814 724-3100

Private and 4 Year
Arts Areas: Instrumental Music, Vocal Music and Theatre
Performing Series: Allegheny College Public Events Series
Performance Facilities: Allegheny Playshop Theatre; Campus Center Auditorium

MUSIC

Carlton R Woods, Chairman   *Number Of Faculty:* 18   *Number Of Students:* 250
Degrees Offered: BA
Courses Offered: Applied Music; History; Theory; Composition
Technical Training: Piano Tuning   *Financial Assistance:* Work-Study Grants
Performing Groups: Chamber Orchestra; Civic Symphony; Wind Symphony; Brass Choir and Quintet; Jazz Ensemble; Choir
Workshops/Festivals: Brass Festival; Summer Music Festival

THEATRE

William F Walton, Chairman   *Number Of Faculty:* 4
Number Of Students: 30 majors   *Degrees Offered:* BA
Courses Offered: Performance; History
Technical Training: Production; Lighting; Design
Teaching Certification Available   Financial Assistance: Work-Study Grants
Performing Groups: Playshop Theatre; Playshop Children's Theatre

ALLEGHENY COUNTY COMMUNITY COLLEGE
Allegheny Campus, Pittsburgh   Pennsylvania 15212
412 321-0192

County and 2 Year
Arts Areas: Instrumental Music, Vocal Music, Theatre and Visual Arts
Performance Facilities: College Auditorium   *Degrees Offered:* AA Music
Degrees Offered: AA Speech & Theatre

ALLENTOWN COLLEGE OF SAINT FRANCIS DE SALES
Station Ave, Center Valley Pennsylvania 18034
215 282-1100

Private and 4 Year *Arts Areas:* Theatre
Performing Series: Performing Artist Series

THEATRE

Gerard Schubert, Department Head *Degrees Offered:* BA
Financial Assistance: Scholarships and Work-Study Grants

BAPTIST BIBLE COLLEGE
578 Venard Rd, Clarks Summit Pennsylvania 18411
717 587-1172

Private and 4 Year *Arts Areas:* Vocal Music and Theatre
Degrees Offered: AA, BA Church Music
Performing Groups: Choir, Choral Ensembles, Chamber Ensembles

BEAVER COLLEGE
Glenside Pennsylvania 19038, 215 884-3500

Private and 4 Year
Arts Areas: Instrumental Music, Vocal Music, Theatre and Visual Arts
Performing Series: Artist Concert Series
Performance Facilities: Theatre Art Center

MUSIC

William V Frabizio, Chairman *Number Of Faculty:* 7
Number Of Students: 72 *Degrees Offered:* BA
Technical Training: Independent Study *Teaching Certification Available*
Financial Assistance: Scholarships and Work-Study Grants
Performing Groups: Orchestra, Vocal Ensembles, String Ensembles, Wind Ensembles, Chorus

THEATRE

Judith Elder, Chairman *Number Of Faculty:* 3 *Number Of Students:* 40
Degrees Offered: BA
Financial Assistance: Scholarships and Work-Study Grants
Performing Groups: Beaver Theatre Playshop

BLOOMSBURG STATE COLLEGE
Bloomsburg Pennsylvania 17815, 717 389-3817

State and 4 Year
Arts Areas: Instrumental Music, Vocal Music, Theatre, Film Arts, Television and Visual Arts
Performing Series: Arts Council Series
Performance Facilities: Haas Center; Carver Hall

THEATRE

Michael McHale, Director of Theatre *Number Of Faculty:* 4
Number Of Students: 35 *Degrees Offered:* BA; BS in Education
Courses Offered: Acting; Directing; History; Playwriting
Technical Training: Production; Lighting; Scene Design; Costuming
Teaching Certification Available *Performing Groups:* Bloomsburg Players

BRYN MAWR COLLEGE
Merion Ave, Bryn Mawr Pennsylvania 19010
215 525-1000

Private and 4 Year
Arts Areas: Instrumental Music, Vocal Music and Theatre

(continued on next page)

Performing Series: Concert Series
Performing Arts Program fully coordinated with Haverford College

DANCE

Barbara Lember, Chairman   **Number Of Faculty:** 1   **Number Of Students:** 50
Technical Training: Dancers - In - Residence Program
Financial Assistance: Scholarships
Workshops/Festivals: Dancers - In - Residence conduct workshops in area public schools

MUSIC

Robert Goodale, Chairman   **Number Of Faculty:** 5   **Number Of Students:** 97
Degrees Offered: BMus, MMus, DMA
Technical Training: Independent Study, Junior Year Abroad Program
Financial Assistance: Internships, Assistantships, Scholarships and Work-Study Grants
Performing Groups: Orchestra, Chorale, Band, Choral Ensemble, String Ensemble, Wind Ensemble
Workshops/Festivals: Visiting Performers Workshops

THEATRE

Robert A Butman, Chairman   **Number Of Faculty:** 2   **Number Of Students:** 75
Courses Offered: Acting, Directing, Designing, Costuming
Technical Training: Performance Emphasis, Theatre Productions are Extracurricular
Performing Groups: Summer Theatre

BUCKNELL UNIVERSITY
Lewisburg   Pennsylvania 17837, 717 523-1271
Private and 4 Year
Arts Areas: Instrumental Music, Vocal Music, Theatre and Visual Arts
Performing Series: Performing Artists Series, Rock Concert Series
Performance Facilities: Little Theatre

MUSIC

Thomas E Warner, Chairman   **Number Of Faculty:** 11   **Number Of Students:** 60
Degrees Offered: BA, BA MusEd   **Technical Training:** Opera
Teaching Certification Available
Financial Assistance: Scholarships and Work-Study Grants
Performing Groups: Orchestra, Chorus, Bands, Glee Club, String Ensembles
Workshops/Festivals: Opera Workshop

THEATRE

Harvey M Powers Jr, Chairman   **Number Of Faculty:** 4
Number Of Students: 50   **Degrees Offered:** BA
Teaching Certification Available
Financial Assistance: Scholarships and Work-Study Grants
Performing Groups: Cap & Dagger

BUCKS COUNTY COMMUNITY COLLEGE
Swamp Rd, Newtown   Pennsylvania 18940
215 968-5861
County and 2 Year
Arts Areas: Dance, Instrumental Music, Vocal Music, Theatre, Film Arts, Television, Visual Arts and Speech
Performing Series: College Auditorium

MUSIC

Gerald C Nowak, Coordinator   **Number Of Faculty:** 7
Number Of Students: 200   **Degrees Offered:** AA
Financial Assistance: Work-Study Grants
Performing Groups: Wind Ensemble; Jazz Band; Choral; Stage Band; Chamber Singers; Choir

(continued on next page)

THEATRE

William Brenner, Chairperson   **Number Of Faculty:** 3
Number Of Students: 50   **Degrees Offered:** AA

CALIFORNIA STATE COLLEGE
California   Pennsylvania 15419, 412 938-4000
State and 4 Year
Arts Areas: Dance, Instrumental Music, Vocal Music, Theatre, Film Arts, Television, Visual Arts and Radio
Performance Facilities: Steele Auditorium; Dixon Hall Stage 2; Learning and Research Center Auditorium

MUSIC

Paul Dolinar, Chairman   **Number Of Faculty:** 8
Degrees Offered: BS in Education
Courses Offered: Survey; Introduction and Fundamentals; Applied Music; Literature
Teaching Certification Available
Financial Assistance: Assistantships and Work-Study Grants
Performing Groups: College Choir; Choral Ensemble; Stage, Concert, and Marching Bands
Workshops/Festivals: High School Chorus Days

THEATRE

Dr Roger C Emelson, Chairman   **Number Of Faculty:** 5
Degrees Offered: BA; BS in Education (Communication); MA (Communication)
Courses Offered: Introduction; Voice; Movement; Acting; Directing; History and Literature
Technical Training: Design; Lighting; Costume Design and Construction
Teaching Certification Available
Financial Assistance: Assistantships and Work-Study Grants
Performing Groups: College Players; Theatre for Children & Youth; Theatre Now; Student Revue

CARLOW COLLEGE
3333 Fifth Ave, Pittsburgh   Pennsylvania 15213
412 683-4800
Private, 4 Year and Roman Catholic
Arts Areas: Instrumental Music, Vocal Music and Theatre

MUSIC

John R Lively, Chairperson   **Degrees Offered:** BA; BA Music Ed
Financial Assistance: Scholarships and Work-Study Grants

THEATRE

Richard Shoen, Chairperson   **Degrees Offered:** BA
Teaching Certification Available

CARNEGIE - MELLON UNIVERSITY
Schenley Park, Pittsburgh   Pennsylvania 15213
412 578-2900
Private and 4 Year
Arts Areas: Instrumental Music, Vocal Music and Theatre
Performance Facilities: Kresge Theatre; Alumni Concert Hall; Mellon Institute Auditorium; Studio Theatre

MUSIC

Robert E Page, Head   **Number Of Faculty:** 59   **Number Of Students:** 225
Degrees Offered: BFA; MFA; D Music Ed; Performance or Concentration in Instrument, Voice, or Composition
Courses Offered: Applied Music; History; Conducting; Form and Analysis; Composition; Literature and Repertoire
Teaching Certification Available
Performing Groups: CMU Trio Series; Baroque Ensemble; Carnegie-Mellon Philharmonic Orchestra; Kiltie

(continued on next page)

Band; Cameron Choir; Jazz Band; Contemporary Ensemble
Workshops/Festivals: Dalcroze International Eurhythmics Workshop; Annual String Symposium; Opera Workshop

THEATRE

Walter Eysselinck, Head   *Number Of Faculty:* 25 Full-time
Number Of Students: 264   *Degrees Offered:* BFA; MFA
Courses Offered: Acting; Voice and Speech; Movement and Dance; Production; History; Makeup; Directing; Technical Production; Costume Design; Light Design; Stage Design; Scene Painting
Performing Groups: The Park Players; Carnegie - Mellon Theatre Company

CEDAR CREST COLLEGE
Allentown   Pennsylvania 18104, 215 437-4471
Private, 4 Year and Women's College
Arts Areas: Dance, Instrumental Music, Vocal Music, Theatre and Visual Arts
Performing Series: Concert Series
Performance Facilities: College Center Theatre; Alumnae Hall Auditorium; Dance Studio (Lees Hall)

DANCE

Doris Hannan, Professor of Physical Education, Chairperson
Number Of Faculty: 1   *Number Of Students:* 89
Degrees Offered: (Cooperative program with Boston University) BA or BS from Cedar Crest; EdM from BU
Courses Offered: Dance Workshop; Folk, Modern Dance, and Ballet
Financial Assistance: Scholarships and Work-Study Grants
Performing Groups: Dance Workshop
Workshops/Festivals: Biannual residency by professional dance company, with masterclasses, lecture/demonstrations, and concert

MUSIC

Wilbur Hollman, Professor of Music, Chairman   *Number Of Faculty:* 3
Number Of Students: 108   *Degrees Offered:* BA
Courses Offered: Applied Music; History; Theory
Teaching Certification Available
Financial Assistance: Scholarships, Work-Study Grants and Loans
Performing Groups: Concert Choir; Madrigals; The Valley Camerata; Masterworks Chorale

THEATRE

Marianna Loosemore, Professor of Drama and Speech, Chairperson
Number Of Faculty: 3   *Number Of Students:* 115   *Degrees Offered:* BA
Courses Offered: BA in Drama/Speech with Acting/Directing or Design/Technical Emphasis
Teaching Certification Available
Financial Assistance: Scholarships, Work-Study Grants and Loans
Performing Groups: Buskin Society; Alpha Psi Omega
Artists-In-Residence/Guest Artists: James Hoskins, Guest Director

CHATHAM COLLEGE
Woodland Rd, Pittsburgh   Pennsylvania 15232
412 441-8200
Private and 4 Year
Arts Areas: Dance, Instrumental Music, Vocal Music, Theatre, Film Arts, Television and Visual Arts
Performing Series: Contemporary Arts Program
Performance Facilities: Play Room; Chapel

MUSIC

Russell J Wichmann, Chairman   *Number Of Faculty:* 6
Number Of Students: 80   *Degrees Offered:* BA
Courses Offered: Materials of Music; Music Journalism; History of Music
Teaching Certification Available

(continued on next page)

Financial Assistance: Scholarships and Work-Study Grants
Performing Groups: Instrumental Ensembles; Chorus; Orchestra; Laboratory School of Music

THEATRE

Jerry Wenneker, Chairman   **Number Of Faculty:** 5   **Number Of Students:** 50
Degrees Offered: BA   **Courses Offered:** Acting; History; Literature
Teaching Certification Available
Financial Assistance: Scholarships and Work-Study Grants
Performing Groups: Chatham Players   **Workshops/Festivals:** Theatre Workshops

---

CHESTNUT HILL COLLEGE
Philadelphia   Pennsylvania 19118, 215 247-4210
Private and 4 Year
Arts Areas: Instrumental Music, Vocal Music and Visual Arts

MUSIC

Sister Marie Therese, Asst Professor of Music, Chairman
Number Of Faculty: 10   **Degrees Offered:** BS in Music Ed; BA in Music
Teaching Certification Available
Financial Assistance: Scholarships and Work-Study Grants
Performing Groups: Orchestra; String Ensembles; Chorus
Artists-In-Residence/Guest Artists: Sister Mary Julia, SSJ, Artist-in-Residence

---

CHEYNEY STATE COLLEGE
Cheyney   Pennsylvania 19319, 215 399-6880
State and 4 Year
Arts Areas: Instrumental Music, Vocal Music, Theatre and Visual Arts

MUSIC

D Jack Moses, Chairman   **Degrees Offered:** BA
Teaching Certification Available
Financial Assistance: Scholarships and Work-Study Grants
Performing Groups: Choir, Band, Vocal & Instrumental Ensembles

THEATRE

Edythe S Bagley, Director

CLARION STATE COLLEGE - CLARION CAMPUS
Wood St, Clarion   Pennsylvania 16214
814 226-6000
State and 4 Year
Arts Areas: Instrumental Music, Vocal Music, Theatre, Television and Visual Arts
Performing Series: Performing Artist Series

MUSIC

Robert VanMeter, Chairman   **Number Of Faculty:** 10   **Number Of Students:** 150
Degrees Offered: BA, BA MusEd   **Teaching Certification Available**
Financial Assistance: Work-Study Grants
Performing Groups: Bands, String Ensembles, Wind Ensembles, Brass Ensemble, Choir, Orchestra, Madrigals

THEATRE

Bob Copeland, Chairman   **Number Of Faculty:** 4   **Number Of Students:** 40
Degrees Offered: BA   **Teaching Certification Available**
Financial Assistance: Scholarships and Work-Study Grants
Workshops/Festivals: Summer Drama Workshop

CLARION STATE COLLEGE - VENANGO CAMPUS
Oil City   Pennsylvania 16301, 814 676-6591
    State and 4 Year   *Arts Areas:* Instrumental Music and Vocal Music
    Degrees Offered: BA MusEd   *Teaching Certification Available*
    Performing Groups: Chorus, Chamber Ensembles, Band

COLLEGE MISERICORDIA
Dallas   Pennsylvania 18612, 717 675-2181
    Private and 4 Year
    Arts Areas: Dance, Instrumental Music, Vocal Music, Theatre and Visual Arts
    Performing Series: Cultural Events Series
    Performance Facilities: Walsh Auditorium

DANCE

Alexei Yudenich, Director   *Number Of Faculty:* 1   *Number Of Students:* 200
Dance program under auspices of Music Department
Courses Offered: Classical Ballet, Choreography
Performing Groups: Dance Theater   *Workshops/Festivals:* Dance Workshop
Degrees Offered: BMus, MusEd; BA Applied Music; MMus, MusEd
Teaching Certification Available
Financial Assistance: Scholarships and Work-Study Grants
Performing Groups: College Chorus, Madrigal Singers, Laboratory Orchestra, Folk Group
Workshops/Festivals: Music Education Workshops

THEATRE

Walter C J Andersen, Chairman   *Number Of Faculty:* 2
Number Of Students: 7   *Degrees Offered:* BA Theatre Arts
Teaching Certification Available   *Financial Assistance:* Work-Study Grants
Performing Groups: Misericordia Players
Workshops/Festivals: Annual Dramatic Production, Annual Children's Theater

COMBS CONSERVATORY OF MUSIC
Philadelphia   Pennsylvania 19119, 215 848-7500
    Private and 4 Year   *Arts Areas:* Instrumental Music and Vocal Music

MUSIC

Charles Showard, Chairman   *Degrees Offered:* BA, BA MusEd, MA, PhD
Technical Training: Composition, Therapy, Organ
Teaching Certification Available   *Financial Assistance:* Scholarships
Performing Groups: String Instruments, Violin Ensembles, Voice Ensembles, Piano, Orchestra, Bands

CURTIS INSTITUTE OF MUSIC
1726 Locust St, Philadelphia   Pennsylvania 19103
215 893-5252
    Private   *Arts Areas:* Instrumental Music and Vocal Music
    Performance Facilities: Curtis Hall

MUSIC

John de Lancie, Director   *Number Of Faculty:* 65   *Number Of Students:* 155
Degrees Offered: BM; MM in Composition
Courses Offered: Applied Music (Voice and Instruments); Theory Fundamentals; Counterpoint; Harmony;
Analysis; Solfege
Financial Assistance: Scholarships
Performing Groups: String Quartet; Wind Quartet; Curtis Symphony Orchestra

DICKINSON COLLEGE
Carlisle   Pennsylvania 17013, 717 243-5121
   Private and 4 Year
   Arts Areas: Instrumental Music, Vocal Music, Theatre, Visual Arts and Radio
   Performing Series: Concert Series

MUSIC

Truman C Bullard, Chairman   *Number Of Faculty:* 5   *Number Of Students:* 75
Degrees Offered: BA   *Technical Training:* Independent Study
Financial Assistance: Scholarships and Work-Study Grants
Performing Groups: Orchestra, Choral Group, Concerts, Band

THEATRE

David Brubaker, Chairman   *Number Of Faculty:* 3   *Number Of Students:* 45
Degrees Offered: BA   *Technical Training:* Independent Study
Financial Assistance: Scholarships and Work-Study Grants
Performing Groups: The Mermaid Players

DREXEL UNIVERSITY
32nd & Chestnut Sts, Philadelphia   Pennsylvania 19104
215 895-2000
   Private and 4 Year
   Arts Areas: Instrumental Music, Vocal Music, Theatre, Television and Visual Arts
   Performing Series: Orchestra Society of Philadelphia Series
   Performance Facilities: Mandell Theatre; Grand Hall; Main Auditorium; Stein Auditorium

MUSIC

Dr Wallace Heaton, Chairman   *Number Of Faculty:* 3
Number Of Students: 350
Courses Offered: Introduction; Harmony; Acoustics; Music Reading; Applied Music
Technical Training: Acoustics   *Financial Assistance:* Work-Study Grants
Performing Groups: Glee Club; Madrigal Singers; Varsity Singers; Band; Colonial Ensemble; Chamber Groups; Orchestra; Jazz Ensemble
Workshops/Festivals: DU Spring Music Festival

THEATRE

Adelle S Rubin, Director; Michael L Rabbitt, Designer/Theatre Manager
Number Of Faculty: 2   *Number Of Students:* 100
Courses Offered: Acting; Scene Design; Lighting Design; Individual Programs
Financial Assistance: Work-Study Grants   *Performing Groups:* Drexel Players

DUQUESNE UNIVERSITY
Pittsburgh   Pennsylvania 15219, 412 434-6220
   Private and 4 Year
   Arts Areas: Instrumental Music, Vocal Music, Theatre, Television and Radio

MUSIC

Dr Robert F Egan, Dean   *Number Of Faculty:* 60   *Number Of Students:* 470
Degrees Offered: BSMus; BSMusEd; MSMus, MSMusEd
Teaching Certification Available
Financial Assistance: Internships, Assistantships, Scholarships and Work-Study Grants
Performing Groups: Concerts, Opera, Chorus, Orchestra, Instrumenta; Groups
Workshops/Festivals: Instrumental Music Conference

THEATRE

Samuel S Meli, Chairman   *Number Of Faculty:* 4   *Number Of Students:* 72
Degrees Offered: BA   *Teaching Certification Available*

(continued on next page)

Financial Assistance: Scholarships and Work-Study Grants
Performing Groups: Red Masquers

EAST STROUDSBURG STATE COLLEGE
East Stroudsburg   Pennsylvania 18301, 717 424-3506
State and 4 Year
Arts Areas: Dance, Instrumental Music, Vocal Music, Theatre, Film Arts, Television, Visual Arts and Radio Station
Performance Facilities: Auditorium; Lecture Halls; Gallery

DANCE

Dr Mary Jane Wolbers, Professor   **Number Of Faculty:** 1
Degrees Offered: BS in Dance Education   **Teaching Certification Available**
Financial Assistance: Work-Study Grants
Workshops/Festivals: Dance Workshop; Dance Festival

MUSIC

Dr Raymond Vanderslice, Professor   **Number Of Faculty:** 7
Degrees Offered: BA   **Financial Assistance:** Work-Study Grants
Performing Groups: Band; College Choir; Treble Choir; Madrigals; Wind Ensemble
Workshops/Festivals: Festival of Arts & Letters

THEATRE

Dr Joseph Brennan, Professor   **Number Of Faculty:** 7
Number Of Students: 250   **Degrees Offered:** BA
Teaching Certification Available   **Financial Assistance:** Work-Study Grants
Performing Groups: Theater Group; Children's Theater Forensics Club
Workshops/Festivals: Festival of Arts & Letters; Summer Theater Festival
Artists-In-Residence/Guest Artists: Robert Miller, Pianist

EASTERN BAPTIST COLLEGE
Fairview Dr, Saint Davids   Pennsylvania 19087
215 688-3300
Private and 4 Year
Arts Areas: Instrumental Music, Vocal Music, Theatre and Visual Arts
Performing Series: Cultural Series

MUSIC

David Manness, Assistant Professor   **Number Of Faculty:** 9
Number Of Students: 126   **Degrees Offered:** BA   **Technical Training:** Opera
Financial Assistance: Scholarships and Work-Study Grants
Performing Groups: Choral Group, Orchestra, String Ensembles, Wind Ensembles

THEATRE

Glenn Loos, Chairman   **Number Of Faculty:** 3   **Number Of Students:** 42
Financial Assistance: Scholarships   **Performing Groups:** Les Jongleurs

---

EDINBORO STATE COLLEGE
Edinboro   Pennsylvania 16444, 814 732-2000
State and 4 Year
Arts Areas: Instrumental Music, Vocal Music, Theatre, Film Arts, Television and Visual Arts
Performing Series: Guest Artists Series; Edinboro Summer Festival
Performance Facilities: Memorial Auditorium; Old Union Hall

MUSIC

Dr Donald Panhorst, Chairman, Music and Drama Department
Number Of Faculty: 23   **Number Of Students:** 220

(continued on next page)

Degrees Offered: BA; BS in Music Ed; MEd in Music
Teaching Certification Available
Financial Assistance: Assistantships and Work-Study Grants

THEATRE

Dr Donald Panhorst, Chairman, Music and Drama Department
Number Of Faculty: 4   **Number Of Students:** 30   **Degrees Offered:** BA
Financial Assistance: Assistantships and Work-Study Grants

ELIZABETHTOWN COLLEGE
Elizabethtown   Pennsylvania 17022, 717 367-1151
Private and 4 Year
Arts Areas: Instrumental Music, Vocal Music, Theatre, Television, Visual Arts and Radio
Performing Series: Concert Series

· MUSIC

Dr Carl N Schull, Chairman   **Number Of Faculty:** 14   **Number Of Students:** 50
Degrees Offered: BA, BA MusicEd
Technical Training: Junior Year Abroad Program
Teaching Certification Available
Financial Assistance: Scholarships and Work-Study Grants
Performing Groups: Chorus, Choral Ensembles, Instrumental Ensembles, Orchestra, Band

THEATRE

Donald E Smith, Chairman   **Number Of Faculty:** 2   **Number Of Students:** 20
Degrees Offered: BA   **Technical Training:** Junior Year Abroad Program
Teaching Certification Available
Financial Assistance: Scholarships and Work-Study Grants
Performing Groups: Sock & Buskin, Religious Drama in Area Churches

---

FRANKLIN AND MARSHALL COLLEGE
Lancaster   Pennsylvania 17601, 717 291-3911
Private and 4 Year
Arts Areas: Dance, Instrumental Music, Vocal Music, Theatre, Film Arts and Visual Arts
Performing Series: Artists-in-Concert Series
Performance Facilities: Green Room Theatre; Hensel Hall; The Other Room Theatre; The College Center

MUSIC

Hugh Allen Gault, Chairman   **Number Of Faculty:** 2   **Number Of Students:** 30
Financial Assistance: Scholarships, Work-Study Grants and Loans
Performing Groups: College Choir; Ensemble; Orchestra

THEATRE

Gordon M Wickstrom, Chairman   **Number Of Faculty:** 4
Number Of Students: 60   **Degrees Offered:** BA
Financial Assistance: Scholarships, Work-Study Grants and Loans
Performing Groups: Green Room Theatre Arts Society; The Other Room Theater

---

GENEVA COLLEGE
Beaver Falls   Pennsylvania 15010, 412 846-5100
Private and 4 Year
Arts Areas: Instrumental Music, Vocal Music and Visual Arts
Performing Series: Guest Artist & Lecture Series

MUSIC

Harold W Greig, Chairman   **Number Of Faculty:** 10   **Number Of Students:** 150
Degrees Offered: BA

(continued on next page)

Technical Training: Study Abroad Program, Independent Study
Financial Assistance: Scholarships and Work-Study Grants
Performing Groups: Wind Ensembles, String Ensembles, Chorus, Singing Groups, Orchestra

THEATRE

Dr Arthur Fleser, Chairman   **Number Of Faculty:** 2   **Number Of Students:** 35
Financial Assistance: Scholarships and Work-Study Grants
Performing Groups: Frill & Dagger

GETTYSBURG COLLEGE

Gettyburg   Pennsylvania 17325, 717 334-3131
   Private and 4 Year
   Arts Areas: Instrumental Music, Vocal Music, Theatre, Visual Arts and Radio
   Performing Series: Performing Artists Series

MUSIC

Parker B Nagnild, Chairman   **Number Of Faculty:** 10
Number Of Students: 140   **Degrees Offered:** BS MusEd
Technical Training: Independent Study
Financial Assistance: Scholarships and Work-Study Grants
Performing Groups: Orchestra, Choral Groups, Bands, Instrumental Groups

THEATRE

Emile O Schumidt, Chairman   **Number Of Faculty:** 2   **Number Of Students:** 28
Degrees Offered: BA   **Technical Training:** Independent Study
Financial Assistance: Scholarships and Work-Study Grants
Performing Groups: Owl & Nightingale

GROVE CITY COLLEGE

Grove City   Pennsylvania 16127, 412 458-6600 Ext 217
   Private and 4 Year
   Arts Areas: Dance, Instrumental Music, Vocal Music, Theatre, Film Arts and Television
   Performance Facilities: Ketler Auditorium; Crawford Auditorium; College Arena; Little Theatre;
   Recital Hall
   Number Of Faculty: 2   **Performing Groups:** Marquettes

MUSIC

Oscar A Cooper   **Number Of Faculty:** 10   **Number Of Students:** 80
Degrees Offered: BMus   **Courses Offered:** Full degree program in Mus Ed
Teaching Certification Available   **Financial Assistance:** Scholarships
Performing Groups: Choir; Orchestra; Marching Band; Concert Band; Touring Choir; Woodwind
Ensemble; Jazz Ensemble

THEATRE

Dr James Dixon, Chairman   **Number Of Faculty:** 3   **Degrees Offered:** BA
Courses Offered: Communication Arts   **Teaching Certification Available**
Financial Assistance: Scholarships   **Performing Groups:** Theta Alpha Phi

HARCUM JUNIOR COLLEGE

Bryn Mawr   Pennsylvania 19010, 215 525-4100
   Private and 2 Year   **Arts Areas:** Theatre
   Performing Series: Concert - Lecture Series
   Performance Facilities: College Auditorium
   Degrees Offered: AA Drama & Speech
   Performing Groups: Drama Club, Student Performances

HARRISBURG AREA COMMUNITY COLLEGE
3300 Cameron St, Harrisburg   Pennsylvania 17110
717 236-9533

County and 2 Year
Arts Areas: Instrumental Music, Vocal Music, Theatre and Visual Arts
Performance Facilities: Rose Lehrman Arts Center   **Degrees Offered:** AA

HAVERFORD COLLEGE
Haverford   Pennsylvania 19041, 215 649-9600

Private and 4 Year
Arts Areas: Instrumental Music, Vocal Music and Visual Arts
Performing Series: "Weekly Collection" Series

MUSIC

Number Of Faculty: 3   **Number Of Students:** 30   **Technical Training:** Opera
Financial Assistance: Scholarships and Work-Study Grants
Performing Groups: Chamber Music Groups, Orchestra, Instrumental Ensembles, Choral Groups

THEATRE

Robert A Butman, Chairman   **Number Of Faculty:** 2   **Number Of Students:** 20

HEDGEROW THEATRE SCHOOL
Rose Valley Rd, Moylan   Pennsylvania 19065
215 566-9892

Private and Special   **Arts Areas:** Theatre
Performance Facilities: Hedgerow Theatre

THEATRE

Rose Schulman, Director of Theatre Education   **Number Of Faculty:** 7
Number Of Students: 75

IMMACULATA COLLEGE
Immaculata   Pennsylvania 19345, 215 647-4400

Private and 4 Year
Arts Areas: Instrumental Music, Vocal Music, Theatre and Visual Arts
Performing Series: IC Cultural Series
Performance Facilities: Alumnae Hall Performing Arts Center; College Lecture Hall

MUSIC

Sr Maureen Stephen, IHM, Chairman   **Number Of Faculty:** 10
Number Of Students: 80   **Degrees Offered:** BM; BA
Teaching Certification Available
Financial Assistance: Scholarships, Work-Study Grants and Talent Grants
Workshops/Festivals: Intercollegiate Choral Festivals; International String Conference; Spring Orchestra
Concert

THEATRE

Sr Marie Hubert, Chairman   **Number Of Faculty:** 1   **Number Of Students:** 30
Courses Offered: Speech; Oral Communication; Children's Theatre; Workshop
Financial Assistance: Scholarships, Work-Study Grants and Talent Grants
Performing Groups: Cue & Curtain Players; Children's Theatre

INDIANA UNIVERSITY OF PENNSYLVANIA
Indiana   Pennsylvania 15701, 412 357-2100

State and 4 Year
Arts Areas: Dance, Instrumental Music, Vocal Music, Theatre, Film Arts, Television and Visual Arts
Performing Series: Artists Series

(continued on next page)

Performance Facilities: Orendorff Auditorium; Fisher Auditorium; Pratt Auditorium ; Zink Hall Dance Studio; Waller Theater; McVitty Auditorium

MUSIC

Dr Richard Knab, Chairperson   *Number Of Faculty:* 30
Number Of Students: 300   *Degrees Offered:* BA; BS; BFA; MA; MEd
Courses Offered: Applied Music; Music Education
Teaching Certification Available
Financial Assistance: Internships, Assistantships, Scholarships, Work-Study Grants and State Employment
Performing Groups: Brass Group; Chamber Group; University Chorale; Symphony Band; Glee Club; Marching Band; Music Theater; Percussion Ensemble; University Chamber Orchestra; University Symphony Orchestra; String Ensemble; Wind Ensemble; Women's Chorus; Woodwind Ensemble; Oratorio Chorus
Workshops/Festivals: Summer School Workshops

THEATRE

Donald Eisen, Chairperson   *Number Of Faculty:* 3   *Number Of Students:* 40
Degrees Offered: BA; BFA
Courses Offered: Theater Education and Professional Theater Preparation Courses
Teaching Certification Available
Financial Assistance: Internships, Assistantships, Scholarships, Work-Study Grants and State Employment
Workshops/Festivals: Theater-By-The-Grove Summer Season

JUNIATA COLLEGE
Huntingdon   Pennsylvania 16652, 814 643-4310 Ext 59
Private and 4 Year
Arts Areas: Instrumental Music, Vocal Music, Theatre, Film Arts and Visual Arts
Performing Series: Juniata College Artists Series
Performance Facilities: Oller Hall

MUSIC

Prof Bruce Hirsch, Chairman   *Number Of Faculty:* 3
Number Of Students: 205   *Degrees Offered:* BA
Performing Groups: Concert Choir, Chamber Singers, Band, Stage Band, Collegium Musicum, Woodwind, Brass, String Ensembles
Workshops/Festivals: Annual Concert Tour

THEATRE

Prof Bruce Davis, Chairman   *Number Of Faculty:* 3   *Number Of Students:* 90
Degrees Offered: BA   *Performing Groups:* Masque

KEYSTONE JUNIOR COLLEGE
LaPlume   Pennsylvania 18440, 717 945-5141 Ext 31
Private and 2 Year   *Arts Areas:* Theatre
Performance Facilities: George Winterstein Experimental Theater

THEATRE

George Winterstein, Chairman   *Number Of Faculty:* 1
Number Of Students: 40   *Degrees Offered:* AA
Financial Assistance: Work-Study Grants   *Performing Groups:* KJC Players

---

KING'S COLLEGE
133 N River, Wilkes-Barre   Pennsylvania 18711
717 824-9931
Private and 4 Year   *Arts Areas:* Theatre and Television

(continued on next page)

THEATRE

Carl Wagner, Director   **Number Of Faculty:** 3   **Number Of Students:** 120
Degrees Offered: BA in Theater
Courses Offered: Stagecraft; Acting; Design; Lighting; Speech; Directing

---

KUTZTOWN STATE COLLEGE
College Hill, Kutztown   Pennsylvania 19530
215 683-3511
State and 4 Year
Arts Areas: Dance, Instrumental Music, Vocal Music, Theatre, Film Arts, Television and Visual Arts
Performing Series: Concert - Lecture Series
Performance Facilities: Schaeffer Auditorium and Little Theatre; Sheridan Art Gallery

MUSIC

Dr Frank H Siekmann, Chairman   **Number Of Faculty:** 10
Number Of Students: 35
Degrees Offered: BA in Music History; BS in Education, Music Concentration
Courses Offered: Music Theory; Performance; History
Teaching Certification Available
Financial Assistance: Assistantships and Work-Study Grants
Performing Groups: Concert and Marching Band; College Choir; Women's Choir; Jazz Band; College Orchestra; Woodwind Ensemble; Brass Ensemble; Percussion Ensemble; Recorder Ensemble

THEATRE

Dr Annette E Mazzaferri, Chairperson, Department of Speech and Theatre
Number Of Faculty: 9   **Number Of Students:** 65
Degrees Offered: BA in Speech and Theatre, Related Arts
Teaching Certification Available
Financial Assistance: Assistantships and Work-Study Grants
Performing Groups: Reader's Theatre; Alpha Psi Omega
Workshops/Festivals: Annual Invitational Reader's Theatre

LA SALLE COLLEGE
20th St & Olney Ave, Philadelphia   Pennsylvania 19141
215 951-1000
Private and 4 Year
Arts Areas: Instrumental Music, Vocal Music, Theatre, Film Arts, Television and Visual Arts
Performing Series: Concert and Lecture Series
Performance Facilities: College Union Theatre; College Union Ballroom; College Union Music Room

MUSIC

Dr George K Diehl, Chairman, Fine Arts Department   **Number Of Faculty:** 4
Degrees Offered: BA
Courses Offered: History; Theory; Composition; Applied; Orchestration
Financial Assistance: Scholarships and Work-Study Grants
Performing Groups: La Salle Singers

LEBANON VALLEY COLLEGE
College Ave, Annville   Pennsylvania 17003
717 867-3561
Private and 4 Year
Arts Areas: Instrumental Music, Vocal Music and Visual Arts
Performing Series: Performing Artist Series

MUSIC

Robert Smith, Chairman   **Number Of Faculty:** 22   **Number Of Students:** 185
Degrees Offered: BA, BA MusEd   **Teaching Certification Available**

(continued on next page)

Financial Assistance: Scholarships and Work-Study Grants
Performing Groups: Band, Orchestra, Chorale, Chamber Ensemble, Choir
Workshops/Festivals: High School Summer Band Clinics

LEHIGH UNIVERSITY
Bethlehem   Pennsylvania 18015, 215 691-7000
Private and 4 Year
Arts Areas: Instrumental Music, Vocal Music, Theatre and Visual Arts
Degrees Offered: BA Music
Financial Assistance: Scholarships and Work-Study Grants
Performing Groups: Instrumental & Vocal Ensembles

THEATRE

H Barrett Davis, Chairman   *Performing Groups:* Mustard & Cheese Drama Club

LINCOLN UNIVERSITY
Lincoln University   Pennsylvania 19352, 315 932-8300
Private and 4 Year
Arts Areas: Instrumental Music, Vocal Music and Visual Arts

MUSIC

Orrin Clayton Suthern, II, Chairman   *Number Of Faculty:* 5
Number Of Students: 14   *Degrees Offered:* BA
Financial Assistance: Scholarships and Work-Study Grants
Performing Groups: Orchestra, Choral Group

THEATRE

Louis S Putnam, Chairman   *Number Of Faculty:* 3   *Number Of Students:* 42
Financial Assistance: Scholarships and Work-Study Grants
Performing Groups: Lincoln University Players

LOCK HAVEN STATE COLLEGE
Lock Haven   Pennsylvania 17745, 717 748-5351
State and 4 Year
Arts Areas: Dance, Instrumental Music, Vocal Music and Theatre
Performing Series: Lock Haven Artist Series
Performance Facilities: John Sloan Fine Arts Center; Price Auditorium

MUSIC

Dr John I Schwarz Jr, Chairman   *Number Of Faculty:* 7
Number Of Students: 78   *Degrees Offered:* BA
Teaching Certification Available
Financial Assistance: Scholarships and Work-Study Grants
Performing Groups: College Choir; College Singers; Marching Band; Concert Band; Orchestra; String Ensemble; Brass Ensemble; Jazz Ensemble
Workshops/Festivals: Fine Arts Festival

THEATRE

Dr Denys J Gary, Chairman   *Number Of Faculty:* 4   *Number Of Students:* 41
Degrees Offered: BA in Fine Arts - Theatre; BS in Secondary Ed Theatre - Communications
Teaching Certification Available
Financial Assistance: Scholarships and Work-Study Grants
Performing Groups: College Players   *Workshops/Festivals:* Fine Arts Festival

LYCOMING COLLEGE
Williamsport   Pennsylvania 17701, 717 326-1951
Private and 4 Year
Arts Areas: Instrumental Music, Vocal Music, Theatre and Visual Arts
Performing Series: Performing Artists Series, Concert Series

MUSIC

Number Of Faculty: 6   *Number Of Students:* 102   *Degrees Offered:* BA
Technical Training: Independent Study
Financial Assistance: Scholarships and Work-Study Grants
Performing Groups: Orchestra, Choral Group, Instrumental Ensembles
Workshops/Festivals: Intercollegiate Music Competition

THEATRE

Robert F Falk, Chairman   *Number Of Faculty:* 3   *Number Of Students:* 51
Degrees Offered: BA   *Technical Training:* Independent Study
Financial Assistance: Scholarships and Work-Study Grants
Performing Groups: Theatre Players

MANOR JUNIOR COLLEGE
Fox Chase Manor, Jenkintown   Pennsylvania 19046
215 885-2360 Ext 2
Private and 2 Year   *Arts Areas:* Vocal Music
Michael Dlaboha, Chairman   *Number Of Faculty:* 1   *Number Of Students:* 50

MANSFIELD STATE COLLEGE
Mansfield   Pennsylvania 16933, 717 662-4478
State and 4 Year
Arts Areas: Instrumental Music, Vocal Music, Theatre, Film Arts, Television and Visual Arts
Performing Series: Fine Arts Series
Performance Facilities: Allen Hall; Butler Music Center; Straughn Auditorium

MUSIC

Dr James Keen, Chairman   *Number Of Faculty:* 29   *Number Of Students:* 275
Degrees Offered: BA; BS; BM; MA; MS; M Ed
Courses Offered: Theory; History and Literature; Conducting; Music Education; Applied Music (Voice and Instruments)
Teaching Certification Available
Financial Assistance: Assistantships, Scholarships and Work-Study Grants
Performing Groups: Bands I, II, III; Mountie Marching Band; Orchestra I, II; Chorus I, II, III; Piano Ensemble; Percussion Ensemble; Opera Workshop; Woodwind Ensemble; Brass Ensemble; The Mansfieldians; Concert Jazz Ensemble; Horn and String Ensemble; Chamber Singers

THEATRE

Dr A Vernon Lapps, Chairman   *Number Of Faculty:* 4   *Number Of Students:* 60
Degrees Offered: AA and BS in Communications (Theatre)
Courses Offered: Voice and Articulation; Stagecraft; Production; Acting; Makeup; Readers Theatre; Directing; Costuming; Stage Lighting; Scene Design; History; Theory; Playwriting
Teaching Certification Available
Financial Assistance: Assistantships, Scholarships and Work-Study Grants
Performing Groups: MSC Players; Readers Theatre
Workshops/Festivals: Spring Communications/Theatre Festival for High School Students

MARYWOOD COLLEGE
2300 Adams Ave, Scranton   Pennsylvania 18509
717 343-6521
Private and 4 Year
Arts Areas: Instrumental Music, Vocal Music, Theatre, Film Arts, Television and Visual Arts
Performance Facilities: Fine Arts Theatre; Comerford Theatre; Performing Arts Studio

MUSIC

Miss Jane McGowty, Chairman   *Number Of Faculty:* 14
Number Of Students: 80   *Degrees Offered:* BM; MA in Music/Church Music
Courses Offered: Applied Music; Music Education; Theory
Financial Assistance: Assistantships, Scholarships and Work-Study Grants
Performing Groups: Audubon Quartet; Marywood Choir, Orchestra, Band
Workshops/Festivals: Marywood Summer Music Camp

THEATRE

Dr George F Perry, Chairman
Number Of Faculty: 2 Theatre; 6 Communication Arts   *Number Of Students:* 135
Degrees Offered: BA; BS
Courses Offered: Stage Mime and Movement; Acting; Dance for Theatre; Production; Directing; Costume and Makeup
Technical Training: Profession Field Training
Teaching Certification Available
Financial Assistance: Assistantships, Scholarships and Work-Study Grants
Performing Groups: The Marywood Players
Artists-In-Residence/Guest Artists: Mary Franey, Artist-in-Residence

---

MERCYHURST COLLEGE
501 E 38th St, Erie   Pennsylvania 16501
814 864-0681
Private and 4 Year
Arts Areas: Dance, Instrumental Music, Vocal Music, Theatre and Visual Arts
Performance Facilities: Weber Hall Dance Studio and Little Theatre; Zurn Recital Hall

DANCE

Kenneth Miller, Director   *Number Of Faculty:* 2   *Number Of Students:* 35
Degrees Offered: BA
Courses Offered: Classical Ballet; Modern Dance; Jazz; Choreography

MUSIC

Dr Louis Mennini, Director   *Number Of Faculty:* 8
Degrees Offered: BA in Music
Courses Offered: Applied Music, Foundation and Advanced
Teaching Certification Available
Financial Assistance: Scholarships and Work-Study Grants
Performing Groups: College Chorus; Chorale; Light Opera Company

THEATRE

Dennis Andres, Director   *Number Of Faculty:* 3   *Number Of Students:* 23
Degrees Offered: BA
Courses Offered: Acting-Directing Specialization; Technical Theatre Specialization
Technical Training: Scene and Lighting Design
Financial Assistance: Scholarships and Work-Study Grants
Performing Groups: Little Theatre Players

MESSIAH COLLEGE

Grantham   Pennsylvania 17027, 717 766-2511

Private and 4 Year
Arts Areas: Instrumental Music, Vocal Music, Theatre and Visual Arts
Performing Series: Cultural Series

MUSIC

Dr Ronald L Miller, Chairman   *Number Of Faculty:* 10
Number Of Students: 60
Degrees Offered: BA in Music; BA in Sacred Music; BS in Music Ed
Teaching Certification Available
Financial Assistance: Scholarships and Work-Study Grants
Performing Groups: Wind Ensemble; Chamber Orchestra; Choral Society; Oratorio Society; Messiah College Singers; Stage Band

THEATRE

Dr Norman Bert, Chairman   *Number Of Faculty:* 1   *Number Of Students:* 70
Degrees Offered: BA   *Courses Offered:* Acting; Directing; Technical
Teaching Certification Available
Financial Assistance: Scholarships and Work-Study Grants
Performing Groups: Platform Arts Society
Workshops/Festivals: Fine Arts Festival (Spring)

MILLERSVILLE STATE COLLEGE

Millersville   Pennsylvania 17551, 717 872-5411

State and 4 Year
Arts Areas: Instrumental Music, Vocal Music, Theatre, Film Arts, Television and Visual Arts
Performing Series: Cultural Affairs Series
Performance Facilities: Lyte Auditorium; Rafters Theatre

MUSIC

Karl E Moyer, Chairman, Assoc Professor of Music   *Number Of Faculty:* 14
Number Of Students: 80   *Degrees Offered:* BS in Music Ed
Courses Offered: Fundamentals; Theory; Applied Music (Voice and Instruments); Eurhythmics; History and Literature; Music Reading; Style and Form; Pedagogy; Orchestration
Teaching Certification Available
Financial Assistance: Scholarships and Work-Study Grants
Performing Groups: College Choir; Chamber Choir; Madrigal Singers; Women's Chorus; College - Community Orchestra; Black & Gold Band; Symphonic Band; Stage Band; Woodwind Quintet; Brass Choir; String Ensemble
Workshops/Festivals: Band Festival

THEATRE

Robert H Fogg, Chairman, Asst Professor of Speech   *Number Of Faculty:* 7
Number Of Students: 15   *Degrees Offered:* BS in Education (Communications)
Courses Offered: Introductory Techniques; Production; History; Acting; Stagecraft; Directing; Appreciation
Teaching Certification Available
Financial Assistance: Scholarships and Work-Study Grants
Performing Groups: Citamard Players

MORAVIAN COLLEGE

Bethlehem   Pennsylvania 18018, 215 865-0741

Private and 4 Year
Arts Areas: Instrumental Music, Vocal Music, Theatre and Visual Arts
Performing Series: Concert Series   *Number Of Faculty:* 13
Number Of Students: 175   *Degrees Offered:* BA
Technical Training: Independent Study   *Teaching Certification Available*

(continued on next page)

Financial Assistance: Scholarships and Work-Study Grants
Performing Groups: Orchestra, Strings, Wind Ensembles, Choral Groups

THEATRE

Eugene Jacobson, Chairman   ***Number Of Faculty:*** 2   ***Number Of Students:*** 32
Degrees Offered: BA   ***Technical Training:*** Independent Study
Teaching Certification Available
Financial Assistance: Scholarships and Work-Study Grants
Performing Groups: Blackfriars

MOUNT ALOYSIUS JUNIOR COLLEGE
Cresson   Pennsylvania 96630, 814 886-4131
Private and 2 Year
Arts Areas: Instrumental Music, Vocal Music and Visual Arts
Performance Facilities: College Auditorium

MUSIC

Ronald L Dekker, Chairman   ***Degrees Offered:*** AA Music
Performing Groups: Vocal and Instrumental Ensembles, Choir

MUHLENBERG COLLEGE
Allentown   Pennsylvania 18104, 215 433-3191
Private and 4 Year
Arts Areas: Instrumental Music, Vocal Music, Theatre and Visual Arts
Performing Series: Concert Series
Performance Facilities: Center for the Arts Theatre and Recital Hall

MUSIC

Dr Charles S McClain, Chairman   ***Number Of Faculty:*** 11
Number Of Students: 54   ***Degrees Offered:*** BA
Courses Offered: Theory; History; Church Music; Applied Music (Voice and Instruments)
Financial Assistance: Scholarships and Work-Study Grants
Performing Groups: Chapel Choir; College Choir; Orchestra; Instrumental Ensembles; Opera
Workshops/Festivals: Festival of the Arts; Opera Workshop

THEATRE

Dr Patrick J Chmel, Director of College Theatre   ***Number Of Faculty:*** 2
Number Of Students: 47   ***Degrees Offered:*** BA
Courses Offered: Acting; Directing; Scene Design; History
Teaching Certification Available
Financial Assistance: Scholarships and Work-Study Grants
Performing Groups: Muhlenberg College Theatre; Muhlenberg Musical Association; Religious Drama Group

---

NEW SCHOOL OF MUSIC
301 S 21st St, Philadelphia   Pennsylvania 19103
215 732-3966
Private and 4 Year   ***Arts Areas:*** Instrumental Music
Performance Facilities: Recital Hall

MUSIC

Max Aronoff, Director   ***Number Of Faculty:*** 34   ***Number Of Students:*** 250
Degrees Offered: BM   ***Courses Offered:*** Theoretical Courses; Applied Music
Financial Assistance: Scholarships and Work-Study Grants
Performing Groups: Curtis String Quartet; New School of Music Orchestra

NORTHAMPTON COUNTY AREA COMMUNITY COLLEGE
3835 Green Pond Rd, Bethlehem   Pennsylvania 18017
215 865-5351 Ext 298
County and 2 Year   *Arts Areas:* Vocal Music, Theatre and Television
Performance Facilities: Theater; Lab Theater

MUSIC

Robert Schanck, Chairman, Professor of Music   *Number Of Faculty:* 1
Number Of Students: 20   *Degrees Offered:* AA in Liberal Arts
Financial Assistance: Work-Study Grants   *Performing Groups:* NCACC Choir

THEATRE

Norman Roberts, Chairman, Professor of Speech/Theater   *Number Of Faculty:* 1
Number Of Students: 30   *Degrees Offered:* AA in Liberal Arts
Courses Offered: Introduction to Theatre; Acting; Directing; Technical Theater
Financial Assistance: Work-Study Grants
Workshops/Festivals: Summer Theater Workshop

PENN HALL JUNIOR COLLEGE AND PREPARATORY SCHOOL
Chambersburg   Pennsylvania 17201, 717 263-3311
Private and 2 Year
Arts Areas: Instrumental Music, Vocal Music, Theatre, Television and Visual Arts
Performing Series: Cultural Arts Series
Performance Facilities: College Auditorium
Degrees Offered: AA *Financial Assistance:* Scholarships

PENNSYLVANIA STATE UNIVERSITY
University Park   Pennsylvania 16802, 814 865-2591
State and 4 Year
Arts Areas: Dance, Instrumental Music, Vocal Music, Theatre, Film Arts, Television and Visual Arts
Performing Series: University Artist Series
Performance Facilities: Playhouse Theatre, Pavilion Theatre, Recreation Hall, Recital Hall;
Schwab Auditorium, University Auditorium

DANCE

Dance program under the auspices of College of Health, PE & Recreation Departments

MUSIC

Robert W Baisley, Chairman   *Number Of Faculty:* 22
Number Of Students: 105   *Degrees Offered:* BA, BFA, MA, MFA
Performing Groups: Alard Quartet, Thalia Trio, Chapel Choirs, Symphonic Wind Ensemble, Men's Glee
Club, University Symphony Orchestra, Penn State Singers, University Concert Choir, Musica da Camera,
Brass Chorale

THEATRE

Douglas N Cook, Chairman Theatre & Film   *Number Of Faculty:* 22
Number Of Students: 348   *Degrees Offered:* BA, BFA, MA, MFA
Technical Training: BFA option in Theatre Production
Financial Assistance: Assistantships, Scholarships and Work-Study Grants
Performing Groups: Jazz Dance Company, The Arts Company, Children's Theatre Ensemble, University
Theatre Productions, Five O'Clock Theatre Productions, The Festival Theatre Company
Workshops/Festivals: Community Theatre Festival, High School Drama Workshop, Penn State Film
Festival, Festival of American Theatre, Workshops in Performance and Production

PHILADELPHIA COLLEGE OF BIBLE
1800 Arch St, Philadelphia   Pennsylvania 19103
215 561-8600

Private and 4 Year   *Arts Areas:* Instrumental Music and Vocal Music
Performing Series: Artist - Lecture Series
Performance Facilities: Robinson Memorial Auditorium; Simpson Recital Hall

MUSIC

Alfred E Lunde, Chairman   *Number Of Faculty:* 8   *Number Of Students:* 70
Degrees Offered: BM in Church Music, Performance, and Composition
Financial Assistance: Scholarships and Work-Study Grants
Performing Groups: Choir; Orchestra; Wind Ensemble; Handbell Choir; Chamber Singers; Brass Ensemble; Oratorio Society

PHILADELPHIA COLLEGE OF THE PERFORMING ARTS
313 Broad St, Philadelphia   Pennsylvania 19107
215 735-9635

Private and 4 Year
Arts Areas: Dance, Instrumental Music and Vocal Music
Performing Series: Concert Series

MUSIC

Number Of Faculty: 100   *Number Of Students:* 300
Degrees Offered: AA; BM; BM/B Music Ed; MM in Opera Singing; MFA in Opera Directing
Teaching Certification Available
Financial Assistance: Scholarships, Work-Study Grants and Private and Federal Grants, Loans, PCPA Tuition Remission Grants

UNIVERSITY OF PITTSBURGH
5th & Bigelow Sts, Pittsburgh   Pennsylvania 15260
412 624-4141

Private and 4 Year
Arts Areas: Dance, Instrumental Music, Vocal Music, Theatre and Visual Arts
Performing Series: Performing Artists Series; Committee on the Arts Series
Performance Facilities: Stephen Foster Memorial Theatre; Henry Clay Frick Fine Arts Auditorium; Studio Theatre; Trees Hall Dance Studio

DANCE

Margaret Skrinar, Director   *Number Of Faculty:* 5   *Number Of Students:* 200
Degrees Offered: BA; MA; MS; MEd; PhD
Courses Offered: Composition; Improvisation; Repertoire; Rhythmic Analysis; Teaching Methods; Anatomy and Kinesiology
Teaching Certification Available   *Financial Assistance:* Assistantships
Performing Groups: Pittsburgh Dance Alloy; Pitt Dance Ensemble
Workshops/Festivals: American College Dance Festival; Northeast Region Anatomy and Kinesiology for Dancers

MUSIC

Dr A Wayne Slawson, Chairman   *Number Of Faculty:* 10
Number Of Students: 90   *Degrees Offered:* BA; MA; DMA
Teaching Certification Available
Financial Assistance: Internships, Assistantships, Scholarships and Work-Study Grants
Performing Groups: Choral Groups; Orchestra; Symphony; String, Wind, and Brass Ensembles; Jazz Ensembles

(continued on next page)

THEATRE

Attilio Favorini, Chairman   **Number Of Faculty:** 10
Number Of Students: 160   **Degrees Offered:** BA; MA; PhD
Teaching Certification Available
Financial Assistance: Internships, Assistantships, Scholarships and Work-Study Grants
Performing Groups: Student Studio Theater; Children's Theater; 99-Cent Floating Theater

---

POINT PARK COLLEGE
Wood St & Blvd of the Allies, Pittsburgh   Pennsylvania 15222
412 391-4100

Private and 4 Year
Arts Areas: Dance, Theatre, Film Arts, Television and Visual Arts
Performance Facilities: Playhouse Performing Arts Center

DANCE

Nicolas Petrov, Director   **Number Of Faculty:** 12   **Number Of Students:** 230
Degrees Offered: BA; BFA
Courses Offered: Degree Programs in Ballet, Jazz, Modern Dance; Tap; Folk; Character
Financial Assistance: Assistantships, Scholarships, Work-Study Grants and Basic Grants, PHEAA, PCS
Performing Groups: Point Park College Dance Company
Workshops/Festivals: Dance Workshop

THEATRE

James Prescott, Director   **Number Of Faculty:** 11   **Number Of Students:** 100
Degrees Offered: BA; BFA
Courses Offered: Acting; Directing; Technical/Design; Musical Theatre
Teaching Certification Available
Financial Assistance: Assistantships, Scholarships, Work-Study Grants and Basic Grants, PHEAA, PCS
Performing Groups: Playhouse Jr; Point Park College Theatre Company
Workshops/Festivals: Theatre Workshop

SAINT VINCENT COLLEGE
Latrobe   Pennsylvania 15650, 412 539-9761

Private and 4 Year
Arts Areas: Instrumental Music, Vocal Music, Theatre, Film Arts and Visual Arts
Performing Series: SVC Concert Series
Performance Facilities: Kennedy Auditorium; Science Center Amphitheatre

MUSIC

Joseph Bronder, Chairman   **Number Of Faculty:** 3   **Number Of Students:** 20
Degrees Offered: BA; BM
Courses Offered: Applied Music; Music Education; Liturgical Music
Teaching Certification Available
Financial Assistance: Scholarships and Work-Study Grants
Performing Groups: SVC Camerata

THEATRE

Joseph Reilly, Director   **Number Of Faculty:** 2   **Number Of Students:** 10
Degrees Offered: BA   **Teaching Certification Available**
Financial Assistance: Scholarships and Work-Study Grants
Performing Groups: SVC Players

SETON HILL COLLEGE
Greensburg   Pennsylvania 15601, 412 834-2200

Private and 4 Year
Arts Areas: Instrumental Music, Vocal Music, Theatre and Visual Arts

(continued on next page)

MUSIC

Sister Helen L Muha, SC, Chairman   **Number Of Faculty:** 6
Number Of Students: 40   **Degrees Offered:** BMus
Teaching Certification Available
Performing Groups: Wind Ensemble, Choral Ensemble, Band
Workshops/Festivals: Annual Arts Festival

THEATRE

Eugene A Saraconi, Chairman   **Number Of Faculty:** 4   **Number Of Students:** 50
Degrees Offered: BA   **Teaching Certification Available**
Financial Assistance: Scholarships and Work-Study Grants
Performing Groups: Theatre Players
Workshops/Festivals: Drama Festival, Annual Arts Festival

SLIPPERY ROCK STATE COLLEGE
Slippery Rock   Pennsylvania 16057, 412 794-7263
State and 4 Year
Arts Areas: Dance, Instrumental Music, Vocal Music, Theatre, Film Arts and Television
Performance Facilities: Miller Auditorium

MUSIC

Alan B Hersh, Chairman   **Number Of Faculty:** 14   **Degrees Offered:** BA
Technical Training: Music Therapy   **Financial Assistance:** Work-Study Grants
Performing Groups: Bands, Choirs, Orchestras, Faculty Ensembles

THEATRE

Dr Theodore Walwik, Chairman   **Number Of Faculty:** 13
Number Of Students: 100   **Degrees Offered:** BA, BS Ed
Teaching Certification Available   **Financial Assistance:** Work-Study Grants
Performing Groups: Slippery Rock SC Players
Workshops/Festivals: Summer Theatre, High School Theatre Workshop

---

SUSQUEHANNA UNIVERSITY
University Ave, Selinsgrove   Pennsylvania 17870
717 374-0101
Private, 4 Year and Lutheran
Arts Areas: Instrumental Music, Vocal Music, Theatre and Visual Arts
Performing Series: Artist Series
Performance Facilities: Weber Chapel Auditorium; Benjamin Apple Theatre; Seibert Recital Hall

MUSIC

James B Steffy, Professor and Department Head   **Number Of Faculty:** 18
Number Of Students: 140 Majors
Degrees Offered: BM in Music Ed, Applied Music, or Church Music; BA in Music
Courses Offered: Applied Music; Literature and Theory; Orchestration; Conducting; Music Education
Teaching Certification Available
Financial Assistance: Scholarships, Work-Study Grants and Grants and Loans
Performing Groups: Chamber Orchestra; Symphonic Band; Marching Band; University Choir; Chapel
Choir; Festival Chorus; Musical Show Orchestra; Ensembles
Workshops/Festivals: Opera Workshop

THEATRE

Larry D Augustine, Department Head, Communications and Theatre Arts Department
Number Of Faculty: 3   **Number Of Students:** 52 Majors
Degrees Offered: BA in Communications and Theatre Arts
Courses Offered: History; Stagecraft; Acting; Oral Interpretation; Scene Design and Lighting; Directing;
Programming and Production; Theory and Criticism
Teaching Certification Available

(continued on next page)

Financial Assistance: Scholarships, Work-Study Grants and Grants and Loans
Performing Groups: University Theatre; Susquehanna University Players; Musical Theatre

---

SWARTHMORE COLLEGE
Swarthmore   Pennsylvania 19081, 215 544-7900
Private and 4 Year
Arts Areas: Instrumental Music, Vocal Music, Theatre and Visual Arts
Performing Series: Concert Series

MUSIC

Peter G Swing, Chairman   *Number Of Faculty:* 7   *Number Of Students:* 65
Degrees Offered: BA   *Technical Training:* Theory
Financial Assistance: Scholarships and Work-Study Grants
Performing Groups: Orchestra, Chorus, Band

THEATRE

Carol L Thompson, Chairman   *Number Of Faculty:* 2   *Number Of Students:* 20
Financial Assistance: Scholarships and Work-Study Grants
Performing Groups: Little Theatre Club

TEMPLE UNIVERSITY
Broad & Montgomery Sts, Philadelphia   Pennsylvania 19122
215 787-7000
State-Related
Arts Areas: Dance, Instrumental Music, Vocal Music, Theatre, Film Arts, Television, Visual Arts and Radio
Performing Series: Temple Theatre Series
Performance Facilities: Tomlinson Theater; Presser Hall; Annenberg Hall;
Randall Lab Theater; Stage Three, Temple Center City; Thomas Hall

DANCE

John Gamble, Chairman   *Number Of Faculty:* 25   *Number Of Students:* 420
Degrees Offered: BFA or Education in Dance; MEd; PhD in Ed
Courses Offered: Applied Courses (Modern Ballet, Jazz, Ethnic)
Teaching Certification Available
Financial Assistance: Assistantships, Scholarships, Work-Study Grants and Loans
Performing Groups: zero, great chazey, Sybyl

MUSIC

Allen Garrett, Dean, College of Music   *Number Of Faculty:* 93
Number Of Students: 650   *Degrees Offered:* BM; MM
Teaching Certification Available
Financial Assistance: Internships, Assistantships, Scholarships, Work-Study Grants and Fellowships
Performing Groups: Choirs; Chamber Ensembles; Bands; Contemporary Performing Ensembles; Orchestra;
Wind Ensemble; Baroque Ensemble
Workshops/Festivals: Summer Workshops; Music Ed Workshops; Piano Master Classes

THEATRE

David Hale, Chairman   *Number Of Faculty:* 17   *Number Of Students:* 205
Degrees Offered: BA; MFA
Courses Offered: BA Degree - General Theater; MFA - Specialties Acting, Design/Technical Courses,
Production, Playwriting
Financial Assistance: Internships, Assistantships, Scholarships, Work-Study Grants and Fellowships
Workshops/Festivals: ATA/ATCF Regional Festival
Artists-In-Residence/Guest Artists: Robert Smith, Kenneth Cavander, and Davey Marlin-Jones, Directors,
Theater Department

THIEL COLLEGE
Greenville   Pennsylvania 16125, 412 588-7700
  Private and 4 Year
  Arts Areas: Instrumental Music, Vocal Music and Visual Arts
  Performing Series: Artist - Lecture Series

MUSIC

  Number Of Faculty: 5   *Number Of Students:* 75   *Degrees Offered:* BA
  Technical Training: Independent Study, Junior Year Abroad Program
  Teaching Certification Available
  Financial Assistance: Scholarships and Work-Study Grants
  Performing Groups: Orchestra, Chorus, String Ensemble, Wind Ensembles, Band

THEATRE

  Emmet W Bongar, Chairman   *Number Of Faculty:* 2   *Number Of Students:* 30
  Technical Training: Independent Study, Junior Year Abroad Program
  Teaching Certification Available
  Financial Assistance: Scholarships and Work-Study Grants

UNITED WESLEYAN COLLEGE
1414 E Cedar St, Allentown   Pennsylvania 18103
215 439-8709
  Private and 4 Year   *Arts Areas:* Instrumental Music and Vocal Music
  Performance Facilities: College Auditorium

MUSIC

  Mrs Beverly Collins, Asst Professor, Chairman   *Number Of Faculty:* 2
  Number Of Students: 10   *Degrees Offered:* AS; BS; BA in Sacred Music
  Financial Assistance: Work-Study Grants and BEOG, SEOG
  Performing Groups: Instrumental Ensemble; Choir

UNIVERSITY OF PENNSYLVANIA
Philadelphia   Pennsylvania 19104, 215 243-5000
  Private and 4 Year
  Arts Areas: Instrumental Music, Vocal Music, Theatre and Visual Arts
  Performing Series: Spectacular Series
  Performance Facilities: Annenberg Center, Dance Studio

DANCE

  Malvena Taiz, Chairman   *Number Of Students:* 300
  Degrees Offered: BA, Philosophy & History of Dance
  Performing Groups: University of Pennsylvania Dance Group
  Workshops/Festivals: Dance Council

MUSIC

  Dr Laurence Bernstein, Chairman   *Number Of Faculty:* 13
  Number Of Students: 55   *Degrees Offered:* BMus, MMus, PhD Musicology
  Teaching Certification Available
  Financial Assistance: Internships, Assistantships, Scholarships and Work-Study Grants
  Performing Groups: University Symphony Choral Society, Collegium Musicum, Choir
  Workshops/Festivals: Summer Workshops (Medieval)

THEATRE

  Janice Silberman, Chairman   *Number Of Students:* 200
  Technical Training: Training for Performance
  Financial Assistance: Internships, Assistantships, Scholarships and Work-Study Grants
  Performing Groups: The Penn Players
  Workshops/Festivals: Directing Workshops, Acting Workshop

VILLANOVA UNIVERSITY

Villanova   Pennsylvania 19085, 215 527-2100

Private and 4 Year   *Arts Areas:* Theatre

THEATRE

James I Christy, Chairman   *Degrees Offered:* BA, MA
Financial Assistance: Scholarships and Work-Study Grants
Performing Groups: Theatre Group

WASHINGTON AND JEFFERSON COLLEGE

Lincoln St, Washington   Pennsylvania 15301
412 222-4400

Arts Areas: Instrumental Music, Vocal Music and Theatre

MUSIC

William M Hudgins, Associate Professor of Music, Chairman
Number Of Faculty: 3   *Degrees Offered:* BA
Financial Assistance: Scholarships and Work-Study Grants
Performing Groups: Wind Ensemble; Choir; Brass Choir; Saxophone Quartet
Workshops/Festivals: W & J Arts Festival

THEATRE

Robert L Brindley, Professor of Communications, Chairman
Number Of Faculty: 1   *Degrees Offered:* BA

WEST CHESTER STATE COLLEGE

West Chester   Pennsylvania 19380, 215 436-1000

State and 4 Year

Arts Areas: Dance, Instrumental Music, Vocal Music, Theatre, Film Arts, Television and Visual Arts
Performing Series: All Star Series; College Union Program Board Series
Performance Facilities: Philips Memorial Auditorium; New Main Auditorium; Swope Auditorium
Studio Theatre; Turks Head Playhouse

DANCE

Melvin M Lorback, Chairperson, Department of Physical Education
Dance Program is under the auspices of the School of Health, Physical Education and Recreation
Number Of Faculty: 3   *Number Of Students:* 5 Majors
Degrees Offered: BS in Health and Physical Education with Dance Concentration
Courses Offered: Technique; Choreography; History; Production
Teaching Certification Available
Financial Assistance: Assistantships, Scholarships and Work-Study Grants
Performing Groups: Theatre Dance Group
Workshops/Festivals: Dance Production Workshops I & II; Summer Dance Workshop

MUSIC

Charles A Sprenkle, Dean, School of Music   *Number Of Faculty:* 60
Number Of Students: 950
Degrees Offered: BS in Music Ed; BA in Music; BM in Performance; MM; MA in Music History
Courses Offered: Theory; Composition; Fine Arts; Music History; Music Education; Applied Music
Teaching Certification Available
Financial Assistance: Assistantships, Scholarships and Work-Study Grants
Performing Groups: Marching Band; Symphonic Band; Concert Band; College String Orchestra; Wind
Ensemble; Symphony Orchestra; Instrumental Ensembles; Chamber Music Groups; Criterion (Jazz Lab
Band); Concert Choir; Mixed Choir; Chamber Choir; Men's Chorus; Women's Chorus; Mixed Chorus;
Music Antiqua; Opera Chorus; Women's Glee Club
Workshops/Festivals: High School Music Workshop; Music Education Workshop; Marching Band and
Band Front Conference and Workshop; Piano Teachers Workshop; PMEA Music Education Workshop

(continued on next page)

THEATRE

Dr William M Morehouse, Chairman   **Number Of Faculty:** 12
Number Of Students: 75
Degrees Offered: BA in Speech Communication, Theatre Arts; BS in Education, Communication Concentration
Teaching Certification Available
Financial Assistance: Assistantships, Scholarships and Work-Study Grants
Performing Groups: Little Theatre; WCSC Musical Theatre Company
Workshops/Festivals: Summer Drama Festival; Summer Drama Workshop

WESTMINSTER COLLEGE
New Wilmington   Pennsylvania 16142, 412 946-6710
Private and 4 Year
Arts Areas: Instrumental Music, Vocal Music, Theatre, Television and Visual Arts
Performing Series: Celebrity Series, Chamber Music Series
Performance Facilities: Beeghly Theatre, Orr Auditorium

MUSIC

Dr Clarence Martin, Chairman   **Number Of Faculty:** 12
Number Of Students: 100   **Degrees Offered:** BMus, BA
Teaching Certification Available
Financial Assistance: Scholarships and Work-Study Grants
Performing Groups: Concert Choir, Orchestra, Symphonic Band, Vesper Choir
Workshops/Festivals: Pennsylvania Music Educators Workshop

THEATRE

Dr Walter E Scheid, Chairman   **Number Of Faculty:** 6
Number Of Students: 75   **Degrees Offered:** BA
Teaching Certification Available
Financial Assistance: Scholarships and Work-Study Grants
Performing Groups: Westminster College Players

WILKES COLLEGE
184 S River St, Wilkes Barre   Pennsylvania 18703
717 824-4651
Private and 4 Year
Arts Areas: Instrumental Music, Vocal Music and Visual Arts
Performing Series: Concert & Lecture Series

MUSIC

William R Gasbarro, Chairman   **Number Of Faculty:** 11
Number Of Students: 150   **Degrees Offered:** BA, BA MusEd
Technical Training: Opera, Independent Study
Teaching Certification Available
Financial Assistance: Scholarships and Work-Study Grants
Performing Groups: Orchestra, Instrumental Groups, Chorus

THEATRE

Alfred Groh, Chairman   **Number Of Faculty:** 4   **Number Of Students:** 56
Financial Assistance: Scholarships and Work-Study Grants
Performing Groups: Cue & Curtain

WILSON COLLEGE
Chambersburg   Pennsylvania 17201, 717 264-4141
Private and 4 Year
Arts Areas: Dance, Instrumental Music, Vocal Music and Visual Arts
Performing Series: Concerts & Lectures Series
Performance Facilities: Art Galleries & Art Studios; Thomson Hall; Lair Hall

(continued on next page)

DANCE

Ms Trina Collins, Artist-in-Residence   *Number Of Faculty:* 1
Degrees Offered: BA; BS   *Courses Offered:* Major in Fine Arts/Modern Dance
Financial Assistance: Work-Study Grants and Loans; Grants
Performing Groups: "Orchesis" - Modern Dance Club

MUSIC

Glen Gould, Professor   *Number Of Faculty:* 2   *Degrees Offered:* BA; BS
Courses Offered: Theory; History; Applied   *Teaching Certification Available*
Financial Assistance: Work-Study Grants and Loans; Grants
Performing Groups: Choir; Instrumental Ensemble
Artists-In-Residence/Guest Artists: Ze'eva Cohen Solo Dance Repertory; Concord String Quartet

---

YORK COLLEGE OF PENNSYLVANIA
Country Club Rd, York   Pennsylvania 17405
717 846-7788
Private and 4 Year
Arts Areas: Instrumental Music, Vocal Music, Theatre, Film Arts, Television and Visual Arts
Performing Series: Concert Series; Candlelight Concerts; Student Recitals
Performance Facilities: Theatre; Gymnasium

DANCE

Courses Offered: Ballet; Square; Classical
Financial Assistance: Scholarships and Work-Study Grants

MUSIC

Heinz Hosch, Chairman   *Number Of Faculty:* 8   *Number Of Students:* 120
Degrees Offered: BA; AA   *Teaching Certification Available*
Financial Assistance: Internships, Scholarships and Work-Study Grants
Performing Groups: Concert Band; Stage Band; Madrigal Singers; Concert Choir

THEATRE

Dr Richard Batteiger, Chairman   *Number Of Faculty:* 3
Number Of Students: 100   *Degrees Offered:* BA; AA
Teaching Certification Available
Financial Assistance: Internships, Scholarships and Work-Study Grants
Performing Groups: Masked Media Players; York Little Theatre
Artists-In-Residence/Guest Artists: Elly Stone; Concordia Choir; Maryland Dance Theatre

BARRINGTON COLLEGE
Middle Highway, Barrington   Rhode Island 02806
401 246-1200 Ext 146
   Private and 4 Year
   Arts Areas: Dance, Instrumental Music, Vocal Music, Theatre and Visual Arts
   Performing Series: General Student Recital Series; Faculty & Guest Recital Series; Blue & Gold Series
   Performance Facilities: Oliver Recital Hall; Easton Hall; Hubbard Hall.

MUSIC

William I Han, Director   *Number Of Faculty:* 5 Full-time, 22 Part-time
Number Of Students: 100
Degrees Offered: BA Music/Music Business; BMus Performance, Choral Music, Music Education;
Theory/Comprehension
Technical Training: Private Lessons & Performing Groups
Teaching Certification Available
Financial Assistance: Scholarships and Work-Study Grants
Performing Groups: Concert Band; College Symphony; Stage Band; Brass, Woodwind, String Ensembles;
College Choir; Oratorio; Madrigal; Small Vocal Ensembles
Workshops/Festivals: "Arts for the Handicapped"; Ethnomusicology Workshop; Early Music Seminar; "Lute
Society of America" Seminar; Choral School

THEATRE

Part of School of Music Program   *Number Of Faculty:* 2 Part-time
Number Of Students: 9 - 23   *Courses Offered:* Music Drama Workshop
Technical Training: Private Lessons; Coaching
Financial Assistance: Scholarships and Work-Study Grants
Performing Groups: Music Drama

BROWN UNIVERSITY
Providence   Rhode Island 02912, 401 863-1000
   Private and 4 Year
   Arts Areas: Dance, Instrumental Music, Vocal Music and Theatre
   Performing Series: Performing Arts Series
   Performance Facilities: Faunce House Theatre; Lyman Theatre; Faunce House Art Gallery Theatre;
Churchill House Theatre

DANCE

Julie Strandberg, Director
Dance program under auspices of Theatre Department
Number Of Faculty: 1   *Number Of Students:* 75
Courses Offered: Basic Dance; Intermediary Dance; Choreography
Performing Groups: Brown Modern Dance Group

MUSIC

Dr David Laurent, Chairman   *Number Of Faculty:* 12
Number Of Students: 1500   *Degrees Offered:* BA; MA; PhD Ethnic Musicology
Technical Training: Electronic Studies; Intergrated Undergraduate Degree
Teaching Certification Available
Financial Assistance: Internships, Assistantships, Scholarships and Work-Study Grants
Performing Groups: Wind Ensemble; Football Band; Concert Band; Brown University Symphony
Orchestra; Chorus; Concert Choir
Workshops/Festivals: Performance Practice Program

THEATRE

James O Barnhill, Director of Theatre; Dr Don B Wilmeth, Executive Officer
Theatre Program under auspices of English Department

(continued on next page)

Number Of Faculty: 8   **Number Of Students:** 450
Degrees Offered: BA Theatre Arts & Dramatic Literature
Technical Training: Acting; Scene Design; Directing; Dance; Technical Theatre
Performing Groups: Sock & Buskin; Brownbrokers; Rites & Reason; Production Workshop

PROVIDENCE COLLEGE
River Ave, Providence   Rhode Island 02918
401 865-1000
Private and 4 Year   **Arts Areas:** Theatre

MUSIC

Robert B Haller, Chairman

THEATRE

R L Peekington, Chairman   **Degrees Offered:** BA
Financial Assistance: Scholarships and Work-Study Grants
Performing Groups: Pyramid Players

RHODE ISLAND COLLEGE
600 Mt Pleasant Ave, Providence   Rhode Island 02908
401 831-6600
State and 4 Year
Arts Areas: Instrumental Music, Vocal Music, Theatre and Visual Arts
Performing Series: Fine Arts Series

MUSIC

Raymond Smith, Chairman   **Number Of Faculty:** 10   **Number Of Students:** 190
Degrees Offered: Ba; BA Mus Ed; MA Teaching   **Technical Training:** Opera
Teaching Certification Available
Financial Assistance: Assistantships, Scholarships and Work-Study Grants
Performing Groups: Choral Group; Orchestra; Chamber Music Ensemble; Instrumental Ensembles
Workshops/Festivals: Recitals

THEATRE

Edward A Scheff, Chairman   **Number Of Faculty:** 10   **Number Of Students:** 190
Degrees Offered: BA Speech and Theatre   **Teaching Certification Available**
Financial Assistance: Assistantships, Scholarships and Work-Study Grants
Performing Groups: Rhode Island College Theatre

UNIVERSITY OF RHODE ISLAND
Kingston   Rhode Island 02881, 401 792-1000
State and 4 Year
Arts Areas: Instrumental Music, Vocal Music, Theatre and Visual Arts
Performance Facilities: Edwards Auditorium; Fine Arts Center Will Theatre and Recital Hall; Keaney
Auditorium

MUSIC

Albert C Giebler, Chairman   **Number Of Faculty:** 12 Full-time, 10 Part-time
Number Of Students: 89   **Degrees Offered:** BA; BMus
Courses Offered: Classical Guitar; Voice; Piano or Organ; Orchestral Instruments; Musical History &
Literature; Music Theory & Composition; Music Ed
Teaching Certification Available
Financial Assistance: Assistantships, Scholarships and Work-Study Grants
Performing Groups: Symphony Orchestra; Marching Band; Concert Choir; Chorus; Chamber Music
Ensembles; Symphonic Wind Ensemble
Workshops/Festivals: Elementary School Music Workshop; Repair of String Instrument Workshop; Summer
Concert Series; URI Summer Festival of the Arts; Spring Interdisciplinary Arts Festival

(continued on next page)

THEATRE

James W Flannery, Chairman   **Number Of Faculty:** 7 Full-time, 2 Part-time
Number Of Students: 60   **Degrees Offered:** BA; BFA
Courses Offered: Acting; Design; Technical Studies; Theatre Studies
Technical Training: Make-up; Scenic Design; Costuming; Lighting
Financial Assistance: Assistantships, Scholarships and Work-Study Grants
Performing Groups: University Theatre; Summer Ensemble
Workshops/Festivals: Springs Arts Festival; URI Festival of the Arts (summer)
Artists-In-Residence/Guest Artists: Michael Grando - Mime; R I String Quartet

---

ROGER WILLIAMS COLLEGE
Bristol   Rhode Island 02809, 401 253-1000
Private and 4 Year   **Arts Areas:** Dance and Theatre
Performance Facilities: Student Center; Coffeehouse Theatre

DANCE

Ms Kelli Davis, Area Coordinator   **Number Of Faculty:** 1
Number Of Students: 39
Courses Offered: Intro to Dance Techniques; Elementary Modern Jazz Technique; Theatre Dance Styles I & II; Introduction to Choreography

MUSIC

Will Ayton, Area Coordinator   **Number Of Faculty:** 1
Number Of Students: 47
Courses Offered: Music in Baroque Era; Music in the Romantic Area; Instrumental and/or Voice Lessons; Fundamentals of Music I & II; History of Music I & II; Evolution of Jazz; Music in the Theatre

THEATRE

William Grandgeorge, Area Coordinator   **Number Of Faculty:** 2
Number Of Students: 47   **Degrees Offered:** BA
Courses Offered: Intro to Theatre; Intro to Acting; Creative Acting; Scene Design & Construction; Costume Construction Workshop; Lighting Design & Execution; Mime Workshop; Theatrical Make-up Workshop; Professional Theatre Direction; World Drama I & II; Theatre Practice; Stage Management; Fashion & Design; Costume Design & Construction; Modern Drama; Theatre of Shakespeare
Teaching Certification Available   **Performing Groups:** Coffeehouse Theatre
Artists-In-Residence/Guest Artists: M O V E, a professional company of dancers

---

SALVE REGINA COLLEGE
Ochre Point Ave, Newport   Rhode Island 02840
401 847-6650
Private and 4 Year   **Arts Areas:** Instrumental Music and Vocal Music
Number Of Faculty: 2   **Number Of Students:** 20   **Degrees Offered:** BA
Teaching Certification Available
Financial Assistance: Assistantships, Scholarships and Work-Study Grants
Performing Groups: Orchestra; Bands; Choir; Recitals; String Ensembles

ALLEN UNIVERSITY

1530 Harden St, Columbia South Carolina 29204
803 256-4287

Private and 4 Year
Arts Areas: Instrumental Music, Vocal Music, Theatre and Visual Arts
Degrees Offered: BA *Teaching Certification Available*
Financial Assistance: Scholarships and Work-Study Grants
Performing Groups: Vocal & Instrumental Ensembles
Degrees Offered: BA in Speech *Teaching Certification Available*
Financial Assistance: Scholarships and Work-Study Grants

ANDERSON COLLEGE

316 Boulevard, Anderson South Carolina 29621
803 226-6181 Ext 244

Private and 2 Year
Arts Areas: Instrumental Music, Vocal Music, Theatre and Visual Arts
Performing Series: Performing Arts Series
Performance Facilities: Auditorium; Recital Hall

MUSIC

Perry Carroll, Chairman, Fine Arts Division *Number Of Faculty:* 7
Number Of Students: 35 *Degrees Offered:* AFA
Financial Assistance: Scholarships and Work-Study Grants
Performing Groups: College Choir; Brass Ensemble; Stage Band; Interaction Singers; Bell Choir
Workshops/Festivals: Fine Arts Festival; Anderson Community Concert Association

THEATRE

Jack Bilbo, Chairman *Number Of Faculty:* 1 *Degrees Offered:* AA

BAPTIST COLLEGE AT CHARLESTON

Box 10087, Charleston South Carolina 29411
803 797-4011

Private and 4 Year *Performing Series:* 2,3,4,7
Performance Facilities: College Auditorium

MUSIC

Olive J Yost, Chairman *Degrees Offered:* BA
Teaching Certification Available *Financial Assistance:* Scholarships
Performing Groups: Instrumental & Vocal Ensembles

THEATRE

Degrees Offered: BA *Teaching Certification Available*
Financial Assistance: Scholarships *Performing Groups:* College Drama

BENEDICT COLLEGE

Columbia South Carolina 29204, 803 779-4930

Private and 4 Year
Arts Areas: Instrumental Music, Vocal Music and Visual Arts
Number Of Faculty: 6 *Number Of Students:* 102 *Degrees Offered:* BA
Financial Assistance: Scholarships
Performing Groups: Orchestra; Chorus; Band; Various Ensembles

THEATRE

William C West, Chairman *Number Of Faculty:* 3 *Number Of Students:* 51
No Degree Program Offered *Performing Groups:* Dramatic Dlub

BOB JONES UNIVERSITY
Wade Hampton Blvd, Greenville   South Carolina 29614
803 242-5100 Ext 238
Private and 4 Year
Arts Areas: Instrumental Music, Vocal Music, Theatre, Film Arts, Television and Visual Arts
Performing Series: University Concert, Opera, & Drama Series
Performance Facilities: Rodeheaver Auditorium; Founder's Memorial Amphitorium; Concert Center; War Memorial Chapel

MUSIC

Gail A Gingery, Chairman   *Number Of Faculty:* 42   *Number Of Students:* 300
Degrees Offered: BA; BS; MA
Courses Offered: Music Education; Sacred Music; Voice; Piano; Piano Pedagogy; Organ
Teaching Certification Available
Financial Assistance: Assistantships and Work - Loan Scholarships
Performing Groups: Choirs; Concert Chorale; Oratorio Chorus; Opera Chorus; Symphony Orchestra; Symphonic Band; Woodwind Choir; French Horn, Trumpet Ensembles; Trombone Choir
Workshops/Festivals: Annual Sacred Music Workshop; Annual Christian High School Music Festival & Contests

THEATRE

DeWitt Jones, Chairman, Division of Speech
Katherine Stenholm Chiarman, Division of Cinema
Number Of Faculty: 34   *Number Of Students:* 188   *Degrees Offered:* BA; BS
Courses Offered: Speech Education; Interpretative Speech; Public Speaking; Radio/TV; Cinema
Technical Training: Broadcast Engineering   *Teaching Certification Available*
Financial Assistance: Assistantships and Work - Loan Scholarships
Performing Groups: University Classic Players; Unusual Films (the production unit of our Division of Cinema)

CENTRAL WESLEYAN COLLEGE
Central   South Carolina 29630, 803 639-2453 Ext 38
Private and 4 Year   *Arts Areas:* Instrumental Music and Vocal Music
Performance Facilities: Folger Fine Arts Auditorium

MUSIC

Joel F Reed, Assistant Professor   *Number Of Faculty:* 4
Number Of Students: 30   *Degrees Offered:* BA MusEd; BA Church Music
Teaching Certification Available
Performing Groups: Concert Choir; Chamber Choir; Pep Band; Brass Ensemble

---

CLAFLIN COLLEGE
College Ave, Orangeburg   South Carolina 29115
803 534-2710
Private and 4 Year
Arts Areas: Instrumental Music, Vocal Music and Visual Arts
Number Of Faculty: 5   *Number Of Students:* 75   *Degrees Offered:* BA Mus Ed
Teaching Certification Available
Financial Assistance: Scholarships and Work-Study Grants
Performing Groups: Chorale; Band; Chorus

COASTAL CAROLINA COLLEGE OF THE UNIVERSITY OF SOUTH CAROLINA
Conway   South Carolina 29526, 803 347-3161
State and 4 Year
Arts Areas: Instrumental Music, Vocal Music, Theatre and Visual Arts
Performance Facilities: Lecture Hall; Theater

(continued on next page)

MUSIC

Carolyn Cox, Assistant Professor   **Number Of Faculty:** 3
Number Of Students: 20   **Degrees Offered:** BA or BS in Music Ed; BGS
Courses Offered: Theory; History; Piano; Guitar; Voice; Organ; Literature
Technical Training: Piano; Voice; Organ; Guitar
Teaching Certification Available
Financial Assistance: Assistantships, Scholarships and Work-Study Grants
Performing Groups: Coastal Carolina Concert Choir; Coastal Carolina Choral Ensemble
Workshops/Festivals: Christmas Concert; Spring Concert; Spring Tour

THEATRE

Michael Fortner, Director   **Number Of Faculty:** 2   **Number Of Students:** 10
Degrees Offered: BGS; BA in English with Dramatic Lit Emphasis
Courses Offered: Acting; Speech; Stagecraft; Graphics; Directing
Technical Training: Makeup; Theater Laboratory; Lighting
Financial Assistance: Assistantships, Scholarships and Work-Study Grants
Performing Groups: Upstage Company

COKER COLLEGE
Hartsville   South Carolina 29550, 803 332-1381
Private and 4 Year
Arts Areas: Dance, Instrumental Music, Vocal Music, Theatre, Film Arts and Visual Arts
Performance Facilities: Margaret Coker Lawton Music Building Recital Hall

DANCE

Nancy Zupp, Chairman   **Number Of Faculty:** 2   **Number Of Students:** 14
Degrees Offered: BA
Courses Offered: Modern Technique; Choreography; Pedagogy; Performing Company
Financial Assistance: Scholarships and Federal and State Grants, Loans, Campus Work

MUSIC

Kenneth L Wilmont, Chairman   **Number Of Faculty:** 4   **Number Of Students:** 35
Degrees Offered: BA in Music and Music Ed   **Teaching Certification Available**
Financial Assistance: Scholarships and Federal and State Grants, Loans, Campus Work

THEATRE

Robert Bloodworth, Chairman   **Number Of Faculty:** 1   **Number Of Students:** 10
Degrees Offered: BA in Drama
Financial Assistance: Scholarships and Federal and State Grants, Loans, Campus Work

---

COLUMBIA COLLEGE
Columbia   South Carolina 29203, 803 754-1100
Private and 4 Year
Arts Areas: Instrumental Music, Vocal Music, Theatre and Visual Arts

MUSIC

Dr James L Caldwell, Chairman   **Number Of Faculty:** 12
Number Of Students: 70   **Degrees Offered:** BA
Financial Assistance: Scholarships and Work-Study Grants

THEATRE

Degrees Offered: BA Drama-Speech   **Teaching Certification Available**
Financial Assistance: Scholarships and Work-Study Grants
Performing Groups: Columbia College Players

CONVERSE COLLEGE
E Main St, Spartanburg   South Carolina 29301
803 585-6421
   Private and 4 Year
   Arts Areas: Instrumental Music, Vocal Music and Visual Arts
   Performing Series: Concert Series

MUSIC

Henry Janiec, Chairman   *Number Of Faculty:* 21   *Number Of Students:* 150
Degrees Offered: BA; MA   *Teaching Certification Available*
Financial Assistance: Scholarships and Work-Study Grants
Performing Groups: Orchestra; Band; Chorus; Spartanburg Symphony Orchestra

THEATRE

Hayward Ellis, Chairman   *Number Of Faculty:* 4   *Number Of Students:* 44
Degrees Offered: BA   *Teaching Certification Available*
Financial Assistance: Scholarships and Work-Study Grants
Performing Groups: Palmetto Players

ERSKINE COLLEGE
Due West   South Carolina 29639, 803 379-2131
   Private and 4 Year
   Arts Areas: Instrumental Music, Vocal Music and Theatre
   Performing Series: Erskine Fine Arts Series; Convocation Series
   Performance Facilities: Memorial Hall; Lesesne Auditorium; Main Street Theatre

MUSIC

Don L Lester, Chairman   *Number Of Faculty:* 4   *Degrees Offered:* BA
Courses Offered: Theory; Materials & Methods; Conducting; Applied Music
Teaching Certification Available
Financial Assistance: Scholarships and Work-Study Grants
Performing Groups: Instrumental Ensemble; Choral

THEATRE

John Bruce Carlock, Jr, Director   *Number Of Faculty:* 1
Number Of Students: 20
Courses Offered: Modern Drama; Theatre Arts; Play Production; Theatre Workshops
Technical Training: Stagecraft; Costumes; Make-up; Set Construction; Acting
Financial Assistance: Scholarships and Work-Study Grants
Performing Groups: Erskine Players; Alpha Psi Omega

FURMAN UNIVERSITY
Greenville   South Carolina 29613, 803 294-2185
   Private and 4 Year
   Arts Areas: Dance, Instrumental Music, Vocal Music, Theatre and Visual Arts
   Performing Series: Furman - Greenville Fine Arts Series
   Performance Facilities: McAlister Auditorium; Playhouse Theatre; Daniel Recital Hall

DANCE

Brenda McCuthen, Instructor in Health & Physical Education
Number Of Faculty: 1   *Number Of Students:* 130
Degrees Offered: BA major in Health & Physical Education
Courses Offered: Modern; Folk; Square; Ethnic
Performing Groups: Furman Dance Theatre
Workshops/Festivals: National Endowment for the Arts - Dance Touring Program

(continued on next page)

MUSIC

Dr Milburn Price, Chairman   **Number Of Faculty:** 24
Number Of Students: 190   **Degrees Offered:** BMus
Courses Offered: Instrumental; Vocal; Church Music
Teaching Certification Available
Financial Assistance: Scholarships and Work-Study Grants

THEATRE

Dr James S Slaugher, Chairman   **Number Of Faculty:** 4   **Degrees Offered:** BA
Teaching Certification Available   **Financial Assistance:** Scholarships and Work-Study Grants

LANDER COLLEGE
Stanley Ave, Greenwood   South Carolina 29646
803 229-8213

State and 4 Year
Arts Areas: Dance, Instrumental Music, Vocal Music, Theatre and Visual Arts
Performing Series: Lander - Greenwood Fine Arts Series
Performance Facilities: Barksdale Physical Education Center; Lander College Auditorium

DANCE

Number Of Faculty: 1   **Number Of Students:** 15
Degrees Offered: BA Theatre & Dance   **Teaching Certification Available**
Financial Assistance: Scholarships and Work-Study Grants

MUSIC

Number Of Faculty: 8   **Number Of Students:** 100   **Degrees Offered:** BA MusEd
Teaching Certification Available
Financial Assistance: Scholarships and Work-Study Grants
Workshops/Festivals: Band clinics during summer

THEATRE

Number Of Faculty: 4   **Number Of Students:** 50   **Degrees Offered:** BA
Teaching Certification Available
Financial Assistance: Scholarships and Work-Study Grants
Workshops/Festivals: The Proposition Company Workshop
Artists-In-Residence/Guest Artists: Alan Schneider; Thomas Reichner

LIMESTONE COLLEGE
College Dr, Gaffney   South Carolina 29340
803 489-7151

Private and 4 Year
Arts Areas: Instrumental Music, Vocal Music, Theatre and Visual Arts
Performing Series: Limestone College/City of Gaffney Fine Arts Series
Performance Facilities: Fullerton Auditorium; Carroll Auditorium

MUSIC

William F Malambri, Division Chairman   **Number Of Faculty:** 9
Number Of Students: 75   **Degrees Offered:** BA in Mus Ed & Applied Music
Teaching Certification Available
Financial Assistance: Scholarships and Work-Study Grants
Performing Groups: College Chorus; College Wind Ensemble; College Jazz Ensemble
Workshops/Festivals: Summer Band Camps; Host to South Carolina Band Festival on a rotating basis

THEATRE

William F Malambri, Division Chairman   **Number Of Faculty:** 2
Number Of Students: 15   **Degrees Offered:** BA

(continued on next page)

Teaching Certification Available
Financial Assistance: Scholarships and Work-Study Grants
Performing Groups: Alpha Psi Omega

NEWBERRY COLLEGE
Newberry   South Carolina 29108, 803 276-5010
Private and 4 Year
Arts Areas: Instrumental Music, Vocal Music, Theatre and Visual Arts

MUSIC

Milton W Moore, Chairman   **Number Of Faculty:** 7   **Number Of Students:** 98
Degrees Offered: BA Mus Ed, Applied Music   **Teaching Certification Available**
Financial Assistance: Scholarships and Work-Study Grants
Performing Groups: Chorus; Instrumental Ensembles; Chorale Ensembles

THEATRE

D C Sanderson, Chairman   **Number Of Faculty:** 4   **Number Of Students:** 54
Degrees Offered: BA Drama-Speech   **Teaching Certification Available**
Financial Assistance: Scholarships and Work-Study Grants
Performing Groups: Newberry College

PRESBYTERIAN COLLEGE
S Broad St, Clinton   South Carolina 29325
803 833-2820
Private and 4 Year
Arts Areas: Instrumental Music, Vocal Music, Theatre and Visual Arts
Number Of Faculty: 3   **Number Of Students:** 42   **Degrees Offered:** BA
Teaching Certification Available   **Financial Assistance:** Work-Study Grants
Performing Groups: Instrumental Ensembles; Chorale; Orchestra

THEATRE

Dale O Rains, Chairman   **Number Of Faculty:** 2   **Number Of Students:** 28
Degrees Offered: BA   **Teaching Certification Available**
Financial Assistance: Scholarships
Performing Groups: Presbyterian College Players

SOUTH CAROLINA STATE COLLEGE
College Ave, Orangeburg   South Carolina 29117
803 536-7000
State and 4 Year
Arts Areas: Dance, Instrumental Music, Vocal Music, Theatre, Television and Visual Arts
Performance Facilities: Martin Luther King Jr Auditorium; Henderson - Davis Theatre
Smith - Hammond - Middleton Memorial Center
Financial Assistance: Scholarships
Performing Groups: S C State College Dancers - under auspices of the Department of Health & Physical
Education; The Henderson - Davis Players Dance Theatre is under the Dramatic Arts area

MUSIC

Dr E C Christian, Chairman   **Number Of Faculty:** 14
Number Of Students: 150   **Degrees Offered:** BA Mus Ed
Courses Offered: Vocal; Instrumental   **Teaching Certification Available**
Financial Assistance: Scholarships
Performing Groups: SC State College Marching 101 Band; Orchestra; Jazz Ensemble; Wind Ensemble;
Collegiate Chorale; Men's & Women's Choirs

THEATRE

Dr H D Flowers, II, Director   **Number Of Faculty:** 5
Number Of Students: 90   **Degrees Offered:** BA Drama

(continued on next page)

Teaching Certification Available   **Financial Assistance:** Scholarships
Performing Groups: The Henderson - Davis Players; The Henderson - Davis Players Children's Theatre; The S C Stage College Summer Theatre Company
Workshops/Festivals: The Invitational Interscholastic Speech & Drama Festival
Artists-In-Residence/Guest Artists: Rod Rogers Dance Co; Columbia, S C Philharmonic Orchestra; The National Players; National Theatre Co; Piedmont Chamber Orchestra; Abbey Lincoln

UNIVERSITY OF SOUTH CAROLINA
The Horsehoe, Columbia   South Carolina 29208
803 777-3101
State and 4 Year
Arts Areas: Dance, Instrumental Music, Vocal Music and Theatre
Performing Series: Performing Arts & Drama Series
Performance Facilities: Drayton Hall; Longstreet Theatre; Fraser Hall

MUSIC

Dr William J Moody, Chairman   **Number Of Faculty:** 32
Number Of Students: 275
Degrees Offered: BA Music, Music Ed; MA Music, Music Ed
Financial Assistance: Scholarships and Work-Study Grants
Performing Groups: Concert Choir; Various Chamber Groups; Opera Workshop

THEATRE

Patti P Gillespie, Chairman   **Number Of Faculty:** 9
Number Of Students: 210   **Degrees Offered:** BA; MA
Technical Training: Stagecraft
Financial Assistance: Scholarships and Work-Study Grants
Performing Groups: University Theatre; Dance '78
Workshops/Festivals: American College Theatre Festival

WINTHROP COLLEGE
Oakland Ave, Rock Hill   South Carolina 29733
803 323-2211
State and 4 Year
Arts Areas: Dance, Instrumental Music, Vocal Music, Theatre and Visual Arts
Performing Series: Cinema Series; Concert Series; Music Faculty Series; Fine Arts Association Series; Film Series
Performance Facilities: James F Byrnes Auditorium; Johnson Auditorium; Kinard Auditorium; Tillman Auditorium

DANCE

Joanne M Lund, Coordinator of Modern Dance   **Number Of Faculty:** 2
Number Of Students: 128
Courses Offered: Folk; Social; Square; Beginning, Intermediate & Advanced Modern Dance; Program Production; Theory of Dance; Dance Appreciation; Choreography I, II, III
Technical Training: Modern Dance; limited opportunity in Folk Dance
Teaching Certification Available   **Performing Groups:** Dance Theatre
Workshops/Festivals: Annual Fall Studio Workshop; Annual Community Christmas Program; Annual Spring Concert; Contributor - Annual Children's Art Festival (Rock Hill)

MUSIC

Jess T Casey, Dean   **Number Of Faculty:** 25   **Number Of Students:** 1,008
Degrees Offered: BM; BME; BA; MM; MME
Courses Offered: Introduction to the History of Music; Theory; Voice; Piano; Guitar; Jazz Ensemble; Concert Band; Opera Workshop; History of Music; Conduction Brass, Woodwind & String Instruments; Counterpoint; Contemporary Music; Appreciation of Jazz; Worship & Music; Styles of Music
Technical Training: Music Education - Choral & Instrumental; Performance (piano, voice, organ, winds & strings)
Teaching Certification Available

(continued on next page)

Financial Assistance: Assistantships, Scholarships and Work-Study Grants
Performing Groups: Winthrop Chorale; Winthrop Chorus; Winthrop Singers; Opera Workshop; Conducting Laboratory; Concert Band; Jazz Ensemble
Workshops/Festivals: All State Honors Chorus; Northern Regional Piano Festival; All County Band Festival

THEATRE

Earl J Wilcox, Chairman   ***Number Of Faculty:*** 3   ***Number Of Students:*** 124
Degrees Offered: BA in Speech/Drama (interdisciplinary program)
Courses Offered: Drama Appreciation; Acting I, II; Creative Drama; Play Directing; Technical Theatre; Directing II; History of Theatre; Art of the Film; Children's Theatre
Technical Training: Acting; Directing; Technical Theatre (scenery, lighting & sound, costuming, make-up); Children's Theatre
Financial Assistance: Assistantships and Work-Study Grants
Performing Groups: Winthrop Theatre
Workshops/Festivals: Palmetto Drama Festival

AUGUSTANA COLLEGE
29th & Summit, Sioux Falls   South Dakota 57102
605 336-5526
>Private and 4 Year
>*Arts Areas:* Dance, Instrumental Music, Vocal Music, Theatre, Television, Visual Arts and Radio
>*Performing Series:* Concert & Lecture Series
>*Performance Facilities:* Kresge Recital Hall; Chapel-Auditorium; Alumni Auditorium

DANCE

Mrs Clara Lee, Chairman, Department of Speech, Drama and Communication
Number Of Faculty: 2   *Number Of Students:* 17
Courses Offered: Classical and Contemporary Ballet
Technical Training: All aspects of ballet, ethnic and folk dance
Financial Assistance: Scholarships

MUSIC

Dr Walter May, Chairman   *Number Of Faculty:* 22   *Number Of Students:* 110
Degrees Offered: BA
Courses Offered: Music Education, Instrumental Techniques, Music Theory, Music History, Conducting, Applied Music
Technical Training: Conducting, Pedagogy and Performance, Class and Private Applied Music, Choral and Instrumental Ensembles
Teaching Certification Available
Financial Assistance: Scholarships and Work-Study Grants
Performing Groups: College Choir; Collegiate Chorale; Madrigal Singers; Concert Band; Varsity Band; College Orchestra; Brasswind Choir; Northlanders Jazz Ensemble; Brass Quintet
Workshops/Festivals: Concert Band Festival; Jazz on the Upper Great Plains Festival; Augustana Orchestra Festival

THEATRE

Mrs Clara Lee, Chairman, Department of Speech, Drama and Communication
Number Of Faculty: 3   *Number Of Students:* 45   *Degrees Offered:* BA
Courses Offered: Stagecraft; Acting; Scene Design; Costuming; Lighting; Play Production; History of Drama; Theater Practice
Teaching Certification Available   *Financial Assistance:* Scholarships
Performing Groups: Little Theatre Company; Viking Varieties Show Cast

---

BLACK HILLS STATE COLLEGE
1200 University Ave, Spearfish   South Dakota 57783
605 642-6011
>State and 4 Year
>*Arts Areas:* Instrumental Music, Vocal Music, Theatre and Visual Arts

MUSIC

Victor Weidensee, Chairman, Fine Arts Division   *Number Of Faculty:* 7
Number Of Students: 125   *Degrees Offered:* BA Ed; BS; BA
Teaching Certification Available
Financial Assistance: Scholarships and Work-Study Grants
Performing Groups: Jazz Ensemble; Wind Ensemble; Concert Choir; Blackhills Singers; Small Ensembles

THEATRE

Al Sandau, Director of Theatre   *Number Of Faculty:* 2
Number Of Students: 20   *Degrees Offered:* BS; BA; BS in Ed
Teaching Certification Available

DAKOTA STATE COLLEGE
Madison   South Dakota 57042, 605 256-3551 Ext 231
   State and 4 Year
   Arts Areas: Instrumental Music, Vocal Music, Theatre and Visual Arts
   Performance Facilities: Kennedy Hall

MUSIC

Dr Marles Preheim, Chairman   *Number Of Faculty:* 5   *Number Of Students:* 30
Degrees Offered: BS   *Teaching Certification Available*
Financial Assistance: Scholarships and Work-Study Grants

THEATRE

David Johnson, Chairman   *Number Of Faculty:* 4   *Number Of Students:* 25
Degrees Offered: BS   *Teaching Certification Available*
Financial Assistance: Scholarships and Work-Study Grants
Performing Groups: Annual Speech-Drama Symposium

DAKOTA WESLEYAN UNIVERSITY
Mitchell   South Dakota 57301, 605 996-6511
   Private and 4 Year
   Arts Areas: Instrumental Music, Vocal Music and Theatre
   Performance Facilities: University Auditorium; Art Center; City Auditorium (Corn Palace)

MUSIC

Paul N Scheuerle, Chairman   *Number Of Faculty:* 5   *Number Of Students:* 35
Degrees Offered: BA Music; BA Music Ed; BMusEd
Courses Offered: Theory; Music History; Music Education; Applied Music
Technical Training: Practicum   *Teaching Certification Available*
Financial Assistance: Scholarships and Work-Study Grants
Performing Groups: Concert Choir; Chamber Band; Pep Bands; Various Enembles; Highlanders; Prairie
Winds Woodwind Quintet; Brass Quintet
Workshops/Festivals: Band Reading Clinic of New Music; Marching Festival; Elementary Methods
Workshop

THEATRE

Mike Turchen, Chairman   *Number Of Faculty:* 2   *Number Of Students:* 30
Degrees Offered: BA Communication/Theatre
Courses Offered: Communications; Acting; Directing; Production
Technical Training: Practicum   *Teaching Certification Available*
Financial Assistance: Scholarships and Work-Study Grants
Performing Groups: University Players
Workshops/Festivals: Children's Theatre Workshop

HURON COLLEGE
Huron   South Dakota 57350, 605 352-8721
   Private and 4 Year
   Arts Areas: Instrumental Music, Vocal Music, Theatre and Visual Arts

MUSIC

Dr Michael Rudd, Chairman   *Number Of Faculty:* 4   *Number Of Students:* 35
Degrees Offered: BA   *Teaching Certification Available*
Financial Assistance: Scholarships   *Performing Groups:* Band; Choir
Number Of Faculty: 1   *Number Of Students:* 15   *Degrees Offered:* BA
Teaching Certification Available   *Financial Assistance:* Scholarships

MOUNT MARTY COLLEGE
1100 W 5th, Yankton   South Dakota 57078
605 668-1011

Private and 4 Year
Arts Areas: Instrumental Music, Vocal Music, Theatre and Visual Arts
Performance Facilities: Marian Auditorium; Rencalli Center; Gregg Hall

MUSIC

John A Lyons, Music Department Chairman   *Number Of Faculty:* 5
Number Of Students: 25   *Degrees Offered:* BA
Teaching Certification Available
Financial Assistance: Scholarships and Work-Study Grants
Performing Groups: Mixed Chorus; Band

THEATRE

Kaarin Johnston, Theatre Department Chairman   *Number Of Faculty:* 2
Number Of Students: 15   *Degrees Offered:* BA
Technical Training: Broadcasting; Film   *Teaching Certification Available*
Financial Assistance: Scholarships and Work-Study Grants

NORTHERN STATE COLLEGE
Jay and 12th St, Aberdeen   South Dakota 57401
605 622-3011

State and 4 Year
Arts Areas: Instrumental Music, Vocal Music, Theatre and Visual Arts
Performing Series: College - Civic Symphony; Stage One - Professional Summer Theater
Performance Facilities: Johnson Fine Arts Center

MUSIC

Lonn Sweet, Chairman Department of Music   *Number Of Faculty:* 8
Number Of Students: 125   *Degrees Offered:* BA; BS
Courses Offered: Teacher Training, Liberal Arts
Technical Training: Instrument Repair   *Teaching Certification Available*
Financial Assistance: Assistantships, Scholarships, Work-Study Grants and Grants
Performing Groups: Collegiate Choir; Women's Choir; Northern Singers; College - Civic Symphony;
Marching Band; Concert Band; Jazz Band; Many smaller Vocal and Instrumental Ensembles

THEATRE

Richard Norquist, Chairman Theater Department   *Number Of Faculty:* 2
Number Of Students: 50   *Degrees Offered:* BS; BA
Courses Offered: Teacher Training, Liberal Arts
Technical Training: Theater Technician   *Teaching Certification Available*
Financial Assistance: Assistantships, Scholarships, Work-Study Grants and Grants
Workshops/Festivals: Stage One - Professional Summer Theater

SIOUX FALLS COLLEGE
1501 S Prairie, Sioux Falls   South Dakota 57101
605 336-2850

Private and 4 Year
Arts Areas: Instrumental Music, Vocal Music, Theatre, Television and Visual Arts
Performance Facilities: Fine Arts Center: Auditorium; Intimate Theatres

MUSIC

Kerchal Armstrong, Professor of Music   *Number Of Faculty:* 5
Number Of Students: 60   *Degrees Offered:* BA
Teaching Certification Available
Financial Assistance: Scholarships and Work-Study Grants

(continued on next page)

Performing Groups: Madrigals; Concert Choir; Concert Band; Jazz Band; Various Ensembles
Workshops/Festivals: Madrigal Dinners Festival; Summer Workshops

THEATRE

Perry Patterson, Professor of Theatre   *Number Of Faculty:* 2
Number Of Students: 30   *Degrees Offered:* BA
Courses Offered: Theatre; Speech; Radio; Television
Technical Training: Radio; Television   *Teaching Certification Available*

THE UNIVERSITY OF SOUTH DAKOTA
Vermillion   South Dakota 57069, 605 677-5481
State and 4 Year
Arts Areas: Dance, Instrumental Music, Vocal Music, Theatre, Film Arts, Television and Visual Arts
Performing Series: American Theatre Association International Artists and Scholars Service
Performance Facilities: Slagle Auditorium; Warren M Lee Center for the Fine Arts - Theatre I, Recital Hall, Arena Theatre

MUSIC

Frank Aiello, Chairman   *Number Of Faculty:* 16   *Number Of Students:* 150
Degrees Offered: BFA Applied Music, MusEd; MM Applied Music, Mus Lit, MusEd, History of Musical Instruments
Courses Offered: Vocal; Instrumental; Music Theory
Teaching Certification Available
Financial Assistance: Assistantships, Scholarships, Work-Study Grants and BEOG Grants
Performing Groups: Symphonic Band; Marching Band; Wind Ensemble; Percussion Ensemble; Tuba Ensemble; Brass Choir; Stage Bands; Orchestra; Choir; Madrigal - Chamber Singers; Mens Chorus; Womens Chorus; Opera Workshop
Workshops/Festivals: Instrumental Clinic; Youth Festival; Stage Band Clinic; Piano Workshop; Choral Clinic

THEATRE

Dr Vincent L Angotti, Chairman/Producer
Number Of Faculty: 6 Full-time, 2 Part-time   *Number Of Students:* 70
Degrees Offered: BFA Theatre/Drama, Preprofessional Theatre Training, Theatre Education, Theatre/Voice
Courses Offered: Acting; Design (Costume, Lighting, Scenic); Directing; Dramatic Literature; Dramatic Theory/Criticism; Movement
Technical Training: Playwriting; Technical Theatre; Theatre History Dance
Teaching Certification Available
Financial Assistance: Internships, Assistantships, Scholarships and Work-Study Grants
Performing Groups: Theatre I; Arena; Traveling Theatre for Youth; American Theatre Student League; Missouri River Players
Workshops/Festivals: American College Theatre Festival; Brian Way Creative Dramatics ; Touring Theatre; Sioux City Community Theatre Classes; Summer High School Workshops

---

SOUTH DAKOTA STATE UNIVERSITY
Brookings   South Dakota 57007, 605 688-6619
State and 4 Year
Arts Areas: Dance, Instrumental Music, Vocal Music, Theatre, Film Arts, Television and Visual Arts
Performing Series: Harding Artist - Lecture Series; FO Butler Enrichment Series; Fine Arts Festival Series
Performance Facilities: South Dakota Memorial Art Center; Lincoln Center; Pugsley Center; Sylvan Theatre

DANCE

Marilyn Richardson, Coordinator   *Number Of Faculty:* 3
Number Of Students: 36   *Degrees Offered:* BA; BS
Teaching Certification Available
Financial Assistance: Internships, Scholarships and Work-Study Grants

(continued on next page)

Performing Groups: Modern Dance Club
Workshops/Festivals: Dance Workshops; Annual Dance Production

MUSIC

Dr Warren Hatfield, Chairman   **Number Of Faculty:** 13
Number Of Students: 125   **Degrees Offered:** BA; BS; BME
Courses Offered: Applied; Ensemble; General; Theory; Literature; Music Education; Pedagogy
Technical Training: Synthesizer   **Teaching Certification Available**
Financial Assistance: Internships, Assistantships, Scholarships and Work-Study Grants
Performing Groups: Symphony Orchestra; Marching and Symphonic Bands; Pep Band; Chamber Singers;
Concert Choir; Statesmen; Oratorio Chorus; Jazz Bands
Workshops/Festivals: Summer Music Camps; Improvisation Workshop; Piano Teachers' Workshop; Vocal
Workshop Musical Production Workshop; Band Directors' Workshop; Marching Band Workshop

THEATRE

Dr James Johnson, Director   **Number Of Faculty:** 4   **Number Of Students:** 28
Degrees Offered: BA; MA
Technical Training: Stagecraft; Scene Design; Lighting
Teaching Certification Available
Financial Assistance: Internships, Assistantships, Scholarships and Work-Study Grants
Performing Groups: Summer Repertory Theatre; Children's Theatre; Readers' Theatre
Workshops/Festivals: High School Drama Workshop; Cottontail Capers (Variety Show)

UNIVERSITY OF SOUTH DAKOTA AT SPRINGFIELD
Springfield   South Dakota 57062, 605 369-2265
State and 4 Year
Arts Areas: Instrumental Music, Vocal Music, Theatre and Visual Arts
Performance Facilities: Auditorium, Main Hall; Music Center

MUSIC

Warren Erickson, Associate Professor
Degrees Offered: AA Music Merchandising, Music
Courses Offered: Instrumental and Vocal Ensembles; Instrumental Lessons; Band; Choir; Harmony; Lit;
Brass; Woodwind; Percussion
Technical Training: Instrument Repair and Sales
Financial Assistance: Scholarships and Work-Study Grants
Performing Groups: Choral and Instrumental Ensembles

THEATRE

Virgil Petrik, Director of Humanities Division
Courses Offered: Drama Activity; Acting; Beginning Directing
Financial Assistance: Scholarships and Work-Study Grants
Performing Groups: Student/Community Theatre Group

SOUTHERN STATE COLLEGE
Springfield   South Dakota 57062, 605 369-2201
State and 4 Year
Arts Areas: Instrumental Music, Vocal Music, Theatre and Visual Arts

MUSIC

Degrees Offered: BA Mus; BA MusEd   **Teaching Certification Available**
Financial Assistance: Scholarships and Work-Study Grants

THEATRE

Virgil D Petrick, Chairman   **Degrees Offered:** BA Speech
Teaching Certification Available
Financial Assistance: Scholarships and Work-Study Grants
Performing Groups: College Theatre

YANKTON COLLEGE
12th & Douglas Ave, Yankton   South Dakota 57078
605 665-3661
   Private and 4 Year
   Arts Areas: Instrumental Music, Vocal Music, Theatre and Visual Arts

MUSIC

Dr J Laiten Weed, Director   *Number Of Faculty:* 7   *Number Of Students:* 56
Degrees Offered: BA Applied Music; BMusEd; B Sacred Music
Teaching Certification Available   Financial Assistance: Scholarships
Performing Groups: Yankton College Conservatory Orchestra

THEATRE

Ambrose P Schenk, Chairman   *Number Of Faculty:* 3   *Number Of Students:* 37
Degrees Offered: BA   *Teaching Certification Available*
Financial Assistance: Scholarships   *Performing Groups:* College Theatre

AUSTIN PEAY STATE UNIVERSITY
Clarksville   Tennessee 37040, 615 648-7676

State and 4 Year
Arts Areas: Instrumental Music, Vocal Music, Theatre and Visual Arts
Performance Facilities: Margaret Fort Trahern Art-Drama Bldg

MUSIC

Thomas W Cowan, Chairman   *Number Of Faculty:* 15   *Number Of Students:* 103
Degrees Offered: BA; BS; MMusEd   *Teaching Certification Available*
Financial Assistance: Assistantships and Scholarships
Performing Groups: Symphony; Choir; Dance Bands; Marching Band

THEATRE

Joe Flippo, Chairman   *Number Of Faculty:* 5   *Number Of Students:* 54
Degrees Offered: BA; BS   *Teaching Certification Available*
Financial Assistance: Scholarships   *Performing Groups:* Clarksville Drama

---

BELMONT COLLEGE
1900 Belmont Blvd, Nashville   Tennessee 37203
615 383-7001

Private and 4 Year
Arts Areas: Instrumental Music, Vocal Music and Theatre
Performing Series: Friends of Chamber Music Series
Performance Facilities: Massey Auditorium; Harton Concert Hall

MUSIC

Number Of Faculty: 22   *Number Of Students:* 100   *Degrees Offered:* BA; BMus
Technical Training: Church Music; Music Education; Music Therapy; Music Business
Teaching Certification Available
Financial Assistance: Scholarships and Work-Study Grants
Performing Groups: Oratorio Chorus; Chorale; Chapel Choir; Band; Instrumental & Vocal Chamber Groups

THEATRE

Dr Jerry L Warren, Chairman   *Number Of Faculty:* 3   *Number Of Students:* 25
Degrees Offered: BA   *Teaching Certification Available*
Financial Assistance: Scholarships and Work-Study Grants

BETHEL COLLEGE
Cherry St, McKenzie   Tennessee 38201
901 352-5321

Private and 4 Year
Arts Areas: Instrumental Music, Vocal Music, Theatre and Visual Arts

MUSIC

Frank Doole, Chairman   *Number Of Faculty:* 3   *Number Of Students:* 32
Degrees Offered: BA MusEd   *Teaching Certification Available*
Financial Assistance: Scholarships and Work-Study Grants
Performing Groups: Ensembles; Group Singing; Orchestra

THEATRE

Paul B Brown, Chairman   *Number Of Faculty:* 1   *Number Of Students:* 15
Degrees Offered: BA Speech   *Teaching Certification Available*
Financial Assistance: Scholarships and Work-Study Grants
Performing Groups: Gold Masquers

BRYON COLLEGE
Dayton   Tennessee 37321, 615 775-2041
 Private and 4 Year   *Arts Areas:* Instrumental Music and Vocal Music
 Performing Series: Concert Series

MUSIC

J James Greasby, Chairman
 Degrees Offered: BA Applied Music; BA MusEd; BA Music Theory
 Teaching Certification Available   *Financial Assistance:* Scholarships
 Performing Groups: Band; Choir

CARSON - NEWMAN COLLEGE
Russell St, Jefferson City   Tennessee 37760
615 475-9061 Ext 265
 Private and 4 Year
 Arts Areas: Instrumental Music, Vocal Music, Theatre and Visual Arts
 Performing Series: Carson - Newman Concert - Lecture Series
 Performance Facilities: Gentry Auditorium; Phoenix II Workshop Theatre

MUSIC

Louis Ball, Coordinator Music Department   *Number Of Faculty:* 12
 Number Of Students: 120   *Degrees Offered:* BMus
 Courses Offered: Music Education; Church; Applied Music
 Teaching Certification Available
 Financial Assistance: Scholarships and Work-Study Grants
 Performing Groups: A Cappella Choir; Concert Band; Male Chorus; Womens Chorus; Madrigals Lyric
Theatre; Brass & Woodwind Ensembles; Vocal - Jazz Ensemble
 Workshops/Festivals: Church Music Workshop - Annually

THEATRE

John Welton, Drama Coach   *Number Of Faculty:* 3   *Number Of Students:* 20
 Degrees Offered: BA   *Courses Offered:* Speech - Drama Major
 Teaching Certification Available
 Financial Assistance: Scholarships and Work-Study Grants

CHRISTIAN BROTHERS COLLEGE
650 E Parkway S, Memphis   Tennessee 38104
901 278-0100
 Private and 4 Year
 Arts Areas: Vocal Music, Theatre, Film Arts and Visual Arts
 Performance Facilities: College Auditorium

MUSIC

Brother Vincent Malham, Music Director   *Number Of Faculty:* 2
 Number Of Students: 30
 Courses Offered: Introduction to Music I; Music, Concert Chorus; CBC Singers; Studies in Music
Literature; Studies in American Music; Special Studies in Music
 Financial Assistance: Scholarships and Work-Study Grants
 Performing Groups: Concert Chorus; CB Singers; Community
 Workshops/Festivals: Fall Music Festival; Christmas Concert; Music Revue

THEATRE

Brother Thomas Schumacher, Director   *Number Of Faculty:* 5
 Number Of Students: 35 - 50
 Courses Offered: Introduction to the Theatre; Acting; Play Production; Play Production Workshop; History
of the Theatre; Theatre Practicum

(continued on next page)

Financial Assistance: Scholarships and Work-Study Grants
Performing Groups: Theatre Guild
Artists-In-Residence/Guest Artists: Brother Vincent Malham and Brother Laurence Walther "Brothers in Concert"

CLEVELAND STATE COMMUNITY COLLEGE
Norman Chapel Rd, Cleveland   Tennessee 37311
615 472-7141 Ext 294
State and 2 Year   **Arts Areas:** Instrumental Music and Vocal Music

MUSIC

Tom Boles, Chairman   **Number Of Faculty:** 1 Full-time, 3 Part-time
Number Of Students: 50   **Degrees Offered:** AA; AS
Courses Offered: Music Theory; Music Appreciation; Music Literature; Public School Music; Chorus; Chamber Choir; Instrumental Ensemble; Stage Band; Brass Class; Instrumental; Voice; Piano; Organ
Financial Assistance: Scholarships and Work-Study Grants
Workshops/Festivals: Woodwind Class; String Class; Music Theatre Workshop

COLUMBIA STATE COMMUNITY COLLEGE
Columbia   Tennessee 38401, 615 388-0120 Ext 242
2 Year   **Arts Areas:** Instrumental Music, Vocal Music, Theatre and Film Arts
Performance Facilities: Auditorium; Gymnasium; Cafeteria

MUSIC

Number Of Faculty: 2   **Number Of Students:** 30 - 50   **Degrees Offered:** AS
Financial Assistance: Scholarships and Work-Study Grants
Performing Groups: College Chorus   **Workshops/Festivals:** Spring Arts Festival

THEATRE

Number Of Faculty: 1   **Number Of Students:** 30   **Degrees Offered:** AS
Financial Assistance: Scholarships and Work-Study Grants
Performing Groups: Disturbing the Peace Players
Workshops/Festivals: Spring Arts Festival

CUMBERLAND COLLEGE
Lebanon   Tennessee 37087, 615 444-2562
Private and 2 Year
Arts Areas: Instrumental Music, Vocal Music and Visual Arts
Performance Facilities: Auditorium

MUSIC

Bert Coble, Director of Music & Chairman of the Music Department
Number Of Faculty: 8   **Degrees Offered:** A Music
Financial Assistance: Scholarships and Work-Study Grants
Performing Groups: College Singers; Band; Show Choir; Handbell Choir; Community Choir
Workshops/Festivals: Dinner At Cumberland; High School Concerts

DAVID LIPSCOMB COLLEGE
Granny White Pike, Nashville   Tennessee 37203
615 269-5661
Private and 4 Year
Arts Areas: Instrumental Music, Vocal Music, Theatre and Visual Arts

MUSIC

Frances H Hill, Chairman   **Number Of Faculty:** 6   **Number Of Students:** 47
Degrees Offered: BA Mus, MusEd, Applied Music   **Teaching Certification Available**
Financial Assistance: Scholarships and Work-Study Grants
Performing Groups: Concerts; Instrumental Ensembles; Band; Recitals

(continued on next page)

THEATRE

Jerry Henderson, Chairman   **Number Of Faculty:** 5   **Number Of Students:** 89
Degrees Offered: BA Speech   **Teaching Certification Available**
Financial Assistance: Scholarships and Work-Study Grants
Performing Groups: Footlighters

DYERSBURG STATE COMMUNITY COLLEGE
1516 Nichols Ave, Dyersburg   Tennessee 38024
901 285-6910
State and 2 Year
Arts Areas: Instrumental Music, Vocal Music and Theatre
Degrees Offered: AA

EAST TENNESSEE STATE UNIVERSITY
ETSU Station, Johnson City   Tennessee 37601
615 929-4317
State and 4 Year
Arts Areas: Dance, Instrumental Music, Vocal Music, Theatre, Film Arts, Television and Visual Arts
Performing Series: Performing Arts Series
Performance Facilities: D P Culp University Center Auditorium; Gilbreath Theatre; University Musical Hall

DANCE

Dr Sid Rice, Chairman of Physical Education Department
Number Of Faculty: 3   **Number Of Students:** 400
Courses Offered: Contemporary Dance; Folk Dance; Dance Techniques; Square Dancing and Social Dancing
Technical Training: Teaching of Folk Dancing
Teaching Certification Available
Financial Assistance: Scholarships and Work-Study Grants
Performing Groups: Senior Orchesis; Junior Orchesis
Workshops/Festivals: Folk Dance Workshops

MUSIC

Dr James E Stafford, Chairman   **Number Of Faculty:** 16
Number Of Students: 160   **Degrees Offered:** BA Mus; BA MusEd; BS MusEd
Courses Offered: Instrumental and Vocal Music
Technical Training: Conducting; Concert Performance in Voice and Instruments
Teaching Certification Available
Financial Assistance: Scholarships and Work-Study Grants
Performing Groups: Opera Theatre; Marching Band; Symphonic Band; Jazz Band; Brass Choir; University Choir; Woodwind Choir

THEATRE

Dr Paul A Walwick, Chairman   **Number Of Faculty:** 3   **Number Of Students:** 75
Degrees Offered: BA Speech; MA Speech; BS Speech
Courses Offered: Principles of Acting; Creative Dramatics; Stagecraft; History of Theatre; Dramatic Literature; Make-up; Stage Lighting; Theatre Laboratory; Costuming
Technical Training: Lighting; Design; Costuming; Sound; Make-up; Properties
Teaching Certification Available
Financial Assistance: Scholarships and Work-Study Grants
Performing Groups: University Theatre; Reader's Theatre; Children's Theatre
Workshops/Festivals: High School Drama Workshop; Speech and Theatre Festival; Dramatic Tournament

FISK UNIVERSITY
17th Ave N, Nashville   Tennessee 37203
615 329-9111 Ext 226

Private and 4 Year
Arts Areas: Dance, Instrumental Music, Vocal Music, Theatre, Film Arts and Visual Arts
Performing Series: University Concert Series
Performance Facilities: Fisk University Little Theatre

DANCE

Number Of Faculty: 1   *Number Of Students:* 50   *Financial Assistance:* Work-Study Grants

MUSIC

Oscar M Henry, Chairman   *Number Of Faculty:* 9   *Number Of Students:* 100
Degrees Offered: BA; BA; BM (in Applied Music); MA
Teaching Certification Available
Financial Assistance: Scholarships and Work-Study Grants
Performing Groups: University Choir; Jubilee Singers; Orchestrated Crowd; Woodwind Ensemble; Black Mass Choir

THEATRE

Gladys I Forde, Chairman   *Number Of Faculty:* 6   *Number Of Students:* 45
Degrees Offered: BA   *Teaching Certification Available*
Financial Assistance: Work-Study Grants
Performing Groups: Fisk University Stagecrafters

FREE WILL BAPTIST COLLEGE
3606 W End Ave, Nashville   Tennessee 37205
615 297-4676

Private and 4 Year   *Arts Areas:* Vocal Music and Theatre
Degrees Offered: BA in Music
Performing Groups: Choir; Instrumental & Vocal Concerts

FREED-HARDEMAN COLLEGE
158 E Main St, Henderson   Tennessee 38340
901 989-4611

Private and 2 Year   *Performing Series:* 2,3,4,7

MUSIC

Kelley B Doyle, Chairman   *Degrees Offered:* AA   *Financial Assistance:* Scholarships

Degrees Offered: AA Speech   *Financial Assistance:* Scholarships   *Performing Groups:* Thespians

GEORGE PEABODY COLLEGE FOR TEACHERS
21st Ave S, Nashville   Tennessee 37203
615 327-8121

Private, 4 Year and Graduate
Arts Areas: Dance, Instrumental Music, Vocal Music, Theatre, Film Arts and Visual Arts
Performance Facilities: Hill Auditorium; Human Development Laboratory Auditorium

DANCE

Dr Ida Long Rogers, Director, Programs for Educational Support Personnel
Number Of Faculty: 1   *Number Of Students:* 10   *Degrees Offered:* BS
Teaching Certification Available
Financial Assistance: Internships, Assistantships, Scholarships and Work-Study Grants
Performing Groups: Modern Dance Group

(continued on next page)

MUSIC

Dr Larry Peterson, Director, School of Music   *Number Of Faculty:* 19
Number Of Students: 200   *Degrees Offered:* BS; BME; MS; MME; EdS; EdD; PhD
Technical Training: Commercial Music   *Teaching Certification Available*
Financial Assistance: Internships, Assistantships, Scholarships and Work-Study Grants
Performing Groups: Choir, Vanderbilt - Peabody Marching Band; Collegium Musicum; Madrigalians;
Vanderbilt - Peabody Jazz Ensemble; Peabody Orchestra

JACKSON STATE COMMUNITY COLLEGE
PO Box 2467, Jackson   Tennessee 38301
901 424-3520
 State and 2 Year
 Arts Areas: Instrumental Music, Vocal Music, Theatre and Television
 Performance Facilities: Gymatorium; Student Center; Music Room; Science Auditorium; TV Studio

MUSIC

Donnie J Adams, Associate Professor   *Number Of Faculty:* 3
Number Of Students: 27   *Degrees Offered:* AA
Courses Offered: Vocal; Keyboard; Instrumental
Financial Assistance: Scholarships
Performing Groups: College Chorus; College Band; Stage Band

THEATRE

Dr C D Culver, Chairperson, Division of Humanities   *Number Of Faculty:* 1
Number Of Students: 12   *Degrees Offered:* AA; AS
Courses Offered: Introduction to Theatre; Acting; Play Production

---

JOHNSON BIBLE COLLEGE
Kimberlin Heights Station, Knoxville   Tennessee 37920
615 573-4517
 Private   *Arts Areas:* Instrumental Music and Vocal Music
 Performance Facilities: Chapel; Auditorium

MUSIC

Michael Dunn, Chairman   *Number Of Faculty:* 5   *Number Of Students:* 20
Degrees Offered: B Church Music   *Courses Offered:* History; Theory; Applied
Financial Assistance: Internships, Scholarships and Work-Study Grants

---

KNOXVILLE COLLEGE
901 College St, Knoxville   Tennessee 37921
615 546-0751
 Private and 4 Year
 Arts Areas: Instrumental Music, Vocal Music and Theatre
 Performing Series: Lyceum Series

MUSIC

Walter Harris, Chairman   *Number Of Faculty:* 7   *Number Of Students:* 68
Degrees Offered: BA; BS MusEd   *Teaching Certification Available*
Financial Assistance: Scholarships and Work-Study Grants
Performing Groups: Band   *Degrees Offered:* BA Speech
Teaching Certification Available
Financial Assistance: Scholarships and Work-Study Grants
Performing Groups: Garnet Masque

LAMBUTH COLLEGE
Jackson   Tennessee 38301, 901 427-6743
> Private and 4 Year   *Arts Areas:* Dance and Theatre
> *Performance Facilities:* Lambuth Theatre

DANCE

Jesse B Byrum, Chairman   *Number Of Faculty:* 1   *Number Of Students:* 20
Degrees Offered: BA   *Teaching Certification Available*
Financial Assistance: Scholarships and Work-Study Grants
Workshops/Festivals: High School Fine Arts Tournament

LANE COLLEGE
545 Lane Ave, Jackson   Tennessee 38301
901 424-4600
> Private and 4 Year   *Arts Areas:* Instrumental Music and Vocal Music

MUSIC

Kenneth C Sampson, Chairman   *Number Of Faculty:* 2   *Number Of Students:* 33
Degrees Offered: BA
Financial Assistance: Scholarships and Work-Study Grants
Performing Groups: Marching Band

LEE COLLEGE
Ocoee St, Cleveland   Tennessee 37311
615 472-2111 Ext 212
> Private and 4 Year
> *Arts Areas:* Instrumental Music, Vocal Music and Visual Arts
> *Performance Facilities:* 2 Auditoriums; Hall

MUSIC

Jim Burns, Chairman Department of Music & Fine Arts   *Number Of Faculty:* 8
Number Of Students: 115   *Degrees Offered:* BA Mus; BM Ed
Technical Training: Church Music; Music Ed   *Teaching Certification Available*
Financial Assistance: Scholarships and Work-Study Grants
Performing Groups: Lee Singers; Ladies at Lee; Campus Choir; Concert Band

LEMOYNE - OWEN COLLEGE
807 Walker Ave, Memphis   Tennessee 38126
901 948-6626 Ext 31
> Private and 4 Year
> *Arts Areas:* Instrumental Music, Vocal Music, Theatre and Visual Arts
> *Performing Series:* Affilate Artists, Inc. of New York

MUSIC

Mildred D Green, Chairman   *Number Of Faculty:* 2
Performing Groups: College Choir; Instrumental Ensemble
Workshops/Festivals: The Affiliate Artist Program; Musical Festival for Spring

THEATRE

I D Thompson, Chairman   *Number Of Faculty:* 1   *Number Of Students:* 75
Performing Groups: LeMoyne-Owen Players
Workshops/Festivals: Spring Arts Festival; National Assn of Dramatics & Speech Arts

LINCOLN MEMORIAL UNIVERSITY
Harrogate   Tennessee 37752, 615 869-3622
  Private and 4 Year
  Arts Areas: Instrumental Music, Vocal Music, Theatre and Visual Arts

MUSIC

Robert Brown, Chairman   *Number Of Faculty:* 2   *Number Of Students:* 30
Degrees Offered: BA   *Teaching Certification Available*
Financial Assistance: Scholarships and Work-Study Grants
Performing Groups: Choir; Band; Ensembles

THEATRE

Donald Loughrie, Chairman   *Number Of Faculty:* 2   *Number Of Students:* 34
Degrees Offered: BA   *Teaching Certification Available*
Financial Assistance: Scholarships and Work-Study Grants   *Performing Groups:* Drama Club

MARTIN COLLEGE
Pulaski   Tennessee 38478, 615 363-1567
  Private and 2 Year
  Arts Areas: Instrumental Music, Vocal Music and Visual Arts
  Degrees Offered: AA   *Financial Assistance:* Scholarships

MARYVILLE COLLEGE
Maryville   Tennessee 37801, 615 982-6412
  Private and 4 Year
  Arts Areas: Instrumental Music, Vocal Music, Theatre and Visual Arts
  Performing Series: Performing Artists Concerts

MUSIC

Dr Harry H Hartec, Chairman   *Number Of Students:* 62   *Degrees Offered:* BA
Teaching Certification Available
Financial Assistance: Scholarships and Work-Study Grants
Performing Groups: Band; Chorus   *Number Of Faculty:* 2
Number Of Students: 29   *Degrees Offered:* BA
Teaching Certification Available
Financial Assistance: Scholarships and Work-Study Grants
Performing Groups: Maryville College Players

MEMPHIS STATE UNIVERSITY
Memphis   Tennessee 38152, 901 454-2081
  State and 4 Year
  Arts Areas: Dance, Instrumental Music, Vocal Music, Theatre, Film Arts, Television and Visual Arts
  Performance Facilities: Harris Music Auditorium; Speech and Drama Theatre

DANCE

Number Of Faculty: 5   *Number Of Students:* 400   *Degrees Offered:* BS Ed
Courses Offered: Modern Dance; Folk & Social Dance; Rhythms
Technical Training: Materials & Methods in Dance
Teaching Certification Available
Performing Groups: Orchesis Modern Dance Club; Folk Dance Company

MUSIC

Dr William Gaver, Chairman   *Number Of Faculty:* 33
Number Of Students: 210   *Degrees Offered:* DMA; BA; BMus
Courses Offered: Music Theory and Composition; Music History, Literature, and Appreciation; Sacred Music; Applied Music
Teaching Certification Available

(continued on next page)

Financial Assistance: Internships, Assistantships, Scholarships and Work-Study Grants
Performing Groups: Band; Orchestra; Choral; Faculty and Student Ensembles; Jazz Band; Memphis State University Opera Theatre
Workshops/Festivals: New Music; Baroque Music; Band Festival; Jazz Festival; High School Days

THEATRE

Dr John Sloan, Chairman   **Number Of Faculty:** 12   **Number Of Students:** 240
Degrees Offered: BA; BFA; MA; MFA
Courses Offered: Theatre; Radio; Television; Film
Technical Training: Available through Instructional Television Center and the Division of Engineering Technology
Teaching Certification Available
Financial Assistance: Internships, Assistantships, Scholarships and Work-Study Grants
Performing Groups: "Evening of Soul" Company; "Moving Line" Touring Company; WTGR
Workshops/Festivals: Red Balloon Players; High School Festivals; "Lunchbox Theatre"

MIDDLE TENNESSEE STATE UNIVERSITY
Murfreesboro   Tennessee 37130, 615 898-2300
State and 4 Year
Arts Areas: Instrumental Music, Vocal Music, Theatre and Visual Arts

MUSIC

Neil H Wright, Chairman   **Number Of Faculty:** 17   **Number Of Students:** 131
Degrees Offered: B Mus; MA; MA Teaching   **Teaching Certification Available**
Financial Assistance: Work-Study Grants
Performing Groups: Woodwind Ensemble; Brass Ensemble; Jazz Ensemble; Concert Choir; Marching Band; Concert Band; Orchestra; Madrigal Singers; Choral Union
Workshops/Festivals: Summer Instrumental Classes

THEATRE

Dr Larry V Lowe, Professor   **Number Of Faculty:** 4   **Number Of Students:** 50
Degrees Offered: BA; BS   **Teaching Certification Available**
Financial Assistance: Work-Study Grants
Performing Groups: University Theatre Players; The Variety Touring Show
Workshops/Festivals: Tennessee Speech and Drama League

MILLIGAN COLLEGE
Milligan College   Tennessee 37682, 615 929-0116
Private and 4 Year
Arts Areas: Instrumental Music, Vocal Music and Theatre
Performing Series: Milligan College Concert Series
Performance Facilities: Seeger Memorial Chapel; Small Auditorium - Derthick Hall

MUSIC

John Andrew Dowd, Music Department Chairman   **Number Of Faculty:** 6
Number Of Students: 54   **Degrees Offered:** BS
Courses Offered: Theory; Music Literature and History; Music Education; Conducting; Applied Music
Teaching Certification Available
Financial Assistance: Scholarships and Work-Study Grants
Performing Groups: Concert Choir; Chorale; Band
Workshops/Festivals: Annual Madrigal Dinner; Christmas Festival

THEATRE

Dr Ira Read, Chairman   **Number Of Faculty:** 1   **Number Of Students:** 60
Courses Offered: Speech Communication; Theatre Arts
Teaching Certification Available
Financial Assistance: Scholarships and Work-Study Grants

MOTLOW STATE COMMUNITY COLLEGE
Box 860, Tullahoma   Tennessee 37388
615 455-8511
   State and 2 Year   *Arts Areas:* Instrumental Music and Vocal Music
   Degrees Offered: AA   *Financial Assistance:* Scholarships

SCARRITT COLLEGE FOR CHRISTIAN WORKERS
19th and Grand Ave, Nashville   Tennessee 37203
615 327-2700
   Private and 4 Year
   Arts Areas: Instrumental Music, Vocal Music and Theatre
   Performance Facilities: Fondren Theater; Wightman Chapel

MUSIC

Dr Carlton Young, Professor   *Number Of Faculty:* 10
Number Of Students: 25   *Degrees Offered:* MA
Courses Offered: Voice Class; Music Leadership in the Church; Instruments in Church Education; The
Church & Music; Church Music Education for Children; Hymnology
Financial Assistance: Scholarships, Work-Study Grants and Student Loans
Performing Groups: Chapel Choir; Chamber Singers
Workshops/Festivals: Oktoberfest; Whightman Meetings; Christmas Concert with other Nashville
Universities; Workshop on Worship; Music & Children in the Local Church

THEATRE

James H Warren, Associate Professor   *Number Of Faculty:* 2
Number Of Students: 106   *Degrees Offered:* BA
Courses Offered: Speech and the Christian Worker; Multimedia and Worship; Staging & Producing Plays;
Musicals in the Church
Financial Assistance: Scholarships and Work-Study Grants
Performing Groups: Scarritt College Players
Workshops/Festivals: Exploring Drama with Old Americans

SOUTHERN MISSIONARY COLLEGE
Collegedale   Tennessee 37315, 615 396-4267
   Private and 4 Year
   Arts Areas: Instrumental Music, Vocal Music, Television, Visual Arts and Radio
   Performing Series: Artist - Adventure Series
   Performance Facilities: Health - PE Center; Miller Hall; Collegedale SDA Church

MUSIC

Dr Marvin L Robertson, Chairman   *Number Of Faculty:* 16
Number Of Students: 50   *Degrees Offered:* BMusEd; BA; AS
Teaching Certification Available
Financial Assistance: Scholarships and Work-Study Grants
Performing Groups: Concert Band; Orchestra; College Choir; Collegiate Chorale; Die Meistersinger Male
Chorus; Wind Ensemble
Workshops/Festivals: Artist - Adventure Series; Chapel Series; Workshops as Available

(continued on next page)

Financial Assistance: Scholarships and Work-Study Grants
Performing Groups: Instrumental Ensembles; Band; Choir; Singing Groups

THEATRE

R S Hill, Chairman   **Number Of Faculty:** 1
Performing Groups: Southwestern Players; Center Players

SOUTHWESTERN AT MEMPHIS

2000 N Parkway, Memphis   Tennessee 38112
901 274-1800 Ext 385
Private and 4 Year
Arts Areas: Instrumental Music, Vocal Music, Theatre and Visual Arts
Performing Series: Faculty Concert Series
Performance Facilities: Hardie Auditorium; Theater Six

MUSIC

Charles Mosby, Chairman   **Number Of Faculty:** 18 College, 10 Prep
Number Of Students: 80 College, 325 Adult & Prep   **Degrees Offered:** BA; BM
Teaching Certification Available
Financial Assistance: Scholarships, Work-Study Grants and As specified by Financial Aid Office
Performing Groups: Chamber Orchestra; Southwestern Singers; First Generation; Madrigal Singers;
Renaissance Ensemble
Workshops/Festivals: Baroque Festival; Renaissance Festival

THEATRE

Betty M Ruffin, Chairman   **Number Of Faculty:** 1 Full-time, 2 Part-time
Number Of Students: 20   **Degrees Offered:** BA
Courses Offered: Acting; Directing; Theatre Arts; Theatre History; Playwriting; Stage Movement
Teaching Certification Available
Financial Assistance: Scholarships, Work-Study Grants and Financial Aid
Performing Groups: New Southwestern Players
Workshops/Festivals: Renaissance Festival (annually); Workshop by Ellis Rabb
Artists-In-Residence/Guest Artists: Ellis Rabb

THE UNIVERSITY OF THE SOUTH

Sewanee   Tennessee 37375, 615 598-5931
Private and 4 Year
Arts Areas: Dance, Instrumental Music, Vocal Music, Theatre and Visual Arts
Performing Series: University Concert Series; Purple Masque; Sewanee Summer Music Center Concerts
Performance Facilities: Auditorium; Chapel; Bell Carillon

DANCE

Marian England, Assistant Director Women's Athletics   **Number Of Faculty:** 1
Number Of Students: 40   **Courses Offered:** Ballet
Financial Assistance: Scholarships and Work-Study Grants
Performing Groups: Sewanee Ballet

MUSIC

Dr Joseph M Running, Professor of Music
Number Of Faculty: 3 Full-time, 2 Part-time   **Number Of Students:** 100
Degrees Offered: BA
Courses Offered: Appreciation; History; Church Music; Counterpoint; Conducting
Technical Training: Piano; Organ; Cello; Voice; Carillon
Financial Assistance: Scholarships and Work-Study Grants
Performing Groups: Choir; Band; Madrigal Group
Workshops/Festivals: Sewanee Summer Music Center

(continued on next page)

THEATRE

Robert H Wilcox, Instructor   **Number Of Faculty:** 1½
Number Of Students: 40 - 50
Courses Offered: Acting; Directing; Stage Design; History; Theory
Financial Assistance: Scholarships and Work-Study Grants
Performing Groups: Purple Masque

TENNESSEE STATE UNIVERSITY
3500 Centennial Blvd, Nashville   Tennessee 37203
615 329-9500

State and 4 Year
Arts Areas: Instrumental Music, Vocal Music, Theatre and Visual Arts
Performing Series: Concert Series

MUSIC

Dr Edward C Lewis, Jr, Chairman   **Number Of Faculty:** 14
Number Of Students: 120   **Degrees Offered:** BA Mus; BA MusEd
Teaching Certification Available   Financial Assistance: Scholarships
Performing Groups: Various Ensembles; Band; Chorus
Degrees Offered: BA Drama-Speech   **Teaching Certification Available**
Financial Assistance: Scholarships

TENNESSEE TECHNOLOGICAL UNIVERSITY
Cookeville   Tennessee 38501, 615 526-0721

State and 4 Year
Arts Areas: Instrumental Music, Vocal Music and Visual Arts

MUSIC

James A Wattenbarger, Chairman   **Number Of Faculty:** 17
Number Of Students: 250   **Degrees Offered:** BA MusEd
Teaching Certification Available
Financial Assistance: Scholarships and Work-Study Grants
Performing Groups: Chorus; Symphony Orchestra

TENNESSEE TEMPLE COLLEGE
1815 Union Ave, Chattanooga   Tennessee 37404
615 698-6021 Ext 241

Private and 4 Year   **Arts Areas:** Instrumental Music and Vocal Music

MUSIC

Mrs Fred Brown, Chairman   **Number Of Faculty:** 15   **Number Of Students:** 177
Degrees Offered: BA Music
Financial Assistance: Scholarships and Work-Study Grants
Performing Groups: Concert Choir; Weigle Singers; Singing Men of Temple; Ladies Chorale; Glee Club; Band; Vocal Ensembles

---

TENNESSEE WESLEYAN COLLEGE
PO Box 40, Athens   Tennessee 37303
615 745-5290

Private and 4 Year
Arts Areas: Instrumental Music, Vocal Music, Theatre and Visual Arts

MUSIC

Lynn D McGill, Chairman   **Number Of Faculty:** 3   **Number Of Students:** 25
Degrees Offered: BA   **Teaching Certification Available**
Financial Assistance: Scholarships and Work-Study Grants

(continued on next page)

Performing Groups: Choir   **Number Of Faculty:** 2   **Number Of Students:** 27
Teaching Certification Available
Financial Assistance: Scholarships and Work-Study Grants
Performing Groups: Komos

UNIVERSITY OF TENNESSEE AT CHATTANOOGA
Chattanooga   Tennessee 37401, 615 755-4011
State and 4 Year
Arts Areas: Instrumental Music, Vocal Music, Theatre, Film Arts and Visual Arts

MUSIC

Dr Peter E Gerschefski, Head   **Number Of Faculty:** 24
Number Of Students: 250   **Degrees Offered:** BS; BA; BMus
Courses Offered: Applied Music; Sacred Music; Theory & Composition; Music Education
Teaching Certification Available
Financial Assistance: Scholarships and Work-Study Grants
Performing Groups: University Orchestra; University Band; 2 Stage Bands; Wind Ensemble; Singing Mocs; Chattanooga Singers; Chamber Singers; Choral Union; 6 Ensembles
Workshops/Festivals: 2 - 3 Workshops per year

THEATRE

David W Wiley, Head   **Number Of Faculty:** 4   **Number Of Students:** 400
Degrees Offered: BA
Courses Offered: Design and Technology; Acting and Directing; History and Literature
Financial Assistance: Scholarships and Work-Study Grants
Performing Groups: UTC Theatre Company; Student Production Group
Workshops/Festivals: High School Theatre and Speech Festival

UNIVERSITY OF TENNESSEE, KNOXVILLE
Cumberland Ave, Knoxville   Tennessee 37916
615 974-2591
State and 4 Year
Arts Areas: Dance, Instrumental Music, Vocal Music and Theatre
Performing Series: Concert - Lecture Series
Performance Facilities: Clarence Brown Theatre; Carousel Theatre; Music Hall; University Center

DANCE

Richard Croskey, Coordinator   **Number Of Faculty:** 5
Number Of Students: 300   **Degrees Offered:** Minor Offered
Courses Offered: Ballet; Modern; Jazz; Tap; Social Dance; Folk & Square
Technical Training: Beginning classes in Ballet, Modern and Tap
Financial Assistance: Work-Study Grants
Performing Groups: New Repertory Dance Company
Workshops/Festivals: Summer Workshops

MUSIC

William Starr, Interim Head   **Number Of Faculty:** 49
Number Of Students: 400   **Degrees Offered:** BS; BA; MMus; MMus; MA; MS
Courses Offered: Theory; Music History; Applied Composition
Technical Training: Electronic Music   **Teaching Certification Available**
Financial Assistance: Assistantships, Scholarships and Work-Study Grants
Performing Groups: Marching & Concert Bands; Opera Theatre; Chamber Ensemble; Concert Choir; Glee Clubs; UT Singers; University Symphony; Trombone Choir; Brass Choir; Percussion Ensemble; Jazz Ensemble
Workshops/Festivals: Summer Festivals; Opera Workshops

THEATRE

Dr Ralph G Allen, Head   **Number Of Faculty:** 12   **Number Of Students:** 150
Degrees Offered: BA; MA

(continued on next page)

Courses Offered: Performance; Technical Theatre; Design; Theatrical History; Dramatic Theory and Criticism; Scenery; Costume and Light Designing
Technical Training: Opera with Music Department and development of professional theatre company
Financial Assistance: Assistantships, Scholarships and Work-Study Grants
Performing Groups: Clarence Brown Company and the Major Company
Workshops/Festivals: Guest Artist Workshops

UNIVERSITY OF TENNESSEE, MARTIN
Martin   Tennessee 38237, 901 587-7133
State and 4 Year
Arts Areas: Dance, Instrumental Music, Vocal Music, Theatre and Visual Arts
Performance Facilities: Performing Arts Theatre

DANCE

Caroline Byrum, Chairman, Physical Education Department
Technical Training: Modern, Practical Study of Modern Dance Movements; Beginning Dance Techniques; Beginning Dance Composition

MUSIC

Michael Hunon, Acting Chairman   **Number Of Faculty:** 15
Number Of Students: 1,382   **Degrees Offered:** BS Ed with Major in MusEd; BA
Technical Training: Electronic Music; Opera
Teaching Certification Available
Financial Assistance: Scholarships and Work-Study Grants
Performing Groups: Jazz Lab Band; Today's People (USO Group): Marching Bands; Concert Bands; Chamber Music
Workshops/Festivals: Opera Workshop; State Marching Band Festival; Music Festivals

THEATRE

William Snyder, Chairman   **Number Of Faculty:** 8
Technical Training: Production; Performance; Acting; Improvisation; Stage Craft; Playwriting
Performing Groups: Vanguard Theatre   **Workshops/Festivals:** Theatre Workshop

TREVECCA NAZARENE COLLEGE
333 Murfreesboro Rd, Nashville   Tennessee 37210
615 244-6000 Ext 374
Private and 4 Year
Arts Areas: Instrumental Music, Vocal Music, Theatre, Television and Visual Arts
Performing Series: Cultural Events Series
Performance Facilities: Wakefield Fine Arts Building; Wakefield Auditorium

MUSIC

Dr Barbara McClain, Chairperson   **Number Of Faculty:** 7
Degrees Offered: BA; BS
Courses Offered: Theory; History; Literature; Music Education; Performance
Technical Training: Performance Individual and Group Lessons
Teaching Certification Available
Financial Assistance: Scholarships and Work-Study Grants
Performing Groups: Concert Choir; Chapel Choir; Choral Society; Concert Band; Chamber Music Ensemble; Handbell Choir; Marching Band; Orchestra
Workshops/Festivals: Individual Workshops for each Performing Group

TUSCULUM COLLEGE
Tusculum Station, Greenville   Tennessee 37743
615 639-2701
Private and 4 Year
Arts Areas: Instrumental Music, Vocal Music, Theatre and Visual Arts
Performing Series: Cultural Events Series

(continued on next page)

Performance Facilities: College Auditorium ***Degrees Offered:*** BA
Financial Assistance: Scholarships and Work-Study Grants
Performing Groups: Vocal & Instrumental Ensembles

THEATRE

David F Behan, Chairman ***Number Of Faculty:*** 2 ***Number Of Students:*** 30
Degrees Offered: BA
Financial Assistance: Scholarships and Work-Study Grants
Performing Groups: Pioneer Players

UNION UNIVERSITY
Jackson Tennessee 38301, 901 422-2576

Private and 4 Year
Arts Areas: Instrumental Music, Vocal Music, Theatre and Visual Arts
Performing Series: Concert-Lecture Series
Performance Facilities: University Auditorium

MUSIC

Dr Kenneth R Hartley, Chairman ***Number Of Faculty:*** 10
Number Of Students: 80
Degrees Offered: BA MusEd, Applied Music, Music Literature, Sacred Music
Teaching Certification Available
Financial Assistance: Scholarships and Work-Study Grants

THEATRE

Number Of Faculty: 1 ***Number Of Students:*** 20
Performing Groups: Union University Players

VANDERBILT UNIVERSITY
21st Ave & West End, Nashville Tennessee 37235
615 322-2561

Private and 4 Year ***Arts Areas:*** Theatre
Performing Series: Chamber Music Series

THEATRE

Cecil D Jones, Chairman ***Number Of Faculty:*** 5 ***Number Of Students:*** 27
Degrees Offered: BA
Financial Assistance: Scholarships and Work-Study Grants
Performing Groups: Vanderbilt University Theatre

ABILENE CHRISTIAN UNIVERSITY
Box 8274, Abilene   Texas 79601
915 677-1977 Ext 462

Private and 4 Year
Arts Areas: Instrumental Music, Vocal Music, Theatre, Television and Visual Arts
Performing Series: ACU Fine Arts Series
Performance Facilities: Auditorium; Theater; Recital Hall; Coliseum

MUSIC

Dr M L Daniels, Head   *Number Of Faculty:* 14   *Number Of Students:* 110
Degrees Offered: BA; BM Ed   *Courses Offered:* Instrumental and Vocal Music
Teaching Certification Available
Financial Assistance: Assistantships, Scholarships and Work-Study Grants
Performing Groups: Symphonic Band; Concert Band; Jazz Ensembles; A Cappella Chorus; Choralaires; Varsity Chorus; Womens Chorus; Orchestra; Various Ensembles
Workshops/Festivals: Summer Band Camp

ALVIN JUNIOR COLLEGE
Alvin   Texas 77511, 713 658-5311

County and 2 Year
Arts Areas: Instrumental Music, Vocal Music and Theatre
Number Of Faculty: 1   *Number Of Students:* 52   *Degrees Offered:* AA Music
Financial Assistance: Scholarships and Work-Study Grants
Performing Groups: Concert Choir; Stage Band; College Singers; Grand Chorus

THEATRE

Jo Bernett, Chairman   *Number Of Faculty:* 1   *Number Of Students:* 52
Financial Assistance: Scholarships and Work-Study Grants
Performing Groups: AJC THeatre

AMARILLO COLLEGE
Box 447, Amarillo   Texas 79105
806 376-5641

County and 2 Year
Arts Areas: Dance, Instrumental Music, Vocal Music and Theatre

MUSIC

Prof Hoffman, Chairman
Degrees Offered: AA Music, Applied, Composition & Theory, MusEd
Performing Groups: Band; Choir; Madrigal Singers; Stage Band
Workshops/Festivals: Opera Workshop

THEATRE

Prof McDonough, Chairman Speech Arts
Degrees Offered: AA in Theatre & Speech   *Performing Groups:* Drama Group

ANGELO STATE UNIVERSITY
San Angelo   Texas 76901, 915 942-2085

State and 4 Year
Arts Areas: Instrumental Music, Vocal Music, Theatre and Visual Arts

MUSIC

Dr Charles Robison, Head, Department of Art and Music
Number Of Faculty: 9 Full-time, 4 Part-time   *Number Of Students:* 250

(continued on next page)

Degrees Offered: BA MusEd; BME; MME   **Teaching Certification Available**
Financial Assistance: Scholarships and Work-Study Grants
Performing Groups: Marching Band; Symphonic Band; Concert Band; Orchestra; Stage Band; Concert Chorale; Chamber Choir; Treble Chorus; Entertainers

---

AUSTIN COLLEGE
900 N Grand Ave, Sherman   Texas 75090
214 892-9101
Private and 4 Year
Arts Areas: Dance, Instrumental Music, Vocal Music, Theatre, Television and Visual Arts
Performing Series: Sherman Symphony; Community Series; A Cappella Choir; College Theatre
Performance Facilities: Wynne Chapel; Richardson Center Auditorium; Ida Green Theatre; Arena Theatre; Craig Hall Auditorium

DANCE

Number Of Faculty: 1   **Number Of Students:** 15
BA, MA under Communication Arts Department; there is no dance department

MUSIC

Bruce Glenn Lunkley, Chairman   **Number Of Faculty:** 7
Number Of Students: 35   **Degrees Offered:** BA; MA
Teaching Certification Available
Financial Assistance: Scholarships and Work-Study Grants
Performing Groups: A Cappella Choir; Choral Union; Civic Orchestra; Choir; Concert Wind Ensemble; Brass Ensemble; Woodwind Ensemble
Workshops/Festivals: Musicians Conference; Choir, Ensemble Tours; Community Series; Stringed Instrument Repair Workshop

THEATRE

Harry Thompson, Chairman   **Number Of Faculty:** 4   **Number Of Students:** 60
Degrees Offered: BA; MA   **Teaching Certification Available**
Financial Assistance: Scholarships and Work-Study Grants
Performing Groups: College Theatre
Workshops/Festivals: Fine Arts Festival; Community Plays

BAYLOR UNIVERSITY
Waco   Texas 76703, 817 755-3601
Private and 4 Year
Arts Areas: Dance, Instrumental Music, Vocal Music, Theatre, Television and Visual Arts
Performing Series: Distinguished Artist Series
Performance Facilities: Waco Hall; Roxy Grove Hall; Weston Theater; Theater One
Number Of Faculty: 1   **Number Of Students:** 40

MUSIC

Daniel Sternberg, Dean   **Number Of Faculty:** 50   **Number Of Students:** 450
Degrees Offered: BMus; BME; MM
Courses Offered: Applied Music; Theory; Literature; History; Conducting
Teaching Certification Available
Financial Assistance: Assistantships, Scholarships and Work-Study Grants
Performing Groups: Oratorio Chorus; Chamber Singers; Chapel Choir; Concert Choir; A Cappela Choir; Symphony Orchestra; Marching Band; Concert Band; Jazz Ensemble; Collegium Musicum

THEATRE

Bill G Cook, Chairman   **Number Of Faculty:** 7   **Number Of Students:** 75
Degrees Offered: BA; BS Ed; BFA; MA
Courses Offered: Directing; Design; Acting; History; Criticism
Teaching Certification Available

(continued on next page)

Financial Assistance: Assistantships, Scholarships and Work-Study Grants
Performing Groups: University Theater
Workshops/Festivals: High School One Act Play Workshop; Children Theater Tour Production

BEE COUNTY COLLEGE
Route 1, Beeville   Texas 78102
512 358-3130

County and 2 Year
Arts Areas: Dance, Instrumental Music, Vocal Music, Theatre and Visual Arts

MUSIC

James L Lee, Division Chairman   **Number Of Faculty:** 2
Number Of Students: 50   **Degrees Offered:** AA; AS
Financial Assistance: Scholarships and Work-Study Grants
Performing Groups: College Concert Band; Stage Band; Concert Choir; Singers
Workshops/Festivals: Piano Workshop; Organ Workshop; Elementary Music Workshop
Number Of Faculty: 2   **Number Of Students:** 30   **Degrees Offered:** AA; AS
Financial Assistance: Scholarships and Work-Study Grants
Performing Groups: Cactus Company   **Workshops/Festivals:** Drama Workshops

BISHOP COLLEGE
3837 Simpson & Stuart Sts, Dallas   Texas 75241
214 376-4311

Private and 4 Year
Arts Areas: Instrumental Music, Vocal Music, Theatre, Television and Visual Arts
Performance Facilities: Carr P Collins Chapel

DANCE

Ann Williams, Physical Education Department   **Number Of Students:** 50
Technical Training: Modern Dance; Jazz; Performance on TV; Production for TV (minor TV presentation with Music and Drama Departments)
Financial Assistance: Assistantships, Scholarships and Work-Study Grants
Performing Groups: Bishop College Dance Troup
Workshops/Festivals: Workshop with Guest Artists; Spring Festival produced by senior students

MUSIC

Dr J Harrison Wilson, Chairman   **Number Of Faculty:** 9
Number Of Students: 210   **Degrees Offered:** BMusEd; BA Music
Technical Training: Jazz   **Teaching Certification Available**
Financial Assistance: Internships, Scholarships and Work-Study Grants
Performing Groups: Concert Choir; Concert Band; Marching Band; Lab Band; Male Glee Club
Workshops/Festivals: Church Music; Festival with High School Students

THEATRE

Dr Jack Gilber, Chairman   **Number Of Faculty:** 3   **Number Of Students:** 40
Degrees Offered: BA Drama - Speech   **Teaching Certification Available**
Financial Assistance: Scholarships and Work-Study Grants
Performing Groups: Readers Theatre; Richard B Harrison Theatre

BLINN COLLEGE
College Ave, Brenham   Texas 77833
713 836-9319

County and 2 Year
Arts Areas: Instrumental Music, Vocal Music and Visual Arts
Number Of Faculty: 2   **Number Of Students:** 46
Degrees Offered: AA Music, MusEd   **Performing Groups:** Band; Chorus
Number Of Faculty: 4   **Number Of Students:** 52   **Degrees Offered:** AA Drama

BRAZOSPORT COLLEGE
PO Drawer 955, Brazosport   Texas 77541
713 265-6131

County and 2 Year   *Arts Areas:* Dance and Theatre

THEATRE

Tom Kinney, Chairman   *Number Of Faculty:* 1   *Number Of Students:* 35
Performing Groups: Drama Group

CENTRAL TEXAS COLLEGE
Hwy 190 W, Killeen   Texas 76541
817 526-1210

County and 2 Year
Arts Areas: Instrumental Music, Vocal Music, Theatre, Television and Visual Arts
Number Of Faculty: 2   *Number Of Students:* 46   *Degrees Offered:* AA Music
Performing Groups: 3,4

CISCO JUNIOR COLLEGE
Cisco   Texas 76437, 817 442-2567

State and 2 Year
Arts Areas: Instrumental Music, Vocal Music and Theatre
Number Of Faculty: 1   *Number Of Students:* 50
Financial Assistance: Scholarships   *Performing Groups:* Wrangler Belles

MUSIC

Wyley M Peebles, Chairman   *Number Of Faculty:* 3   *Number Of Students:* 75
Degrees Offered: AAA; AA
Courses Offered: Theory; Literature; Band; Choir; Winds; Voice; Piano; Organ
Financial Assistance: Scholarships and Work-Study Grants
Performing Groups: Band; Stage Band; College Singers; Madrigal Singers

THEATRE

Wyley M Peebles, Chairman   *Number Of Faculty:* 2   *Number Of Students:* 20
Degrees Offered: AA
Courses Offered: Acting; Rehearsal and Performance; Make-up; Technical Theatre
Financial Assistance: Scholarships and Work-Study Grants
Performing Groups: College Players   *Workshops/Festivals:* UIL Contests

COLLEGE OF THE MAINLAND
8001 Palmer Hwy, Texas City   Texas 77590
713 938-1211 Ext 214

2 Year
Arts Areas: Instrumental Music, Vocal Music, Theatre and Visual Arts
Performing Series: Mainland Community Theatre Series
Performance Facilities: Arena Theatre; College Center and Learning Resources Center Teaching Auditorium

MUSIC

Larry Stanley, Chairman, Division of Arts & Humanities
Number Of Faculty: 4   *Number Of Students:* 50   *Degrees Offered:* AA
Courses Offered: Instrumental; Vocal   *Financial Assistance:* Scholarships
Performing Groups: Lab Band; Jazz Band; COM Singers
Workshops/Festivals: Gulf Coast Swing Choir Festival

THEATRE

Jack Westin, Theatre Coordinator Division of Arts & Humanities
Number Of Faculty: 1   *Number Of Students:* 30   *Degrees Offered:* AA

(continued on next page)

Courses Offered: Theatre Workshop; Introduction to Theatre; Stagecraft; Acting; History of Theatre
Financial Assistance: Scholarships
Performing Groups: Mainland Community Theatre
Workshops/Festivals: Acting Workshops; Set Design Workshops; Lighting and Make-up Workshops

COOKE COUNTY JUNIOR COLLEGE
Box 815, Gainesville   Texas 76240
817 668-7731
County and 2 Year
Arts Areas: Instrumental Music, Vocal Music and Theatre
Performance Facilities: College Auditorium

MUSIC

Glenn Wilson, Chairman   **Number Of Faculty:** 1   **Number Of Students:** 35
Degrees Offered: AA music   **Performing Groups:** Band; Chorus; Madrigal Singers

THEATRE

Paul Hutchins, Chairman   **Performing Groups:** Drama Club

CORPUS CHRISTI STATE UNIVERSITY
6300 Ocean Dr
PO Box 6010, Corpus Christi   Texas 78411
512 991-6810 Ext 259
State and Upper Level
Arts Areas: Instrumental Music, Vocal Music, Theatre, Film Arts, Television and Visual Arts
Performing Series: Arts and Humanities Noon Series
Performance Facilities: Auditorium; Gallery

MUSIC

Dr Miriam Wagenschein, Dean, College of Arts and Humanities
Number Of Faculty: 4 Full-time, 29 Part-time   **Number Of Students:** 45
Degrees Offered: BMus
Courses Offered: Music Education; Music Performance; Keyboard Pedagogy
Teaching Certification Available
Financial Assistance: Scholarships and Work-Study Grants
Performing Groups: Orchestra; Choir; Band; Chamber Singers; Stage Band; Opera Workshop; Percussion Ensemble; Brass Choir; Chamber Music Groups
Workshops/Festivals: Workshops: Building the Voice; Woodwind Teaching and Performance; Woodwind Repair and Maintenance; Marching Band Techniques & Arranging

THEATRE

Dr Miriam Wagenschein, Dean, College of Arts & Humanities
Number Of Faculty: 3   **Number Of Students:** 10   **Degrees Offered:** BA; MA
Courses Offered: Theory; Theatre; RTV; Film
Teaching Certification Available
Financial Assistance: Scholarships and Work-Study Grants
Workshops/Festivals: Fine Arts Festival

DALLAS BAPTIST COLLEGE
3000 Florina, Dallas   Texas 75211
214 331-8311 Ext 318
4 Year
Arts Areas: Instrumental Music, Vocal Music, Theatre, Film Arts, Television and Visual Arts
Performing Series: Studio Group (Instrumental); Wind Ensemble; A Cappella Choir; DBC Chorale
Gateway Players (Drama)

MUSIC

Dr Wesley Coffman, Coffman   **Number Of Faculty:** 8   **Number Of Students:** 100

(continued on next page)

Degrees Offered: BA or BS in MusEd, Church Mus, Applied
Teaching Certification Available
Financial Assistance: Scholarships and Work-Study Grants
Performing Groups: Studio Group (Instrumental); Wind Ensemble; A Cappella Choir; DBC Chorale
Workshops/Festivals: Fine Arts Festival in Spring; Music Education Workshop; Metroplex Honor Chorus & Band

THEATRE

Dr Carl Marder III, Chairman of Theatre   **Number Of Faculty:** 2
Number Of Students: 100   **Degrees Offered:** BA or BS in Drama, Speech or Media
Teaching Certification Available
Financial Assistance: Scholarships and Work-Study Grants
Performing Groups: Gateway Players
Workshops/Festivals: Forensic Contest; Fine Arts Festival

DALLAS BIBLE COLLEGE
8733 LaPrada, Dallas   Texas 75228
214 328-7171

Private and 4 Year   **Arts Areas:** Instrumental Music and Vocal Music
Performance Facilities: College Chapel

MUSIC

Wm D Haas, Director of Music & Promotion   **Number Of Students:** 20
Degrees Offered: BS Mus - Christian Ed
Financial Assistance: Scholarships, Work-Study Grants and BEOG

DALLAS THEATER CENTER
3636 Turtle Creek Blvd, Dallas   Texas 75219
214 526-0107

Private and 2 Year   **Arts Areas:** Theatre
Performance Facilities: Kilita Humphreys Theater; Down Center Stage

THEATRE

Dr Paul Baker, Chairman   **Number Of Faculty:** 36   **Number Of Students:** 90
Degrees Offered: MFA
Courses Offered: Complete Dramatic Program; Teen - Children Theater
Financial Assistance: Scholarships   **Performing Groups:** Mime Troupe
Workshops/Festivals: New Play Festival
Professional Apprentice program in conjunction with Academic

DEL MAR COLLEGE
Corpus Christi   Texas 78404, 512 882-6231 Ext 211
City and 2 Year
Arts Areas: Instrumental Music, Vocal Music, Theatre and Visual Arts
Performing Series: Cultural Program Series; Faculty Concert Series
Performance Facilities: Wolfe Recital Hall; Del Mar Auditorium
Courses Offered: Folk and Modern Dance

MUSIC

Merton B Johnson, Dean of Fine Arts   **Number Of Faculty:** 23
Number Of Students: 135   **Degrees Offered:** AA
Courses Offered: Theory; Music Literature; Applied; Methods; Band; Orchestra; Choir; Chamber; Opera; Stage Band; Jazz Improvisation; Appreciation
Financial Assistance: Assistantships, Scholarships and Work-Study Grants
Performing Groups: Faculty Piano Trio and Woodwind Quintet; Choir; Band; Orchestra; Piano Accompaniment; Percussion Ensemble; Brass Choir; Chamber Singers; Piano Chamber Music; Woodwind Quintet; String Chamber Music; Brass Quintet; Flute Choir; Guitar Chamber; Stage Band; Chorale
Workshops/Festivals: Numerous Public School Events; Contempory Music Festival

(continued on next page)

Number Of Faculty: 1 Part-time   **Number Of Students:** 22
Program is offered in conjunction with Corpus Christi State University
Courses Offered: Introduction to Theatre; Acting; Oral Interpretation
Financial Assistance: Assistantships, Scholarships and Work-Study Grants

DOMINICAN COLLEGE
2401 Holcombe Blvd, Houston   Texas 77021
713 747-2700
Private and 4 Year
Arts Areas: Instrumental Music, Vocal Music and Visual Arts

MUSIC

Dawn Crawford, Chairman   **Degrees Offered:** BA Mus Applied; BA MusEd

EAST TEXAS BAPTIST COLLEGE
1209 N Grove, Marshall   Texas 75670
214 935-7963
Private and 4 Year
Arts Areas: Instrumental Music, Vocal Music, Theatre and Visual Arts
Performing Series: Fine Arts Series

MUSIC

Robert L Spencer, Chairman   **Number Of Faculty:** 8   **Number Of Students:** 80
Degrees Offered: BMusEd; BA Music   **Teaching Certification Available**
Financial Assistance: Scholarships and Work-Study Grants

THEATRE

Mark Blakeney, Chairman   **Number Of Faculty:** 2   **Number Of Students:** 30
Degrees Offered: BA Speech   **Teaching Certification Available**
Financial Assistance: Scholarships and Work-Study Grants

EAST TEXAS STATE UNIVERSITY
Commerce   Texas 75428, 214 468-2291
State and 4 Year   **Arts Areas:** Instrumental Music and Vocal Music
Performing Series: Forum Arts
Performance Facilities: Concert Hall; University Auditorium; American Ballroom

MUSIC

Robert W House, Head   **Number Of Faculty:** 20
Degrees Offered: BMus; BM Ed; BM Theory-Comp; BM Lit
Courses Offered: Applied; Theory; Composition; Music Literature; Music Education
Teaching Certification Available
Financial Assistance: Assistantships, Scholarships and Work-Study Grants
Performing Groups: University Singers; Chorale; Chamber Singers; Opera Ensemble; Piano Ensemble;
Band; Brass Choir; Woodwind Choir; Brass Ensemble; Woodwind Ensemble; Trombone Choir; Horn Choir;
Jazz Ensemble; Improvisation Ensemble; Percussion Ensemble; Flute Choir; Tuba Ensemble
Workshops/Festivals: Piano Workshop; Composition Clinic; Band Workshop; Elementary Music Workshop

THEATRE

Curtis L Pope, Head of Department   **Number Of Faculty:** 8
Number Of Students: 180   **Degrees Offered:** BS; BA; MA; MS
Courses Offered: Acting; Directing; History; Design; Lighting; Playwriting; Dance; Costuming
Technical Training: Scenic Design; Costuming; Lighting; Technical Theatre
Teaching Certification Available
Financial Assistance: Assistantships, Scholarships and Work-Study Grants
Performing Groups: University Playhouse; Theatre-for-Children; Environmental Theatre; Summer Theatre
Workshop

EASTFIELD COLLEGE
3737 Motley Dr, Mesquite   Texas 75150
214 746-3100
　　County and 2 Year
　　Arts Areas: Instrumental Music, Vocal Music, Theatre and Visual Arts
　　Performing Series: The 20th Century Music Festival
　　Performance Facilities: Performance Hall

MUSIC

Dr John Stewart, Humanities Chairman   *Number Of Faculty:* 7
Degrees Offered: AA
Financial Assistance: Scholarships and Work-Study Grants
Performing Groups: Jazz Band; Concert Band; Jazz Vocal Ensemble; Concert Choir

THEATRE

Robert Erwin, Theatre Director   *Number Of Faculty:* 1
Number Of Students: 25   *Degrees Offered:* AA
Financial Assistance: Scholarships and Work-Study Grants
Performing Groups: Eastfield Theatre Group

EL CENTRO COLLEGE
Main & Lamar St, Dallas   Texas 75202
214 746-2311
　　County and 2 Year
　　Arts Areas: Instrumental Music, Vocal Music, Theatre and Visual Arts
　　Performing Series: Student Activities sponsor Lyceum Series & guest artists
　　Performance Facilities: Corner Theatre

MUSIC

Number Of Faculty: 3   *Degrees Offered:* AA
Financial Assistance: Scholarships and Work-Study Grants
Performing Groups: Chorus

DANCE

Number Of Faculty: 2   *Performing Groups:* Drama Group Performances

FORT WORTH CHRISTIAN COLLEGE
7517 Bogart Dr, Ft Worth   Texas 76118
817 281-6504
　　Private and 2 Year
　　Arts Areas: Instrumental Music, Vocal Music, Theatre and Visual Arts
　　Degrees Offered: AA Mus   *Degrees Offered:* AA Drama
　　Financial Assistance: Work-Study Grants

FRANK PHILLIPS COLLEGE
Box 111, Borger   Texas 79006
806 274-5311
　　County and 2 Year
　　Arts Areas: Instrumental Music, Vocal Music and Theatre
　　Performance Facilities: College Auditorium   *Degrees Offered:* AA Music
　　Performing Groups: Vocal and Instrumental Ensembles

THEATRE

John Banvard, Chairman   *Performing Groups:* Dran

GRAYSON COUNTY COLLEGE
6101 Hwy 691, Denison   Texas 75020
214 893-6834 Ext 52
>County and 2 Year
>*Arts Areas:* Instrumental Music, Vocal Music, Theatre, Television and Visual Arts
>*Performing Series:* Recital Series
>*Performance Facilities:* Fine Arts Auditorium; Nursing Auditorium; Student Center; Dinner Theatre;
>Library (Recitals)

MUSIC

>Dr Charles McAdams, Director Division of Fine Arts   *Number Of Faculty:* 5
>*Degrees Offered:* AA   *Courses Offered:* Music
>*Technical Training:* Piano Tuning; Piano Repair
>*Financial Assistance:* Scholarships, Work-Study Grants and BEOG
>*Performing Groups:* Viking Choir; Voyagers; Viking Stage Band; Brass Ensemble
>*Workshops/Festivals:* Baroque Music Festival

THEATRE

>Dr Charles McAdams, Director Division of Fine Arts   *Number Of Faculty:* 1
>*Degrees Offered:* AA   *Courses Offered:* Drama
>*Financial Assistance:* Scholarships and Work-Study Grants
>*Performing Groups:* Viking Players

HARDIN - SIMMONS UNIVERSITY
Abilene   Texas 79601, 915 677-7281
>Private and 4 Year
>*Arts Areas:* Instrumental Music, Vocal Music, Theatre and Visual Arts
>*Performance Facilities:* Woodward Dellis Recital Hall; Van Ellis Theater

MUSIC

>Dr T W Dean, Dean School of Music   *Number Of Faculty:* 17
>*Number Of Students:* 190   *Degrees Offered:* BMus; BMusEd; MMus; MMusEd
>*Technical Training:* Electronic Music   *Teaching Certification Available*
>*Financial Assistance:* Assistantships, Scholarships and Work-Study Grants
>*Performing Groups:* University Symphony; Concert Band; Cowboy Band; University Chorale; Concert
>Choir; Madrigal Singers; Singers Ho!; Singing Men; Jazz Ensemble; Opera Workshop
>*Workshops/Festivals:* College and High School Choral Festival

THEATRE

>Dr Jerry Reynolds, Chairman   *Number Of Faculty:* 3   *Number Of Students:* 45
>*Degrees Offered:* BA Speech and/or Drama; MA Speech and/or Drama
>*Courses Offered:* Acting; Production; Technical; Lighting
>*Teaching Certification Available*
>*Financial Assistance:* Assistantships, Scholarships and Work-Study Grants
>*Performing Groups:* Drama; Musical Comedy; Reader's Theater
>*Workshops/Festivals:* Annual High School Speech Festival

HENDERSON COUNTY JUNIOR COLLEGE
Athens   Texas 75751, 214 675-6319
>State and 2 Year
>*Arts Areas:* Dance, Instrumental Music, Vocal Music and Theatre
>*Performing Series:* Fine Arts Series
>*Performance Facilities:* Auditorium; Student Union Ballroom

DANCE

>Pam Tiner, Director of Cardettes   *Number Of Faculty:* 1
>*Number Of Students:* 65   *Degrees Offered:* AA

(continued on next page)

Courses Offered: Cardettes and Modern Dance
Financial Assistance: Scholarships and Work-Study Grants
Performing Groups: Cardettes

MUSIC

Hubert Wilbur, Chairman   **Number Of Faculty:** 4   **Number Of Students:** 100
Degrees Offered: AA
Courses Offered: Fundamentals of Music; Music Appreciation; Theory
Financial Assistance: Scholarships and Work-Study Grants
Performing Groups: Band; Stage Band; Choir; Cardinal Singers
Workshops/Festivals: Band Festival; Select Band

THEATRE

George Oliver, Director of Theatre   **Number Of Faculty:** 1
Number Of Students: 30   **Degrees Offered:** AA
Courses Offered: Elementary Dramatics; History of the Theatre; Intermediate Acting; Stagecraft
Financial Assistance: Scholarships and Work-Study Grants
Workshops/Festivals: Cardinal Forensic and Drama Workshop

HIGH SCHOOL FOR THE PERFORMING AND VISUAL ARTS
3517 Austin St, Houston   Texas 77004
713 522-7811
City and grades 10-12
Arts Areas: Dance, Instrumental Music, Vocal Music, Theatre, Film Arts, Television and Visual Arts

DANCE

Mary Martha Lappe, Coordinator   **Number Of Faculty:** 2
Number Of Students: 100
Courses Offered: Ballet; Modern Dance; Composition; Pointe Technique; Jazz; Character Dance; Tap; Dance History; Dance Production; Dance Photography; Dance Journalism; Survey of Dance; Rhythmic Analysis

MUSIC

Edward Trongone, Coordinator (Instrumental); Jean Galloway, Coordinator (Vocal)
Number Of Faculty: 5   **Number Of Students:** 200
Courses Offered: Orchestra; Stage Band; Chorale; Girls' Ensemble; Madrigal Singers; Theory; Sight Singing; Piano Lab; Composition; Improvisation; Music Literature; Music History

THEATRE

Lela Blount, Coordinator   **Number Of Faculty:** 3   **Number Of Students:** 100
Courses Offered: Basic Design; Architectural Design; Introduction to the Theatre; Acting; Directing; Technical Theatre; Mime; Choreography; Fencing; Playwriting; Creative Children's Theatre; History of the Theatre; Make-up; Costume; Production

---

HILL JUNIOR COLLEGE
Hillsboro   Texas 77036, 817 582-2555
County and 2 Year
Arts Areas: Instrumental Music, Vocal Music, Theatre and Visual Arts
Number Of Faculty: 3   **Number Of Students:** 69   **Degrees Offered:** AA Music
Financial Assistance: Scholarships and Work-Study Grants
Performing Groups: Hill College Symphonic Wind Ensemble; Jazz Lab Band; Jazz Ensemble; Hill Chorale

THEATRE

Jack Smith, Chairman   **Number Of Faculty:** 1   **Number Of Students:** 23
Degrees Offered: AA
Financial Assistance: Scholarships and Work-Study Grants
Performing Groups: Hill Players

HOUSTON BAPTIST UNIVERSITY
7502 Fondren Rd, Houston   Texas 77074
713 774-7661
Private and 4 Year
Arts Areas: Instrumental Music, Vocal Music, Theatre and Visual Arts
Performance Facilities: Denham Hall; Mabee Theatre; Anderson Student Center; Sharp Gymnasium

MUSIC

Dr Gary Horton, Chairman Department of Fine Arts   *Number Of Faculty:* 8
Number Of Students: 300   *Degrees Offered:* BA; BS; BME
Courses Offered: Theory; History; Literature; Music Education; Church Music; Applied Music; Ensembles; Senior Seminar
Teaching Certification Available
Financial Assistance: Scholarships and Work-Study Grants
Performing Groups: University Singers; Chapel Choir; University Orchestra; Stage Band; Concert Band; Theatre Men; Bell Canto Singers
Workshops/Festivals: Opera Workshop; Fine Arts Festival; Percussion Arts Workshop

THEATRE

Dr James Taylor, Chairman Department of Communication and Theatre Arts
Number Of Faculty: 2   *Number Of Students:* 35   *Degrees Offered:* BA; BS
Courses Offered: Applied Theatre; Drama Appreciation; History of Theatre; Acting; Directing; Contemporary Theatre; Theatre and Church; Scene Construction; Phonetics; Speech; Theatre in Public Schools; Scene Design; Lighting; History American Theatre; Special Topics; Senior Seminar
Teaching Certification Available
Financial Assistance: Scholarships and Work-Study Grants
Performing Groups: Gallery Theatre Players
Workshops/Festivals: Student One-Act Plays

UNIVERSITY OF HOUSTON, CENTRAL CAMPUS
4800 Calhoun, Houston   Texas 77004
713 749-1011
State and 4 Year
Arts Areas: Dance, Instrumental Music, Vocal Music, Theatre, Film Arts, Television and Visual Arts
Performance Facilities: Cullen Auditorium; Attic Theatre; Dudley Recital Hall; Lyndall Wortham Theatre; Lab Theatre

MUSIC

Milton Katims, Artistic Director   *Number Of Faculty:* 48
Number Of Students: 462
Degrees Offered: BMus in Perf, Theory, Comp, Music Lit, MusEd; BA Mus; MM in Perf, Theory, Comp, Mus Lit, Conducting
Teaching Certification Available
Financial Assistance: Assistantships, Scholarships and Work-Study Grants
Performing Groups: University Chorus; Concert Chorale; Today's Generation; UH Symphony Orchestra; Concert Band; Marching Band; Wind Ensemble; Jazz Ensemble; Collegium Musicum

THEATRE

Sidney Berger, Chairman   *Number Of Faculty:* 8   *Number Of Students:* 150
Degrees Offered: BA; MA; MFA
Courses Offered: Acting; Directing; Stage Movement; Stagecraft; Mime
Technical Training: Stagecraft; Lighting; Scene Design; Costume Construction
Teaching Certification Available
Financial Assistance: Assistantships, Scholarships and Work-Study Grants
Performing Groups: Mime Troupe
Workshops/Festivals: Houston Shakespeare Festival

UNIVERSITY OF HOUSTON, DOWNTOWN COLLEGE
1 Main St, Houston   Texas 77002
713 749-1011

State and 4 Year   *Arts Areas:* Vocal Music, Theatre and Visual Arts
Performance Facilities: Auditorium; Two Galleries

MUSIC

Number Of Faculty: 1   *Number Of Students:* 75 - 125
Financial Assistance: Scholarships and Work-Study Grants
Performing Groups: UHDC; Chorus

THEATRE

Number Of Faculty: 1   *Number Of Students:* 75 - 125   *Courses Offered:* Acting; Theatre History
Artists-In-Residence/Guest Artists: John Biggers

HOWARD COLLEGE, BIG SPRING
N Birdwell Lane, Big Spring   Texas 79720
915 267-6311 Ext 44

County and 2 Year
Arts Areas: Instrumental Music, Vocal Music, Theatre, Television and Visual Arts
Performing Series: Community Concert Series
Performance Facilities: Howard College Auditorium

MUSIC

Mary Skalicky, Chairman   *Number Of Faculty:* 2   *Degrees Offered:* AA
Financial Assistance: Scholarships and Work-Study Grants
Performing Groups: College Choir; Stage Band (Combo); Choraliers; Resident Duo-Pianists
Workshops/Festivals: Fine Arts Festival; Opera Workshop

THEATRE

John Gordon, Instructor   *Number Of Faculty:* 1   *Degrees Offered:* AA
Financial Assistance: Scholarships and Work-Study Grants
Performing Groups: Hawk Players   *Workshops/Festivals:* Fine Arts Festival

HOWARD PAYNE COLLEGE
Brownwood   Texas 76801, 915 656-2502

Private and 4 Year
Arts Areas: Instrumental Music, Vocal Music, Theatre and Visual Arts

MUSIC

George Baker, Chairman   *Number Of Faculty:* 12   *Number Of Students:* 125
Degrees Offered: BA; BMus; BMusEd   *Teaching Certification Available*
Financial Assistance: Scholarships and Work-Study Grants

THEATRE

Alex Reeve, Chairman   *Number Of Faculty:* 6   *Number Of Students:* 120
Degrees Offered: BA   *Technical Training:* Children's Theatre
Teaching Certification Available
Financial Assistance: Scholarships and Work-Study Grants

HUSTON - TILLOTSON COLLEGE
1820 E 8th St, Austin   Texas 78702
512 476-7421

Private and 4 Year
Arts Areas: Instrumental Music, Vocal Music and Visual Arts
Performing Series: Cultural Entertainment Committee Series

(continued on next page)

MUSIC

Dorothy N Cashan, Chairman   **Number Of Faculty:** 3   **Number Of Students:** 45
Degrees Offered: BA MusEd   **Teaching Certification Available**
Financial Assistance: Scholarships and Work-Study Grants

THEATRE

Number Of Faculty: 2   **Number Of Students:** 30   **Degrees Offered:** BA
Financial Assistance: Scholarships and Work-Study Grants
Performing Groups: Theatre Lab

INCARNATE WORD COLLEGE
4301 Broadway, San Antonio   Texas 78209
512 826-3292
Private and 4 Year
Arts Areas: Instrumental Music, Vocal Music, Theatre and Visual Arts

MUSIC

Sister Judith Ann Gibson, Chairman   **Number Of Faculty:** 6
Number Of Students: 40   **Degrees Offered:** BMus
Teaching Certification Available
Financial Assistance: Scholarships and Work-Study Grants
Performing Groups: College Chorale; Piano Ensemble

THEATRE

Sister Germaine Corbin, Chairman   **Number Of Faculty:** 3
Number Of Students: 30   **Degrees Offered:** BA   **Teaching Certification Available**
Financial Assistance: Scholarships and Work-Study Grants
Performing Groups: Readers Theatre; Children's Theatre

JACKSONVILLE COLLEGE
Jacksonville   Texas 75766, 214 506-2518
Private and 2 Year   **Arts Areas:** Instrumental Music and Vocal Music
Performance Facilities: College Auditorium
Courses Offered: AA Music; Individual Instruction; Tranfer Programs

KILGORE COLLEGE
1100 Broadway, Kilgore   Texas 75662
214 984-8531 Ext 229
State and 2 Year
Arts Areas: Dance, Instrumental Music, Vocal Music, Theatre and Visual Arts
Performance Facilities: Van Cliburn Auditorium; Dodson Auditorium; Faculty Lounge; Fine Arts Foyer

MUSIC

Wallace Read, Chairman   **Number Of Faculty:** 7   **Degrees Offered:** AA
Financial Assistance: Assistantships, Scholarships and Work-Study Grants
Performing Groups: Grand Chorus; Chorale; Madrigal Singers; Swing Choir; Ranger Band; Stage Band
Number Of Faculty: 2   **Degrees Offered:** AA
Financial Assistance: Assistantships, Scholarships and Work-Study Grants
Workshops/Festivals: One-Act Play Festival; One-Act Play District and Regional Contests

LAMAR UNIVERSITY
Beaumont   Texas 77710, 713 838-7121
State and 4 Year
Arts Areas: Dance, Instrumental Music, Vocal Music, Theatre and Visual Arts
Performing Series: Setzev Center Fine Arts Series; College of Fine Arts Series
Performance Facilities: University Theatre; McDonald Gymnasium

(continued on next page)

DANCE

Belle Holm, Head, Department Women's Physical Education
Number Of Faculty: 4 **Number Of Students:** 50
Performing Groups: Lamar Ballet Company; Lamar Modern and Jazz Dance Company

MUSIC

Dr George Parks, Head **Number Of Faculty:** 17 **Number Of Students:** 160
Degrees Offered: BMus; BMusEd; BS; MMus; MMusEd
Teaching Certification Available
Financial Assistance: Assistantships and Scholarships
Performing Groups: Grand Choir; Jazz Band; Symphony Orchestra; Opera Company; Concert Choir;
Symphonic Band; Marching Band; Concert Band
Workshops/Festivals: Summer High School Band Camp

THEATRE

Dr Walker James, Director of Theatre **Number Of Faculty:** 4
Number Of Students: 35 **Degrees Offered:** BS; BA
Teaching Certification Available
Financial Assistance: Assistantships and Scholarships
Performing Groups: Cardinal Theatre; Children's Theatre
Workshops/Festivals: Summer High School Drama Workshops

LAREDO JUNIOR COLLEGE
West Washington St, Laredo Texas 78040
512 724-7982
City and 2 Year
Arts Areas: Dance, Instrumental Music, Vocal Music, Theatre and Visual Arts
Performance Facilities: Kazeen College Center; Maravillo Gymnasium

MUSIC

Lura Davidson, Music Instructor **Number Of Faculty:** 2
Number Of Students: 187 **Degrees Offered:** AA
Courses Offered: Music Lit; Music Theory; Music Fundamentals
Financial Assistance: Scholarships and Work-Study Grants
Performing Groups: LJC Dance Band; Choir and Voice Ensembles; Orchesis Dance Club
Workshops/Festivals: Childrens Creative Workshop; Spring Concert of Dance; National Guild for Piano
Competition; High School Choral Clinic

THEATRE

Stanley Kielson, Speech and Drama Chairperson **Number Of Faculty:** 1
Number Of Students: 65 **Degrees Offered:** AA
Courses Offered: Introduction to Theater; Acting Techniques; Acting; Stagecraft
Financial Assistance: Scholarships and Work-Study Grants
Performing Groups: Arena Theater

LEE COLLEGE
Lee Dr & Golf St, Baytown Texas 77520
713 427-5611
City and 2 Year
Arts Areas: Instrumental Music, Vocal Music, Theatre, Film Arts and Visual Arts
Performing Series: Cultural Events Series
Performance Facilities: College Auditorium **Number Of Faculty:** 5
Degrees Offered: AA Music
Financial Assistance: Scholarships and Work-Study Grants
Performing Groups: Brass Ensemble; Percussion Ensemble; Piano Ensemble; Lee Collegians Stage Band;
Woodwind Ensemble; LEEsure Singers; College Concert Choir; Lee College Concert Band; Baytown
Community Orchestra

(continued on next page)

Number Of Faculty: 1   **Degrees Offered:** AA Drama & Speech
Financial Assistance: Scholarships and Work-Study Grants
Performing Groups: College Drama group

LON MORRIS COLLEGE
LMC Station, Jacksonville   Texas 75766
214 586-2471
Private and 2 Year
Arts Areas: Dance, Instrumental Music, Vocal Music and Theatre
Performance Facilities: College Arena; Proscenium
Dance courses are offered as part of the overall theatre curriculum

MUSIC

Robert Fordyce, Chairman   **Number Of Faculty:** 2   **Number Of Students:** 25
Degrees Offered: AA   **Courses Offered:** Voice; Piano; Organ; Direction
Financial Assistance: Scholarships and Work-Study Grants
Performing Groups: Girls' Sextet; Boys' Quartet; Stella Russell Singers; College Choir
Workshops/Festivals: Symphony and other Concerts

THEATRE

Ruth Alexander, Chairman   **Number Of Faculty:** 3   **Number Of Students:** 61
Degrees Offered: AA
Financial Assistance: Scholarships and Work-Study Grants
Performing Groups: Touring Companies; Masque & Wig Players
Workshops/Festivals: High School Contests; Student-directed One Acts

LUBBOCK CHRISTIAN COLLEGE
Lubbock   Texas 79407, 806 792-3221
Private and 4 Year
Arts Areas: Instrumental Music, Vocal Music, Theatre and Visual Arts
Performance Facilities: Moody Auditorium (1250 seats); Maddox-Pugh Educational Center
Center-in-the-Round

MUSIC

Dr Wayne Hinds, Chairman   **Number Of Faculty:** 5   **Number Of Students:** 75
Degrees Offered: BA Music   **Teaching Certification Available**
Financial Assistance: Scholarships
Performing Groups: Band; Orchestra; Piano Ensemble; Chorus; A Cappella Choir
Workshops/Festivals: Spring Festival

THEATRE

June Bearden, Chairman   **Number Of Faculty:** 3   **Number Of Students:** 50
Degrees Offered: AA; BA Speech   **Teaching Certification Available**
Financial Assistance: Scholarships
Performing Groups: La Compania (chapter of Delta Psi Omega)

MARY HARDIN - BAYLOR COLLEGE
MH-B Station, Belton   Texas 76513
817 939-5811 Ext 73
Private and 4 Year
Arts Areas: Instrumental Music, Vocal Music, Theatre and Visual Arts

MUSIC

Jerry R Hill, DME   **Number Of Faculty:** 11   **Number Of Students:** 95
Degrees Offered: BA; BFA; BS; BMus
Courses Offered: Piano; Voice; Organ; Instruments
Teaching Certification Available
Financial Assistance: Scholarships and Work-Study Grants

(continued on next page)

Performing Groups: String Ensemble; Brass Ensemble; Stage Band; Vocal Ensemble; Master Choir
Workshops/Festivals: Piano Workshop; Choir Camp; Church Music Camp; Choral Clinic

THEATRE

Charles G Taylor, Assistant Professor   *Number Of Faculty:* 1
Number Of Students: 10   *Degrees Offered:* BA; BFA
Financial Assistance: Scholarships and Work-Study Grants
Performing Groups: Alpha Psi Omega
Workshops/Festivals: American College Theatre Association; Interscholastic Forensics Tournament; High School Invitational Forensics; Area One-Act Play Contest (High School)

MCLENNAN COMMUNITY COLLEGE
1400 College Dr, Waco   Texas 76708
817 756-6551
County and 2 Year
Arts Areas: Instrumental Music, Vocal Music, Theatre and Visual Arts
Performance Facilities: Theatre; Student Center

MUSIC

Bill Haskett, Chairman, Fine Arts Department
Number Of Faculty: 6 Full-time, 6 Part-time   *Number Of Students:* 100
Degrees Offered: AA
Courses Offered: Concert Band; Improvisation; Stage Band; Ensemble; Class Piano; Theory; Basic Music; Fundamentals for Music Teachers; Music Literature; Recital; Italian; French and German Diction; Choir; Applied Music
Financial Assistance: Scholarships and Work-Study Grants
Performing Groups: The McLennan Singers; Concert Band; Stage Bands; Brass, Percussion, Voice, Jazz and Woodwind Ensembles
Workshops/Festivals: Solo and Ensemble; Instrumental, Choral, Piano and Stage Band Competition for area public schools

THEATRE

James Henderson, Instructor of Drama   *Number Of Faculty:* 1
Number Of Students: 25   *Degrees Offered:* AA
Courses Offered: Rehersal; Performance; Theatre Workshop; Voice; Interpretation; Acting; Technical Production; World of Drama; Stage Production; Costume; Set Design and Construction

---

MCMURRY COLLEGE
S 14th & Sayles Blvd, Abilene   Texas 79605
915 692-4130 Ext 295
Private and 4 Year
Arts Areas: Instrumental Music, Vocal Music and Theatre
Performing Series: College Series
Performance Facilities: Radford Auditorium; Recital Hall; Moody Theater

MUSIC

David S Blackburn, Chairman   *Number Of Faculty:* 10
Number Of Students: 85   *Degrees Offered:* BMus; BA; BMusEd
Teaching Certification Available
Financial Assistance: Scholarships and Work-Study Grants
Performing Groups: Chapel Choir; Chanters Concert Choir; Morning Star; Concert Band; Jazz Ensemble
Workshops/Festivals: Opera Workshop

THEATRE

Kim Stone, Chairman   *Number Of Faculty:* 2   *Number Of Students:* 35
Degrees Offered: BA; BS   *Teaching Certification Available*
Financial Assistance: Scholarships and Work-Study Grants
Workshops/Festivals: UIL Sponsor & Theater Workshop

MIDLAND COLLEGE
3600 N Garfield, Midland   Texas 79701
915 684-7851 Ext 180
  2 Year
  Arts Areas: Instrumental Music, Vocal Music, Theatre, Television and Visual Arts
  Performance Facilities: Midland Community Theatre; Academic/Fine Arts Complex

MUSIC

Robert J LaFontaine, Music Director
Number Of Faculty: 2 Full-time, 6 Part-time   *Number Of Students:* 160
Degrees Offered: AA
Financial Assistance: Scholarships and Work-Study Grants
Performing Groups: Chamber Singers; Choir; Glee Clubs; Band; Wind Ensemble; Opera Workshop
Workshops/Festivals: Spring Fine Arts Festival   *Number Of Faculty:* 2

MIDWESTERN STATE UNIVERSITY
3400 Taft Blvd, Wichita Falls   Texas 76308
817 692-6611
  State and 4 Year
  Arts Areas: Instrumental Music, Vocal Music, Theatre and Visual Arts
  Performing Series: Artist - Lecture Series
  Performance Facilities: Arena Theatre; Proscenium Theatre; Band Hall; Recital Hall; Fine Arts Theatre

MUSIC

Don Maxwell, Chairman   *Number Of Faculty:* 16   *Number Of Students:* 750
Degrees Offered: BMusEd; BMus; BA; MMusEd; MMus
Courses Offered: Instrumental Music; Piano; Vocal; Composition
Teaching Certification Available
Financial Assistance: Assistantships, Scholarships and Work-Study Grants
Performing Groups: University Band; University Stage Band; Jazz Ensemble; University Choir; University Chorale; University Symphony Orchestra
Workshops/Festivals: Summer Band Camp

THEATRE

June E Kable, Chairman   *Number Of Faculty:* 6   *Number Of Students:* 120
Degrees Offered: BA; BS Ed; MA
Courses Offered: Acting; Directing; Costume Construction; Scene Design and Construction; Make-up
Teaching Certification Available
Financial Assistance: Assistantships, Scholarships and Work-Study Grants
Performing Groups: Repertory Theatre; Midwestern State University Theatre

MOUNTAIN VIEW COLLEGE
4849 W Illinois Ave, Dallas   Texas 75211
214 746-4132
  County and 2 Year
  Arts Areas: Dance, Instrumental Music, Vocal Music, Theatre and Visual Arts
  Performing Series: Recital Series
  Performance Facilities: Mountain View College Performance Hall; Mountain View College Arena Theatre

DANCE

Jane Quetin, Chairman   *Number Of Faculty:* 1   *Number Of Students:* 15
Degrees Offered: AA   *Financial Assistance:* Work-Study Grants
Performing Groups: Concert Dancers   *Workshops/Festivals:* Dance Concert

MUSIC

Mark Hettle, Chairman   *Number Of Faculty:* 15   *Number Of Students:* 80
Degrees Offered: AA

(continued on next page)

Financial Assistance: Scholarships and Work-Study Grants
Performing Groups: Lab Bands; Symphonic Wind Ensemble; Brass Quintet; Mixed Ensemble; Male Ensemble; Female Ensemble; Choir
Workshops/Festivals: Jazz Festival; Comprehensive Musicianship Workshop; Piano Solo Competition; Piano Concerto Competition; Original Student Composition Competition

THEATRE

Rod Wilson, Chairman   **Number Of Faculty:** 3   **Number Of Students:** 40
Degrees Offered: AA   **Technical Training:** Lights; Sound
Financial Assistance: Work-Study Grants
Workshops/Festivals: High School One-Act Play Festival

NAVARRO COLLEGE
Highway 31 W, Corsicana   Texas 75110
214 874-6501 Ext 264
County and 2 Year
Arts Areas: Instrumental Music, Vocal Music, Theatre, Television and Visual Arts
Performance Facilities: Beene Music Hall; Leighton B Dawson Auditorium

MUSIC

Frank Sargent, Chairman, Department of Music   **Number Of Faculty:** 3
Number Of Students: 115   **Degrees Offered:** AA
Courses Offered: Theory; Music Appreciation; Music Literature; Music Education
Technical Training: Instrumental; Keyboard; Vocal
Financial Assistance: Scholarships and Work-Study Grants
Performing Groups: Marching Band; Concert Band; Lab Band; College Choir; Chamber Singers; Community Chorus
Workshops/Festivals: Homecoming Marching Band Festival

NORTH TEXAS STATE UNIVERSITY
Denton   Texas 76203, 817 788-2477
State and 4 Year
Arts Areas: Dance, Instrumental Music, Vocal Music, Theatre, Film Arts, Television and Visual Arts
Performance Facilities: Coliseum; University Theater; Music Recital Hall; Main Auditorium

DANCE

Dr Irma Caton, Director   **Number Of Faculty:** 4   **Number Of Students:** 40
Degrees Offered: BS; MS   **Courses Offered:** Technique; Theory; Composition
Technical Training: Ballet; Modern; Jazz; Tap; Social; Folk; Square
Teaching Certification Available
Financial Assistance: Graduate Assistantships
Performing Groups: University Dance Company; Dance Theatre of the Southwest - Professional

MUSIC

Marceau C Myers, Dean   **Number Of Faculty:** 80   **Number Of Students:** 1500
Degrees Offered: BMus; BA; MMus; MMusEd; DMA; PhD
Courses Offered: Band; Choir; Applied; Jazz; Literature; Theory; Teaching of Music; Church Music; Voice
Technical Training: Instrument Repair   **Teaching Certification Available**
Financial Assistance: Assistantships, Scholarships and Work-Study Grants
Performing Groups: Music Laboratory; A Cappella Choir; Chapel Choir; Men's Chorus; Women's Chorus; Grand Chorus; Symphony Orchestra; Symphonic Wind Ensemble; Concert Band; Marching Band; University

THEATRE

Imogene Dickey, Acting Director   **Number Of Faculty:** 4
Number Of Students: 150   **Degrees Offered:** BA; MA; MS
Courses Offered: Acting; History of the Theatre; Readers Theatre; Speech

(continued on next page)

Technical Training: Make-up; Costuming; Stagecraft; Lighting; Design; Scenic Design; Production Design
Teaching Certification Available
Financial Assistance: Assistantships, Scholarships and Work-Study Grants
Performing Groups: University Players; Alpha Psi Omega; Summer Repertory Company

ODESSA COLLEGE
PO Box 3752, Odessa   Texas 79760
915 337-5381

City/County 2 Year   **Arts Areas:** Instrumental Music and Vocal Music
Performing Series: Fine Arts Series
Performance Facilities: Odessa College Auditorium; Odessa College Theatre

DANCE

Pat Martin, Chairman   **Number Of Faculty:** 1   **Number Of Students:** 15
Financial Assistance: Scholarships and Work-Study Grants

MUSIC

Jack W Hendrix, Chairman   **Number Of Faculty:** 10   **Number Of Students:** 55
Degrees Offered: AA
Courses Offered: Reed Making; Prep Theory; Prep Applied Music
Technical Training: Applied Music
Financial Assistance: Scholarships and Work-Study Grants
Performing Groups: A Cappella Choir; Madrigals; Symphonic Wind Ensemble; Concert Band; Recorder
Consort; Vocal and Instrumental Ensembles
Workshops/Festivals: Jr High Choir; Sr High Choral; Band

THEATRE

Wally Jackson, Chairman   **Number Of Faculty:** 2   **Number Of Students:** 25
Degrees Offered: AA
Financial Assistance: Scholarships and Work-Study Grants
Performing Groups: Drama Productions; Annual Musical Production
Workshops/Festivals: UIL Workshops; Recruiting Workshops

OUR LADY OF THE LAKE COLLEGE
411 SW 24th St, San Antonio   Texas 78207
512 434-6711

Private and 4 Year
Arts Areas: Instrumental Music, Vocal Music, Theatre and Visual Arts

MUSIC

Jule Adele Espey, Chairman   **Number Of Faculty:** 8   **Number Of Students:** 28
Degrees Offered: BMus; BMusEd; BA Music   **Teaching Certification Available**
Financial Assistance: Scholarships and Work-Study Grants

THEATRE

Richard Slocum, Chairman   **Number Of Faculty:** 7   **Number Of Students:** 98
Teaching Certification Available
Financial Assistance: Scholarships and Work-Study Grants

PAN AMERICAN UNIVERSITY
Edinburg   Texas 78539, 512 381-3471

State and 4 Year
Arts Areas: Instrumental Music, Vocal Music, Theatre, Film Arts, Television and Visual Arts
Performance Facilities: Fine Arts Auditorium; LRC Auditorium

DANCE

Dance program under auspices of Physical Education Department
Technical Training: Folk; Square Dance; Modern Dance; Dances of Latin America

(continued on next page)

MUSIC

Dean R Carty, Head   **Number Of Faculty:** 15   **Number Of Students:** 200
Degrees Offered: BA   **Teaching Certification Available**
Financial Assistance: Scholarships and Work-Study Grants
Performing Groups: Concert Band; Choir; Orchestra; Stage Band; Chamber Music Group
Workshops/Festivals: Opera Workshop

THEATRE

Marian Monta, Head   **Number Of Faculty:** 15   **Number Of Students:** 180
Degrees Offered: BA   **Teaching Certification Available**
Financial Assistance: Scholarships and Work-Study Grants
Workshops/Festivals: Summer Theatre Workshop (PASS)

PANOLA JUNIOR COLLEGE
Carthage   Texas 75633, 214 693-3836
State and 2 Year
Arts Areas: Instrumental Music, Vocal Music and Theatre
Performance Facilities: Q M Martin Auditorium

MUSIC

Robert Reid, Chairman   **Number Of Faculty:** 2   **Degrees Offered:** AA
Financial Assistance: Scholarships and Work-Study Grants
Performing Groups: Stage Band; Choir; Select Singers (Pipers)

THEATRE

Maxine Christian, Chairman   **Number Of Faculty:** 1   **Degrees Offered:** AA
Financial Assistance: Scholarships and Work-Study Grants

PARIS JUNIOR COLLEGE
2400 Clarksville, Paris   Texas 75460
214 785-7661
2 Year and District
Arts Areas: Instrumental Music, Vocal Music, Theatre and Visual Arts
Performance Facilities: Paris Junior College Theatre for the Performing Arts; Henry P Mayer Center for the Musical Arts

MUSIC

Charles Stephens, Music Department Coordinator   **Number Of Faculty:** 3
Number Of Students: 80   **Degrees Offered:** AA
Courses Offered: Applied Music; Voice; Theory; Music Literature; Appreciation; Workshop; Instrumental Ensemble; Jazz Ensemble; Chorus; Madrigals; Music for Public School Teachers
Financial Assistance: Scholarships, Work-Study Grants and BEOG
Performing Groups: Madrigal Singers; College Chorale; CIvic Chorus; Instrumental Ensemble
Workshops/Festivals: Fine Arts Festival

THEATRE

Ray Karrer, Chairman   **Number Of Faculty:** 2   **Number Of Students:** 25
Degrees Offered: AA
Courses Offered: Introduction to Theatre; Acting; Stagecraft; Voice; Make-up
Technical Training: Stagecraft; Make-up; Production
Financial Assistance: Scholarships and Work-Study Grants
Performing Groups: Le Troupe   **Workshops/Festivals:** Fine Arts Festival

---

PAUL QUINN COLLEGE
Waco   Texas 75704, 817 753-8081
Private and 4 Year   **Arts Areas:** Vocal Music, Theatre and Visual Arts
Performance Facilities: George B Young Auditorium   **Number Of Faculty:** 1

(continued on next page)

Number Of Students: 30
Financial Assistance: Scholarships and Work-Study Grants
Performing Groups: Choir

PRAIRIE VIEW AGRICULTURAL & MECHANICAL COLLEGE
Prairie View   Texas 77445, 713 857-3311

State and 4 Year   **Arts Areas:** Theatre   **Number Of Faculty:** 7
Number Of Students: 154   **Degrees Offered:** BA; BMus; MA; MMus
Teaching Certification Available
Financial Assistance: Scholarships and Work-Study Grants
Workshops/Festivals: Annual Music Workshop

RANGER JUNIOR COLLEGE
Ranger   Texas 76470, 817 647-3234

City and 2 Year
Arts Areas: Instrumental Music, Vocal Music, Theatre and Visual Arts

MUSIC

R B Goleman, Chairman   **Number Of Faculty:** 2   **Number Of Students:** 38
Degrees Offered: AA
Financial Assistance: Scholarships and Work-Study Grants
Performing Groups: Concert Choir; Marching Band; Symphonic Band; Stage Band; Collegiate Singers
Courses Offered: Introduction to Theatre, Acting

RICE UNIVERSITY
6100 S Main, Houston   Texas 77001
713 527-8101

Private and 4 Year
Arts Areas: Instrumental Music, Vocal Music, Theatre and Visual Arts
Performing Series: Music Artist Series; Friends of Music Chamber Series
Performance Facilities: Hamman Hall

MUSIC

Samuel Jones, Dean   **Number Of Faculty:** 29   **Number Of Students:** 100
Degrees Offered: BMus; MMus
Courses Offered: Instrumental Music; Composition; History; Theory; Conducting; Vocal Music
Financial Assistance: Assistantships, Scholarships and Work-Study Grants
Performing Groups: Orchestra; Rice Chorale; The Shepherd Quartet; Faculty Brass Quintet; Woodwind Ensemble; Faculty Woodwind Trio

THEATRE

Neil Havens, Chairman   **Number Of Faculty:** 2   **Number Of Students:** 20
Courses Offered: Introduction to Theatre
Financial Assistance: Assistantships, Scholarships and Work-Study Grants
Performing Groups: The Rice Players
Artists-In-Residence/Guest Artists: Richard Lert; Eudice Shapiro; Frances Bible; Richard Brown; Wayne Crouse; Paul Ellison; Raphael Fliegel; Mary Norris; Ronald Patterson; Albert Tipton; Shirley Trepel; Eric Arbiter; Michael Pickar; Thomas Bacon; Mack Guderian; David Waters; Warren Deck; Beatrice Rose

---

RICHLAND COLLEGE
12800 Abrams Rd, Dallas   Texas 75081
214 746-4550

County and 2 Year
Arts Areas: Dance, Instrumental Music, Vocal Music and Theatre
Performing Series: Community Services Concert Series
Performance Facilities: Performance Hall; Arena Theater

(continued on next page)

DANCE

Phyllis Barger, Instructor   **Number Of Faculty:** 1   **Number Of Students:** 35
Degrees Offered: AA   **Courses Offered:** Beginning Dance for Theater
Financial Assistance: Work-Study Grants

MUSIC

Jerry Wallace, Instructor   **Number Of Faculty:** 22
Number Of Students: 1200   **Degrees Offered:** AA
Courses Offered: Literature; Appreciation; Theory; Fundamentals; Composition; Applied Music; Diction
Technical Training: Theory and Composition; Applied - Instrumental and Vocal
Financial Assistance: Scholarships and Work-Study Grants
Performing Groups: Concert Band; Concert Choir; Stage Band; Select Choir; Madrigals; Brass; Wind; Percussion
Workshops/Festivals: Choral and Instrumental Festival

THEATRE

Bob Dyer, Instructor   **Number Of Faculty:** 9   **Number Of Students:** 200
Degrees Offered: AA
Courses Offered: Voice & Articulation; Scene Study; Light Design; Costume History; History of Theater; Introduction to Theater; Stage-craft; Make-up; Acting; Movement

---

SAINT EDWARDS UNIVERSITY
3001 S Congress, Austin   Texas 78704
512 444-2621

Private and 4 Year
Arts Areas: Instrumental Music, Vocal Music, Theatre and Visual Arts
Performance Facilities: Mary Moody Theatre for the Performing Arts

MUSIC

J P Morgan, Chairman   **Number Of Faculty:** 2   **Number Of Students:** 130
Degrees Offered: Applied, Voice, Piano; Choir; Music for Classroom Teachers
Financial Assistance: Scholarships and Work-Study Grants
Performing Groups: Hilltopper Choir; Omni Singers

THEATRE

Edward Mangam, Chairman   **Number Of Faculty:** 2   **Number Of Students:** 30
Degrees Offered: BA Theatre Arts
Financial Assistance: Scholarships and Work-Study Grants

SAINT MARY'S UNIVERSITY
One Camino Santa Maria, San Antonio   Texas 78284
512 436-3011

Private and 4 Year
Arts Areas: Instrumental Music, Vocal Music, Theatre, Film Arts and Visual Arts
Performance Facilities: Shoestring Cellar; Reinbolt Hall; Continuing Education Center Auditorium

MUSIC

John Moore, Assistant Professor of Music   **Number Of Faculty:** 10
Number Of Students: 190   **Degrees Offered:** BA Mus; BA MusEd
Teaching Certification Available
Financial Assistance: Scholarships and Work-Study Grants
Performing Groups: Choral Ensemble; Stage Band; Brass Ensemble; Woodwind Ensemble; Dixieland Combo

THEATRE

Dr Charles Myler, Chairman   **Number Of Faculty:** 1   **Number Of Students:** 12
Degrees Offered: BA   **Teaching Certification Available**

(continued on next page)

Financial Assistance: Scholarships and Work-Study Grants
Performing Groups: The Shoestring Players

SAINT PHILLIPS COLLEGE
2111 Nevada St, San Antonio   Texas 78203
512 532-4211
County and 2 Year
Arts Areas: Instrumental Music, Vocal Music and Theatre
Performing Series: Concert - Lecture Series
Performance Facilities: College Auditorium   **Degrees Offered:** AA Music
Degrees Offered: AA Drama

UNIVERSITY OF SAINT THOMAS
3812 Montrose Blvd, Houston   Texas 77006
713 522-7911
Private and 4 Year
Arts Areas: Instrumental Music, Vocal Music, Theatre and Film Arts
Performance Facilities: Jones Theatre; Jones Hall

MUSIC

Edgar Martin, Chairman   **Number Of Faculty:** 11   **Degrees Offered:** BMus; BA
Financial Assistance: Scholarships and Work-Study Grants
Performing Groups: The University Singers; Jazz Ensemble; Woodwind Quintet; The Chamber Singers; Brass Ensemble; Litergical Music Ensemble; Guitar Ensemble; New Music Ensemble
Workshops/Festivals: Music at Noon; Spring Scholarship Festival; Evening Concerts

THEATRE

Sam Havens, Chairman   **Number Of Faculty:** 4   **Degrees Offered:** BA Drama
Financial Assistance: Scholarships and Work-Study Grants

SAM HOUSTON STATE UNIVERSITY
Sam Houston Ave, Huntsville   Texas 77341
713 295-6211 Ext 2968
State and 4 Year
Arts Areas: Dance, Instrumental Music, Vocal Music, Theatre, Television and Visual Arts
Performance Facilities: Main Stage; Showcase Theatre; Recital Halls; Old Main Auditorium; University Coliseum

DANCE

Dr Mary Ella Montague, Chairman   **Number Of Faculty:** 3
Number Of Students: 321   **Degrees Offered:** BA Ed; BA
Courses Offered: Tap; Jazz; Ballet; Social; Ballroom; Modern; Folk; Square
Technical Training: Lighting; Costuming; Set Design
Teaching Certification Available   **Financial Assistance:** Work-Study Grants
Performing Groups: The Sam Houston Performing Dance Group
Workshops/Festivals: The Fine Arts Symposium; High School Dance Symposium; Annual Concert

MUSIC

Dr Fisher Tull, Chairman   **Number Of Faculty:** 33   **Number Of Students:** 400
Degrees Offered: BMusEd; BMus; MA; MMusEd
Courses Offered: Conducting; Percussion; Strings; Improvisation; Pedagogy; Piano; Theory; Musicianship; Elements of Jazz Arranging; Junior Composition; Style Analysis; Seminar in Composition; History; Impressionistic Harmony; Music Appreciation; Opera Literature
Teaching Certification Available
Financial Assistance: Internships, Assistantships, Scholarships and Work-Study Grants
Performing Groups: A Cappella Choir; Women's Chorus; Band; Jazz Band; Symphony Orchestra; Madrigal Singers; Grand Chorus; Brass Choir; Singing Men; Opera Workshop
Workshops/Festivals: High School Competitions; Contemporary Music Festival; Jazz Festival; Band Camp; Drum Major Camp

(continued on next page)

THEATRE

Dr James Miller, Chairman, Speech and Drama   *Number Of Faculty:* 6
Number Of Students: 130   *Degrees Offered:* BFA; BA Ed; BA
Courses Offered: Introduction to Theatre; Make-up; Theatre Speech; History of Costume; History of Theatre; Scene Design; Lighting; Play Directing
Teaching Certification Available
Financial Assistance: Internships, Assistantships, Scholarships and Work-Study Grants
Workshops/Festivals: Theatre Workshops; UIL Workshops

SAN ANTONIO COLLEGE
1300 San Pedro Ave, San Antonio   Texas 78284
512 734-5381
City and 2 Year
Arts Areas: Instrumental Music, Vocal Music, Theatre, Film Arts, Television and Visual Arts
Courses Offered: Modern Dance; Folk Dance; Ballroom Dancing

MUSIC

Dr Marjorie T Walthan, Chairman   *Degrees Offered:* AA
Technical Training: Church Music
Financial Assistance: Scholarships and Work-Study Grants
Performing Groups: College Choir; A Cappella Choir; Madrigal Singers; Vocal Ensembles; Chorus; Instrumental Ensembles; Orchestra
Workshops/Festivals: Summer Music Workshop

THEATRE

Reinhold Lucke, Chairman   *Degrees Offered:* AA
Financial Assistance: Scholarships and Work-Study Grants
Performing Groups: College Theatre

SAN JACINTO COLLEGE
Spencer Hwy, Pasadena   Texas 77505
713 479-1501
2 Year and District
Arts Areas: Dance, Instrumental Music, Vocal Music, Theatre and Film Arts
Performance Facilities: Auditorium; Studios; Library

DANCE

Dorothy Brown, Chairman   *Number Of Faculty:* 9   *Number Of Students:* 600
Degrees Offered: AA; AS   *Financial Assistance:* Work-Study Grants and BEOG

MUSIC

Joyce Ghormley, Chairman   *Number Of Faculty:* 5   *Degrees Offered:* AA; AS
Financial Assistance: Scholarships, Work-Study Grants and BEOG

THEATRE

Jerry Powell, Chairman   *Number Of Faculty:* 5   *Number Of Students:* 400
Degrees Offered: AA; AS

SAN JACINTO COLLEGE, NORTH
5800 Uvalde, Houston   Texas 77049
713 458-4050
State and 2 Year
Arts Areas: Dance, Instrumental Music, Vocal Music and Theatre
Performance Facilities: Gym; Lecture Auditorium

DANCE

Dr Maymo Lewis, Chairman, Women's Physical Education   *Number Of Faculty:* 1

(continued on next page)

Number Of Students: 40   **Courses Offered:** Jazz; Tap; Modern Dance
Financial Assistance: Usual forms of student financial aid

MUSIC

Timothy Fleming, Chairman   **Number Of Faculty:** 3   **Number Of Students:** 35
Degrees Offered: AA
Courses Offered: Theory; Ear Training; Choir; Music Literature; Music Fundamentals; Piano; Voice
Financial Assistance: Scholarships and Usual forms of student financial aid
Number Of Faculty: 1   **Degrees Offered:** AA
Courses Offered: Acting; Theatre; Oral Interpretation; Diction

---

SCHREINER COLLEGE
PO Box 4498, Kerrville   Texas 78028
512 896-5411 Ext 11
Private and 2 Year
Arts Areas: Dance, Instrumental Music, Vocal Music, Theatre and Visual Arts

DANCE

Nursel Conrad, Instructor   **Number Of Faculty:** 1   **Number Of Students:** 38
Courses Offered: Ballet
Financial Assistance: Scholarships and Work-Study Grants

MUSIC

Janet Weatherhogg, Instructor   **Number Of Faculty:** 2
Courses Offered: Music Appreciation; Applied; Voice; Choir
Financial Assistance: Scholarships

THEATRE

Claudia Latimer, Instructor   **Number Of Faculty:** 1
Courses Offered: Speech; Drama; Theatre History; Acting
Financial Assistance: Work-Study Grants

SOUTH PLAINS COLLEGE
Levelland   Texas 79336, 806 894-4921 Ext 241
2 Year
Arts Areas: Instrumental Music, Vocal Music, Theatre and Country-Western
Performance Facilities: College Auditorium; Stadium
Courses Offered: Modern Jazz; Folk and Square Dancing; Modern Dance
Dance classes taught under auspices of Physical Education Department
Financial Assistance: Scholarships and Work-Study Grants

MUSIC

Harley Bulls, Chairman   **Number Of Faculty:** 5   **Number Of Students:** 252
Degrees Offered: AA
Courses Offered: Theory; Diction; Literature; Instruments; Country Instruments
Financial Assistance: Scholarships and Work-Study Grants
Performing Groups: Stage Band; Concert Band; Country/Bluegrass Bands; Vocal Ensembles
Workshops/Festivals: Country/Bluegrass Festival

THEATRE

Helen Starr Roberts, Associate Professor   **Number Of Faculty:** 2
Number Of Students: 89   **Degrees Offered:** AA
Courses Offered: Speech; Voice & Articulation; Debate; Oral Interpretation

SOUTH TEXAS JUNIOR COLLEGE
1 Main St, Houston   Texas 77002
713 225-1651

Private and 2 Year   *Arts Areas:* Theatre
Performing Series: Cultural Events Series
Performance Facilities: College Auditorium

THEATRE

Jack Carrol, Chairman   *Performing Groups:* Drama Group

SOUTHERN METHODIST UNIVERSITY
Meadows School of the Arts, Dallas   Texas 75275
214 692-2600

Private and 4 Year
Arts Areas: Dance, Instrumental Music, Vocal Music, Theatre, Film Arts, Television and Visual Arts
Performing Series: League of Professional Theatre Training Schools
Performance Facilities: Bob Hope Theatre; Margo Jones Theatre; Caruth Concert Hall

DANCE

Toni Beck, Chairman   *Number Of Faculty:* 6   *Number Of Students:* 50
Degrees Offered: BFA; MFA
Technical Training: Dance Therapy; Ethnic Dance; Dance Education
Financial Assistance: Internships, Assistantships, Scholarships and Work-Study Grants

MUSIC

Thayne Tolle, Chairman   *Number Of Faculty:* 35   *Number Of Students:* 275
Degrees Offered: BMus; MMus; MSM
Technical Training: Music Therapy; Music Education   *Teaching Certification Available*
Financial Assistance: Internships, Assistantships, Scholarships and Work-Study Grants
Performing Groups: Dallas String Quartet; Dallas Brass Quintet; Dallas Woodwind Ensemble
Workshops/Festivals: Music Education Workshop; Music Camp Workshop; Organ Workshop; Guitar Workshop; Piano Workshop

THEATRE

Number Of Faculty: 14   *Number Of Students:* 100   *Degrees Offered:* BFA; MFA
Technical Training: Arts Administration; Musical Comedy
Teaching Certification Available
Financial Assistance: Internships, Assistantships, Scholarships and Work-Study Grants
Workshops/Festivals: Directors' Colloquium annually; European Theatre Study annually

SOUTHWEST TEXAS JUNIOR COLLEGE
Uvalde   Texas 78801, 512 278-5634

County and 2 Year
Arts Areas: Instrumental Music, Vocal Music and Theatre
Performance Facilities: Imogen Tate Auditorium

MUSIC

Joe Silva, Music Director   *Number Of Faculty:* 1   *Number Of Students:* 40
Degrees Offered: AA   *Courses Offered:* Instrumental Music; Choral Music
Financial Assistance: Scholarships and Work-Study Grants
Performing Groups: Campus Band; Mixed Chorus

THEATRE

Joan Johnson, Director of Theatre   *Number Of Faculty:* 1
Number Of Students: 40   *Degrees Offered:* AA
Financial Assistance: Scholarships and Work-Study Grants
Performing Groups: Palm Players

SOUTHWEST TEXAS STATE UNIVERSITY
San Marcos   Texas 78666, 512 245-2308

State and 4 Year
Arts Areas: Dance, Instrumental Music, Vocal Music, Theatre and Visual Arts
Performing Series: University Arts Series
Performance Facilities: Evans Auditorium; Main Theatre

DANCE

Dr Theodore Keck, Chairman Health and Physical Education
Number Of Faculty: 3   *Number Of Students:* 65
Degrees Offered: BS Ed - Dance Concentration
Teaching Certification Available   *Financial Assistance:* Work-Study Grants
Workshops/Festivals: Summer Dance Workshop

MUSIC

Dr Arlis Hiebert, Chairman   *Number Of Faculty:* 25
Number Of Students: 220   *Degrees Offered:* BMus; BMusEd; MEd
Teaching Certification Available
Financial Assistance: Assistantships, Scholarships and Work-Study Grants
Performing Groups: Band; Orchestra; Choir; Stage Band; Music Theatre; Madrigals; Ensembles
Workshops/Festivals: Summer Band Camp; Music Education Workshop; Pianist's Workshop

THEATRE

Dr John Clifford, Director of Theatre   *Number Of Faculty:* 12
Number Of Students: 140   *Degrees Offered:* BFA; BA; BS Ed; MA
Technical Training: Stagecraft   *Teaching Certification Available*
Financial Assistance: Assistantships, Scholarships and Work-Study Grants
Workshops/Festivals: Technical Theatre Workshops; High School Drama Workshop; SW Theatre
Conference

SOUTHWESTERN ADVENTIST COLLEGE
Keene   Texas 76059, 817 645-8811

Private and 4 Year
Arts Areas: Instrumental Music, Vocal Music and Television

MUSIC

Dr Richard J White, Chairman of Fine Arts Department   *Number Of Faculty:* 7
Number Of Students: 165   *Degrees Offered:* BA; BS; BMus
Courses Offered: Theory; Music Education; Music History and Literature; Applied Music; Ensembles
Teaching Certification Available
Financial Assistance: Scholarships and Work-Study Grants
Performing Groups: Concert Choir; Concert Band; Brass Ensemble
Workshops/Festivals: Annual Music Festival

SOUTHWESTERN ASSEMBLEY OF GOD COLLEGE
1200 Sycamore St, Waxahachie   Texas 75165
214 937-4010

Private and 4 Year
Arts Areas: Instrumental Music, Vocal Music and Theatre
Degrees Offered: BS Church Music; BS Mus
Financial Assistance: Work-Study Grants

SOUTHWESTERN BAPTIST THEOLOGICAL SEMINARY
PO Box 22,000, Fort Worth   Texas 76122
817 923-1921 Ext 311

Private and Graduate
Arts Areas: Instrumental Music, Vocal Music and Church Music
Performance Facilities: Reynolds Auditorium; Truett Auditorium

(continued on next page)

MUSIC

James C McKinney, Dean, School of Church Music   **Number Of Faculty:** 22
Number Of Students: 319   **Degrees Offered:** M Church Mus; MM; DMus Arts
Financial Assistance: Assistantships and Scholarships
Performing Groups: Brass Ensemble; String Ensemble; Woodwind Ensemble; Handbell Choir; Collegium Musicum; Consort Singers; Men's Chorus; Southwestern Singers; Oratorio Chorus; Chapel Choir; Seminary Choir; Opera Workshop
Workshops/Festivals: Southwestern Church Music Workshop

SOUTHWESTERN CHRISTIAN COLLEGE
Terrell   Texas 75160, 214 563-3341
Private and 2 Year   **Arts Areas:** Theatre

MUSIC

A Hugh Granam, Chairman
Performing Groups: Chorale Club; A Cappella Chorus; College Chorus; Local & Instrumental Ensembles

---

SOUTHWESTERN UNIVERSITY AT GEORGETOWN
Georgetown   Texas 38626, 512 863-6511 Ext 329
Private and 4 Year
Arts Areas: Instrumental Music, Vocal Music, Theatre, Television and Visual Arts
Performing Series: The Artist Series
Performance Facilities: Alma Thomas Theatre; Cullen Auditorium; Fine Arts Recital Hall; Lois Perkins Chapel

MUSIC

Ellsworth Peterson, Chairman   **Number Of Faculty:** 9½
Number Of Students: 85   **Degrees Offered:** BMus; BMusEd
Courses Offered: Sacred Music; Applied Music; Music Literature
Teaching Certification Available
Financial Assistance: Internships, Assistantships, Scholarships and Work-Study Grants
Performing Groups: Southwestern Singers; Choir; Extraordinaires; Concert Band; Sinfonietta; Stage Band
Workshops/Festivals: Summer Choral Institute; Opera Theatre; Summer Piano Clinic

THEATRE

Angus Springer, Chairman   **Number Of Faculty:** 3   **Number Of Students:** 26
Degrees Offered: BFA; BA; BS   **Courses Offered:** Theater/Speech
Teaching Certification Available
Financial Assistance: Internships, Assistantships, Scholarships and Work-Study Grants
Performing Groups: Mask & Wig Players
Artists-In-Residence/Guest Artists: Drusilla Huffmaster, Artist in Residence

---

STEPHEN F AUSTIN STATE UNIVERSITY
Nacogdoches   Texas 75962, 713 569-2801
State and 4 Year
Arts Areas: Dance, Instrumental Music, Vocal Music, Theatre, Television and Radio
Performing Series: Fine Arts Series
Performance Facilities: Fine Arts Auditorium; Kennedy Auditorium; Coliseum

DANCE

Margeann McMillan, Dance Department Head   **Number Of Faculty:** 3
Number Of Students: 200   **Degrees Offered:** BA and BS in Physical Education
Courses Offered: Modern; Ballet; Folk   **Teaching Certification Available**
Financial Assistance: Internships, Assistantships and Work-Study Grants
Performing Groups: SFA Dancers

(continued on next page)

MUSIC

Robert Blocker, Music Department Head   **Number Of Faculty:** 21
Number Of Students: 275   **Degrees Offered:** BMus; BFA; MA
Courses Offered: Applied Music; Music Theory; History
Teaching Certification Available
Financial Assistance: Internships, Assistantships, Scholarships and Work-Study Grants
Performing Groups: A Cappella Choir; Orchestra; Band; Grand Chorus; Jazz Band; Brass Quintet;
Percussion Ensemble; Chamber Orchestra; Brass Choir
Workshops/Festivals: Jazz Festival; Elementary Music Workshop; Band Camp

THEATRE

Tom Heino, Head, Department of Theater   **Number Of Faculty:** 5
Number Of Students: 140   **Degrees Offered:** BFA; MA
Courses Offered: Acting; Tech; Theater; Costuming; Lighting
Teaching Certification Available
Financial Assistance: Internships, Assistantships, Scholarships and Work-Study Grants
Performing Groups: Summer Theater; Actors Workshop; SFA Players
Workshops/Festivals: Theater Workshop; Children's Theater; Technical Workshop

---

SUL ROSS STATE UNIVERSITY
Alpine   Texas 79830, 715 837-3461 Ext 256
State and 4 Year
Arts Areas: Instrumental Music, Vocal Music, Theatre, Television and Visual Arts
Performance Facilities: Large Theatre; Little Theatre; Outdoor Theatre

MUSIC

Samuel E Davis, Chairman   **Number Of Faculty:** 5   **Number Of Students:** 300
Degrees Offered: BA; BMus; BMusEd; MEd
Courses Offered: Ensembles; Theory; History; Applied
Teaching Certification Available
Financial Assistance: Assistantships, Scholarships and Work-Study Grants
Performing Groups: Concert Choir; University Chorus; Vocal Ensemble; Orchestra; Concert Band;
Marching Band; Stage Band
Workshops/Festivals: Summer High School Band Camp and Choir Camp

THEATRE

George Bradley, Chairman   **Number Of Faculty:** 3   **Number Of Students:** 50
Degrees Offered: BA; BA Ed
Courses Offered: Acting; Costume; Design; Playwriting; History
Teaching Certification Available
Financial Assistance: Assistantships, Scholarships and Work-Study Grants
Performing Groups: Theatre Players; Big Bend Summer Theatre Players

---

TARLETON STATE UNIVERSITY
Stephenville   Texas 76402, 817 965-5041
State and 4 Year
Arts Areas: Instrumental Music, Vocal Music, Theatre and Visual Arts
Performing Series: Friends of Music

MUSIC

Christian Rosner, Head, Department of Music and Art   **Number Of Faculty:** 7
Number Of Students: 50   **Degrees Offered:** BMusEd
Teaching Certification Available
Financial Assistance: Scholarships and Work-Study Grants
Performing Groups: University Singers; A Cappella Choir; Marching Band; Symphonic Band; Stage Band;
Opera Workshop
Workshops/Festivals: Summer program for Young Band Members

(continued on next page)

THEATRE

Mary Jane Mingus, Assistant Professor   **Number Of Faculty:** 1
Number Of Students: 20
Financial Assistance: Scholarships and Work-Study Grants
Performing Groups: Tarleton Players

TARRANT COUNTY JUNIOR COLLEGE, NORTHEAST CAMPUS
828 Harwood Rd, Hurst   Texas 76053
817 281-7860

County and 2 Year
Arts Areas: Instrumental Music, Vocal Music, Theatre, Film Arts and Visual Arts
Performance Facilities: Northeast Playhouse

MUSIC

Dr J T Matthews, Chairman   **Number Of Faculty:** 22   **Number Of Students:** 200
Degrees Offered: AA Mus, MusEd, Applied Music
Financial Assistance: Scholarships and Work-Study Grants
Performing Groups: 2 Bands; 3 Choirs; Instrumental Ensembles
Workshops/Festivals: Opera Workshop

THEATRE

Dr Cordell Parker, Chairman   **Number Of Faculty:** 3   **Number Of Students:** 50
Degrees Offered: AA
Financial Assistance: Scholarships and Work-Study Grants
Performing Groups: Drama Group

TARRANT COUNTY JUNIOR COLLEGE, SOUTH CAMPUS
5301 Campus Dr, Fort Worth   Texas 76119
817 534-4861

2 Year
Arts Areas: Dance, Instrumental Music, Vocal Music, Theatre, Film Arts and Visual Arts
Performing Series: Concert - Lecture Series; Regular Theatre Season; Regular Music Season
Performance Facilities: Carillon Theatre

MUSIC

Leonard McCormic, Chairman   **Number Of Faculty:** 7 Full-time, 14 Part-time
Number Of Students: 125   **Degrees Offered:** AA
Courses Offered: Theory; Music Literature; Appreciation; Applied; Band; Choir
Financial Assistance: Scholarships and Work-Study Grants
Performing Groups: Studio Band; Chamber String Ensemble; TCJC Singers; Symphonic Band; South Campus Madrigal Singers

THEATRE

Dr Gwendel Mulkey, Chairman   **Number Of Faculty:** 3 Full-time, 6 Part-time
Number Of Students: 50   **Degrees Offered:** AA
Courses Offered: Introduction to Theatre; Stagecraft; Lighting & Set Design; Acting; History of Theatre
Financial Assistance: Scholarships and Work-Study Grants
Performing Groups: Carillon Players; Carillon Puppeteers
Workshops/Festivals: Summer Children's Theatre Program

TEMPLE JUNIOR COLLEGE
2600 S First St, Temple   Texas 76501
817 773-9961 Ext 65

State and 2 Year
Arts Areas: Instrumental Music, Vocal Music, Theatre and Visual Arts
Performance Facilities: TJC Auditorium; TJC Backstage Theatre

(continued on next page)

(Temple JC — cont'd)

MUSIC

Larry Guess, Music Division Director   **Number Of Faculty:** 8
Number Of Students: 200   **Degrees Offered:** AA
Courses Offered: Vocal and Instrumental
Financial Assistance: Scholarships and Work-Study Grants
Performing Groups: Concert Choir; Chamber Singers; Chorale; Pop Ensemble; Concert Band; Stage Band

THEATRE

Wayne I Toone, Chairman   **Number Of Faculty:** 1   **Number Of Students:** 35
Degrees Offered: AA
Courses Offered: Introduction to Theatre; Theatre Activities
Financial Assistance: Scholarships and Work-Study Grants
Performing Groups: College Players

TEXARKANA COLLEGE
1024 Tucker, Texarkana   Texas 75501
214 838-4541
County and 2 Year
Arts Areas: Instrumental Music, Vocal Music, Theatre and Visual Arts
Performance Facilities: College Auditorium   **Number Of Faculty:** 2
Number Of Students: 36   **Degrees Offered:** AA Music
Financial Assistance: Scholarships and Work-Study Grants
Performing Groups: Troubadours; College Choir; Concert Choir; Wind Ensemble; Vocal Ensemble;
Instrumental Ensemble; Stage Band

THEATRE

Mildred Parsons, Chairman   **Number Of Faculty:** 2   **Number Of Students:** 36
Degrees Offered: AA
Financial Assistance: Scholarships and Work-Study Grants
Performing Groups: Texarkana College Players
Workshops/Festivals: Speech & Drama Workshop

TEXAS AGRICULTURAL & INDUSTRIAL UNIVERSITY, KINGSVILLE
Kingsville   Texas 78363, 512 592-6461
State and 4 Year
Arts Areas: Instrumental Music, Vocal Music, Theatre, Television and Visual Arts
Performance Facilities: Dramatics Auditorium

MUSIC

Dr Thomas C Pierson, Chairman   **Number Of Faculty:** 16
Number Of Students: 140   **Degrees Offered:** BA; BMus
Financial Assistance: Scholarships and Work-Study Grants
Performing Groups: Band; Choir; Orchestra; A&I Singers; Brass Choir; Woodwind Ensemble Musical
Theatre; Chamber Orchestra; Musical Theatre; Chamber Orchestra
Workshops/Festivals: Opera Workshop; Jazz Workshop

THEATRE

Dr Randall J Buchanan, Chairman   **Number Of Faculty:** 10
Number Of Students: 220   **Degrees Offered:** BA
Teaching Certification Available
Performing Groups: University Theatre; Children's Theatre
Workshops/Festivals: Drama Workshop

TEXAS CHRISTIAN UNIVERSITY
Fort Worth   Texas 76129, 817 926-2461 Ext 247
Private and 4 Year
Arts Areas: Dance, Instrumental Music, Vocal Music, Theatre, Film Arts, Television and Visual Arts

(continued on next page)

Performing Series: Artist Series; Visiting Artist; Artists in Residence
Performance Facilities: Landreth Auditorium; University Theatre; Edrington Scott Theatre; Granbury Opera House

DANCE

Fernando Schaffenburg, Head, Division of Ballet and Modern Dance
Number Of Faculty: 6   *Number Of Students:* 130   *Degrees Offered:* BFA; MFA
Courses Offered: Ballet Technique; Modern Dance; Character Dance; Choreography; Pantomime; Adagio & Variations; History
Financial Assistance: Assistantships, Scholarships and Work-Study Grants
Performing Groups: TCU Ballet Ensemble; TCU Modern Dance Ensemble; Chi Tau Epsilon Ensemble
Workshops/Festivals: Performances and other projects with the Fort Worth Ballet Association; Master Classes

MUSIC

Dr Michael Winesanker, Chairman, Department of Music   *Number Of Faculty:* 35
Number Of Students: 165   *Degrees Offered:* BMus; BMusEd; BA; MM; MMEd; MA
Courses Offered: Performance; Music Education; Church Music; Theory and Composition; History and Musicology
Teaching Certification Available
Financial Assistance: Assistantships, Scholarships and Work-Study Grants
Performing Groups: University Orchestra; Symphonic Band; Marching Band; Jazz Band; Chorale Union; Concert Chorale; Chapel Choir
Workshops/Festivals: Fine Arts Festival; Kraus Master Class in Piano; Opera Workshop

THEATRE

Dr Kent Gallagher, Chairman   *Number Of Faculty:* 5   *Number Of Students:* 55
Degrees Offered: BFA; BA; BS Ed; MFA; MA
Courses Offered: Acting; Directing; Scenography; Costuming; History; Criticism
Teaching Certification Available
Financial Assistance: Assistantships, Scholarships and Work-Study Grants
Performing Groups: University Players
Workshops/Festivals: Regional Festival; Area Drama Workshop; American College Theatre
Artists-In-Residence/Guest Artists: Mme Lili Kraus; Michael Schneider; Dr Oscar Brockett

---

TEXAS COLLEGE
Tyler   Texas 75701, 214 594-3200
Private and 4 Year
Arts Areas: Instrumental Music, Vocal Music, Theatre and Visual Arts
Performance Facilities: Martin Hall Auditorium

MUSIC

Mrs Sylvon Clayborn, Chairman   *Number Of Faculty:* 6
Number Of Students: 100   *Degrees Offered:* BA Music
Teaching Certification Available
Financial Assistance: Scholarships and Work-Study Grants
Performing Groups: Band; Choral Club   *Workshops/Festivals:* Concert Series

THEATRE

Mrs Pamala Irwin, Chairman   *Number Of Faculty:* 3   *Number Of Students:* 40

TEXAS LUTHERAN COLLEGE
1000 W Court, Seguin   Texas 78155
512 379-4161
Private and 4 Year
Arts Areas: Instrumental Music, Vocal Music, Theatre and Visual Arts
Performance Facilities: Wupperman Little Theater; Chapel of Abiding Presence

(continued on next page)

MUSIC

Dr Thomas S Thomas, Chairman   **Number Of Faculty:** 9
Number Of Students: 150   **Degrees Offered:** BMusEd
Teaching Certification Available
Financial Assistance: Scholarships and Work-Study Grants
Workshops/Festivals: Summer Jr and Sr High School Band Clinic; Summer Choral Clinic

THEATRE

David Rod, Chairman   **Number Of Faculty:** 1   **Number Of Students:** 40
Financial Assistance: Scholarships and Work-Study Grants

TEXAS SOUTHERN UNIVERSITY
3201 Wheeler Ave, Houston   Texas 77004
713 527-7011
State and 4 Year
Arts Areas: Dance, Instrumental Music, Vocal Music, Theatre, Film Arts, Television and Visual Arts
Performance Facilities: Hannah Hall Auditorium; Martin Luther King Center Auditorium

DANCE

Dr Majorie Stuart, Chairperson   **Number Of Faculty:** 6
Number Of Students: 75   **Courses Offered:** Modern; Interpretive; Afro-American
Financial Assistance: Scholarships and Work-Study Grants
Performing Groups: Modern Dance Group

MUSIC

Jack Bradley, Head, Music Department   **Number Of Faculty:** 20
Number Of Students: 200   **Degrees Offered:** BMusEd; BMus; MA; MMusEd
Courses Offered: Voice; Operatic; Choral Ensembles; Winds; Percussion; Musicology
Teaching Certification Available
Financial Assistance: Scholarships and Work-Study Grants
Performing Groups: University Choir; Choral Choir; Jazz Ensemble; Marching Band
Workshops/Festivals: High School Jazz; Music - Educational Workshops; Co-sponsors of National
Association Technical Singing Auditions

THEATRE

Dr Gary Carr, Chairman   **Number Of Faculty:** 6   **Number Of Students:** 38
Degrees Offered: BA; MA
Courses Offered: Theatre Workshop; Voice and Diction; Technical; Playwriting; Scene Design; Theatre
Administration; Modern Drama; History of Movies
Teaching Certification Available   **Financial Assistance:** Scholarships and Work-Study Grants
Performing Groups: Texas Southern University Players
Workshops/Festivals: Annual Spring Production
Artists-In-Residence/Guest Artists: Dr Carlton Molette; Jack Bradley; Dr Arron Horne; Robert L Steele;
Majorie Stuart

TEXAS SOUTHMOST COLLEGE
Brownsville   Texas 78520, 512 546-6232
County and 2 Year
Arts Areas: Dance, Instrumental Music, Vocal Music, Theatre and Visual Arts
Performance Facilities: Jacob Brown Auditorium

MUSIC

Number Of Faculty: 1   **Number Of Students:** 30   **Degrees Offered:** AA
Financial Assistance: Scholarships and Work-Study Grants

THEATRE

Norma Drake, Chairman   **Number Of Faculty:** 1   **Number Of Students:** 30

(continued on next page)

Courses Offered: Introduction to Theatre; Play Production
Financial Assistance: Scholarships and Work-Study Grants
Performing Groups: Curtain Callers

TEXAS TECH UNIVERSITY
Lubbock   Texas 79409, 806 742-5132

State and 4 Year
Arts Areas: Dance, Instrumental Music, Vocal Music, Theatre, Television and Visual Arts
Performing Series: University Artist Series
Performance Facilities: Texas Tech Concert Hall; Auditorium

DANCE

Diana Love Moore, Dance Division Coordinator   *Number Of Faculty:* 2
Number Of Students: 50   *Degrees Offered:* BS; BA
Financial Assistance: Assistantships
Workshops/Festivals: Dance Concert; Summer Dance Workshop; Perform in Musical Productions

MUSIC

Dr Harold L Luce, Music Department Chairman   *Number Of Faculty:* 45
Number Of Students: 415   *Degrees Offered:* BMus; BME; MM; MM Ed; PhD
Teaching Certification Available
Financial Assistance: Assistantships, Scholarships and Work-Study Grants
Performing Groups: Chorus; Band; Orchestra; Ensembles; Faculty Woodwind Quintet; Faculty Brass Quintet
Workshops/Festivals: American Contemporary Music Festival; Music Education Workshop

THEATRE

Dr Richard A Weaver, Director of Theatre   *Number Of Faculty:* 6
Number Of Students: 300   *Degrees Offered:* BA; MFA; MA
Teaching Certification Available
Financial Assistance: Assistantships and Scholarships
Workshops/Festivals: High School Summer Theatre Workshop

TEXAS WESLEYAN COLLEGE
PO Box 3277, Fort Worth   Texas 76105
817 534-0251

Private and 4 Year
Arts Areas: Instrumental Music, Vocal Music, Theatre and Visual Arts
Performing Series: Artist Series; Celebrity Series; Distinguished Alumnus Recital Series
Performance Facilities: Fine Arts Auditorium; Science Center Theater

MUSIC

Dr Donald W Bellah, Chairman Division of Fine Arts
Number Of Faculty: 9 Full-time, 3 Part-time   *Number Of Students:* 65
Degrees Offered: BMusEd
Courses Offered: Theory; Music Literature; String, Brass & Woodwind Instrument Techniques; Choral & Instrumental Conducting; Music Education; Music History; Form & Analysis; Counterpoint; Choral Arranging; Orchestration; Accompanying; Piano Pedagogy; Class Piano; Composition
Teaching Certification Available
Financial Assistance: Scholarships and Work-Study Grants
Performing Groups: Wesleyan Singers; Oratorio Chorus; Wind Ensemble; Orchestra; Lab Band
Workshops/Festivals: Annual Choral Festival for Fort Worth High Schools; Jazz Band Festival

THEATRE

Mason Johnson, Chairman, Speech - Drama Department
Number Of Faculty: 2 Full-time, 1 Part-time   *Number Of Students:* 30
Degrees Offered: BA
Courses Offered: Fundamentals of Speech; Public Speaking; Voice & Diction; Oral Interpretation;

(*continued on next page*)

Discussion & Argumentation; Debating; Phonetics; Interpretation; Speech Correction; Play Production & Acting; Stage Craftsmanship; Costume & Make-up; Stage Lighting; Acoustics & Sound; Shakespeare; History of Theatre; Play Directing
Teaching Certification Available
Financial Assistance: Scholarships and Work-Study Grants
Performing Groups: Texas Wesleyan Players
Workshops/Festivals: One-Act Play Festival

TEXAS WOMEN'S UNIVERSITY
Denton Texas 76204, 817 387-8422
State and 4 Year
Arts Areas: Dance, Instrumental Music, Vocal Music, Theatre, Television and Visual Arts
Performing Series: Concert and Drama Series
Performance Facilities: Main Auditorium

DANCE

Adrian Fisk, Chairman   **Number Of Faculty:** 3   **Number Of Students:** 200
Degrees Offered: BS; BA; MA; PhD
Technical Training: Ballet, Modern Jazz, Tap, Dance Theory - History, Production - Performance, Folk, Ethnological Character
Financial Assistance: Assistantships, Scholarships and Work-Study Grants
Performing Groups: Dance Repertory Theatre
Workshops/Festivals: National Endowment Residencies

MUSIC

Dr Frederick Fox, Chairman   **Number Of Faculty:** 25
Number Of Students: 354
Degrees Offered: BS Applied Music, Music Education, Music Therapy, Piano Pedagogy; MA Applied Music, Music Education, Music Therapy, Church Music, Piano Pedagogy
Teaching Certification Available
Financial Assistance: Assistantships, Scholarships and Work-Study Grants
Performing Groups: Modern Choir, Lass-O Band, Orchestra, Serenaders (Stage Band); Lasso Coraliers
Workshops/Festivals: All Girl Band Festival, Contemporary Music Festival, Opera Workshop

THEATRE

Dr Don Ryan, Chairman   **Number Of Faculty:** 2   **Number Of Students:** 75
Degrees Offered: BS, BA Speech with Concentration in Theatre Broadcasting, Special Education, Speech Therapy
Technical Training: Children's Theater, University Theater, Radio & TV Production
Teaching Certification Available
Financial Assistance: Scholarships and Work-Study Grants
Performing Groups: Readers Theatre, Puppet Tours, University Players

UNIVERSITY OF TEXAS - AUSTIN
Austin Texas 78712, 512 471-1655
State and 4 Year
Arts Areas: Dance, Instrumental Music, Vocal Music, Theatre and Visual Arts
Performing Series: Great Musicians Series; Cultural Entertainment Committee Series
Performance Facilities: Hogg Auditorium; Theatre Room; Batts Auditorium; Ballroom; Recital Hall; Laboratory Theatre; Opera Theatre; B Iden Payne Theatre

DANCE

Lathan Sanford, Advisor   **Number Of Faculty:** 7   **Number Of Students:** 80
Degrees Offered: BFA; BA; MFA; PhD
Courses Offered: Modern; Jazz; Ballet; Dance/Drama
Technical Training: BFA Drama Production (Dance)
Financial Assistance: Scholarships and Work-Study Grants
Workshops/Festivals: TSSEC Dance Contest

(continued on next page)

MUSIC

Daniel Patrylak, Chairman   *Number Of Faculty:* 67   *Number Of Students:* 700
Degrees Offered: BM; BA; MM; MMEd; PhD
Courses Offered: Applied; Theory/Composition; Education; Literature
Teaching Certification Available
Financial Assistance: Assistantships, Scholarships and Work-Study Grants
Performing Groups: Faculty Ensembles; Student Ensembles
Workshops/Festivals: TSSEC Music, Music Education, Choral, Instrumental, Conducting Workshops

THEATRE

Frederick Hunter, Acting Chairman   *Number Of Faculty:* 33
Number Of Students: 285   *Degrees Offered:* BA; BFA; MFA; PhD
Courses Offered: Acting; Directing; Playwriting; Design; Costume; Dance
Teaching Certification Available
Financial Assistance: Assistantships, Scholarships and Work-Study Grants
Performing Groups: Drama 670 Acting
Workshops/Festivals: High School Theatre Workshop; E P Conkle New Play Workshop
Artists-In-Residence/Guest Artists: Michael Finlayson (Drama); Jean Barr; Waldie Anderson; Eugene Kurtz; Amanda Vick Lethco; Robert Snow; Leonard Treasch (Music)

TRINITY UNIVERSITY
715 Stadium Dr, San Antonio   Texas 78284
512 736-8406
Private and 4 Year
Arts Areas: Dance, Instrumental Music, Vocal Music, Theatre, Film Arts, Television and Visual Arts
Performing Series: Abend Musik Series

DANCE

Number Of Faculty: 1   *Number Of Students:* 50

MUSIC

William Thornton, Chairman   *Number Of Faculty:* 11
Number Of Students: 500   *Degrees Offered:* BM; BA; MA
Courses Offered: Theory; Music History; Music Appreciation; Sight Singing; Ear Training; Applied Music
Teaching Certification Available   *Financial Assistance:* Assistantships
Performing Groups: Choir; Community Orchestra; Band; Collegium Musicum; Opera Workshop; Chamber Singers

THEATRE

Dr James Symons, Chairman   *Number Of Faculty:* 11   *Number Of Students:* 150
Degrees Offered: BA; MFA   *Courses Offered:* Theater History; Acting; Speech
Technical Training: Production; Design; Lighting; Costume Construction
Financial Assistance: Assistantships
Performing Groups: Dallas Theater Center
Workshops/Festivals: Evening Drama Workshop; Speech Workshop; Debate Workshop

TYLER JUNIOR COLLEGE
E Fifth St, Tyler   Texas 75701
214 593-4010
   State and 2 Year
   Arts Areas: Instrumental Music, Vocal Music, Theatre and Visual Arts
   Performance Facilities: Wise Auditorium

DANCE

Dance program under auspices of Physical Education Department

MUSIC

J W Johnson, Chairman   **Number Of Faculty:** 7   **Number Of Students:** 275
Degrees Offered: AA   **Financial Assistance:** Scholarships
Performing Groups: Apache Band; Concert Band; Lab Jazz Band; Small Instrumental Ensembles; Concert Chorus; Chamber Singers; Madrical Singers; Pop Vocal Group
Workshops/Festivals: High School District & Regional Instrumental and Vocal Contests

THEATRE

Jean Browne PhD, Chairman   **Number Of Faculty:** 7   **Number Of Students:** 700
Degrees Offered: AA
Courses Offered: Voice & Diction; Oral Interpretation; Acting; Introduction to Theatre; History of Theater; Stage Craft; Forensics
Technical Training: Apprenticeship programs in Costume, Set Construction, Make-up
Financial Assistance: Scholarships
Performing Groups: Las Mascahas Club; Readers Theater
Workshops/Festivals: Forensic Program; High School One-Act Play (UIL); Stage Violence Workshop; Dance Workshop

UNIVERSITY OF DALLAS
Irving   Texas 75061, 214 253-1123
   State and 4 Year   **Arts Areas:** Dance, Theatre and Visual Arts
   Performance Facilities: The Margaret Jonsson Theatre

THEATRE

Judith French, Chairman   **Number Of Faculty:** 4   **Number Of Students:** 80
Degrees Offered: BA Drama   **Teaching Certification Available**
Financial Assistance: Scholarships and Work-Study Grants
Performing Groups: University Theatre
Workshops/Festivals: Texas Catholic Interscholastic League Tournament

UNIVERSITY OF TEXAS, ARLINGTON
Box 19188, UTA Station, Arlington   Texas 76019
214 261-8461
   State and 4 Year
   Arts Areas: Instrumental Music, Vocal Music and Theatre

MUSIC

Prof Mahan, Chairman
Degrees Offered: BA Mus (Instrumental, Choral, Applied)
Teaching Certification Available
Performing Groups: Concert Band; University Chorus; Lab Band; Symphonic Band; Orchestra; Ensemble; Chamber Singers
Workshops/Festivals: Opera Workshops

(continued on next page)

THEATRE

Chapin Ross, Chairman   **Degrees Offered:** Communication BA Drama Option
Teaching Certification Available   Performing Groups: Little Theatre

---

UNIVERSITY OF TEXAS, AUSTIN
Austin   Texas 78712, 512 471-1655
State and 4 Year
Arts Areas: Dance, Instrumental Music, Vocal Music, Theatre, Film Arts, Television and Visual Arts
Performing Series: Solo Artist Series; Chamber Music Celebration; Cultural Entertainment Committee Series
Performance Facilities: Hogg and Batts Auditoriums; Recital Hall; Theatre Room; Laboratory Theatre; Opera Theatre

DANCE

Lathan Sanford, Acting Chairman   **Number Of Faculty:** 7
Number Of Students: 80   **Degrees Offered:** BFA; BA
Courses Offered: Modern; Jazz; Ballet; Dance - Drama
Financial Assistance: Scholarships and Work-Study Grants
Workshops/Festivals: TSSEC Dance Contest

MUSIC

Morris Beachy, Acting Chairman   **Number Of Faculty:** 72
Number Of Students: 700   **Degrees Offered:** BMus; BA; MMus; PhD; DMA
Teaching Certification Available
Financial Assistance: Assistantships, Scholarships and Work-Study Grants
Performing Groups: Faculty Ensembles
Workshops/Festivals: TSSEC Music; Music Education; Choral; Instrumental; Conducting Workshops

THEATRE

Webster Smalley, Chairman   **Number Of Faculty:** 33   **Number Of Students:** 300
Degrees Offered: BA; BRA; MA; MFA; PhD   **Technical Training:** Technical Theatre
Teaching Certification Available
Financial Assistance: Assistantships, Scholarships and Work-Study Grants
Workshops/Festivals: High School One-Act Play Competition; Acting, Combat, Production Workshops

---

UNIVERSITY OF TEXAS, EL PASO
El Paso   Texas 79968, 915 747-5666
State and 4 Year
Arts Areas: Dance, Instrumental Music, Vocal Music, Theatre and Visual Arts

DANCE

Dr R E Henderson, Chairman   **Number Of Faculty:** 3   **Number Of Students:** 9
Degrees Offered: BMus   **Technical Training:** Choreography; Staging
Teaching Certification Available   Financial Assistance: Work-Study Grants
Performing Groups: University - Civic Ballet
Workshops/Festivals: Ten clinics with the Chamizal National Park Service

MUSIC

Dr R E Henderson, Chairman   **Number Of Faculty:** 16 plus 14 part-time
Number Of Students: 156   **Degrees Offered:** BMus; MMusEd
Technical Training: Monotone Clinic; Electronic Production Technique
Teaching Certification Available
Financial Assistance: Scholarships and Work-Study Grants
Performing Groups: One Marching Band; Three Pep Bands; The Golddiggers; Concert Band; Symphonic Wind Ensemble; Lab Jazz Band; Woodwind Ensemble; Brass Ensemble; Symphonic Orchestra; String Ensemble; Opera & Ballet Orchestras; Bell Choir; Classical Guitar Ensemble; Mariachi Ensemble; University-Civic Opera; University Chorale; Chorus; Opera & Oratorio Choirs; Jazz Choir-Band; El Paso Boy Choir in Residence; Chamber Music Ensembles (Student/Faculty); Faculty String Quartet in

(continued on next page)

Residence; Faculty Woodwind Ensemble; Faculty Vocal Groups
Workshops/Festivals: Ten Clinics with the Chamizal Clinic

THEATRE

Dr H N Williams, Chairman   *Number Of Faculty:* 3   *Number Of Students:* 30
Degrees Offered: BA; MA
Technical Training: Theater Design; Lighting; Costume
Teaching Certification Available
Financial Assistance: Assistantships, Scholarships and Work-Study Grants
Performing Groups: University Players; Arabic Theater Mimes
Workshops/Festivals: Summer Workshop

THE VICTORIA COLLEGE
2200 Red River, Victoria   Texas 77901
512 573-3295

County and 2 Year   *Arts Areas:* Dance, Instrumental Music and Vocal Music

MUSIC

Wilbur Collins, Chairman   *Number Of Faculty:* 4   *Number Of Students:* 100
Financial Assistance: Scholarships
Performing Groups: Wind, Brass, Vocal Ensembles

THEATRE

Erline Grizzle, Chairman   *Number Of Faculty:* 1   *Number Of Students:* 25
Financial Assistance: Scholarships   *Performing Groups:* Speech & Drama Club

---

WAYLAND BAPTIST COLLEGE
Plainview   Texas 79072, 806 296-5521 Ext 17

Private
Arts Areas: Instrumental Music, Vocal Music, Theatre, Television and Radio
Performance Facilities: Recital Hall; Band Hall; Auditorium; Black Box Theatre; TV Studios

MUSIC

Corre Berry, Head, Department of Music   *Number Of Faculty:* 8
Number Of Students: 300
Degrees Offered: BMus; BA in Music in Applied, Music Ed, Church Mus
Teaching Certification Available
Financial Assistance: Scholarships and Work-Study Grants
Performing Groups: Spirit of America Singers; Concert Choir; Wayland Singers; Band
Workshops/Festivals: Flag Camp; UIL contests in Band and Vocal

THEATRE

Roland Myers, Acting Head, Department of Speech & Theater
Number Of Faculty: 2   *Number Of Students:* 100   *Degrees Offered:* BA
Teaching Certification Available

WEATHERFORD COLLEGE
308 E Park, Weatherford   Texas 76086
817 594-5471 Ext 36

County and 2 Year
Arts Areas: Instrumental Music, Vocal Music, Theatre, Visual Arts and Speech
Performance Facilities: Small Auditorium; Main Auditorium; Student Center

MUSIC

Myrna Fields, Music Department Chairman   *Number Of Faculty:* 3
Number Of Students: 40   *Degrees Offered:* AA
Financial Assistance: Work-Study Grants

(continued on next page)

Performing Groups: Bell Choir; College Choir; College Band; Stage Band; Country Gold; Chamber Choir
Workshops/Festivals: High School Band; High School Choir

THEATRE

Jim Ramp, Chairman, Department of Speech & Drama   **Number Of Faculty:** 2
Number Of Students: 25   **Degrees Offered:** AA
Courses Offered: Introduction to Acting; Acting Workshop; Introduction to Theatre; Interpretation

WEST TEXAS STATE UNIVERSITY
Canyon   Texas 79016, 806 656-3861
State and 4 Year
Arts Areas: Dance, Instrumental Music, Vocal Music, Theatre, Television and Visual Arts
Performance Facilities: Branding Iron Theatre; Northern Concert - Recital Hall

MUSIC

Dr Harry Haines, Head   **Number Of Faculty:** 25   **Number Of Students:** 325
Degrees Offered: BME; BMus; MA; MM   **Teaching Certification Available**
Financial Assistance: Assistantships, Scholarships and Work-Study Grants
Performing Groups: Band; Orchestra; Chorale; Opera Workshop; Stage Band; Brass Choir
Workshops/Festivals: Choral Music Camp; Instrumental Music Camp; Opera Workshop

THEATRE

Dr Ray Ewing, Head   **Number Of Faculty:** 2   **Number Of Students:** 50
Degrees Offered: BA; BS; MA   **Teaching Certification Available**

WHARTON COUNTY JUNIOR COLLEGE
911 Boling Hwy, Wharton   Texas 77488
713 532-4560 Ext 33
County and 2 Year
Arts Areas: Instrumental Music, Vocal Music, Theatre, Film Arts, Television and Visual Arts
Performance Facilities: Duson - Hansen Fine Arts Theatre

MUSIC

William Wolfe, Music Department Chairman   **Number Of Faculty:** 4
Number Of Students: 300   **Degrees Offered:** AA
Courses Offered: Music Literature; Theory; Music Appreciation; Applied; Ensembles
Financial Assistance: Scholarships and Work-Study Grants
Performing Groups: Marching Band; Concert Band; Stage Bands; Choir; Madrigal Singers; Brass Choir
Workshops/Festivals: Stage Band Festival; Stage Band Workshop; Piano Recital for area Piano Students

THEATRE

Nancy Brown, Theatre Department Chairperson   **Number Of Faculty:** 2½
Number Of Students: 50   **Degrees Offered:** AA
Courses Offered: Rehearsal & Performance; Introduction to the Theatre; Voice and Articulation;
Stagecraft; Acting
Technical Training: Design in Technical Theatre
Financial Assistance: Scholarships and Work-Study Grants
Performing Groups: Readers Theatre; Greenroom Players
Workshops/Festivals: Texas Secondary Theatre Conference Workshop; UIL One-Act Play Contest;
Intercollegiate One-Act Play Contest

WILEY COLLEGE
711 Rosborough Springs Rd, Marshall   Texas 75670
214 938-8341 Ext 49
Private and 4 Year   **Arts Areas:** Instrumental Music and Vocal Music
Performance Facilities: Wiley College Auditorium

(continued on next page)

MUSIC

Ronald O'Neal, Chairman *Number Of Faculty:* 5 *Number Of Students:* 20
Degrees Offered: BA Mus *Teaching Certification Available*
Financial Assistance: Scholarships and Work-Study Grants
Performing Groups: A Cappella Choir

BRIGHAM YOUNG UNIVERSITY
Price   Utah 84602, 801 374-1211 Ext 2818

Private and 4 Year
Arts Areas: Instrumental Music, Vocal Music, Theatre, Film Arts, Television, Visual Arts and Radio
Performing Series: Lyceum Series
Performance Facilities: deJong Concert Hall; Pardoe Theatre; Madsen Hall; Nelke Theatre; Margetts Theatre
Dance is under the auspices of the Physical Education Department

MUSIC

Dr A Harold Goodman, Chairman   *Number Of Faculty:* 43
Number Of Students: 5,000   *Degrees Offered:* BMus; BMusEd; MMus; MMusEd; PhD
Courses Offered: Instrumental Music; Vocal Music; Performance; Theory; Composition
Technical Training: Overseas Study - Opera   *Teaching Certification Available*
Financial Assistance: Internships, Assistantships, Scholarships and Work-Study Grants
Performing Groups: Faculty String Quartet; Woodwind Quintet; A Cappella Choir; Wind Symphony; Synthesis
Workshops/Festivals: Sounds of Summer Music Clinic; International Piano Festival

THEATRE

Dr Charles L Metten, Chairman   *Number Of Faculty:* 17
Number Of Students: 3,500   *Degrees Offered:* BA; BFA; MA; MFA; PhD
Courses Offered: Acting; Child Drama; Costume Design; Designer - Technician; Directing; Musical Theatre; Playwriting; Theatre Arts Education
Teaching Certification Available
Financial Assistance: Internships, Assistantships, Scholarships and Work-Study Grants
Performing Groups: University Theatre; Whittlin' Whistlin' Brigade; Mask Club
Workshops/Festivals: Theatre Workshops

COLLEGE OF EASTERN UTAH
451 E 4th N, Price   Utah 84501
801 637-2120

State and 2 Year
Arts Areas: Dance, Instrumental Music, Vocal Music, Theatre and Visual Arts
Performance Facilities: Geary Theatre

DANCE

Joy Peterson, Chairman   *Number Of Faculty:* 2   *Number Of Students:* 150
Degrees Offered: AA
Courses Offered: (Limited to every other year) Tap and Jazz Dancing; Folk and Square Dancing; Ballroom Dance; Modern Dance; Creative Dance
Financial Assistance: Scholarships and Work-Study Grants

MUSIC

Jay O Andrus, Chairman   *Number Of Faculty:* 4   *Number Of Students:* 110
Degrees Offered: AA
Courses Offered: Music Appreciation; Guitar; Piano; Voice; Band; Choir
Financial Assistance: Scholarships and Work-Study Grants
Performing Groups: Concert Choir; Concert Band; Chamber Choir; Woodwind Quintet
Workshops/Festivals: Utah High School Honor Band

THEATRE

Lee Johnson, Chairman   *Number Of Faculty:* 3   *Number Of Students:* 30
Degrees Offered: AA

(continued on next page)

Courses Offered: Theatre Arts Appreciation; Shakespeare; Modern Plays; Stage Make-up; Play Production; Touring Theatre; Children's Theatre
Financial Assistance: Scholarships and Work-Study Grants
Performing Groups: College Theatre; Community Theatre

DIXIE COLLEGE
225 S 700 E, Saint George   Utah 84770
801 673-4811 Ext 290
State and 2 Year
Arts Areas: Dance, Instrumental Music, Vocal Music, Theatre, Film Arts, Television, Visual Arts and Radio
Performing Series: Southwest '78
Performance Facilities: Proscenium Stage; Arena Theatre; Concert Hall; Recital Halls

DANCE

Pat Roper, Instructor   **Number Of Faculty:** 2   **Number Of Students:** 100
Degrees Offered: AS; AA
Courses Offered: Folk Dance; Square Dance; Modern Dance; Ballet; Social Dance

MUSIC

Ronald L Garner, Music Area Coordinator   **Number Of Faculty:** 7
Number Of Students: 300   **Degrees Offered:** AA; AS
Financial Assistance: Scholarships, Work-Study Grants and Government Grants and Loans
Performing Groups: Program Bureau; Concert Choir; Chamber Choir; College Band; College Orchestra; Brotherhood
Workshops/Festivals: Piano Festival; Band Festival

THEATRE

C Paul Andersen, Director   **Number Of Faculty:** 5   **Number Of Students:** 200
Degrees Offered: AA; AS
Financial Assistance: Scholarships and Work-Study Grants
Performing Groups: Theatre; Children's Theatre; Touring Theatre; Pioneer Courthouse Players; Old Barn Theatre Company
Workshops/Festivals: Regional High School Drama Competition

SNOW COLLEGE
140 E College Ave, Ephraim   Utah 84627
801 283-4021 Ext 262
State and 2 Year
Arts Areas: Dance, Instrumental Music, Vocal Music and Theatre
Performance Facilities: Auditorium; Lifetime Sports & Physical Education Complex Building

DANCE

Sherri Jensen, Chairman   **Number Of Faculty:** 6   **Number Of Students:** 150
Degrees Offered: AA; AS
Financial Assistance: Scholarships and Work-Study Grants
Performing Groups: Orchesis; Ballet

MUSIC

McLoyd Erickson, Chairman   **Number Of Faculty:** 7   **Number Of Students:** 250
Degrees Offered: AA   **Courses Offered:** Vocal; Instrumental Music; Stage Band
Financial Assistance: Scholarships and Work-Study Grants
Performing Groups: Stage Band; A Cappella Choir; Snow College Singers; String Band; Symphony Group
Workshops/Festivals: Summer Snow Music Festival

THEATRE

Joe Crane, Chairman   **Number Of Faculty:** 2   **Number Of Students:** 82
Degrees Offered: AA   **Courses Offered:** Theatre Arts; Staging; Speech; Scenery

SOUTHERN UTAH STATE COLLEGE
351 W Center, Cedar City   Utah 84720
801 566-4411

State and 4 Year
Arts Areas: Instrumental Music, Vocal Music, Theatre and Visual Arts
Performing Series: Concert Series
Performance Facilities: Southern Utah Auditorium
Degrees Offered: BMus; BMusEd   *Teaching Certification Available*
Financial Assistance: Scholarships and Work-Study Grants
Performing Groups: Symphony; Chorus; Band; Orchestra

THEATRE

Fred C Adams, Chairman   *Number Of Faculty:* 5   *Number Of Students:* 75
Degrees Offered: BA   *Teaching Certification Available*
Financial Assistance: Scholarships and Work-Study Grants
Performing Groups: Campus Community Theatre
Workshops/Festivals: Shakespearean Guild

UTAH STATE UNIVERSITY
UMC 40, Logan   Utah 84322
801 752-4100

State and 4 Year
Arts Areas: Dance, Instrumental Music, Vocal Music, Theatre and Television
Performance Facilities: Utah State and Chase Fine Arts Centers

MUSIC

Prof Irving Wassermann, Chairman   *Number Of Faculty:* 12
Number Of Students: 150
Degrees Offered: BA; BS Mus, MusEd, Applied Music; MA Ed; MA; D Ed
Teaching Certification Available
Financial Assistance: Assistantships, Scholarships and Work-Study Grants
Performing Groups: Symphony Orchestra; Symphonic Band; Varsity Band; Jazz Ensemble; Chorale; Choir
Workshops/Festivals: Jr & Sr High Band Invitationals; Band Festival; Summer Music Clinic

THEATRE

Prof Floyd T Morgan, Chairman   *Number Of Faculty:* 6
Number Of Students: 45
Degrees Offered: BA; BFA Theatre Arts, Theatre Arts Teaching, Theatre Arts - Communications Composite; MA; MFA
Technical Training: Design/Technical Emphasis or Performance Emphasis available to BFA Students
Teaching Certification Available
Financial Assistance: Assistantships, Scholarships and Work-Study Grants
Performing Groups: Utah State Theatre; Workshop Company; Old Lyric Repertory Co (Member of URTA)
Workshops/Festivals: Old Lyric Repertory Company

UNIVERSITY OF UTAH
College of Fine Arts, Salt Lake City   Utah 84112
801 581-6764

State and 4 Year
Arts Areas: Dance, Instrumental Music, Vocal Music, Theatre, Film Arts and Visual Arts
Performance Facilities: Pioneer Memorial Theatre; Kingsbury Hall; Student Theatres

DANCE

Mattlyn Gavers, Chairman   *Number Of Faculty:* 6   *Number Of Students:* 150
Degrees Offered: BFA; MFA; MA
Financial Assistance: Assistantships and Scholarships

(continued on next page)

Performing Groups: Ballet Showcase; Ballet Ensemble
Workshops/Festivals: Summer Workshop

MUSIC

Dr Forrest D Stoll, Acting Chairman   **Number Of Faculty:** 50
Number Of Students: 400   **Degrees Offered:** BMus; MMus; PhD
Technical Training: Electronic Music   **Teaching Certification Available**
Financial Assistance: Assistantships, Scholarships and Work-Study Grants
Performing Groups: Bands; Symphony Orchestra; Jazz Ensembles; Chamber Groups; Opera Workshop; Choral Groups
Workshops/Festivals: Contemporary Festivals; Workshops in Jazz, Choral, Band, Orchestra, String Trombone and Piano; Teacher Seminars

THEATRE

Dr Keith M Engar, Chairman   **Number Of Faculty:** 45
Degrees Offered: BFA; MFA; PhD
Courses Offered: Performance; Children's Theatre; Musical Theatre; Theatre Design; Arts Administration
Performing Groups: Pioneer Memorial Theatre Company; Puppetry Group
Workshops/Festivals: Summer Children's Theatre; Touring Company of State of Utah; U of U Players at Lagoon

---

WEBER STATE COLLEGE
3750 Harrison Blvd, Ogden   Utah 84408
801 399-5941
4 Year
Arts Areas: Dance, Instrumental Music, Vocal Music, Theatre, Film Arts, Television and Visual Arts
Performance Facilities: Weber State College Fine Arts Center

DANCE

Dr Wallace Nalder, Recreation, and Dance, Health Education, Physical Education
Number Of Faculty: 3   **Number Of Students:** 20
Performing Groups: Orchesis; Folk; Modern; Rhythmic for Elementary Education Social, Square, Ballet
Workshops/Festivals: Rhythmic Activity for Elementary Education; Orchesis Concerts sponsored by Students

MUSIC

Dr Herbert Cecil, Chairman   **Number Of Faculty:** 11
Number Of Students: 100   **Degrees Offered:** BA; BS
Teaching Certification Available
Financial Assistance: Scholarships and Work-Study Grants
Performing Groups: Woodwind Ensemble; String Ensemble; A Cappella Choir; WSC Chorale; Weber State Singers; Voce Coeds; Trombone Choir; Symphony String Orchestra; Symphony Band; Stage Band; Percussion Ensemble
Workshops/Festivals: High School Music Festival

THEATRE

Dr T Leonard Rowley, Chairman   **Number Of Faculty:** 5
Number Of Students: 50   **Degrees Offered:** BS; BA
Teaching Certification Available
Financial Assistance: Scholarships and Work-Study Grants
Performing Groups: Weber State Theatre; Commedia Players
Workshops/Festivals: High School Drama Festival

WESTMINISTER COLLEGE
1840 S 13th St E, Salt Lake City   Utah 84105
801 484-1651
Private and 4 Year
Arts Areas: Instrumental Music, Vocal Music, Theatre and Visual Arts

(continued on next page)

Performing Series: Performing Artists Concert Series
Performance Facilities: Westminister Theatre

MUSIC

Kenneth Kuchler, Chairman   **Number Of Faculty:** 4   **Number Of Students:** 65
Degrees Offered: BMus   **Teaching Certification Available**
Financial Assistance: Scholarships and Work-Study Grants
Performing Groups: College-Community Symphony Orchestra; Concert Choir; Chorale Ensemble; Chamber Ensemble

THEATRE

Jay W Lees, Chairman   **Number Of Faculty:** 2   **Number Of Students:** 35
Degrees Offered: BA; BFA   **Teaching Certification Available**
Financial Assistance: Assistantships, Scholarships and Work-Study Grants
Performing Groups: Westminister Players

BENNINGTON COLLEGE
Bennington   Vermont 05201, 802 442-5401 Ext 212
  Private and 4 Year
  Arts Areas: Dance, Instrumental Music, Vocal Music, Theatre, Visual Arts and Black Music
  Performing Series: Lecture and Concert Series
  Performance Facilities: Carriage Barn; Barn Studio Theatre

DANCE

  Barbara Roan, Rotating Chairman   *Number Of Faculty:* 9
  Number Of Students: 74   *Degrees Offered:* BA; MA
  Courses Offered: Dance Technique; Performance; Modern Dance; Design & Lighting for Dance;
  Labanotation; Stagecraft; Sound
  Financial Assistance: Work-Study Grants   *Performing Groups:* Dance Company
  Workshops/Festivals: Winter Tour

MUSIC

  Jack Glick, Rotating Chairman and Bill Dixon, Black Music Division
  Number Of Faculty: 11   *Degrees Offered:* BA; MA
  Courses Offered: Experimental Orchestra; Composer's Laboratory; Choral Music; Chamber Music; Piano
  Improvisation; Twentieth Century Harmony; Score Analysis; Conducting and Orchestration; Electronic
  Music; Accoustics; Individual Instruments and Voice
  Financial Assistance: Work-Study Grants
  Performing Groups: Concerts; Orchestra; Chorus; Instrumental Ensembles
  Workshops/Festivals: Weekly Workshops; Weekly Faculty Concert

THEATRE

  Laurence O'Dwyer, Rotating Chairman   *Number Of Faculty:* 6
  Degrees Offered: BA; MA
  Courses Offered: Playwriting; Directing; Acting; Lighting; Design; Voice and Speech; Stagecraft; Puppetry;
  Costume Design
  Financial Assistance: Work-Study Grants   *Performing Groups:* Repertory
  Workshops/Festivals: Children's Theatre Workshop

CASTLETON STATE COLLEGE
Castleton   Vermont 05735, 802 468-5611
  State and 4 Year
  Arts Areas: Dance, Instrumental Music, Vocal Music, Theatre and Visual Arts
  Performing Series: Artist Series; Weekly Events Series
  Performance Facilities: Fine Arts Center

DANCE

  Mrs Harold Abraham, Chairman   *Number Of Faculty:* 2
  Number Of Students: 80   *Degrees Offered:* BA Theatre Arts; BS Theatre Arts
  Technical Training: Technical Theatre   *Teaching Certification Available*
  Financial Assistance: Work-Study Grants   *Performing Groups:* Dance Ensemble
  Workshops/Festivals: Artist-in-Residence Performances; Master Classes

MUSIC

  Dr Robert Aborn, Chairman   *Number Of Faculty:* 3   *Degrees Offered:* BA; BS
  Technical Training: Applied Music   *Teaching Certification Available*
  Financial Assistance: Work-Study Grants
  Performing Groups: Small instrumental Ensemble Groups; Chorus; Wind Ensemble (includes community
  members)

(continued on next page)

THEATRE

Byron Avery, Chairman   **Number Of Faculty:** 3   **Number Of Students:** 200
Degrees Offered: BA; BS
Technical Training: Technical Production; Stagecraft; Lighting; Scene Design
Financial Assistance: Work-Study Grants   **Performing Groups:** Players
Workshops/Festivals: Regional ATA; AAE; Vermont Council on the Arts; State One-Acts

---

GODDARD COLLEGE
Plainfield   Vermont 05667, 802 454-8311
Private and 4 Year
Arts Areas: Instrumental Music, Vocal Music, Theatre, Film Arts and Visual Arts
Performing Series: Concert Lecture Series
Performance Facilities: The Haybarn Theatre

DANCE

Dana Wolfe-Louis Montez de Oca, Chairman   **Number Of Students:** 50
Degrees Offered: BA   **Technical Training:** Ballet; Modern Dance
Financial Assistance: Scholarships and Work-Study Grants
Performing Groups: Dance Ensembles

MUSIC

Lois Harris, Instructor   **Number Of Faculty:** 3   **Number Of Students:** 35
Degrees Offered: BMus; BMusEd   **Teaching Certification Available**
Financial Assistance: Scholarships and Work-Study Grants
Performing Groups: Concerts; Chorus; Orchestra; Instrumental Ensembles

THEATRE

Paul Vila, Chairman   **Number Of Faculty:** 3   **Number Of Students:** 35
Degrees Offered: BA   **Teaching Certification Available**
Financial Assistance: Scholarships and Work-Study Grants
Performing Groups: Goddard Players

GREEN MOUNTAIN COLLEGE
Poultney   Vermont 05764, 802 287-9313
Private and 2 Year
Arts Areas: Instrumental Music, Vocal Music, Theatre and Visual Arts
Performance Facilities: College Auditorium   **Degrees Offered:** AA Music
Performing Groups: Vocal & Instrumental Ensembles

THEATRE

Saul Elkin, Chairman   **Number Of Faculty:** 2   **Number Of Students:** 30
Performing Groups: Thespian Art Players

JOHNSON STATE COLLEGE
Johnson   Vermont 05656, 802 635-2356
State and 4 Year
Arts Areas: Instrumental Music, Vocal Music and Visual Arts
Performing Series: Johnson Friends of the Arts; Concert and Lecture Series
Performance Facilities: Dibden Center for the Arts

DANCE

Rebecca Smith, Chairman   **Number Of Faculty:** 1   **Number Of Students:** 50
Technical Training: Contemporary Modern Dance
Performing Groups: The Johnson Dancers
Workshops/Festivals: Daniel Nagrin Workshop Course

(continued on next page)

MUSIC

Dr John Duffy, Chairman   **Number Of Faculty:** 11   **Number Of Students:** 95
Degrees Offered: BA   **Technical Training:** Opera Workshops; Electronic Music
Teaching Certification Available
Financial Assistance: Scholarships and Work-Study Grants
Performing Groups: Opera Theatre; Chorale Ensemble; Instrumental Ensembles
Workshops/Festivals: Opera Workshop; Vermont Symphony Orchestra

THEATRE

Ralph Carter, Chairman   **Number Of Faculty:** 4   **Number Of Students:** 25
Technical Training: Instruction in Basic Theatre
Teaching Certification Available   **Performing Groups:** Johnson Players

LYNDON STATE COLLEGE
Lyndonville   Vermont 05851, 802 626-3335
State and 4 Year
Arts Areas: Instrumental Music, Vocal Music, Theatre and Visual Arts
Performing Series: Cooperation Performing Series; Northeast Kingdon Series
Performance Facilities: Alexander Twilight Theatre

DANCE

Carol Goldstein, Chairman   **Technical Training:** Dance Therapy

MUSIC

Melissa Brown, Chairman   **Number Of Faculty:** 20   **Number Of Students:** 200
Degrees Offered: BMus   **Teaching Certification Available**
Financial Assistance: Scholarships and Work-Study Grants
Performing Groups: Athenaeum Players

THEATRE

Phillip Anderson, Chairman   **Number Of Faculty:** 3   **Number Of Students:** 125
Degrees Offered: BA   **Teaching Certification Available**
Financial Assistance: Scholarships and Work-Study Grants
Performing Groups: Twilight Players; Tours
Workshops/Festivals: Summer Theatre Workshop with Professionals

MARLBORO COLLEGE
Marlboro   Vermont 05344, 812 254-2393
Private and 4 Year
Arts Areas: Instrumental Music, Vocal Music, Theatre and Visual Arts
Performing Series: Cultural Events Series
Performance Facilities: Marlboro Performing Arts Center

MUSIC

Blanche H Moyse, Instructor   **Number Of Faculty:** 3   **Number Of Students:** 25
Degrees Offered: BA; BS   **Technical Training:** Jr Year Abroad Program; Opera
Financial Assistance: Scholarships and Work-Study Grants
Performing Groups: Choral Groups; Chamber Music
Workshops/Festivals: Bach Festival

THEATRE

Geoffry Brown, Director   **Number Of Faculty:** 2   **Number Of Students:** 25
Degrees Offered: BA   **Technical Training:** Acting; Directing; Playwriting; Film
Financial Assistance: Scholarships and Work-Study Grants
Performing Groups: Theatre Workshop (Associated with the Marlboro General Theatre Co)
Workshops/Festivals: Summer Theatre Festival

MIDDLEBURY COLLEGE

Middlebury   Vermont 05753, 802 388-2763

Private and 4 Year
Arts Areas: Dance, Instrumental Music, Vocal Music, Theatre and Visual Arts
Performing Series: Middlebury College Concert Series
Performance Facilities: Wright Theatre

DANCE

Christine Lister, Dance Instructor   **Number Of Faculty:** 1
Number Of Students: 110   **Degrees Offered:** BA Mus with emphasis in Dance
Performing Groups: Middlebury College Performing Dance Ensemble

MUSIC

George B Todd, Chairman   **Number Of Faculty:** 5
Number Of Students: 200-250   **Degrees Offered:** BA Mus
Technical Training: Applied Music Instruction in Piano, Organ, Voice, Flute, Classical Guitar, Violin, Viola, Recorder
Teaching Certification Available
Performing Groups: Middlebury College Choir; Middlebury Orchestra; Middlebury Contemporary Chamber Ensemble

THEATRE

Erie Volkert, Director   **Number Of Faculty:** 3   **Number Of Students:** 200
Degrees Offered: BA English and Drama   **Teaching Certification Available**

NORWICH UNIVERSITY

Northfield   Vermont 05663, 802 485-5011 Ext 257

Private, 4 Year and Coed Military College
Arts Areas: Instrumental Music, Vocal Music and Theatre
Performance Facilities: Dole Auditorium

MUSIC

Robert Allee, Director of University Bands   **Number Of Faculty:** 2
Courses Offered: Music Literature; Applied; Choir; Theory; Instrumental Ensemble; Band; Orchestra
Financial Assistance: Scholarships and Work-Study Grants
Performing Groups: Vermont Symphonic; Vermont Philharmonic; Grenadiers; Choir; Regimental Band

THEATRE

Carleton Berry, Associate Professor of Theater & Speech
Number Of Faculty: 1
Financial Assistance: Scholarships and Work-Study Grants
Performing Groups: Pegasus Players

SAINT MICHAEL'S COLLEGE

56 College Parkway, Winooski   Vermont 05404
802 655-2000 Ext 2449

Private and 4 Year
Arts Areas: Instrumental Music, Vocal Music, Theatre and Visual Arts
Performing Series: Concert and Lecture Series
Performance Facilities: McCarthy Arts Center Theatre; McCarthy Arts Center Recital; Herrouet Theatre

MUSIC

Donald A Rathgeb, Chairman, Fine Arts Department   **Number Of Faculty:** 2
Number Of Students: 40
Degrees Offered: BA in Fine Arts, Mus; BA in Fine Arts, MusEd
Courses Offered: History; Theory; Practical
Teaching Certification Available

(continued on next page)

Financial Assistance: Scholarships and Work-Study Grants
Performing Groups: Wind Ensemble; Glee Club; Jazz Ensemble; Chorale

THEATRE

Donald A Rathgeb, Chairman, Fine Arts Department   **Number Of Faculty:** 2
Number Of Students: 40   **Degrees Offered:** BA in Fine Arts, Drama
Courses Offered: History; Literature; Acting; Directing; Technical
Teaching Certification Available
Financial Assistance: Scholarships and Work-Study Grants
Performing Groups: Fine Arts Department; Drama Club
Workshops/Festivals: Saint Michael's Playhouse; Summer Theatre

---

UNIVERSITY OF VERMONT
Burlington   Vermont 05401, 802 656-3430
State and 4 Year
Arts Areas: Dance, Instrumental Music, Vocal Music, Theatre, Film Arts, Television and Visual Arts
Performing Series: George Bishop Lane Series
Performance Facilities: Royall Tyler Theatre

MUSIC

William Metcalfe, Acting Chairman   **Number Of Faculty:** 24
Number Of Students: 72   **Degrees Offered:** BA Mus; BS MusEd; MA; MA Teaching
Teaching Certification Available   **Financial Assistance:** Work-Study Grants
Performing Groups: Choir; Band; Brass Ensemble; Orchestra; Stage Band; Choral Union; Madrigals; Small Ensembles; UVM Baroque Ensemble; ConBrio Chamber Ensemble
Workshops/Festivals: High School Summer Music Session; International Music Educators' Conference; Vermont Mozart Festival; Interstate Wind Festival

THEATRE

Edward Feidner, Chairman   **Number Of Faculty:** 5   **Number Of Students:** 600
Degrees Offered: BA   **Teaching Certification Available**
Financial Assistance: Work-Study Grants
Performing Groups: Spring Touring Group
Workshops/Festivals: Champlain Shakespeare Festival

WINDHAM COLLEGE
Putney   Vermont 05346, 802 387-5511
Private and 4 Year   **Arts Areas:** Dance, Theatre and Visual Arts
Performing Series: Windham Summer Repertory Theatre
Performance Facilities: Mainstage; Studio Theatre; Dance Studio

DANCE

Mollie Burke, Chairman   **Number Of Faculty:** 1   **Number Of Students:** 30
Degrees Offered: BFA
Courses Offered: Beginning; Intermediate; Improvisation; Composition; Tutorials
Financial Assistance: Scholarships, Work-Study Grants and Federal Programs

THEATRE

Orvis Rigsby, Assistant Professor   **Number Of Faculty:** 2
Number Of Students: 25   **Degrees Offered:** BFA
Courses Offered: Literature; Technical; Design; Acting; Directing; Contractuals; Playwriting
Teaching Certification Available
Financial Assistance: Scholarships and Work-Study Grants
Performing Groups: Patchwork Players   **Workshops/Festivals:** WSRT

BLUEFIELD COLLEGE
Bluefield   Virginia 24605, 304 327-7137
   Private and 4 Year   *Arts Areas:* Vocal Music and Theatre

MUSIC

J P Jardine, Chairman   *Number Of Faculty:* 3   *Degrees Offered:* AA; BA
Courses Offered: Appreciation; Theory; History; Applied
Teaching Certification Available
Financial Assistance: Scholarships and Work-Study Grants
Performing Groups: Choir

THEATRE

Dr Michael Garrett, Chairman   *Number Of Faculty:* 1
Courses Offered: Drama; Appreciation; Practicum in Theatre
Financial Assistance: Scholarships and Work-Study Grants

BRIDGEWATER COLLEGE
E College St, Bridgewater   Virginia 22812
703 828-2501
   Private and 4 Year
   Arts Areas: Instrumental Music, Vocal Music and Visual Arts
   Performing Series: Concert-Lecture Series
   Performance Facilities: College Auditorium

MUSIC

Philip E Trout, Chairman   *Number Of Faculty:* 5   *Number Of Students:* 50
Degrees Offered: BA   *Teaching Certification Available*
Financial Assistance: Scholarships and Work-Study Grants
Performing Groups: Vocal and Instrumental Ensembles

CHRISTOPHER NEWPORT COLLEGE
Box 6070, Newport News   Virginia 23606
804 599-7073
   State and 4 Year
   Arts Areas: Dance, Instrumental Music, Vocal Music, Theatre, Film Arts, Visual Arts and Speech
   Performing Series: Fine and Performing Arts Monthly Concert Series; Nancy Ramseur Concert Series
   Performance Facilities: Campus Center Theatre

MUSIC

James R Hines, Chairman   *Number Of Faculty:* 9   *Number Of Students:* 100
Degrees Offered: BFA
Workshops/Festivals: Performing Arts Series; Opera Studio; Workshops

THEATRE

Dr Bruno Koch, Chairman   *Number Of Faculty:* 3   *Number Of Students:* 100
Degrees Offered: BFA   *Teaching Certification Available*
Performing Groups: CNC Players   *Workshops/Festivals:* Education Theatre Series

---

CLINCH VALLEY COLLEGE OF THE UNIVERSITY OF VIRGINIA
Wise   Virginia 24293, 703 328-2431 Ext 264
   State and 4 Year
   Arts Areas: Dance, Instrumental Music, Vocal Music and Theatre
   Performance Facilities: Auditorium

(continued on next page)

MUSIC

D M Donathan, Director   **Number Of Faculty:** 1   **Number Of Students:** 75
Courses Offered: Music Literature; Applied; Music Education
Performing Groups: The CVC Choir
Workshops/Festivals: International Arts Festival

THEATRE

Charles W Lewis, Director   **Number Of Faculty:** 2   **Number Of Students:** 46
Degrees Offered: BA
Courses Offered: Acting; Production; Directing; Playwriting; Practicum; Modern Drama
Performing Groups: CVC Highland Players
Workshops/Festivals: Summer Workshops

COLLEGE OF WILLIAM AND MARY
Williamsburg   Virginia 23185, 804 253-4000
State and 4 Year
Arts Areas: Instrumental Music, Vocal Music, Theatre and Visual Arts
Performing Series: The Concert Series
Performance Facilities: Phi Beta Kappa Memorial Hall

MUSIC

Frank T Lendrim, Department Head   **Number Of Faculty:** 23
Number Of Students: 33   **Degrees Offered:** BA
Teaching Certification Available
Financial Assistance: Scholarships and Work-Study Grants
Performing Groups: Choir; Band; Orchestra; Chorus; Chamber Singers

THEATRE

Patrick H Micken, Department Head   **Number Of Faculty:** 5
Number Of Students: 35   **Degrees Offered:** BA
Teaching Certification Available
Financial Assistance: Scholarships and Work-Study Grants
Performing Groups: William and Mary Theatre; Premiere Theatre

---

EASTERN MENNONITE COLLEGE
Harrisonburg   Virginia 22801, 703 433-2771 Ext 137
Private and 4 Year
Arts Areas: Instrumental Music, Vocal Music, Theatre and Visual Arts
Performing Series: Lecture - Music Series
Performance Facilities: Chapel Auditorium

MUSIC

Willard M Swartley and Kenneth J Nafziger, Co-Chairmen
Number Of Faculty: 5   **Degrees Offered:** BA Mus; BA MusEd
Courses Offered: Theory; Composition; History and Literature; Conducting; Pedagogy; Church Music; Applied
Teaching Certification Available   **Financial Assistance:** Work-Study Grants
Performing Groups: Choir; Instrumental Ensembles

THEATRE

J B Landis, Chairman, English Department
Financial Assistance: Work-Study Grants   **Performing Groups:** Drama Guild

---

EMORY AND HENRY COLLEGE
Emory   Virginia 24327, 703 944-3121
Private and 4 Year   **Arts Areas:** Instrumental Music and Vocal Music
Performing Series: Concert and Lecture Series
Performance Facilities: College Auditorium

(continued on next page)

MUSIC

Charles R Davis, Chairman   **Number Of Faculty:** 4   **Number Of Students:** 32
Degrees Offered: BA   **Financial Assistance:** Scholarships
Performing Groups: Vocal and Instrumental Ensembles

FERRUM COLLEGE
Ferrum   Virginia 24088, 703 365-2121
Private and 4 Year
Arts Areas: Instrumental Music, Vocal Music, Theatre, Television and Visual Arts
Performing Series: Cultural Arts Series; Insight Series
Performance Facilities: Vaughn Memorial Chapel; Educational Building; Swartz Gymnasium; Schoolfield
Building

MUSIC

James E McConnell, Associate Professor of Music   **Number Of Faculty:** 6
Number Of Students: 400   **Degrees Offered:** BA; BS; AA
Courses Offered: Church Music; Organ History and Literature; Church Music in Theory and Practice;
Hymnology
Financial Assistance: Scholarships and Work-Study Grants
Performing Groups: New Ferrum Singers; Voices of Hope; Ferrum College Concert Choir
Workshops/Festivals: Christmas Concert; Tours; Spring Fine Arts Festivals

THEATRE

R Rex Stephenson, Assistant Professor of Drama/Speech   **Number Of Faculty:** 2
Number Of Students: 100   **Degrees Offered:** AA
Courses Offered: Introduction to the Theatre; Fundamentals of Acting; Oral Interpretation and Puppetry;
Principles of Stage Make-up; Play Production; Stagecraft; Television Programming and Production
Workshop; Rehearsal and Performance
Financial Assistance: Scholarships and Work-Study Grants
Performing Groups: Ferrum Players; Jack Tale Players and Jack Tale Storytellers
Workshops/Festivals: Spring Fine Arts Festival; Tours of the state with grant from Commission of the
Arts and Humanitites

HAMPTON INSTITUTE
Hampton   Virginia 23668, 804 727-5000
Private and City
Arts Areas: Dance, Instrumental Music, Vocal Music, Theatre, Film Arts, Television and Visual Arts
Performing Series: Performing Arts Series
Performance Facilities: Ogden Hall; Little Theatre

MUSIC

Willis E Daughtry, PhD, Chairman   **Number Of Faculty:** 15
Number Of Students: 71   **Degrees Offered:** BS; BA
Teaching Certification Available

(continued on next page)

Financial Assistance: Scholarships and Work-Study Grants
Performing Groups: Marching Band; Concert Band; College Choir; Concert Choir; Vocal Ensemble; Brass Ensemble; Jazz Band; Keyboard Ensemble; String Ensemble

THEATRE

Joyce W O'Rouke, Chairman   **Number Of Faculty:** 5   **Number Of Students:** 68
Degrees Offered: BA   **Teaching Certification Available**
Financial Assistance: Scholarships   **Performing Groups:** Hampton Players

HOLLINS COLLEGE

Hollins College   Virginia 24020, 703 362-6333
  Private and 4 Year
  Arts Areas: Dance, Instrumental Music, Vocal Music, Theatre and Visual Arts
  Performing Series: Sallie Gray Shepherd Series

DANCE

Degrees Offered: BA   **Financial Assistance:** Scholarships   **Performing Groups:** Dance Group

MUSIC

Oscar McCollough, Chairman   **Number Of Faculty:** 7   **Number Of Students:** 25
Degrees Offered: BA   **Financial Assistance:** Scholarships
Performing Groups: Band; Ensembles; Choir

THEATRE

G Dean Goodsell, Chairman   **Degrees Offered:** BA
Financial Assistance: Scholarships   **Performing Groups:** Drama Assn

JAMES MADISON UNIVERSITY

Harrisonburg   Virginia 22801, 703 433-6211
  State and 4 Year
  Arts Areas: Dance, Instrumental Music, Vocal Music, Theatre, Film Arts, Television and Visual Arts
  Performing Series: Artist and Lecture Presentations
  Performance Facilities: Latimer - Shaeffer Theatre; Duke Fine Arts Building

DANCE

Dr Earlynn Miller, Coordinator   **Number Of Faculty:** 6
Number Of Students: 60   **Degrees Offered:** BA; MS
Courses Offered: Techniques of Dance Theatre; Methods of Teaching; History; Choreography; Costuming; Management; Publicity; Set Design and Construction; Lighting; Acting; Makeup
Financial Assistance: Assistantships and Work-Study Grants
Performing Groups: James Madison University Dance Theatre; Folk Ensemble; Modern Ensemble; Virginia Dance Theatre

MUSIC

Dr Joseph J Estock, Department Head   **Number Of Faculty:** 31
Number Of Students: 300   **Degrees Offered:** BMusEd; BMus; M MusEd
Technical Training: Music Composition Skills; Electronic Music Performance & Composition; Performance Skills; Learning Theories/Educational Practices
Teaching Certification Available
Financial Assistance: Assistantships, Scholarships and Work-Study Grants
Performing Groups: Marching Band; Concert Band; Chamber Ensembles; Chorus; College Chorale; Concert Choir; Orchestra; Chamber Orchestra; The Madison Singers; University Jazz Ensemble; University Jazz Band; Woodwind Ensembles; Brass Ensembles; Wind Ensemble; Piano Accompanying and Ensemble; Vocal Jazz Choir; Percussion Ensemble; Horn Choir; Trumpet Choir; Flute Choir; Clarinet Choir

THEATRE

Dr Thomas H Arthur, Chairman   **Number Of Faculty:** 6
Number Of Students: 95   **Degrees Offered:** BA

(continued on next page)

Technical Training: Set Design; Construction; Lighting; Acting; Make-up; Costuming; Management; Publicity
Teaching Certification Available
Financial Assistance: Assistantships, Scholarships and Work-Study Grants
Performing Groups: James Madison University Theatre; Experimental Theatre
Workshops/Festivals: Fine Arts Festival

LONGWOOD COLLEGE
Farmville   Virginia 23901, 804 392-9371
State and 4 Year
Arts Areas: Dance, Instrumental Music, Vocal Music, Theatre, Film Arts and Visual Arts
Performing Series: Artists Series
Performance Facilities: Jarman Hall; Molnar Recital Hall

DANCE

Number Of Faculty: 2   **Teaching Certification Available**
Financial Assistance: Scholarships
Performing Groups: Longwood College Company of Dancers

MUSIC

Dr James McCray, Chairman   **Number Of Faculty:** 10   **Number Of Students:** 75
Degrees Offered: BA Mus; BS MusEd
Courses Offered: Theory; Appreciation; History and Literature; Applied; Music Education
Technical Training: Voice Instruction; Applied in Organ, Harpsichord, Piano, Strings, Woodwinds, and Brass
Teaching Certification Available
Financial Assistance: Scholarships and Work-Study Grants
Performing Groups: Concert Choir; Camerata Singers; Instrumental Ensembles
Workshops/Festivals: Christmas Renaissance Dinner; Master Classes in Vocal, Organ, and Piano Performance; Contemporary Music Symposium

THEATRE

Dr Patton Lockwood, Chairman   **Number Of Faculty:** 5
Number Of Students: 72   **Degrees Offered:** BS; BA
Courses Offered: Performance and Technical Skills; Literature and History of the Theatre
Teaching Certification Available
Financial Assistance: Scholarships and Work-Study Grants   **Performing Groups:** The Longwood Players

LYNCHBURG COLLEGE
Lynchburg   Virginia 24504, 804 845-9071
Private and 4 Year
Arts Areas: Instrumental Music, Vocal Music, Theatre and Visual Arts

MUSIC

Robert S Ellinwood, Chairman   **Number Of Faculty:** 5
Number Of Students: 47   **Degrees Offered:** BA Mus, MusEd
Teaching Certification Available
Financial Assistance: Scholarships and Work-Study Grants
Performing Groups: Chorale Groups; Instrumental Ensembles; Band
Workshops/Festivals: Opera Workshop

THEATRE

Robert C Hailey, Chairman   **Degrees Offered:** BA
Teaching Certification Available
Financial Assistance: Scholarships and Work-Study Grants
Performing Groups: Lynchburg College Theatre

LYNCHBURG COLLEGE
Lynchburg   Virginia 24501, 804 845-9071 Ext 301
>   Private and 4 Year
>   **Arts Areas:** Dance, Instrumental Music, Vocal Music, Theatre and Visual Arts
>   **Performing Series:** Fine Arts Series; Theatre Series
>   **Performance Facilities:** Dillard Theatre; Hopwood Auditorium; Helen Wood Recital Hall; Dance Studio

DANCE

James C Fox, Chairman, Department of Physical Education, Health & Recreation
Number Of Faculty: 1
Courses Offered: Modern Dance Technique; Modern Dance Composition; Show Dance; Teaching Modern Dance
Teaching Certification Available
Financial Assistance: Scholarships and Work-Study Grants
Performing Groups: Lynchburg College Company of Modern Dance

MUSIC

Robert S Ellinwood, Chairman   **Number Of Faculty:** 5
Number Of Students: 47   **Degrees Offered:** BA Mus; BA MusEd
Teaching Certification Available
Financial Assistance: Scholarships and Work-Study Grants
Performing Groups: Chorale Groups; Instrumental Ensembles; Band
Workshops/Festivals: Opera Workshop

THEATRE

Robert C Hailey, Chairman   **Degrees Offered:** BA
Teaching Certification Available
Financial Assistance: Scholarships and Work-Study Grants
Performing Groups: Lynchburg College Theatre

MARY BALDWIN COLLEGE
Frederick St, Staunton   Virginia 24401
703 885-0811
>   Private and 4 Year
>   **Arts Areas:** Dance, Instrumental Music, Vocal Music, Theatre, Television and Visual Arts
>   **Performance Facilities:** King Auditorium; Francis Auditorium; Page Terrace

DANCE

Gwendolyn E Walsh, Assistant Professor of Physical Education
Number Of Faculty: 1   **Number Of Students:** 35   **Degrees Offered:** BA
Courses Offered: Ballet; Mime; Folk; Square; Dance History
Technical Training: Physical Education
Financial Assistance: Internships, Assistantships, Scholarships and Work-Study Grants
Workshops/Festivals: Fine Arts Festival

MUSIC

Gordon Page, Professor   **Number Of Faculty:** 2   **Degrees Offered:** BA
Courses Offered: Applied; Introductory Studies in Music; Music as Language; Symphonic Music; Bach; Beethoven; Choral Conducting; Western Music; Colloquium; Directed Inquiry & Research; The American Musical Theater; Directing
Teaching Certification Available
Financial Assistance: Internships, Assistantships, Scholarships and Work-Study Grants
Performing Groups: Choir
Workshops/Festivals: Fine Arts Festival; King Series; Choir Workshop

THEATRE

Virginia R Francisco, Associate Professor   **Number Of Faculty:** 3
Degrees Offered: BA

(continued on next page)

Courses Offered: The World of Theater; Oral Interpretation; Scene Design; Stagecraft; Modern Drama; Costume; Make-up; Lighting; Contemporary Theater in London; Introduction to Shakespeare; Spanish Drama; Perspective; Acting; Medieval Drama; Directing; Theatre History; Greek Tragedy
Teaching Certification Available
Financial Assistance: Internships, Assistantships, Scholarships and Work-Study Grants
Performing Groups: Reader's Theater; Student Plays; Oak Grove; Theater Wagon

MARY WASHINGTON COLLEGE
Fredericksburg   Virginia 22401, 703 373-7250
State and 4 Year
Arts Areas: Dance, Instrumental Music, Vocal Music, Theatre and Visual Arts
Performing Series: Artists Series   **Performance Facilities:** College Auditorium

MUSIC

Degrees Offered: BA Mus   **Financial Assistance:** Scholarships
Performing Groups: Band; Chorus; Orchestra

THEATRE

Roger Kenvin, Chairman   **Number Of Faculty:** 4   **Number Of Students:** 60
Degrees Offered: BA   **Financial Assistance:** Scholarships
Performing Groups: Mary Washington Players

NORFOLK STATE COLLEGE
2401 Corpen Ave, Norfolk   Virginia 23504
703 627-4373
State and 4 Year
Arts Areas: Instrumental Music, Vocal Music, Theatre and Visual Arts
Performing Series: Concert Series   **Performance Facilities:** College Auditorium
Degrees Offered: BA   **Financial Assistance:** Scholarships
Workshops/Festivals: Opera Workshop   **Degrees Offered:** BA   **Financial Assistance:** Scholarships

OLD DOMINION UNIVERSITY
Norfolk   Virginia 23508, 804 489-6000
State and 4 Year
Arts Areas: Dance, Instrumental Music, Vocal Music, Theatre and Visual Arts
Performance Facilities: University Theater; Batten Arts and Letters Auditorium

DANCE

Istvan Ament, Director, ODU Community Ballet   **Number Of Faculty:** 5
Number Of Students: 115
Courses Offered: Classical; Toe & Variation; Modern; Jazz; Character
Financial Assistance: Scholarships   **Performing Groups:** ODU Community Ballet

MUSIC

Harold Protsman, Chairman   **Number Of Faculty:** 13   **Number Of Students:** 145
Degrees Offered: BA; BS
Courses Offered: Orchestra Music; Organ; Piano; Voice; Music History & Composition
Technical Training: Orchestral Instruments; Organ; Voce; Piano
Teaching Certification Available
Financial Assistance: Scholarships and Work-Study Grants
Performing Groups: Brass Quintet; Concert Choir; Jazz Ensemble; Madrigal Singers; Pep Band; Singing Monarchs; Faculty Trio; Symphonic Wind Ensemble
Workshops/Festivals: Brass Instrumentalist Workshop

THEATRE

Paul Dicklin, Director of Theater   **Number Of Faculty:** 2
Number Of Students: 30   **Degrees Offered:** BA Speech

(continued on next page)

Courses Offered: Acting; Appreciation; Play Production; Lighting; Set Design
Financial Assistance: Scholarships and Work-Study Grants
Performing Groups: Old Dominion Players

RADFORD COLLEGE
Norwood St, Radford   Virginia 24142
703 731-5000
State and 4 Year
Arts Areas: Dance, Instrumental Music, Vocal Music, Theatre and Visual Arts
Performing Series: Piedmont Chamber Orchestra; Houston Ballet & Orchestra
Performance Facilities: Preston Hall Auditorium; Porterfield Hall Theatre; Peters Hall

DANCE

Dr Mary Pat Balkus, Chairman   **Number Of Faculty:** 3
Number Of Students: 47   **Degrees Offered:** BS; BA
Courses Offered: Ballet; Social Dance; Tap Dance; Beginning and Introductory Modern Dance; Jazz; Rehearsal and Performance; Introduction to Dance Therapy; Folk and Square Dance; Methods of Teaching Dance; Dance Production; Problems in Dance; Point & Technique; Dance Appreciation; Accompaniment for Movement; Dance for Children; Symposium in Dance; Choreographic Studies in Dance; History and Philosophy of Dance; Independent Study
Financial Assistance: Scholarships and Work-Study Grants
Performing Groups: Radford College Dance Theatre

MUSIC

Eugene C Fellin, Chairman   **Number Of Faculty:** 16   **Number Of Students:** 150
Degrees Offered: BA; BS; BS MA; MS
Courses Offered: Music Education; Performance; Composition; History
Teaching Certification Available
Financial Assistance: Assistantships, Scholarships and Work-Study Grants
Performing Groups: The Radford Orchestra; Highlander Concert Band; Chorale; Concert Choir
Workshops/Festivals: Music Teachers Workshop

THEATRE

Dr James W Hawes, Chairman   **Number Of Faculty:** 3   **Number Of Students:** 39
Degrees Offered: BA; BS
Courses Offered: Acting; Directing; Theatre Design; Costume Design; Technical Theatre; Management; History and Literature; Playwriting
Teaching Certification Available
Financial Assistance: Assistantships, Scholarships and Work-Study Grants
Performing Groups: Radford College Theatre Players

RANDOLPH - MACON COLLEGE
Ashland   Virginia 23005, 804 798-8372
Private and 4 Year
Arts Areas: Dance, Instrumental Music, Vocal Music, Theatre and Visual Arts

MUSIC

R D Ward, Chairman   **Number Of Faculty:** 2   **Number Of Students:** 30
Financial Assistance: Scholarships, Work-Study Grants and Loans
Performing Groups: Chorus; Woodwind Ensemble

THEATRE

David Kilgore, Chairman   **Number Of Faculty:** 1   **Number Of Students:** 25
Financial Assistance: Scholarships, Work-Study Grants and Loans
Performing Groups: Drama Guild

ROANOKE COLLEGE
Salem Virginia 24153, 703 389-2351 Ext 250
> Private and 4 Year
> *Arts Areas:* Instrumental Music, Vocal Music, Theatre, Television and Visual Arts
> *Performing Series:* Roanoke College Concert Series
> *Performance Facilities:* Antrim Chapel

MUSIC

Frank M Williams, Chairman   *Number Of Faculty:* 5   *Number Of Students:* 500
Degrees Offered: BA Fine Arts   *Teaching Certification Available*
Financial Assistance: Scholarships and Work-Study Grants
Performing Groups: Concert Choir; Collegium Musicum: Band; Chapel Choir
Workshops/Festivals: Musical Theatre

THEATRE

Sam R Good, Chairman   *Number Of Faculty:* 1   *Number Of Students:* 300
Degrees Offered: BFA   *Teaching Certification Available*
Financial Assistance: Scholarships and Work-Study Grants
Performing Groups: APO Drama Fraternity   *Workshops/Festivals:* Musical Theatre

SHENANDOAH COLLEGE & CONSERVATORY OF MUSIC
Millwood Pike, Winchester   Virginia 22601
703 667-8714
> Private and 4 Year   *Arts Areas:* Instrumental Music and Vocal Music

MUSIC

Number Of Faculty: 42   *Number Of Students:* 330
Degrees Offered: BMus; MMusEd   *Financial Assistance:* Scholarships
Performing Groups: Musical Ensembles; Chamber Orchestra; Choir

SOUTHERN SEMINARY JUNIOR COLLEGE
Buena Vista   Virginia 24416, 703 261-6181
> Private and 2 Year
> *Arts Areas:* Dance, Instrumental Music, Vocal Music and Theatre
> *Performance Facilities:* Auditorium; Theater; Dance Studio; Concert Room

DANCE

Anne E Mish, Chairman, Division of Physical Education   *Number Of Faculty:* 1
Financial Assistance: Work-Study Grants

MUSIC

Dr Mary M Mahone, Chairman   *Number Of Faculty:* 1   *Number Of Students:* 25
Degrees Offered: AA   *Courses Offered:* Vocal; Piano; Music History; Theory
Financial Assistance: Work-Study Grants
Performing Groups: Choir; Music Collegium

THEATRE

Number Of Faculty: 1   *Number Of Students:* 25   *Degrees Offered:* AA
Financial Assistance: Work-Study Grants   *Performing Groups:* Southern Sem Theater

SULLINS COLLEGE
Bristol   Virginia 24201, 703 699-6112
> Private and 2 Year
> *Arts Areas:* Dance, Instrumental Music, Vocal Music, Theatre and Visual Arts

(continued on next page)

DANCE

Valentina Belova, Chairman   **Degrees Offered:** AA
Financial Assistance: Scholarships

MUSIC

F William Thomas, Chairman   **Degrees Offered:** AA
Financial Assistance: Scholarships
Performing Groups: Vocal & Instrumental Ensembles

THEATRE

James F Cunningham, Chairman   **Degrees Offered:** AA
Financial Assistance: Scholarships   **Performing Groups:** Sullins Players

---

SWEET BRIAR COLLEGE
Sweet Briar   Virginia 24595, 804 381-5422
Private and 4 Year
Arts Areas: Dance, Instrumental Music, Vocal Music, Theatre and Visual Arts
Financial Assistance: Scholarships and Loans
Performing Groups: Sweet Briar Dance Theatre

MUSIC

John R Shannon, Chairman   **Number Of Faculty:** 4   **Number Of Students:** 125
Degrees Offered: BA   **Financial Assistance:** Scholarships and Loans

THEATRE

Joseph Roach, Chairman   **Number Of Faculty:** 3   **Number Of Students:** 80
Degrees Offered: Theatre Arts; Dance Theatre
Courses Offered: History of the Theatre; Dramatic Literature; Theory; Acting; Directing; Dance
Technique; Dance Composition; Dance History
Financial Assistance: Scholarships and Loans
Performing Groups: Paint and Patches

TIDEWATER COMMUNITY COLLEGE, FREDERICK CAMPUS
State Rt 135, Portsmouth   Virginia 23703
804 484-2121 Ext 246
State and 2 Year
Arts Areas: Instrumental Music, Vocal Music and Theatre

MUSIC

Donald Smith, Coordinator of Music   **Number Of Faculty:** 10
Number Of Students: 60   **Degrees Offered:** AA
Courses Offered: Theory; Appreciation; Applied
Financial Assistance: Work-Study Grants
Performing Groups: Tidewater Community College Chorale; Frederick Singers

THEATRE

Gayle E Pipkin, Director of Drama   **Number Of Faculty:** 1
Number Of Students: 30   **Degrees Offered:** AA
Courses Offered: Acting; Directing; History of Theater; Rehearsal and Performance
Financial Assistance: Work-Study Grants

UNIVERSITY OF RICHMOND
University Post Office, Richmond   Virginia 23173
Private and 4 Year
Arts Areas: Dance, Instrumental Music, Vocal Music, Theatre and Visual Arts
Performance Facilities: Camp Memorial Theatre

(continued on next page)

MUSIC

Barbara H McMurty, Chairman   **Number Of Faculty:** 17
Number Of Students: 220
Degrees Offered: BA; BMus; BMus Applied; BMusEd; MMus; MMusEd; MMus Choral Conducting
Teaching Certification Available
Financial Assistance: Scholarships and Work-Study Grants
Performing Groups: Schola Cantorum; University Choir; Band; Orchestra Stage Band

THEATRE

Dr Jerry Tarver, Chairman   **Number Of Faculty:** 5   **Number Of Students:** 65
Degrees Offered: BA   **Teaching Certification Available**
Financial Assistance: Assistantships and Work-Study Grants
Workshops/Festivals: High School Speech and Theatre Institute

---

VIRGINIA COMMONWEALTH UNIVERSITY
910 W Franklin St, Richmond   Virginia 23200
703 770-6357
State and 4 Year
Arts Areas: Instrumental Music, Vocal Music, Theatre and Visual Arts
Performing Series: Concert & Dance Committee
Performance Facilities: University Auditorium

MUSIC

Ronald B Thomas, Chairman   **Number Of Faculty:** 33   **Number Of Students:** 250
Degrees Offered: BMus; BMusEd; MA   **Teaching Certification Available**
Financial Assistance: Scholarships and Work-Study Grants
Performing Groups: Band; Chorus; Orchestra
Workshops/Festivals: Opera Workshop

THEATRE

Kenneth Campbell, Chairman   **Number Of Faculty:** 15
Number Of Students: 205   **Degrees Offered:** BFA; MFA
Teaching Certification Available
Financial Assistance: Scholarships and Work-Study Grants
Performing Groups: University Theatre

VIRGINIA COMMONWEALTH UNIVERSITY
901 W Franklin St, Richmond   Virginia 23284
State and 4 Year
School of the Arts - 325 N Harrison St
Arts Areas: Instrumental Music, Vocal Music, Theatre and Visual Arts
Performance Facilities: University Auditorium; Local Churches; Music Center

MUSIC

Ronald B Thomas, Chairman   **Number Of Faculty:** 33   **Number Of Students:** 250
Degrees Offered: BMus; BMusEd; MA   **Teaching Certification Available**
Financial Assistance: Scholarships and Work-Study Grants
Performing Groups: Band; Chorus; Orchestra
Workshops/Festivals: Opera Workshop

THEATRE

Kenneth Campbell, Chairman   **Number Of Faculty:** 15
Number Of Students: 205   **Degrees Offered:** BFA; MFA
Teaching Certification Available
Financial Assistance: Scholarships and Work-Study Grants
Performing Groups: University Theatre

VIRGINIA INTERMONT COLLEGE
Bristol   Virginia 24201, 703 669-6101
 Private and 4 Year
 Arts Areas: Dance, Instrumental Music, Vocal Music, Theatre and Visual Arts
 Performance Facilities: Fine Arts Center Little Theatre and Recital Hall; Harrison - Jones Memorial Hall

DANCE

Constance Hardinge, Chairman Ballet Program   *Number Of Faculty:* 4
Number Of Students: 60   *Degrees Offered:* BA
Courses Offered: Ballet; Jazz; Ballet Terminology; Dance History; Modern; Teaching of Ballet; Character; Choreography; Variations and Adagio; Classical Ballet based on Russian and Italian techniques
Teaching Certification Available
Financial Assistance: Internships, Assistantships, Scholarships and Work-Study Grants
Performing Groups: Bristol Concert Ballet Company
Workshops/Festivals: "Nutcracker" during the Christmas season; two spring seasons of "Coppelia" and "Showcase" where original choreography is presented

MUSIC

Stephen Hamilton, Chairman   *Number Of Faculty:* 4   *Number Of Students:* 30
Degrees Offered: BA
Courses Offered: Applied; Theory; History & Literature; Music Appreciation; Hymnology; Conducting; Teacher Training
Teaching Certification Available
Financial Assistance: Internships, Assistantships, Scholarships and Work-Study Grants
Performing Groups: Choir; Madrigal Singers; No Names (singing group); Instrumental Ensembles
Workshops/Festivals: Concert Series; Organ, Piano, Vocal, Instrumental Master Classes and Workshops

THEATRE

James L Andre, Chairman   *Number Of Faculty:* 1   *Number Of Students:* 10
Degrees Offered: AA
Courses Offered: Introduction to Theatre; Acting; Stagecraft; History of Theatre; Make-up; Oral Interpretation and Readers Theatre
Financial Assistance: Internships, Assistantships, Scholarships and Work-Study Grants
Performing Groups: VI College Players
Workshops/Festivals: One-Act Play Invitational Festival; Readers Theatre; Annual Festival for High Schools

VIRGINIA POLYTECHNIC INSTITUTE AND STATE UNIVERSITY
Blacksburg   Virginia 24061, 703 951-5200
 State and 4 Year
 Arts Areas: Instrumental Music, Vocal Music, Theatre, Film Arts and Television
 Performing Series: Concert-Lecture Series; Broadway Series; Popular Concert Series; Performing Arts Federation Series
 Performance Facilities: Squires Theatre; Barruss, Brown, and McBryde Auditoriums; PAB Little Theatre

MUSIC

David R Widder, Chairman   *Number Of Faculty:* 15   *Number Of Students:* 62
Degrees Offered: BA
Courses Offered: History; Theory; Composition; Applied; Ensembles
Teaching Certification Available
Financial Assistance: Scholarships and Work-Study Grants
Performing Groups: Chamber Orchestra; New River Valley Symphony; Collegium Musicum; University Symphonic Wind Ensemble; Jazz Ensemble; Concert Band; Marching Virginians; Highty-Tighties; New Virginians; Chamber Choir; Techmen; Opera Workshop; Choral Union; Chamber Groups
Workshops/Festivals: Jazz; Choral; Concert Band

THEATRE

Donald A Drapeau, Chairman   *Number Of Faculty:* 7   *Number Of Students:* 63
Degrees Offered: BA; MFA

(continued on next page)

Courses Offered: History; Literature; Performance; Design/Tech; Arts Administration
Technical Training: Performance; Directing; Design/Tech
Teaching Certification Available
Financial Assistance: Scholarships and Work-Study Grants
Performing Groups: University Theatre; Maroon Mask; Virginia Mime Troupe
Workshops/Festivals: Summer Arts Festival; Dance Workshop; Mime Workshop

VIRGINIA STATE COLLEGE
Petersburg   Virginia 23803, 703 526-5111
    State and 4 Year
    Arts Areas: Instrumental Music, Vocal Music and Visual Arts
    Performing Series: Artists Recitals Series

MUSIC

Dr Howell T Jones, Chairman   **Number Of Faculty:** 17
Number Of Students: 100   **Degrees Offered:** BA
Teaching Certification Available
Financial Assistance: Scholarships and Work-Study Grants
Workshops/Festivals: Opera Workshop

VIRGINIA UNION UNIVERSITY
1500 N Lombardy St, Richmond   Virginia 23220
804 359-9331
    Private and 4 Year   **Arts Areas:** Instrumental Music and Vocal Music
    Performing Series: Concert Series
    Performance Facilities: University Auditorium

MUSIC

Odell Hobbs, Chairman   **Degrees Offered:** BA
Teaching Certification Available   **Financial Assistance:** Scholarships
Performing Groups: Band; Chorus; Glee Club

VIRGINIA WESLEYAN COLLEGE
Wesleyan Dr, Norfolk   Virginia 23502
804 461-3232
    Private and 4 Year
    Arts Areas: Instrumental Music, Vocal Music, Theatre, Film Arts and Visual Arts
    Performing Series: Cultural Events Series
    Performance Facilities: Monumental Chapel

MUSIC

Dr Robert D Clayton, Chairman   **Number Of Faculty:** 1
Number Of Students: 70   **Courses Offered:** Music History; Music Appreciation
Technical Training: Applied   **Teaching Certification Available**
Financial Assistance: Work-Study Grants
Performing Groups: Chorus; Chamber Choir; Instrumental Ensemble

UNIVERSITY OF VIRGINIA
Charlottesville   Virginia 22903, 804 924-3326
    State and 4 Year
    Arts Areas: Dance, Instrumental Music, Vocal Music and Theatre
    Performing Series: Tuesday Evening Concert Series; Artists Series
    Performance Facilities: Cabell Hall Auditorium; Helms Experimental Theater; Culbreth Theater;
    University Hall

(continued on next page)

MUSIC

Walter B Ross, Chairman   **Number Of Faculty:** 12   **Number Of Students:** 3000
Degrees Offered: MA; BA   **Courses Offered:** Theory; History; Ensembles
Technical Training: Conducting
Financial Assistance: Assistantships, Scholarships and Work-Study Grants
Performing Groups: University & Community Orchestra; University Symphonic Band; Men's Glee Club; Women's Chorus; University Singers (Mixed)

THEATRE

George Black, Chairman   **Number Of Faculty:** 12   **Number Of Students:** 120
Degrees Offered: BA; MA; MFA
Financial Assistance: Assistantships, Scholarships and Work-Study Grants
Performing Groups: The Virginia Players; Heritage Repertory Theatre
Workshops/Festivals: ACTF Regional; High School League - Drama Finals

---

WASHINGTON AND LEE UNIVERSITY
Lexington   Virginia 24450, 703 463-9111
Private and 4 Year
Arts Areas: Instrumental Music, Vocal Music, Theatre, Film Arts and Television
Performing Series: Rockbridge Concert - Theatre Series; W & L Concert Guild
Performance Facilities: Lee Chapel; University Theatre; WLUR-FM/Cable Nine Broadcast Studios

MUSIC

Robert Stewart, Chairman   **Number Of Faculty:** 3   **Number Of Students:** 390
Degrees Offered: BA   **Technical Training:** Voice; Applied
Performing Groups: Glee Club; Brass Choir & Percussion Ensemble; Sazeracs

THEATRE

Lee Kahn and Albert C Gordon, Chairmen   **Number Of Faculty:** 3
Number Of Students: 202   **Degrees Offered:** BA
Technical Training: Scenery; Lighting; Props; Costumes; Directing
Performing Groups: University Theatre
Workshops/Festivals: Workshops under Arthur & Margaret Glasgow Endowment

CENTRAL WASHINGTON UNIVERSITY
Ellensburg   Washington 98926, 509 963-1111
State and 4 Year
Arts Areas: Dance, Instrumental Music, Vocal Music, Theatre, Film Arts, Television, Visual Arts and Radio
Performance Facilities: Hertz Hall; McConnell Auditorium; Three-Penny Playhouse; Nicholson Pavilion

DANCE

Courses Offered: Modern Dance; Folk Dance; Ballroom Dance; Tap Dance; Orchesis
Dance offered under the auspices of the Physical Education Department

MUSIC

Dr Joseph Haruda, Chairman   *Number Of Faculty:* 19
Number Of Students: 200   *Degrees Offered:* BMus; BMusEd; MMus; MMusEd
Courses Offered: Jazz History; Introduction to Music; Theory; Applied; Jazz Choir; Ensembles; Chamber Groups; Band; Orchestra; Music History; Composition; Music Education; Honors Program; Psychology and Guidance in Music Education
Teaching Certification Available   *Financial Assistance:* Scholarships
Performing Groups: Vocal Jazz Choir; Woodwind Ensemble; Brass Choir; Chamber Orchestra; Flute Choir; Recorder Chamber Group; Percussion Ensemble; Stage Band; String Ensemble; Central Swingers; Madrigal Singers; Wind Ensemble; Choir; Orchestra; Marching and Concert Band

THEATRE

Dr Milo Smith, Chairman   *Number Of Faculty:* 6   *Number Of Students:* 90
Degrees Offered: BA; BA Ed
Courses Offered: Introduction to Drama; Rehearsal & Performance; Theory; Stagecraft; Design; Make-up; Creative Dramatics; Directing; Lighting; History of Drama; Puppetry; Playwriting; Fashion; Costume Design; Children's Theater; European Theater; Touring Theater; Roman-Greek-American-British Drama
Teaching Certification Available   *Financial Assistance:* Scholarships
Performing Groups: Alpha Psi Omega   *Workshops/Festivals:* Opera Workshop

---

CENTRALIA COLLEGE
PO Box 639, Centralia   Washington 98531
206 736-9391 Ext 258
State and 2 Year
Arts Areas: Instrumental Music, Vocal Music, Theatre, Film Arts and Television
Performance Facilities: Centralia College Theatre

MUSIC

Kenneth Kimball, Chairman   *Number Of Faculty:* 7   *Number Of Students:* 23
Degrees Offered: AA
Technical Training: Private Instruction, Piano, Organ, Brass Instruments, String Instruments, Woodwind Instruments, Voice
Financial Assistance: Work-Study Grants
Performing Groups: Concert Band, Stage Band, Pop Band, Mixed Chorus, Women's Vocal Ensemble, Brass Sextet, Woodwind Quintet

THEATRE

Phillip R Wickstrom, Chairman   *Number Of Faculty:* 1
Number Of Students: 7   *Degrees Offered:* AA
Financial Assistance: Work-Study Grants   *Performing Groups:* The College Players

CORNISH INSTITUTE OF ALLIED ARTS
710 E Roy, Seattle   Washington 98102
206 323-1400

Private and 4 Year
Arts Areas: Dance, Instrumental Music, Vocal Music, Theatre and Visual Arts
Performance Facilities: Cornish Theater

DANCE

Karen Irvin, Chairman   *Number Of Faculty:* 9   *Number Of Students:* 370
Degrees Offered: BFA; BAA   *Courses Offered:* Ballet; Modern Dance
Financial Assistance: Scholarships, Work-Study Grants and NDSL
Performing Groups: Cornish Dance Theater

MUSIC

Martin Friedman, Chairman   *Number Of Faculty:* 54   *Number Of Students:* 325
Degrees Offered: BMus; BAA
Courses Offered: Vocal; Instrumental/Composition; Jazz
Financial Assistance: Scholarships, Work-Study Grants and NDSL
Performing Groups: Chorus; Collegium Musicum; Chamber Music; Jazz; Guitar; Vocal Ensembles
Workshops/Festivals: Opera Workshop; Musical Theater Workshop

THEATRE

Julian Schembri, Chairman   *Number Of Faculty:* 7   *Number Of Students:* 30
Degrees Offered: BFA   *Courses Offered:* Acting
Financial Assistance: Scholarships, Work-Study Grants and NDSL
Performing Groups: Cornish Theater

EASTERN WASHINGTON STATE COLLEGE
Cheney   Washington 99004, 509 359-2225

State and 4 Year
Arts Areas: Dance, Instrumental Music, Vocal Music, Theatre, Film Arts, Television and Visual Arts
Performing Series: EWSC Artist and Lecture Series
Performance Facilities: Showalter Auditorium, College Theatre, Music Recital Hall, Events Building

DANCE

Mrs Edith Bucklin, Orchisis Director   *Number Of Faculty:* 2
Number Of Students: 300   *Degrees Offered:* BA
Courses Offered: Jazz, Ballet, Modern, Folk, Square Dance, Social Dance
Performing Groups: Orchesis
Workshops/Festivals: Dance Symposium, Northwest Dance Symposium, High School Creative Arts Summer
Series

MUSIC

Dr Wendal Jones, Chairman   *Number Of Faculty:* 23
Number Of Students: 1,329   *Degrees Offered:* BA, MA, Ed D
Technical Training: Reed Making, Piano Maintenance
Teaching Certification Available
Financial Assistance: Assistantships, Scholarships and Work-Study Grants
Performing Groups: Percussion Ensemble, Brass Ensemble, Festival Arts Trio, Willowell String Quartet,
Contemporary Music Ensemble, EWSC Symphony Orchestra, Band, Collegians, Madrigals
Workshops/Festivals: Tamarack Festival, High School Creative Arts Summer Series, Choral and Band
Sightreading Workshops, Opera Workshop

THEATRE

Dr R Boyd Devin, Chairman   *Number Of Faculty:* 5   *Number Of Students:* 120
Degrees Offered: BA, BA Ed
Technical Training: Scenery Construction, Scene Design, Stage Lighting, Costume Construction, Costume

(continued on next page)

Design, Stage Management Technique
Teaching Certification Available
Financial Assistance: Internships, Assistantships and Work-Study Grants
Performing Groups: College Theatre Group
Workshops/Festivals: High School Creative Arts Summer Series

FORT WRIGHT COLLEGE OF THE HOLY NAMES
W 4000 Randolph Rd, Spokane   Washington 99204
509 328-2970

Private and 4 Year
Arts Areas: Instrumental Music, Vocal Music, Theatre and Visual Arts
Performing Series: Concert Series

MUSIC

Xavier Mary Courvoisier, SNJM, Chairperson   **Number Of Faculty:** 8
Number Of Students: 130   **Degrees Offered:** BA; BFA; BMusEd
Technical Training: Music Performance in Voice, Piano, Orchestral Instruments, and Classical Guitar
Teaching Certification Available
Financial Assistance: Assistantships, Scholarships and Work-Study Grants
Performing Groups: College - Community Orchestra; Chorus, Voice and Instrumental Ensembles
Workshops/Festivals: Master Classes in Voice and Piano

THEATRE

Robert Welch, Chairman   **Number Of Faculty:** 3   **Number Of Students:** 35
Degrees Offered: BFA; BA
Courses Offered: Acting; Stage Production; Make-up; Voice & Diction; Set Design; Light Design; Actor's Lab; Directing & Performance; Directors' Workshop; Introduction to Theatre; Independent Study
Teaching Certification Available
Financial Assistance: Assistantships, Scholarships and Work-Study Grants
Performing Groups: The Interplayers Ensemble

GONZAGA UNIVERSITY
Spokane   Washington 99258, 509 328-4220

Private and 4 Year
Arts Areas: Dance, Vocal Music, Theatre and Television
Performance Facilities: Gene Russell Theater
Courses Offered: Ballet; Theater Dance

MUSIC

Paul Palmes, Chairman   **Number Of Faculty:** 6   **Number Of Students:** 60
Degrees Offered: BA Mus
Courses Offered: Vocal; Piano; Theory; Music History; Music Appreciation
Technical Training: Piano; Voice   **Financial Assistance:** Work-Study Grants
Performing Groups: "Stepp Sisters" Show Group; Concert Choir; "Ars Nova" Pop Choir; Stage Band
Workshops/Festivals: Stage III; Spring Music Festival; Various Variety Shows

THEATRE

David Hardaway, Director of Theater   **Number Of Faculty:** 2
Number Of Students: 30
Degrees Offered: Communication Arts in Drama; MEd; Communication Arts
Courses Offered: Acting; Directing; History; Literature and Theater
Financial Assistance: Work-Study Grants
Performing Groups: Main Performing Group; Stage III Group

HIGHLINE COMMUNITY COLLEGE
240th & Pacific Hwy, S, Midway   Washington 98031
206 878-3710 Ext 307
>County and 2 Year
>
>**Arts Areas:** Dance, Instrumental Music, Vocal Music, Theatre and Visual Arts
>
>**Performance Facilities:** Lecture Hall; Pavilion; Drama Theatre

DANCE

Number Of Faculty: 6   **Number Of Students:** 90
Courses Offered: Beginning Ballet; Modern Jazz Dance; Dance as Communication

MUSIC

Number Of Faculty: 3   **Number Of Students:** 650   **Degrees Offered:** AA
Courses Offered: Instrumental; Vocal
Performing Groups: String & Brass Ensembles; Choral; Concert Band

THEATRE

Number Of Faculty: 1   **Number Of Students:** 300   **Degrees Offered:** AA
Courses Offered: Acting; Puppetry; Stagecraft

LOWER COLUMBIA COLLEGE
1600 Maple, Longview   Washington 98632
206 577-2354
>State and 2 Year
>
>**Arts Areas:** Instrumental Music, Vocal Music, Theatre, Film Arts and Visual Arts
>
>**Performance Facilities:** Little Theatre

MUSIC

Dr Martin Sherry, Chairman   **Number Of Faculty:** 4   **Number Of Students:** 220
Degrees Offered: AA; AS   **Financial Assistance:** Work-Study Grants

THEATRE

Donald Correll, Chairman   **Number Of Faculty:** 1   **Number Of Students:** 19
Degrees Offered: AA; AS   **Courses Offered:** Introduction to Theatre; Stagecraft
Financial Assistance: Work-Study Grants   **Artists-In-Residence/Guest Artists:** Jan Zach

NORTHWEST COLLEGE
PO Box 579, Kirkland   Washington 98033
206 822-8266 Ext 256
>Private and 4 Year   **Arts Areas:** Instrumental Music and Vocal Music
>
>**Performance Facilities:** Music Center

MUSIC

Dr W Robert Swaffield, Coordinator   **Number Of Faculty:** 12
Number Of Students: 60   **Degrees Offered:** AA; BA Sacred Mus
Financial Assistance: Internships, Scholarships and Work-Study Grants
Workshops/Festivals: Christmas Festival; Spring Concert; Recitals

PACIFIC LUTHERAN UNIVERSITY
Tacoma   Washington 98447, 206 531-6900 Ext 209
>Private and 4 Year
>
>**Arts Areas:** Dance, Instrumental Music, Vocal Music, Theatre, Film Arts, Television and Visual Arts
>
>**Performing Series:** Artist Series; Lecture & Convocation Series; Entertainment Series
>
>**Performance Facilities:** Olson Auditorium; Eastvold Auditorium; Chris Knutzen Hall; Ingram Hall; Xavier Hall

(continued on next page)

DANCE

Katherine Beckman, Chairman   **Number Of Faculty:** 1
Number Of Students: 185-200   **Degrees Offered:** Dance Minor
Courses Offered: Technique (Modern Dance); Rhythms and Dance; Professional Activity; Dance (History and Analysis of Technique); Choreography and Dance Production
Workshops/Festivals: Northwest Dance Festival

MUSIC

Maurice Skones, Chairman   **Number Of Faculty:** 24   **Number Of Students:** 240
Degrees Offered: BA MusEd; BMus; BA Mus; M Mus
Teaching Certification Available   Financial Assistance: Scholarships
Performing Groups: Choir; Oratorio Chorus; Orchestra; Band; Stage Band; String Quartet
Workshops/Festivals: Christmas Festival Concert

THEATRE

Gary B Wilson PhD, Chairperson   **Number Of Faculty:** 8
Number Of Students: 80   **Degrees Offered:** BA; BFA
Courses Offered: Directing; Scene Design; Lighting; Independent Study; Stage Tech; Oral Interpretation;
Technical Training: Crew Work; Design (Set and Light)
Teaching Certification Available   Financial Assistance: Scholarships
Performing Groups: University Theatre; Alpha Psi Omega

UNIVERSITY OF PUGET SOUND
1500 N Warner, Tacoma   Washington 98416
206 756-3100

Private   **Arts Areas:** Instrumental Music, Vocal Music and Theatre
Performing Series: Artist - Lecture Series
Performance Facilities: Inside Theatre

MUSIC

Bruce Rodgers, Director, School of Music   **Number Of Faculty:** 21
Number Of Students: 549   **Degrees Offered:** B Mus; BA; MM
Teaching Certification Available
Financial Assistance: Assistantships, Scholarships and Work-Study Grants
Workshops/Festivals: Summer Workshops

THEATRE

Carol Sloman, Chairman, Department of Communication   **Number Of Faculty:** 3
Number Of Students: 35   **Degrees Offered:** BA
Teaching Certification Available
Financial Assistance: Assistantships, Scholarships and Work-Study Grants
Performing Groups: Inside Theatre; UPStage

SAINT MARTIN'S COLLEGE
Olympia   Washington 98503, 206 491-4700

Private and 4 Year
Arts Areas: Instrumental Music, Vocal Music, Theatre and Visual Arts
Performing Series: Concert and Lecture Series
Performance Facilities: College Auditorium

Number Of Faculty: 6   **Number Of Students:** 55   **Degrees Offered:** BMus, BMusEd
Teaching Certification Available
Financial Assistance: Assistantships, Scholarships and Work-Study Grants

(continued on next page)

THEATRE

Dr W Dickerson, Chairman   **Number Of Faculty:** 4   **Number Of Students:** 40
Degrees Offered: BA   **Teaching Certification Available**
Financial Assistance: Assistantships, Scholarships and Work-Study Grants
Performing Groups: St Martin's Players

SEATTLE PACIFIC UNIVERSITY
3307 3rd Ave W, Seattle   Washington 98119
206 281-2036
Private and 4 Year
Arts Areas: Instrumental Music, Vocal Music, Theatre and Visual Arts
Performance Facilities: McKinley Auditorium; First Free Methodist Church; Demaray Hall Auditorium

MUSIC

Hubert Wash, Acting Director   **Number Of Faculty:** 18
Number Of Students: 145   **Degrees Offered:** BA MusEd; BA
Teaching Certification Available
Financial Assistance: Scholarships, Work-Study Grants and NDSL Loans
Performing Groups: Symphonic Wind Ensemble; Jazz Ensemble; Oratorio; Symphony Orchestra; Concert Band; Seattle Pacific Singers; Concert Choir; Chapel Choir; Christian Consort

THEATRE

James Chapman, Director of Dramatic Arts   **Number Of Faculty:** 3
Number Of Students: 600   **Degrees Offered:** BA
Courses Offered: Acting; Directing; Oral Interpretation; Mime; History of Costume; Playwriting
Teaching Certification Available
Financial Assistance: Scholarships and Work-Study Grants
Performing Groups: Main Stage; Childrens Touring Ensemble; Chancel Players
Workshops/Festivals: Fine Arts Week; Religious Drama Workshop

SEATTLE UNIVERSITY
11 & Spring St, Seattle   Washington 98122
206 626-6336
Private and 4 Year
Arts Areas: Dance, Instrumental Music, Vocal Music, Theatre, Film Arts and Visual Arts

DANCE

Mrs Phyllis Legters, Chairman   **Degrees Offered:** BA
Financial Assistance: Scholarships and Work-Study Grants

MUSIC

Dr Louis Christensen, Chairman   **Number Of Faculty:** 5
Degrees Offered: BA Mus   **Teaching Certification Available**
Financial Assistance: Scholarships and Work-Study Grants

THEATRE

David M Butler, Chairman   **Number Of Faculty:** 5
Teaching Certification Available
Financial Assistance: Scholarships and Work-Study Grants

WALLA WALLA COLLEGE
College Place   Washington 99324, 509 527-2561
Private and 4 Year   **Arts Areas:** Instrumental Music and Vocal Music
Performing Series: Walla Walla Symphony; Walla Walla College Lyceum Series
Performance Facilities: Fine Arts Auditorium ; Columbia Auditorium; Village Hall

(continued on next page)

MUSIC

Dr Harold Lickey, Chairman   **Number Of Faculty:** 8   **Number Of Students:** 120
Degrees Offered: B MusEd; BA   **Teaching Certification Available**
Financial Assistance: Work-Study Grants
Performing Groups: Concert Band; Percussion Ensemble; Schola Cantorum; Concert Choir; Woodwind Ensemble; Brass Choir

---

WASHINGTON STATE UNIVERSITY
Pullman   Washington 99164, 509 335-4581
State and 4 Year
Arts Areas: Instrumental Music, Vocal Music, Theatre, Film Arts, Television and Visual Arts
Performance Facilities: Kimbrough Hall; Bryan Hall; Daggy Theatre; Performing Arts Coliseum; Fine Arts Theatre

MUSIC

H James Schoepflin, Chairman   **Number Of Faculty:** 28
Number Of Students: 230   **Degrees Offered:** B Mus; BA; MA
Courses Offered: Performance; Theory; Composition; Music Education
Teaching Certification Available
Financial Assistance: Assistantships, Scholarships and Work-Study Grants

THEATRE

Director Wadleigh, Chairman   **Number Of Faculty:** 7
Number Of Students: 176
Performing Groups: Comedians; Readers Theatre; Summer Palace

UNIVERSITY OF WASHINGTON
Seattle   Washington 98195, 206 543-2100
State and 4 Year
Arts Areas: Dance, Instrumental Music, Vocal Music and Theatre
Performance Facilities: Penthouse Theatre; Showboat Theatre; Glenn Hughes Playhouse; Meany Hall Mainstage
Number Of Faculty: 4   **Number Of Students:** 40   **Degrees Offered:** BA
Financial Assistance: Scholarships and Work-Study Grants
Performing Groups: University Dance Company

MUSIC

John T Moore, Director, School of Music   **Number Of Faculty:** 60
Number Of Students: 450   **Degrees Offered:** BA; B Mus; DMA; PhD
Teaching Certification Available
Financial Assistance: Assistantships, Scholarships, Work-Study Grants and Hourly Employment
Performing Groups: Chorale; Oratorio Chorus; Madrigals; Singers; Wind Sinfonietta; Contemporary Group; Symphony; Marching Band; Concert Band
Workshops/Festivals: Metro - Music Educators Solo and Ensemble Contest; High School Choral Festival; High School Stage Band Festival; Metropolitan Auditions; Congress of Strings

THEATRE

Paul S Hostetler, Chairman   **Number Of Faculty:** 22
Number Of Students: 300   **Degrees Offered:** BA; BFA; MFA; PhD
Technical Training: Professional Actor Training Program; Directing; Scene Design; Costume Design; Technical Direction
Teaching Certification Available

WESTERN WASHINGTON STATE COLLEGE
High St, Bellingham   Washington 98225
206 676-3000 Ext 3866
State and 4 Year
Arts Areas: Dance, Instrumental Music, Vocal Music and Theatre
Performance Facilities: Main Auditorium; Concert Hall; Old Main Theater; Experimental Theater

DANCE

Dennis Catrell, Chairman
Courses Offered: Ballet; Modern; Modern Jazz; Composition; Labonotation; Theory; History and Philosophy

MUSIC

Phillip Ager, Chairman   *Number Of Faculty:* 18   *Number Of Students:* 188
Degrees Offered: BA; BEd; MA; MEd
Courses Offered: Early, tradition, contemporary, avant-garde, jazz and electronic music through performance, composition and analysis
Teaching Certification Available
Financial Assistance: Assistantships, Scholarships and Work-Study Grants
Performing Groups: College Choir; Concert Choir; Chamber Choirs; Symphonic Band; Wind Ensemble; Jazz Workshop; Jazz Ensembles; College Symphony Orchestra; Chamber Music; Opera; Collegium Musicum
Workshops/Festivals: Seminar in Choral Direction and Literature; Chamber Music Reading; String Teachers Workshop; Birch Bay Band Workshop; Choral Workshop; The Singer and the Choir Director

THEATRE

Dennis Catrell, Chairman, Department of Theater/Dance   *Number Of Faculty:* 9
Number Of Students: 300   *Degrees Offered:* BA; BEd; MA; MEd
Courses Offered: Theory & Production; Design for State; Stagecraft & Lighting; Acting; History; Drafting; Rendering & Models; Costuming; Film Genre; Creative Dramatics; Puppetry; Contemporary; Shakespeare
Teaching Certification Available
Financial Assistance: Assistantships, Scholarships and Work-Study Grants
Performing Groups: Western Theater; Western Youth Theatre Touring Company; Western Summer Stock; Western Dance Theater
Workshops/Festivals: Summer Acting Workshop for High School Students; Puppetry; Creative Dance for Children; Creative Drama; WWSC Drama Directors' Institute; Play Analysis and Theatre Production Planning; Summer Stock; Dance Summer

WHITMAN COLLEGE
345 Boyer Ave, Walla Walla   Washington 99362
509 529-5100
Private and 4 Year
Arts Areas: Instrumental Music, Vocal Music, Theatre and Visual Arts
Performing Series: Fine Arts Series

MUSIC

Kenneth E Schilling, Chairman   *Number Of Faculty:* 8
Number Of Students: 105   *Degrees Offered:* BA Mus, MMusEd
Technical Training: Opera   *Teaching Certification Available*
Financial Assistance: Scholarships and Work-Study Grants
Performing Groups: Sinfonietta, Orchestra, Chorus, Instrumental Ensembles
Workshops/Festivals: Opera Workshop

THEATRE

John R Friemann, Chairman   *Number Of Faculty:* 3   *Number Of Students:* 40
Degrees Offered: BA   *Teaching Certification Available*
Financial Assistance: Scholarships and Work-Study Grants
Performing Groups: Whitman Theatre

WHITWORTH COLLEGE
Spokane   Washington 99251, 509 466-1000
Private and 4 Year
Arts Areas: Instrumental Music, Vocal Music, Theatre and Visual Arts
Performance Facilities: Music Recital Hall; Auditorium

MUSIC

Richard Evans, Coordinator of Music   *Number Of Faculty:* 15
Number Of Students: 200   *Degrees Offered:* BA
Teaching Certification Available
Financial Assistance: Scholarships and Work-Study Grants
Performing Groups: Concert Band; Choir; Madrigals; Chorus; Jazz Ensemble; Orchestra

THEATRE

Albert Gunderson, Coordinator of Theatre   *Number Of Faculty:* 3
Number Of Students: 80   *Degrees Offered:* BA
Teaching Certification Available
Financial Assistance: Scholarships and Work-Study Grants
Performing Groups: Theatre; Readers Theater

ALDERSON - BROADDUS COLLEGE
Philippi   West Virginia 26416, 304 457-1700
> Private and 4 Year
> *Arts Areas:* Instrumental Music, Vocal Music, Theatre and Visual Arts
> *Performing Series:* Cultural Events Series
> *Performance Facilities:* Wilcox Chapel; Funkhauser Auditorium; Memorial Coliseum

MUSIC

Dr Charles Ervin, Chairperson   *Number Of Faculty:* 8
Number Of Students: 60   *Degrees Offered:* BA Mus; BA MusEd
Teaching Certification Available
Financial Assistance: Scholarships and Work-Study Grants
Performing Groups: The A-B Tour Choir; The West Virginians

THEATRE

Dr Kenneth Harris, Chairperson   *Number Of Faculty:* 1   *Degrees Offered:* BA
Teaching Certification Available

BETHANY COLLEGE
Bethany   West Virginia 26032, 304 829-7000
> Private and 4 Year
> *Arts Areas:* Instrumental Music, Vocal Music, Theatre, Television and Visual Arts

MUSIC

George K Hauptfuehrer, Chairman   *Number Of Faculty:* 4
Number Of Students: 50   *Degrees Offered:* BA
Teaching Certification Available   *Financial Assistance:* Scholarships

THEATRE

David J Judy, Chairman   *Number Of Faculty:* 2   *Number Of Students:* 40
Degrees Offered: BA Theatre   *Teaching Certification Available*
Financial Assistance: Scholarships

BLUEFIELD COLLEGE
Bluefield   West Virginia 24605, 703 327-7137
> Private and 4 Year
> *Arts Areas:* Instrumental Music, Vocal Music, Theatre and Visual Arts
> *Performing Series:* Concert Lecture Series
> *Performance Facilities:* Bluefield College Theatre

MUSIC

J P Jardaine, Chairman   *Number Of Faculty:* 2   *Number Of Students:* 23
Degrees Offered: AA Music, Music Ed   *Financial Assistance:* Work-Study Grants
Performing Groups: Bluefield College Choir
Workshops/Festivals: Annual "Messiah" performance

THEATRE

Charles R Hannum, Chairman   *Number Of Faculty:* 1   *Number Of Students:* 10
Degrees Offered: BA   *Teaching Certification Available*
Financial Assistance: Work-Study Grants
Performing Groups: Bluefield College Theatre

CONCORD COLLEGE

Athens   West Virginia 24712, 304 384-3115
    State and 4 Year
    Arts Areas: Instrumental Music, Vocal Music, Theatre and Visual Arts

MUSIC

Edward L Masters, Chairman   *Number Of Faculty:* 7   *Number Of Students:* 72
Degrees Offered: BA Mus   *Teaching Certification Available*
Financial Assistance: Scholarships and Work-Study Grants

THEATRE

Ronald L Burgher, Chairman   *Degrees Offered:* BA
Teaching Certification Available
Financial Assistance: Scholarships and Work-Study Grants
Performing Groups: Concord College Theatre

DAVIS & ELKINS COLLEGE

Sycamore St, Elkins   West Virginia 26241
304 636-1900
    Private and 4 Year   *Arts Areas:* Vocal Music, Theatre and Visual Arts
    Performing Series: Impact; Davis and Elkins Theatre Subscription Season; Second Tuesday Readings
    Performance Facilities: Boiler House Theatre; Studio Theatre

MUSIC

Richard Kadel, Chairman   *Number Of Faculty:* 3   *Number Of Students:* 60
Degrees Offered: BA
Courses Offered: Theory; History; Applied; Appreciation; Music for Elementary Teachers; Chorus;
Madrigal Singers
Financial Assistance: Scholarships and Work-Study Grants
Performing Groups: Chorus; Madrigal Singers; Choral Union

THEATRE

Michael Pedretti, Director of Theatre   *Number Of Faculty:* 3
Number Of Students: 100   *Degrees Offered:* BA; BS
Courses Offered: Acting; Directing; Oral Interpretation; History & Literature
Technical Training: Design; Technical Theatre; Lighting; Make-up; Costumes
Teaching Certification Available
Financial Assistance: Scholarships, Work-Study Grants and Assistantships
Performing Groups: D & E Theatre; Green Room Society; Iota Omega
Workshops/Festivals: Acting/Mime workshops with high schools

FAIRMONT STATE COLLEGE

Locust Ave, Fairmont   West Virginia 26554
304 367-4219 Ext 4219
    State
    Arts Areas: Instrumental Music, Vocal Music, Theatre, Film Arts, Television and Visual Arts
    Performance Facilities: Wallman Hall

MUSIC

Rucgard P Wellock, Chairman   *Number Of Faculty:* 12
Number Of Students: 84   *Degrees Offered:* BA Ed
Courses Offered: Theory; History; Ensembles; Conducting; Applied; Music Education; Electronic
Technical Training: Music Management; Instrument Repairs
Teaching Certification Available
Financial Assistance: Scholarships and Work-Study Grants
Performing Groups: Touring Choir; Symphonic Choir; Chamber Singers; Band; Wind Ensemble;
Symphony Orchestra; Brass Ensemble; Stage Band; Woodwind Ensembles; Tuba Ensemble; Percussion

(continued on next page)

Ensemble
Workshops/Festivals: Choral Festival; Solo and Ensemble Festival

THEATRE

Jo Ann Lough, Chairman   ***Number Of Faculty:*** 7   ***Number Of Students:*** 48
Degrees Offered: BA Ed
Courses Offered: Speech; Debate; Oral Interpretation; Theatre; Technical
Teaching Certification Available
Financial Assistance: Assistantships, Scholarships and Work-Study Grants
Performing Groups: Debate; Oral Interpreation; Theatre: "Masquers" "Summer Town and Gown"
Workshops/Festivals: WV Forensics Association; WV Theatre Association; Theatre Workshops; Children's Theatre

---

GLENVILLE STATE COLLEGE
200 High St, Glenville   West Virginia 26351
304 462-7361
State and 4 Year   ***Arts Areas:*** Vocal Music and Theatre

MUSIC

Degrees Offered: BA   ***Teaching Certification Available***
Financial Assistance: Scholarships
Performing Groups: Instrumental Ensembles, Choir

GREENBRIER COLLEGE
Lewisburg   West Virginia 24901, 304 645-1111
Private and 2 Year
Arts Areas: Dance, Instrumental Music, Vocal Music, Theatre and Television
Degrees Offered: AA
Financial Assistance: Scholarships and Work-Study Grants

MARSHALL UNIVERSITY
Huntington   West Virginia 25701, 304 696-3170
State and 4 Year
Arts Areas: Instrumental Music, Vocal Music, Theatre and Visual Arts
Performing Series: Marshall Artists Series; Baxter Series; Mount Series; Forum Series
Performance Facilities: Keith - Albee Theater; Old Main Auditorium

MUSIC

Wendell Kumlien, Chairman   ***Number Of Faculty:*** 22   ***Number Of Students:*** 216
Degrees Offered: BA; MA   ***Teaching Certification Available***
Financial Assistance: Assistantships, Scholarships and Work-Study Grants
Performing Groups: Orchestra; Marching Band; Symphonic Band; Wind Symphony; Jazz Ensemble; Symphonic Choir; Choral Union; Opera Workshop; University Singers; Collegium Musicum; Brass; Woodwind; Percussion and String Ensembles
Workshops/Festivals: Jazz Festival; Band and Choral Workshops

THEATRE

Dr N B East, Theater Area Coordinator   ***Number Of Faculty:*** 3
Number Of Students: 56   ***Degrees Offered:*** BA; MA
The Theater Department is under the Speech Department. The degrees are in speech with a theater emphasis
Teaching Certification Available
Financial Assistance: Assistantships, Scholarships and Work-Study Grants
Performing Groups: Marshall University Theater
Workshops/Festivals: Regional High School One-Act Play Festival

MORRIS HARVEY COLLEGE
2300 McCorkle Ave SE, Charleston   West Virginia 25304
304 346-9471
>Private and 4 Year
>*Arts Areas:* Instrumental Music, Vocal Music, Theatre and Visual Arts

MUSIC

>Harold E Ewing, Chairman   **Number Of Faculty:** 6   **Number Of Students:** 27
>*Degrees Offered:* BA   *Teaching Certification Available*
>*Financial Assistance:* Scholarships and Work-Study Grants

THEATRE

>Kenneth Slattery, Chairman   **Number Of Faculty:** 2   **Number Of Students:** 25
>*Degrees Offered:* BA   *Teaching Certification Available*
>*Financial Assistance:* Scholarships and Work-Study Grants
>*Performing Groups:* Blackfriars

POTOMAC STATE COLLEGE
Keyser   West Virginia 26726, 304 788-3011
>State and 2 Year
>*Arts Areas:* Instrumental Music, Vocal Music, Theatre and Visual Arts
>*Performance Facilities:* Church - McKee Arts Center

MUSIC

>Charles Whitehill, Chairman   **Number Of Faculty:** 9   **Number Of Students:** 65
>*Degrees Offered:* AA   *Performing Groups:* Band, Stage Band, Chorus, Ensembles

THEATRE

>Tony Whitmore, Chairman   **Number Of Faculty:** 2   **Number Of Students:** 15
>*Degrees Offered:* AA   *Performing Groups:* The Players

SALEM COLLEGE
Salem   West Virginia 26426, 304 782-5011
>Private and 4 Year
>*Arts Areas:* Instrumental Music, Vocal Music, Theatre, Television and Radio

MUSIC

>Ruth Rogers, Chairman   **Number Of Faculty:** 5
>*Degrees Offered:* B Mus; B MusEd
>*Courses Offered:* Theory; Survey; Music Appreciation; Conducting; Directed Study; Education Courses; Arranging; History; Applied
>*Teaching Certification Available*
>*Financial Assistance:* Assistantships, Scholarships and Work-Study Grants
>*Performing Groups:* Concert Choir; Band; String Ensemble; Woodwind Ensemble; Brass Ensemble; Stage Band; Salem Singers; Percussion Ensemble; Recorder Consort

THEATRE

>Venita Zinn, Chairman   **Number Of Faculty:** 8   **Degrees Offered:** BA
>*Courses Offered:* Broadcasting; Drama; Writing/Journalism; Speech
>*Technical Training:* Internships in Broadcasting
>*Teaching Certification Available*
>*Financial Assistance:* Assistantships, Scholarships and Work-Study Grants
>*Performing Groups:* Salem College Theatre Group; Readers Theatre

SHEPHERD COLLEGE

Shepherdstown   West Virginia 25443, 304 876-2511
   State and 2 Year
   Arts Areas: Instrumental Music, Vocal Music, Theatre, Visual Arts and Radio
   Performing Series: College Artist Series
   Performance Facilities: Reynolds Hall

MUSIC

Guy Frank, Professor   *Number Of Faculty:* 6   *Number Of Students:* 60
Degrees Offered: BA MusEd   *Teaching Certification Available*
Financial Assistance: Scholarships and Work-Study Grants
Performing Groups: Band; Choir; Jazz Ensemble; Brass Ensemble; Woodwind Ensemble; Percussion Ensemble; Chamber Singers; Shepherd "Pop" Singers; Recorder Ensemble
Workshops/Festivals: Invitational High School Band Clinic; Invitational Reading Clinic (High School & Jr High School - Instrumental)

THEATRE

George Wilson, Assistant Professor   *Number Of Faculty:* 2
Courses Offered: Speech/Drama Minor; Radio Minor
Financial Assistance: Scholarships and Work-Study Grants
Workshops/Festivals: High School Invitational Drama Festival

WEST LIBERTY STATE COLLEGE

West Liberty   West Virginia 26074, 304 336-5000
   State and 4 Year
   Arts Areas: Instrumental Music, Vocal Music, Theatre and Visual Arts
   Performing Series: West Liberty Concert Series; West Liberty Lecture Series
   Performance Facilities: College Hall; Kelly Theatre; College Union Ballroom

MUSIC

Charles D Boggess, Chairman   *Number Of Faculty:* 16
Number Of Students: 125   *Degrees Offered:* BA
Courses Offered: Teacher Education; Comprehensive
Teaching Certification Available
Financial Assistance: Scholarships, Work-Study Grants and Student Loans
Performing Groups: Concert Choir; Chorus; Concert Band; Stage Band; Marching Band; Woodwind Quintet; Percussion Ensemble; Brass Ensemble
Workshops/Festivals: Region VI WVMEA Solo & Ensemble Festival; Tri-State Marching Band Festival; Tri-State Choral Day; Annual Teacher Education Workshop; Choral Workshop

THEATRE

Vernon D Riemer, Chairman, Department of Oral Communications and Theatre Arts
Number Of Faculty: 6   *Number Of Students:* 100   *Degrees Offered:* BA
Courses Offered: Teacher Education   *Teaching Certification Available*
Financial Assistance: Scholarships, Work-Study Grants and Student Loans
Performing Groups: Hilltop Players; Hilltop Players Professional Company (summer)
Workshops/Festivals: Area Drama Festival; High School Drama Day

WEST VIRGINIA INSTITUTE OF TECHNOLOGY

Montgomery   West Virginia 25136, 304 442-3071
   State and 4 Year   *Arts Areas:* Instrumental Music and Vocal Music
   Number Of Faculty: 3   *Number Of Students:* 27   *Degrees Offered:* BA MusEd
   Teaching Certification Available
   Financial Assistance: Scholarships and Work-Study Grants

WEST VIRGINIA STATE COLLEGE
Institute   West Virginia 25112, 304 766-3194

State and 4 Year

Arts Areas: Instrumental Music, Vocal Music, Theatre, Film Arts, Television and Visual Arts
Performance Facilities: F S Belcher Theatre

MUSIC

Dr Kent Hall, Chairman   *Number Of Faculty:* 6 Full-time, 2 Part-time
Number Of Students: 85
Degrees Offered: BS MusEd, Comprehensive; Associate in Church Music
Teaching Certification Available
Financial Assistance: Scholarships and Work-Study Grants
Performing Groups: Concert Band; Jazz Ensemble; College Singers; Concert Choir; Brass Choir
Workshops/Festivals: Festival of Sacred Music; Jazz Clinic

THEATRE

David Wohl, Director   *Number Of Faculty:* 1   *Number Of Students:* 47
Courses Offered: Acting; Directing; Scene Design; Make-up; Management; History; Basic Production
Technical Training: Lighting; Design; Construction
Financial Assistance: Scholarships and Work-Study Grants
Performing Groups: West Virginia State College Players; Alpha Psi Omega Honorary Drama
Workshops/Festivals: West Virginia Regional High School Drama Festival
Artists-In-Residence/Guest Artists: Peter Nero; Canadian Brass; Woody Herman; National Players

WEST VIRGINIA UNIVERSITY - CREATIVE ARTS CENTER
Morgantown   West Virginia 26505, 304 293-4841

State and 4 Year

Arts Areas: Instrumental Music, Vocal Music, Theatre and Visual Arts
Performance Facilities: Concert Theatre; Studio Theatre; Opera Theatre; Classroom Theatre; Choir Room

MUSIC

Dr C B Wilson, Professor   *Number Of Faculty:* 44   *Number Of Students:* 450
Degrees Offered: BMus; MM; DMA; PhD
Courses Offered: Performance; Music Education; Composition; Music History & Theory
Teaching Certification Available
Financial Assistance: Assistantships, Scholarships and Work-Study Grants
Performing Groups: Bands; Orchestras; Choirs; Percussion Ensembles; Trombone Ensemble; Jazz Ensemble; Opera Workshop; Collegium Musicum
Workshops/Festivals: Summer Fine Arts Camp; String Workshop; Early Music; Marching Band Workshop

THEATRE

Dr John Whitty, Professor   *Number Of Faculty:* 13   *Number Of Students:* 150
Degrees Offered: BA; BFA; MA
Courses Offered: Acting/Directing; Design/Technical Theatre
Financial Assistance: Assistantships, Scholarships and Work-Study Grants
Performing Groups: University Theatre; Puppet - Mobile
Workshops/Festivals: Summer Repertory Theatre; High School Drama Festival

WEST VIRGINIA WESLEYAN COLLEGE
Buckhannon   West Virginia 26201, 304 473-7011 Ext 8044

Private and 4 Year

Arts Areas: Dance, Instrumental Music, Vocal Music and Theatre
Performing Series: Liberal Education Series
Performance Facilities: Atkinson Auditorium

MUSIC

Dr Bobby Loftis, Chairman   *Number Of Faculty:* 8   *Number Of Students:* 100
Degrees Offered: BA, BMusEd   *Teaching Certification Available*

(continued on next page)

Financial Assistance: Scholarships and Work-Study Grants
Performing Groups: Marching Band, Concert Band, Jazz Band, Tour Choir, Chapel Choir, Chorale Women's Glee Club

THEATRE

Charles I Presar, Chairman   **Number Of Faculty:** 7   **Number Of Students:** 30
Degrees Offered: BA   **Technical Training:** Technical Training in Production
Teaching Certification Available   Financial Assistance: Work-Study Grants
Performing Groups: WVWC Theatre, Reader's Theatre, WVWC Children's Theatre
Workshops/Festivals: Summer Workshop for High School Students

ALVERNO COLLEGE
3401 S 39th St, Milwaukee   Wisconsin 53215
414 671-5400 Ext 258
Private and 4 Year
Arts Areas: Instrumental Music, Vocal Music, Theatre and Visual Arts
Performing Series: Society of Fine Arts; Evenings of Chamber Music
Performance Facilities: Alverno College Auditorium; Wehr Hall; Alphonsa Hall

MUSIC

Sister Mary Hueller, Coordinator   **Number Of Faculty:** 20
Number Of Students: 120
Degrees Offered: B Music, Applied Music, Church Music, Music Education, Music Therapy
Courses Offered: Music Theory; Music History & Literature; Courses in Specialized area
Teaching Certification Available
Financial Assistance: Scholarships and Work-Study Grants
Performing Groups: Women's Chorus; Madrigal Singers; Pro Musica; Orchestra; Small Instrument Ensembles
Workshops/Festivals: Piano, Group Piano, Music Education Workshops

THEATRE

Robert Pitman, Coordinator   **Number Of Faculty:** 2   **Number Of Students:** 25
Courses Offered: Theatre Arts
Financial Assistance: Scholarships and Work-Study Grants
Performing Groups: Theatre Alverno

BELOIT COLLEGE
Beloit   Wisconsin 53511, 608 365-3391
Private and 4 Year
Arts Areas: Instrumental Music, Vocal Music, Theatre and Visual Arts
Performing Series: Concert Series

MUSIC

Harlan Snow, Chairman   **Number Of Faculty:** 19   **Number Of Students:** 60
Degrees Offered: BMus   *Teaching Certification Available*
Financial Assistance: Scholarships and Work-Study Grants
Performing Groups: Chamber Ensemble; Brass Ensemble; String Ensemble; Wind Ensemble; Choir; Choral Ensembles; Orchestra

THEATRE

Kork Denmark, Chairman   **Number Of Faculty:** 7   **Number Of Students:** 100
Degrees Offered: BA   *Teaching Certification Available*
Financial Assistance: Scholarships and Work-Study Grants
Performing Groups: Beloit College Players; The Coit Theatre

CARDINAL STRITCH COLLEGE
6801 N Yates Rd, Milwaukee   Wisconsin 53217
414 351-5400 Ext 205
Private and 4 Year
Arts Areas: Instrumental Music, Vocal Music and Visual Arts

MUSIC

Sister Annice Diderich,OSF, Chairman   **Number Of Faculty:** 9
Number Of Students: 20   *Degrees Offered:* BA Applied Music Pedagogy; BA Mus
Courses Offered: Keyboard Skills; Musicianship Courses; Music Literature Courses; Materials; Methods; Applied

(continued on next page)

Financial Assistance: Scholarships and Work-Study Grants
Performing Groups: Vocal Chamber Ensemble (student); Faculty Concerts
Workshops/Festivals: Piano Workshops co-sponsored with Milwaukee Music Teachers' Association

---

CARROLL COLLEGE
100 N East Ave, Waukesha   Wisconsin 53186
414 547-1211
Private and 4 Year
Arts Areas: Instrumental Music, Vocal Music, Theatre, Television and Visual Arts
Performance Facilities: Youmans Little Theatre; Shattuck Chapel - Music Center; Auditorium

MUSIC

Dr Charles G Boyer, Chairman   **Number Of Faculty:** 4
Number Of Students: 175   **Degrees Offered:** BA
Courses Offered: Music Performance; Music Education; Music - Business; Church Music
Teaching Certification Available
Financial Assistance: Internships, Scholarships and Work-Study Grants
Performing Groups: Concert Band; Concert Choir; Carrolleers; Marching Band; Jazz Ensemble; Wind Ensemble; Woodwind, Brass & Percussion Ensembles; Choral Union; Waukesha Area Symphonic Band
Workshops/Festivals: High School Band Clinic; High School Choral Clinic; All-School Arts Festival

THEATRE

David M Molthen, Assistant Professor   **Number Of Faculty:** 2
Number Of Students: 26   **Degrees Offered:** BA
Courses Offered: Pre-professional; Education
Teaching Certification Available
Financial Assistance: Internships, Scholarships and Work-Study Grants
Performing Groups: Carroll Players
Workshops/Festivals: All-School Fine Arts Festival

CARTHAGE COLLEGE
Kenosha   Wisconsin 53141, 414 551-8500
Private and 4 Year
Arts Areas: Instrumental Music, Vocal Music and Theatre
Performing Series: Arts & Lecture Series
Performance Facilities: Wartburg Auditorium; Siebert Chapel; Johnson Recital Hall

MUSIC

Dr Richard Sjoerdsma, Chairman   **Number Of Faculty:** 6 Full-time, 7 Part-time
Number Of Students: 50   **Degrees Offered:** BA Mus
Courses Offered: History; Theory Applied; Music Education
Teaching Certification Available
Financial Assistance: Scholarships and Work-Study Grants
Performing Groups: Brass & Wind Ensemble; Bands; Choral Ensembles; Chorale; Chamber Ensemble; Orchestra

THEATRE

Dr T S Holland, Chairman   **Number Of Faculty:** 5 Full-time; 2 Part-time
Number Of Students: 27
Degrees Offered: BA Speech Communication & Theater Major
Courses Offered: General; Speech Communication; Theater; Applied
Teaching Certification Available
Financial Assistance: Scholarships and Work-Study Grants
Performing Groups: "Speech - Theater Arts Department Presents"

EDGEWOOD COLLEGE
855 Woodrow St, Madison   Wisconsin 53711
608 257-4861
> Private and 4 Year
> *Arts Areas:* Dance, Instrumental Music, Vocal Music, Theatre and Visual Arts
> *Performance Facilities:* Regina Theatre

DANCE

> Mrs Mary Elliott, Chairman   *Number Of Faculty:* 1
> *Financial Assistance:* Work-Study Grants

MUSIC

> Sister Virginia Smith, Chairman   *Number Of Faculty:* 3
> *Number Of Students:* 50 - 100   *Degrees Offered:* BA
> *Courses Offered:* Vocal & Instrumental   *Teaching Certification Available*
> *Financial Assistance:* Scholarships and Work-Study Grants
> *Performing Groups:* Festival Choir; Edgewood College Chorus; Edgewood College Swing Choir
> *Workshops/Festivals:* Spring Arts Festival

THEATRE

> Jewell P Fitzgerald, Chairman   *Number Of Faculty:* 3
> *Number Of Students:* 30 - 50   *Degrees Offered:* BA Performing Arts
> *Technical Training:* Professional Actors Training Program
> *Teaching Certification Available*
> *Financial Assistance:* Assistantships, Scholarships and Work-Study Grants
> *Performing Groups:* Edgewood Players; Studio Theatre; Edgewood Summer Theatre
> *Workshops/Festivals:* Spring Arts Festival

HOLY FAMILY COLLEGE
Manitowoc   Wisconsin 54220, 414 684-6691
> Private and 4 Year
> *Arts Areas:* Instrumental Music, Vocal Music and Visual Arts
> *Number Of Faculty:* 4   *Degrees Offered:* BMusEd
> *Financial Assistance:* Scholarships and Work-Study Grants
> *Performing Groups:* Choir, Band

LAKELAND COLLEGE
Sheboygan   Wisconsin 53081, 414 565-2111
> Private and 4 Year
> *Arts Areas:* Instrumental Music, Vocal Music, Theatre and Visual Arts
> *Performing Series:* Fine Arts Series

MUSIC

> W Henry Ellerbusch, Chairman   *Number Of Faculty:* 4
> *Number Of Students:* 42   *Degrees Offered:* BMus
> *Teaching Certification Available*
> *Financial Assistance:* Scholarships and Work-Study Grants
> *Performing Groups:* Chorus, Band, Various Ensembles

THEATRE

> Dean F Graunke, Chairman   *Number Of Faculty:* 3   *Number Of Students:* 45
> *Degrees Offered:* BA   *Teaching Certification Available*
> *Financial Assistance:* Scholarships and Work-Study Grants
> *Performing Groups:* The Campus Players

LAWRENCE UNIVERSITY

Appleton Wisconsin 54911, 404 739-3681

Private and 4 Year   *Arts Areas:* Instrumental Music and Vocal Music
Performing Series: Artist Series; Chamber Series
Performance Facilities: Harper Hall; Stansbury Theatre; F Theodore Cloak Theatre

MUSIC

Charles Schwartz, Dean of the Conservatory   *Number Of Faculty:* 27
Number Of Students: 173   *Degrees Offered:* BMus
Teaching Certification Available
Financial Assistance: Internships, Assistantships, Scholarships and Work-Study Grants
Performing Groups: Choir; Band; Orchestra; Jazz Ensemble; Percussion Ensemble; Women's Chorus

THEATRE

Richard France, Chairman   *Number Of Faculty:* 4   *Number Of Students:* 31
Degrees Offered: BA Theatre & Drama
Courses Offered: Acting/Directing; History/Literature; Design
Technical Training: Stagecraft; Set, Light & Costume Design   *Teaching Certification Available*
Financial Assistance: Internships, Assistantships, Scholarships and Work-Study Grants
Performing Groups: Lawrence University Theatre Company; Lawrence University Dance Company

MADISON AREA TECHNICAL COLLEGE

211 N Carroll St, Madison Wisconsin 53703
608 266-5100

County and 2 Year
Arts Areas: Dance, Instrumental Music, Vocal Music, Theatre, Film Arts and Visual Arts
Performing Series: Music in Performance
Performance Facilities: Madison Area Technical College Auditorium

DANCE

Number Of Faculty: 1   *Number Of Students:* 50   *Courses Offered:* Dance I & II
Financial Assistance: Work-Study Grants

MUSIC

Roland Johnson, Associate Chairman   *Number Of Faculty:* 10
Number Of Students: 600   *Degrees Offered:* AA
Courses Offered: New College Singers; MATC Concert Chorale; Jazz Ensemble; Contemporary Music
History; Music Appreciation; Symphonic Band; Basis Music Theory; Music Theory I & II; General History
of Music; Music Composition; Music in Performance
Financial Assistance: Work-Study Grants
Performing Groups: New College Singers; Jazz Ensemble; Madison Municipal Band
Workshops/Festivals: New College Singers Swing Choir Festival; New College Singers Supershow

THEATRE

Cynthia Knox, Chairperson   *Number Of Faculty:* 2
Courses Offered: Oral Interpretation; Basic Drama Production   *Financial Assistance:* Work-Study Grants

MARIAN COLLEGE OF FOND DU LAC

45 S National Ave, Fond du Lac Wisconsin 54935
414 921-3900 Ext 217

Private and 4 Year
Arts Areas: Instrumental Music, Vocal Music and Visual Arts

MUSIC

Sister Margaretta Ehrlich, Chairman   *Number Of Faculty:* 2
Courses Offered: Basic Theory & Appreciation; Music Education

(continued on next page)

Performing Groups: Mixed Chorus; Vocal Ensemble; Wind Ensemble; String Ensemble
Workshops/Festivals: Two Annual School Concerts

MARQUETTE UNIVERSITY
615 N 11th St, Milwaukee   Wisconsin 53233
414 244-7504

Private and 4 Year   **Arts Areas:** Dance and Theatre
Performing Series: Concert - Lecture Series
Performance Facilities: Evan P and Marion Helfaer Theatre

DANCE

Sheila Reilly, Chairman   **Number Of Faculty:** 1   **Number Of Students:** 100
Financial Assistance: Assistantships and Work-Study Grants
Performing Groups: Band, Chorus

THEATRE

Michael J Price, Chairman   **Number Of Faculty:** 5   **Number Of Students:** 40
Degrees Offered: BA Theatre Arts; MA
Financial Assistance: Assistantships, Scholarships and Work-Study Grants
Performing Groups: Marquette Theatre Group

MILTON COLLEGE
Milton   Wisconsin 53563, 608 868-2912 Ext 924

Private and 4 Year   **Arts Areas:** Instrumental Music and Vocal Music

MUSIC

Robert Bond, Chairman   **Number Of Faculty:** 8   **Number Of Students:** 80
Degrees Offered: BMus; BMusEd   **Courses Offered:** Instrumental; Voice
Teaching Certification Available

THEATRE

Thom Sabota, Chairman   **Number Of Faculty:** 2   **Number Of Students:** 10
Financial Assistance: Scholarships and Work-Study Grants
Performing Groups: Milton College Players

MOUNT MARY COLLEGE
2900 N Menomonee River Pkwy, Milwaukee   Wisconsin 53222
414 258-4810

Private and 4 Year
Arts Areas: Dance, Instrumental Music, Vocal Music and Theatre
Performance Facilities: College Theater; Rattan Room (Concerts)

DANCE

Joan Gonwa, Instructor   **Number Of Faculty:** 1   **Degrees Offered:** BA
Courses Offered: Beginning & Intermediate Modern Dance; Creative Improvisation
Financial Assistance: Scholarships and Work-Study Grants

MUSIC

Sister Marcia Zofkie, Chairman   **Number Of Faculty:** 7   **Degrees Offered:** BA
Courses Offered: Piano; Choral Conducting & Techniques; Creative Musical Experiences; Chapel Choir; Madrigal Singers; Swing Choir; Voice Class; Recorder; Piano Ensemble; Guitar; Organ, Piano, Strings, Voice
Technical Training: Voice; Applied Instruments
Teaching Certification Available
Financial Assistance: Scholarships and Financial Aid
Workshops/Festivals: Liturgical

(continued on next page)

THEATRE

Sister Catherine McKee, Chairman   *Number Of Faculty:* 4
Degrees Offered: BA
Courses Offered: The Art of Oral Interpretation; Principles of Stage Direction; Voice Enhancement; Public Speaking
Technical Training: Stagecraft; Directing
Financial Assistance: Scholarships and Financial Aid

MOUNT SCENARIO COLLEGE
College Avenue W, Ladysmith   Wisconsin 54848
715 532-5511
   Private and 4 Year
   Arts Areas: Dance, Instrumental Music, Vocal Music, Theatre and Visual Arts
   Performance Facilities: Dance Studio; Fine Arts Center Auditorium; Fine Arts Center Gallery

DANCE

Number Of Faculty: 2
Courses Offered: Dance I; Modern Dance; Ballet; Theatre Dance
Financial Assistance: Scholarships and Work-Study Grants
Performing Groups: Dance Ensemble

MUSIC

Richard Probert, Associate Professor   *Number Of Faculty:* 4
Number Of Students: 29   *Degrees Offered:* BA; BS; BFA
Courses Offered: Music; Music Management; Music Education
Teaching Certification Available
Financial Assistance: Scholarships and Work-Study Grants
Performing Groups: Concert Chorale; Wind Ensemble; Jazz Ensemble

THEATRE

John Reilly, Assistant Professor   *Number Of Faculty:* 1
Number Of Students: 4   *Courses Offered:* Theatre Arts

NORTHLAND COLLEGE
Ashland   Wisconsin 54806, 715 682-4531
   Private and 4 Year
   Arts Areas: Instrumental Music, Vocal Music and Visual Arts
   Performing Series: Arts & Lecture Series; Annual Folk Festival
   Performance Facilities: Alvord Theatre

MUSIC

Don Jackson, Chairman   *Number Of Faculty:* 4 Full-time, 3 Part-time
Number Of Students: 45   *Degrees Offered:* BA
Technical Training: Folk Instrument Building
Teaching Certification Available
Financial Assistance: Scholarships, Work-Study Grants and Performing Awards
Performing Groups: Orchestra; Wind Ensemble; Ancient Instrument Ensemble; Jazz Band; Choir; New Land Singers (Female Vocal); The Vogaeurs (Men's Chorus)
Workshops/Festivals: Spring Band Clinic; Folk Festival; Folk Instrument Workshop

RIPON COLLEGE
Ripon   Wisconsin 54971, 414 748-8106
   Private and 4 Year
   Arts Areas: Dance, Instrumental Music, Vocal Music, Theatre and Visual Arts
   Performing Series: Fine Arts Series; Chamber Music at Ripon
   Performance Facilities: C J Rodman Center for the Arts; Memorial Hall
   Number Of Faculty: 1
   Courses Offered: Fundamentals; Theory & Technique; Dance Composition; Production

MUSIC

Dr Raymond E Stahura, Chairman   *Number Of Faculty:* 4   *Degrees Offered:* BA
Courses Offered: Theory; History; Literature; Applied   *Teaching Certification Available*
Financial Assistance: Scholarships and Work-Study Grants
Performing Groups: Chamber Singers; Brass; Woodwind & String Ensembles; Orchestra; Jazz Ensemble; Symphonic Wind Ensemble; Choral Union

THEATRE

Dr Edmund B Roney, Chairman   *Number Of Faculty:* 3   *Degrees Offered:* BA
Courses Offered: History; Literature; Theory; Applied
Teaching Certification Available   *Financial Assistance:* Scholarships and Work-Study Grants
Performing Groups: Readers' Theatre; Drama Productions

SAINT NORBERT COLLEGE
De Pere   Wisconsin 54115, 414 336-3181 Ext 332
   Private and 4 Year
   Arts Areas: Dance, Instrumental Music, Vocal Music, Theatre, Film Arts, Television and Visual Arts
   Performance Facilities: Abbot Pennings Hall of Fine Arts

DANCE

Number Of Faculty: 1   *Number Of Students:* 20   *Degrees Offered:* BA
Teaching Certification Available
Financial Assistance: Scholarships and Work-Study Grants

MUSIC

Number Of Faculty: 8   *Number Of Students:* 65   *Degrees Offered:* BA, BMus, BMusEd
Teaching Certification Available
Financial Assistance: Scholarships and Work-Study Grants
Performing Groups: Chamber Singers, Oratorio Choir, Stage Band, Swinging Knights, Brass Quintet
Workshops/Festivals: Harvest Music Festival, Piano Teachers' Workshop, Opera Workshop, Summer Theory for High School

THEATRE

Number Of Faculty: 2   *Number Of Students:* 20   *Degrees Offered:* BA
Teaching Certification Available
Financial Assistance: Scholarships and Work-Study Grants

SILVER LAKE COLLEGE
2406 S Alverno Rd, Manitowoc   Wisconsin 54220
414 684-6691 Ext 61
   Private and 4 Year
   Arts Areas: Instrumental Music, Vocal Music and Visual Arts
   Performance Facilities: Fine Arts Theatre; Silver Lake College Chapel

MUSIC

Sister L Zemke, Coordinator   *Number Of Faculty:* 11
Number Of Students: 50   *Degrees Offered:* BMusEd
Teaching Certification Available   *Financial Assistance:* Scholarships and Work-Study Grants

(continued on next page)

Performing Groups: Madrigals; Swing Choir; College Chorus; College Orchestra; Community Chorus; Stage Band; Jazz Ensemble; Vocal Ensemble; Instrumental Ensemble; Recorder Ensemble
Workshops/Festivals: Spring Choral Festival; Organ & Piano Workshops

SYMPHONY SCHOOL OF AMERICA
PO Box 2554, LaCrosse   Wisconsin 54601
608 788-3796

Private and Special   ***Arts Areas:*** Dance and Instrumental Music
Performing Series: Concert Series
Performance Facilities: Dodge State Pk - Wenger Stage; University of Wisconsin, LaCrosse - Fine Arts Building Toland Theatre

DANCE

Number Of Faculty: 2   ***Number Of Students:*** 35   ***Courses Offered:*** Ballet
Financial Assistance: Scholarships
Performing Groups: The Festival Ballet Troupe
Workshops/Festivals: Ballet Workshop

MUSIC

Francesco Italiano, Director   ***Number Of Faculty:*** 21
Number Of Students: 80
Degrees Offered: College credit offered through University of Wisconsin, LaCrosse
Courses Offered: Instrumental; Orchestra; Ensemble
Technical Training: Apprenticeship Training   ***Financial Assistance:*** Scholarships
Performing Groups: Faculty String Quartets; Woodwind & Brass Ensembles
Workshops/Festivals: Symphony of the Hills Festival; Great River Symphony
Artists-In-Residence/Guest Artists: Antonia Brico; Elizabeth Green; David Kraehenbuehl

VITERBO COLLEGE
815 S 9th St, La Crosse   Wisconsin 54601
608 784-0040 Ext 177

Private and 4 Year
Arts Areas: Dance, Instrumental Music, Vocal Music, Theatre and Visual Arts
Performing Series: Viterbo Fine Arts Series; Viterbo Concert Series; Viterbo Film Series
Performance Facilities: Main Theater; Recital Hall; Black Box Theater; Dance Studio

MUSIC

Sister Johanna Seubert, Chairperson   ***Number Of Faculty:*** 13
Number Of Students: 80   ***Degrees Offered:*** BMus
Courses Offered: Theory; Music Literature; History; Applied; Music Ed Courses
Teaching Certification Available
Financial Assistance: Scholarships and Work-Study Grants
Performing Groups: Concert Choir; Chamber Singers; Orchestra; Band; Collegiate Choir; String, Brass, Woodwind, Jazz, Piano

THEATRE

Father Phillip Recher, Chairman   ***Number Of Faculty:*** 3
Number Of Students: 14   ***Degrees Offered:*** BA
Courses Offered: Theatre Education; Theatre Production; Acting/Directing
Teaching Certification Available

UNIVERSITY OF WISCONSIN CENTER, MANITOWOC COUNTY
705 Viebahn St, Manitowoc   Wisconsin 54220
414 682-8251 Ext 55

State and 2 Year
Arts Areas: Instrumental Music, Vocal Music, Theatre and Visual Arts
Performing Series: Lecture & Fine Arts Series   ***Performance Facilities:*** Auditorium

(continued on next page)

MUSIC

Michael J Arendt, Assistant Professor   **Number Of Faculty:** 1
Number Of Students: 60   **Degrees Offered:** AA; AS
Courses Offered: Band; Chorus; Jazz Ensemble; Orchestra
Technical Training: Music Theory; Fundamentals; Literature; Applied
Financial Assistance: Scholarships and Work-Study Grants
Performing Groups: U W Center Jazz Ensemble; Symphonic Band
Workshops/Festivals: Clinics; Spring, Summer & Winter Concerts

THEATRE

David H Semmes, Assistant Professor   **Number Of Faculty:** 1
Number Of Students: 40   **Degrees Offered:** AA; AS
Courses Offered: Production Courses, History; Management; Interpretation
Technical Training: Production Courses
Financial Assistance: Scholarships and Work-Study Grants
Performing Groups: Theatre Production; Summer Theatre
Workshops/Festivals: University Summer Playhouse; UW Center System Annual Festival

---

WISCONSIN COLLEGE CONSERVATORY
1584 N Prospect Ave, Milwaukee   Wisconsin 53202
414 276-4350

Private and 4 Year
Arts Areas: Dance, Instrumental Music and Vocal Music

MUSIC

Gerald Stanick, Chairman   **Number Of Faculty:** 28   **Number Of Students:** 100
Degrees Offered: BMus, MMus   **Teaching Certification Available**
Financial Assistance: Scholarships and Work-Study Grants

UNIVERSITY OF WISCONSIN, RIVER FALLS
River Falls   Wisconsin 54022, 715 425-3911

State, 4 Year and Graduate School
Arts Areas: Instrumental Music, Vocal Music, Theatre, Television and Visual Arts
Performance Facilities: Recital Hall; Kleinpell Fine Arts Building Theatre; Kleinpell Fine Arts Building

MUSIC

Dr Elliot Wold, Chairman   **Number Of Faculty:** 14   **Number Of Students:** 210
Degrees Offered: BS Mus; BA Mus; BMusEd
Courses Offered: Theory; Performance; Education; (Vocal & Instrumental)
Technical Training: Piano Technology   **Teaching Certification Available**
Financial Assistance: Internships, Scholarships and Work-Study Grants
Performing Groups: Concert Choir; Chamber Band; Symphony Band; Chamber Singers; Marching Band;
New Music Ensemble; Vocal & Instrumental Ensembles
Workshops/Festivals: Fine Arts Festival

THEATRE

Dr Jerald Carstens, Chairman, Department of Speech   **Number Of Faculty:** 8
Number Of Students: 65
Degrees Offered: BS Speech; BA Speech; BS Sec Ed Speech
Courses Offered: Theatre; Education   **Teaching Certification Available**
Financial Assistance: Internships, Scholarships and Work-Study Grants
Performing Groups: Masquers; St Croix Valley Summer Theatre
Workshops/Festivals: Fine Arts Festival

UNIVERSITY OF WISCONSIN, EAU CLAIRE
Eau Claire   Wisconsin 54701, 715 836-2637

State and 4 Year

Arts Areas: Dance, Instrumental Music, Vocal Music, Theatre, Television and Visual Arts
Performing Series: Artist Series; Chamber Series
Performance Facilities: Earl S Kjer Theater; Riverside Experimental Theater; Gantner Concert Hall;
Recital Halls

DANCE

Dance program under auspices of Department of Physical Education
Courses Offered: Folk, Modern, Square Dance
Performing Groups: Orchesis (Dance Society)

MUSIC

Dr M M Schimke, Chairman   *Number Of Faculty:* 32   *Number Of Students:* 336
Degrees Offered: BMus; BMusEd; MST; MAT
Courses Offered: Organ; Music Therapy; Instrumental Teaching; Vocal Teaching; Vocal; Piano;
Instrumental
Teaching Certification Available
Financial Assistance: Scholarships and Work-Study Grants
Performing Groups: Chamber Orchestra; Orchestra; Concert Choir; Women's Glee Club; Statesmen (Men's
Glee Club); Oratorio; Symphony Band; Concert Band; Jazz Ensembles; Brass Choir; Wind Ensemble
Workshops/Festivals: Choral Workshop; Jazz Festival; Contemporary Symposium; Voice Clinic; Wind
Clinic; State Music Festival

THEATRE

Dr Fred Whited, Jr, Chairman, Speech Department
Theatre program under auspices of Speech Department
Number Of Faculty: 19   *Number Of Students:* 43   *Degrees Offered:* BA
Courses Offered: Stage Design; Costume Design; Acting; Directing; Producting; Children's Stagecraft;
Lighting; Voice & Diction; History; Practicum
Financial Assistance: Scholarships and Work-Study Grants
Workshops/Festivals: Five major productions and two Theatre for Young Audience productions each year,
in addition to a semi-professional summer stock season

UNIVERSITY OF WISCONSIN, GREEN BAY
University Circle Dr, Green Bay   Wisconsin 54302
414 465-2348

State and 4 Year

Arts Areas: Dance, Instrumental Music, Vocal Music, Theatre and Visual Arts
Performance Facilities: University Theatre

DANCE

Nikolai Makaroff, Chairman   *Number Of Faculty:* 2   *Number Of Students:* 150
Degrees Offered: BA, MA   *Teaching Certification Available*
Financial Assistance: Work-Study Grants

MUSIC

Robert Bauer, Chairman   *Number Of Faculty:* 9   *Number Of Students:* 300
Degrees Offered: BA, MA
Technical Training: Music Education, Music Merchandising, Music Repair
Teaching Certification Available   *Financial Assistance:* Work-Study Grants
Performing Groups: Wind Ensemble, Jazz Ensemble, Concert Choir, University Singers, Oratorio Choir,
Brass Choir
Workshops/Festivals: Jazz Festival; Summer Music Clinics

(continued on next page)

THEATRE

Russell Whaley, Chairman **Number Of Faculty:** 5 **Number Of Students:** 250
Degrees Offered: BA, MA
Technical Training: Technical Theater, Ballet, Acting, Directing
Teaching Certification Available **Financial Assistance:** Work-Study Grants
Workshops/Festivals: Children's Theatre Workshpop, Radio/TV/Film Workshop, Summer Workshop

---

UNIVERSITY OF WISCONSIN, LA CROSSE
1725 State St, La Crosse Wisconsin 54601
608 785-8000
State and 4 Year
Arts Areas: Dance, Instrumental Music, Vocal Music, Theatre, Film Arts, Television and Visual Arts
Performing Series: UW - L Lectures & Concerts Series (Forum Series & Recitalist Series)
Performance Facilities: Toland Theatre; Main Auditorium; Cartwright Center

DANCE

Eileen Muth, Director
Dance program under auspices of Physical Education Department
Number Of Faculty: 4 **Number Of Students:** 900
Courses Offered: Dance Appreciation; Fundamentals of Dance; Square & Ethnic Dance; Modern Dance; Children's Dance; Dance Composition
Performing Groups: Orchesis Group; L--X(Ethnic Dance Club); Square Dance Club
Workshops/Festivals: Workshops for High School students in modern dance technique, gymnastics, and other dance forms

MUSIC

William V Estes, Chairman **Number Of Faculty:** 20 **Number Of Students:** 170
Degrees Offered: BS; BS Ed; BA
Courses Offered: Vocal & Instrumental Sequences
Teaching Certification Available
Financial Assistance: Scholarships and Work-Study Grants
Performing Groups: Marching Chiefs; Tribe Jazz Band; The Collegiates Show Choir; Stage Choir; Stage Band; Orchestra; Choral Ensembles; Brass Ensemble; Wind Ensembles; Chamber Groups
Workshops/Festivals: Symphony School of America; Choral & Instrumental Seminars; Opera Workshop

THEATRE

Thomas Wirkus, Chairman, Speech/Theater **Number Of Faculty:** 5
Number Of Students: 60 **Degrees Offered:** BA; BS
Technical Training: Courses and Laboratories in Design, Construction, Make-up, Costuming, Lighting & Management
Financial Assistance: Scholarships and Work-Study Grants
Performing Groups: University Theater; Studio Theater; Children's Theater; Touring Theater (summer)
Workshops/Festivals: "Call to Coffee" workshops, in conjunction with Wisconsin Theatre Association; High School Clinics once or twice yearly
Artists-In-Residence/Guest Artists: Jean Kraft; The National Opera Company; The Rubin - Swerdlow Duo; Thom Mason; Milwaukee Symphony Orchestra

---

UNIVERSITY OF WISCONSIN, MADISON
Madison Wisconsin 53706, 608 262-1234
State and 4 Year
Arts Areas: Dance, Instrumental Music, Vocal Music, Theatre, Film Arts, Television, Visual Arts and Radio
Performance Facilities: Vilas Thrust Theatre, Vilas Experimental Theatre, Wisconsin Union Theatre

DANCE

Louis Kloepper, Chairman **Number Of Faculty:** 12 **Number Of Students:** 250
Dance program under auspices of Women's Physical Education Department
Degrees Offered: BA Performing & Choreography, Teaching, Dance Therapy; MA; PhD
Technical Training: Three year undergraduate Dance Therapy Program
Teaching Certification Available

(continued on next page)

Financial Assistance: Scholarships and Work-Study Grants
Performing Groups: UW Repertory Dance Theatre, Ann Nassif Dance Theatre, Young Choreographers Concert, Visiting Artist Concert

MUSIC

Dale Gilbert, Chairman   **Number Of Faculty:** 60   **Number Of Students:** 500
Degrees Offered: BMus Musicology, Applied, Theory; BMusEd; MMus Applied Composition, Theory MMusEd; PhD Music History, Theory
Teaching Certification Available
Financial Assistance: Assistantships, Scholarships and Work-Study Grants
Performing Groups: Wind Ensemble, Symphonic Band, Concert Band, Varsity Band, UW Symphony Orchestra, Chamber Orchestra, Concert Choir, Women's Chorus, Choral Union, Chorale, Masters Singers, Chamber Singers, Collegium Musicum, Black Music Ensemble, Jazz Ensemble, Contemporary Chamber Ensemble

THEATRE

Ordean Ness, Chairman   **Number Of Faculty:** 15   **Number Of Students:** 185
Degrees Offered: BA, MA, MFA, PhD   **Technical Training:** Technical Theatre
Teaching Certification Available
Financial Assistance: Assistantships, Scholarships and Work-Study Grants
Performing Groups: University Theatre

UNIVERSITY OF WISCONSIN, MARSHFIELD/WOOD COUNTY CENTER
2000 W 5th St, Marshfield   Wisconsin 54449
715 387-1147
State and 2 Year
Arts Areas: Dance, Instrumental Music, Vocal Music and Theatre
Performing Series: Lecutre & Concert Series
Performance Facilities: UW Center - Marshfield/Wood County Theatre

MUSIC

Number Of Faculty: 2   **Degrees Offered:** AA
Courses Offered: Orchestra; Band; Chorus; Jazz Ensemble; Vocal Ensemble; Music Theory I & II; Music Literature & Appreciation; Music History & Literature; Instrumental; Piano; Voice
Financial Assistance: Scholarships and Work-Study Grants
Performing Groups: Jazz Ensemble; Swing Choir; Campus Band; Campus Choir; Orchestra

THEATRE

Number Of Faculty: 1   **Degrees Offered:** AA
Courses Offered: Introduction to Theatre; Theatre Laboratory
Financial Assistance: Scholarships and Work-Study Grants
Performing Groups: Campus Community Players

THE UNIVERSITY OF WISCONSIN, MILWAUKEE
SCHOOL OF FINE ARTS
Milwaukee   Wisconsin 53201, 414 963-4762
State and 4 Year
Arts Areas: Dance, Instrumental Music, Vocal Music, Theatre, Film Arts and Visual Arts
Performing Series: Summer Evenings of Music; Pabst Theater Concert Series
Performance Facilities: Fine Arts Theatre; Recital Hall; Studio Theatre; Engelmann Auditorium

DANCE

Gloria Gustafson, Chairman   **Number Of Faculty:** 10
Number Of Students: 110   **Degrees Offered:** BFA
Courses Offered: Ballet; Contemporary; Afro-American; Pointe; Partnering; Composition; Music
Teaching Certification Available   **Financial Assistance:** Scholarships and Work-Study Grants
Performing Groups: Fine Arts Dance Theatre; Fine Arts Student Dance Ensemble

(continued on next page)

MUSIC

Dr Emanuel Rubin, Chairman   **Number Of Faculty:** 51
Number Of Students: 450   **Degrees Offered:** BFA; BFA MusEd; MMus; MMusEd
Technical Training: Performance Skills; Theoretical Constructs of Musical Composition; Learning Theories/Educational Practices; Electronic Music
Teaching Certification Available
Financial Assistance: Scholarships and Work-Study Grants
Performing Groups: Symphony Orchestra; Wind Symphony; Symphony Band; Jazz Ensemble; University Band; Women's Chorus; Oratorio Chorus; Concert Choir; Madrigal Singers; Collegium Musicum; Musica Intima; New Music Ensemble; Opera Theatre
Workshops/Festivals: Christmas Festival of Courtly Music; High School Honor Band; Vocal Honors Day; State Solo & Ensemble Festival

THEATRE

Sanford Robbins, Chairman   **Number Of Faculty:** 20   **Number Of Students:** 150
Degrees Offered: BFA; MFA
Technical Training: Professional training in Acting, Costume Construction, Technical Theatre, Design for Performance
Financial Assistance: Assistantships, Scholarships and Work-Study Grants
Performing Groups: University Theatre Productions

UNIVERSITY OF WISCONSIN, OSHKOSH
Oshkosh   Wisconsin 54901, 414 424-4422
State and 4 Year
Arts Areas: Dance, Instrumental Music, Vocal Music, Theatre, Film Arts, Television and Visual Arts
Performing Series: Lecture Series; Concert Series
Performance Facilities: Music Hall; Frederick March Theatre; Experimental Theatre

DANCE

Phyllis Roney, Chairperson   **Number Of Faculty:** 3   **Number Of Students:** 710
Degrees Offered: BSEd   **Courses Offered:** Folk, Square, Social, Modern Dance
Workshops/Festivals: Community Arts Festival

MUSIC

John M Minniear, Chairman   **Number Of Faculty:** 32   **Number Of Students:** 250
Degrees Offered: BA; BS; BMus; BMusEd; MST; BMus Therapy; BMus Merchandising
Courses Offered: Performance; Music Education; Music Therapy
Teaching Certification Available
Financial Assistance: Internships, Assistantships, Scholarships and Work-Study Grants
Performing Groups: University Choir; Bel Canto Chorus; Chamber Choir; Titan Band; Regimental Band; Symphonic Winds; Jazz Bands I & II; Percussion Ensemble; Collegium Trio; Brass Quintet; String Quartet; Opera
Workshops/Festivals: Suzuki Pre-School/Elementary String Program; Prep Music Program; Wimebagoland Summer Music Festival; All - Star Clinics in Woodwine, Brass, Strings, Vocal, Jazz Education

THEATRE

Gloria Lind, Coordinator   **Number Of Faculty:** 5   **Number Of Students:** 150
Degrees Offered: BA; BS; MST
Courses Offered: Theatre Arts Emphasis; Drama Education Emphasis
Technical Training: Scenic; Lighting; Costume Design
Teaching Certification Available
Financial Assistance: Internships, Assistantships, Scholarships and Work-Study Grants
Workshops/Festivals: Festivals; Community Arts Festival

UNIVERSITY OF WISCONSIN, PARKSIDE
Kenosha   Wisconsin 53140, 414 553-2121
> State and 4 Year
> *Arts Areas:* Instrumental Music, Vocal Music, Theatre, Television and Visual Arts
> *Performing Series:* Professional productions, Lecture - Fine Arts Series, Student Activities Series
> *Performance Facilities:* Communications Arts Theatre, Art Gallery

MUSIC

Dr August Wegnec, Chairman   *Number Of Faculty:* 19
Number Of Students: 120   *Degrees Offered:* BA
Teaching Certification Available
Financial Assistance: Scholarships and Work-Study Grants
Performing Groups: Choir, Chorale, Recorder Consort, Chamber Singers, Jazz Ensemble, Concert Band, Orchestra, Woodwind Ensemble, Brass Ensemble, Chamber Ensemble

THEATRE

Tom Reiner, Coordinator   *Number Of Faculty:* 3   *Number Of Students:* 70
Degrees Offered: BA   *Technical Training:* Scene Design
Teaching Certification Available   *Financial Assistance:* Work-Study Grants
Performing Groups: The Players

THE UNIVERSITY OF WISCONSIN, PLATTEVILLE
Platteville   Wisconsin 53818, 608 342-1100
> State and 4 Year
> *Arts Areas:* Instrumental Music, Vocal Music, Theatre and Television
> *Performing Series:* Concert Series
> *Performance Facilities:* Little Theatre; Beaux Arts; Fieldhouse

MUSIC

Roland Anfinson, Chairman   *Number Of Faculty:* 11
Degrees Offered: BS MusEd; MS Teaching; BS or BA in Music
Courses Offered: Theory; History & Literature; Music Appreciation; Twentieth Century American Music; Methods & Conducting; Techniques
Teaching Certification Available
Financial Assistance: Assistantships, Scholarships and Work-Study Grants
Performing Groups: Wind Ensemble; Symphony Band; Marching Band; Jazz Ensembles; Orchestra; Mixed Choir; Men's Glee Club; Women's Glee Club; Swing Choir; Brass, String, Percussion, Woodwind Ensembles
Workshops/Festivals: Piano Teachers Workshops; Cello Forum; Summer Music Camp; Choral Festival; Choral - Drama Festival; Jazz Ensemble Festival; Guitar Workshop

THEATRE

Roger Gottschalk, Chairman, Fine Arts   *Number Of Faculty:* 2
Number Of Students: 25   *Degrees Offered:* Minor in Theatre
Courses Offered: Theatre Production; Theatre History; Dramatic Literature
Teaching Certification Available
Financial Assistance: Scholarships and Work-Study Grants
Performing Groups: Summer Shakespeare Festival

UNIVERSITY OF WISCONSIN, SHEBOYGAN
PO Box 719, Lower Falls Rd, Sheboygan   Wisconsin 53081
414 458-5566 Ext 70
> State and 2 Year
> *Arts Areas:* Dance, Instrumental Music, Vocal Music, Theatre, Film Arts, Television and Visual Arts
> *Performing Series:* Special Events Committee
> *Performance Facilities:* Fine Arts Theatre

(continued on next page)

DANCE

Kay Foster, Chairman **Number Of Faculty:** 1 **Number Of Students:** 20

MUSIC

William Hughes, Chairman **Number Of Faculty:** 2 **Number Of Students:** 200
Financial Assistance: Scholarships **Performing Groups:** Jazz Ensemble
Workshops/Festivals: High School Music Students and Directors

THEATRE

Dean F Graunke, Chairman **Number Of Faculty:** 2 **Number Of Students:** 100
Degrees Offered: AA
Financial Assistance: Scholarships and Work-Study Grants
Performing Groups: Delta Psi Omega, Reader's Theatre, UW-S Players
Workshops/Festivals: Annual District Drama Festival for High Schools, University Drama Workshop

---

UNIVERSITY OF WISCONSIN, STEVENS POINT
2100 Main St, Stevens Point Wisconsin 54481
715 346-0123
State and 4 Year
Arts Areas: Dance, Instrumental Music, Vocal Music, Theatre, Film Arts, Television and Visual Arts
Performing Series: Arts & Lectures Series
Performance Facilities: Jenkins Theatre; Michelsen Concert Hall

DANCE

Seldon Faulkner, Chairman **Number Of Faculty:** 3 **Number Of Students:** 125
Courses Offered: Ballet; Modern Social; Composition
Teaching Certification Available **Financial Assistance:** Work-Study Grants
Performing Groups: International Folke Dancers Group

MUSIC

Julius E Erlenbach, Chairman **Number Of Faculty:** 30
Number Of Students: 350
Degrees Offered: BMus; BMus Applied; BMus Theory/Composition; BMus Literature; MS Teaching;
MMusEd
Courses Offered: Music History; Music Literature; Music Theory; Private Applied Music
Technical Training: Piano tuning & repair **Teaching Certification Available**
Financial Assistance: Scholarships and Work-Study Grants
Performing Groups: Symphonic Wind Ensemble; Symphonic Band; University Choir; University Concert
Choir; Mid - Americans (Swing Choir); Madrigal Singers; Symphony Orchestra; University Jazz Ensemble;
University Percussion Ensemble; Wisconsin Arts Woodwind Quintet; University Brass Ensemble; University
String Ensemble
Workshops/Festivals: Annual Band Reading Clinic; Choral Clinic; Madrigal Dinner; Point Music Camp;
Point Piano Camp; Suzuki Talent Education Institute; Opera Workshop Perfrmances; Percussion Clinic

THEATRE

Seldon Faulkner, Chairman **Number Of Faculty:** 9 **Number Of Students:** 225
Degrees Offered: BS; BA
Courses Offered: Lighting; Design; Costuming; Directing; Acting; Scenic
Technical Training: Scenic; Lighting; Stage Design
Teaching Certification Available
Financial Assistance: Scholarships and Work-Study Grants
Performing Groups: University Theatre
Workshops/Festivals: Wisconsin State Forensics Debates - annually; Workshops
Artists-In-Residence/Guest Artists: Oregon Mime Theatre; 5 x 2 Dance Company

UNIVERSITY OF WISCONSIN, SUPERIOR
Superior   Wisconsin 54880, 715 392-8101 Ext 369
State and 4 Year
Arts Areas: Dance, Instrumental Music, Vocal Music, Theatre, Film Arts, Television and Visual Arts
Performing Series: University Theatre, Showcase Theatre
Performance Facilities: Paul E Holden Fine And Applied Arts Center

DANCE

Dr Glenn Gerdes, Chairman   *Number Of Faculty:* 1   *Number Of Students:* 30
Degrees Offered: AA, BA, BS, Minor in Dance
Teaching Certification Available   *Financial Assistance:* Work-Study Grants
Performing Groups: University Dance Theatre
Workshops/Festivals: Fine Arts Festival

MUSIC

Dr Joseph Meidt, Chairman   *Number Of Faculty:* 18   *Number Of Students:* 150
Degrees Offered: BMus, BS, BS, MS Teaching, MA Teaching
Technical Training: Instrumental, Vocal, Orchestral, Organ, Carillon
Teaching Certification Available
Financial Assistance: Assistantships, Scholarships and Work-Study Grants
Performing Groups: University Orchestra, University Choral Society; Concert Band, Marching Band, Male Glee Club, Jazz Lab Band, Duluth - Superior Symphony
Workshops/Festivals: Fine Arts Festival, Saturday Conservatory, 4-H Fine Arts Fair

THEATRE

Dr Bill Stock, Communications Arts Chairman   *Number Of Faculty:* 7
Number Of Students: 100   *Degrees Offered:* AA, BA, BFA, BS, MA
Technical Training: Production, Direction, Acting, Management
Teaching Certification Available
Financial Assistance: Internships, Assistantships, Scholarships and Work-Study Grants
Performing Groups: University Theatre, Experimental Theatre, Showcase Productions, Children's Theatre, Consortium Touring Theatre
Workshops/Festivals: Fine Arts Festival, Mime, Touring Theatre, Children's Theatre, 4-H Fine Arts Fair, Wisconsin High School Forensics Workshop and Institutes

UNIVERSITY OF WISCONSIN, WHITEWATER
800 W Main St, Whitewater   Wisconsin 53190
414 472-1221
State and 4 Year
Arts Areas: Dance, Instrumental Music, Vocal Music, Theatre, Television and Visual Arts
Performing Series: Performing Arts Series
Performance Facilities: Barnett Theatre; Experimental Theatre; Hyer Auditorium; Williams Center

DANCE

Mercedes Fernadez, Director
Dance program under auspices of Theatre Department
Number Of Faculty: 1   *Number Of Students:* 30
Degrees Offered: BA Dance Minor   *Teaching Certification Available*
Financial Assistance: Scholarships and Work-Study Grants
Performing Groups: Modern Dance Company

MUSIC

Dr Dennis Rohrs, Chairman   *Number Of Faculty:* 20   *Number Of Students:* 200
Degrees Offered: BA; MST; MAT   *Teaching Certification Available*
Financial Assistance: Scholarships and Work-Study Grants
Performing Groups: Band; Orchestra; Jazz Ensemble; Choral; Quartets; Quintets; Trios; Mixed Chorus; Madrigals; University - Community Chorus
Workshops/Festivals: High School Summer Music Camp; Music Directors Workshop

(continued on next page)

THEATRE

Gene Wilson, Chairman   ***Number Of Faculty:*** 7   ***Number Of Students:*** 60
Degrees Offered: BA   ***Teaching Certification Available***
Financial Assistance: Scholarships and Work-Study Grants
Performing Groups: University Players; Children's Theatre; Touring Theatre

CASPER COLLEGE
125 College Dr, Casper   Wyoming 82601
307 268-2110
   County and 2 Year
   Arts Areas: Dance, Instrumental Music, Vocal Music, Theatre, Film Arts, Television and Visual Arts

DANCE

Carroll McKee, Drama Director   *Number Of Faculty:* 2
Number Of Students: 60   *Degrees Offered:* AA
Courses Offered: Modern Dance; Social & Folk Dancing; Square Dancing
Financial Assistance: Scholarships and Work-Study Grants

MUSIC

Dr Thomas Kinser, Chairman, Fine Arts   *Number Of Faculty:* 8
Number Of Students: 90   *Degrees Offered:* AA
Technical Training: On-the-job training with area bands and symphony
Financial Assistance: Scholarships and Work-Study Grants
Performing Groups: Jazz, Percussion, String, Brass, Vocal, Woodwind Ensembles; Concert Chord; Concert Band; Casper Symphony Orchestra; Casper Chamber Orchestra; Casper Youth Symphony
Workshops/Festivals: State High School Jazz Band Festival

THEATRE

Carroll McKee, Director   *Number Of Faculty:* 2   *Number Of Students:* 80
Degrees Offered: AA
Financial Assistance: Scholarships and Work-Study Grants
Performing Groups: Penthouse Theatre

CENTRAL WYOMING COLLEGE
Riverton   Wyoming 82501, 307 856-9291 Ext 67
   County and 2 Year
   Arts Areas: Instrumental Music, Vocal Music and Theatre
   Performance Facilities: College Theatre; Dobler Reading Room; College Gym

MUSIC

Bob Dahlberg, Instructor   *Number Of Faculty:* 2   *Number Of Students:* 12
Degrees Offered: AA Music
Courses Offered: Theory I & II; Intro to Music; Music History; Class Piano & Guitar; Chorus; Ensembles; Applied Music; Musical Theater
Financial Assistance: Scholarships and Work-Study Grants
Performing Groups: Chorus; Vocal; Piano; Instrumental Ensembles
Workshops/Festivals: District Festivals for High Schools; Clinics for Public School Teachers & Students; Piano Teachers Workshops

THEATRE

Robert C Kirtley, Director   *Number Of Faculty:* 1   *Number Of Students:* 8
Degrees Offered: AA
Courses Offered: Acting; Stagecraft; Into to Theatre; Theatre Practice; Oral Interpretation
Technical Training: Stage Construction; Stage Lighting; Prop Construction; Make-up
Financial Assistance: Scholarships and Work-Study Grants
Performing Groups: College Theatre; Children's Theatre; Delta Psi Omega; Musical Theatre
Workshops/Festivals: Children's Theatre Workshop; Improvisation Workshop

NORTHWEST COMMUNITY COLLEGE
231 W 6th St, Powell   Wyoming 82435
State and 2 Year
Arts Areas: Instrumental Music, Vocal Music, Theatre, Film Arts and Visual Arts
Performance Facilities: Liberal Arts Auditorium

Number Of Faculty: 3   **Number Of Students:** 45   **Degrees Offered:** AA
Courses Offered: Appreciation; Theory; Applied; Harmony; Electronic
Financial Assistance: Scholarships and Work-Study Grants
Performing Groups: Symphonic Wind Ensemble; Civic String Orchestra; Stage Band; Northwest Winds

Number Of Faculty: 1   **Number Of Students:** 20   **Degrees Offered:** AA
Courses Offered: Theatre; Acting; Stagecraft; Play Production
Financial Assistance: Scholarships and Work-Study Grants
Performing Groups: College Theatre; Children's Theatre

WESTERN WYOMING COMMUNITY COLLEGE
2500 College Dr, Rock Springs   Wyoming 82901
307 382-2121
County and 2 Year   **Arts Areas:** Instrumental Music and Vocal Music
Degrees Offered: AA   **Teaching Certification Available**
Financial Assistance: Scholarships and Work-Study Grants

UNIVERSITY OF WYOMING
Laramie   Wyoming 82070, 307 766-4121
State and 4 Year
Arts Areas: Instrumental Music, Vocal Music, Film Arts, Television, Visual Arts and Radio
Performing Series: Cultural Affairs Committee
Performance Facilities: Fine Arts Center Concert Hall

DANCE

Margaret Mains, Chairman   **Number Of Faculty:** 1   **Number Of Students:** 100
Technical Training: Modern, Folk, Social, Classical Ballet
Performing Groups: Orchesis
Workshops/Festivals: Workshops for Elementary Schools

MUSIC

David Tomatz, Chairman   **Number Of Faculty:** 15   **Number Of Students:** 210
Degrees Offered: BMus, BMusEd, MMus Applied, MMus, MMusEd
Technical Training: Opera, Electronic Music
Teaching Certification Available
Financial Assistance: Internships, Assistantships, Scholarships and Work-Study Grants
Performing Groups: Opera Theatre, Symphony Orchestra, Choral Ensemble, Instrumental Ensembles
Workshops/Festivals: Western Arts Music Festival; Chamber, Voice, and Opera Workshops

THEATRE

E C Reynolds, Chairman   **Number Of Faculty:** 12   **Number Of Students:** 170
Degrees Offered: BA, BFA, MFA   **Teaching Certification Available**
Financial Assistance: Internships, Assistantships, Scholarships and Work-Study Grants
Performing Groups: University Theatre

CATEGORICAL INDEX

CATEGORICAL

Dance

ADELPHI UNIVERSITY, 346
AGNES SCOTT COLLEGE, 105
UNIVERSITY OF AKRON COLLEGE OF FINE AND APPLIED ARTS, 408
UNIVERSITY OF ALABAMA, BIRMINGHAM, 1
UNIVERSITY OF ALASKA, ANCHORAGE, 7
ALBANO BALLET AND PERFORMING ARTS ACADEMY, INC, 70
ALFRED UNIVERSITY, 347
ALICE LLOYD COLLEGE, 197
ALL NEWTON MUSIC SCHOOL, 228
ALLAN HANCOCK COLLEGE, 17
AMARILLO COLLEGE, 512
AMBASSADOR COLLEGE, 17
AMERICAN MUSICAL AND DRAMATIC ACADEMY, INC, 347
THE AMERICAN UNIVERSITY ACADEMY FOR THE PERFORMING ARTS, 81
APPALACHIAN STATE UNIVERSITY, 387
ARIZONA STATE UNIVERSITY, 8
UNIVERSITY OF ARIZONA, 8
UNIVERSITY OF ARKANSAS, MONTICELLO, 13
UNIVERSITY OF ARKANSAS, LITTLE ROCK, 14
AUGUSTANA COLLEGE, 491
AUSTIN COLLEGE, 513
AVILA COLLEGE, 290
BAKERSFIELD COLLEGE, 18
BARAT COLLEGE, 125
BARD COLLEGE, 348
BARRINGTON COLLEGE, 480
BAY PATH JUNIOR COLLEGE, 229
BAYLOR UNIVERSITY, 513
BEE COUNTY COLLEGE, 514
BEMIDJI STATE COLLEGE, 269
BENEDICTINE COLLEGE, 181
BENNETT COLLEGE, 348
BENNETT COLLEGE, 387
BENNINGTON COLLEGE, 558
BEREA COLLEGE, 198
BERRY COLLEGE, 107
BOISE STATE UNIVERSITY, 120
BOSTON CONSERVATORY OF MUSIC, 231
BOWDOIN COLLEGE, 216
BOWIE STATE COLLEGE, 219
BOWLING GREEN STATE UNIVERSITY, 410
BRADFORD COLLEGE, 232
BRAINERD COMMUNITY COLLEGE, 270
BRAZOSPORT COLLEGE, 515
BRENAU COLLEGE, 107
UNIVERSITY OF BRIDGEPORT, 71
BRONX COMMUNITY COLLEGE, 349
BROOKDALE COMMUNITY COLLEGE, 329
BROOKLYN COLLEGE SCHOOL OF PERFORMING ARTS, 349
BROWARD COMMUNITY COLLEGE, 86
BROWN UNIVERSITY, 480

BUCKS COUNTY COMMUNITY COLLEGE, 454
BUNKER HILL COMMUNITY COLLEGE, 233
BUTLER UNIVERSITY JORDAN COLLEGE OF MUSIC, 154
THE CALIFORNIA INSTITUTE OF THE ARTS, 19
CALIFORNIA STATE COLLEGE, 455
CALIFORNIA STATE UNIVERSITY, CHICO, 22
CALIFORNIA STATE UNIVERSITY, FRESNO, 23
CALIFORNIA STATE UNIVERSITY, FULLERTON, 23
CALIFORNIA STATE UNIVERSITY, LONG BEACH, 24
CALIFORNIA STATE UNIVERSITY, LOS ANGELES, 25
CALIFORNIA STATE UNIVERSITY, SACRAMENTO, 26
UNIVERSITY OF CALIFORNIA, DAVIS, 26
UNIVERSITY OF CALIFORNIA, IRVINE, 27
UNIVERSITY OF CALIFORNIA, SAN DIEGO, 28
UNIVERSITY OF CALIFORNIA, SANTA CRUZ, 28
CALVIN COLLEGE, 251
CANADA COLLEGE, 28
CAPE COD CONSERVATORY OF MUSIC AND ARTS, 233
CARLETON COLLEGE, 271
CASE WESTERN RESERVE UNIVERSITY, 411
CASPER COLLEGE, 610
CASTLETON STATE COLLEGE, 558
THE CATHOLIC UNIVERSITY OF AMERICA, 81
CECIL COMMUNITY COLLEGE, 219
CEDAR CREST COLLEGE, 456
CENTENARY COLLEGE OF LOUISANA, 206
CENTRAL CONNECTICUT STATE COLLEGE, 71
CENTRAL METHODIST COLLEGE, 290
CENTRAL MISSOURI STATE UNIVERSITY, 291
CENTRAL STATE UNIVERSITY, 432
CENTRAL WASHINGTON UNIVERSITY, 577
CHATHAM COLLEGE, 456
CHOWAN COLLEGE, 389
CHRISTOPHER NEWPORT COLLEGE, 563
UNIVERSITY OF CINCINNATI COLLEGE-CONSERVATORY OF MUSIC, 412
THE CITY COLLEGE, CITY UNIVERSITY OF NEW YORK, 351
CLATSOP COMMUNITY COLLEGE, 442
CLEVELAND INSTITUTE OF MUSIC, 413
CLEVELAND MUSIC SCHOOL SETTLEMENT, 413
CLEVELAND STATE UNIVERSITY, 414
CLINCH VALLEY COLLEGE OF THE UNIVERSITY OF VIRGINIA, 563
COKER COLLEGE, 485
COLBY COLLEGE, 217
COLBY COLLEGE, 325
COLGATE UNIVERSITY, 353
COLLEGE OF DU PAGE, 128
COLLEGE OF EASTERN UTAH, 553
COLLEGE OF GREAT FALLS, 309
COLLEGE MISERICORDIA, 458
COLLEGE OF NOTRE DAME, 30
COLLEGE OF SAINT BENEDICT, 271
COLLEGE OF SAINT CATHERINE, 271
COLLEGE OF SAINT FRANCIS, 128
COLLEGE OF SAINT ROSE, 353

COLLEGE OF SAINT TERESA, 272
COLLEGE OF SAN MATEO, 30
COLLEGE OF SANTA FE, 342
COLLEGE OF THE SEQUOIAS, 31
COLLEGE OF THE SISKIYOUS, 31
THE COLLEGE OF WHITE PLAINS OF PACE UNIVERSITY, 354
COLORADO COLLEGE, 61
COLORADO MOUNTAIN COLLEGE WEST CAMPUS, 61
COLORADO STATE UNIVERSITY, 62
COLORADO WOMEN'S COLLEGE, 63
UNIVERSITY OF COLORADO, BOULDER, 63
COLUMBIA COLLEGE, 291
COLUMBIA UNIVERSITY, BARNARD COLLEGE, 354
COLUMBUS COLLEGE, 108
COMMUNITY COLLEGE OF BALTIMORE, 220
COMMUNITY MUSIC CENTER, 32
COMMUNITY MUSIC SCHOOL OF BUFFALO, 355
COMPTON COMMUNITY COLLEGE, 32
CONCORDIA COLLEGE, 273
CONNECTICUT COLLEGE, 72
UNIVERSITY OF CONNECTICUT, 72
CORNELL UNIVERSITY, 355
CORNISH INSTITUTE OF ALLIED ARTS, 578
COTTEY COLLEGE, 292
CREIGHTON UNIVERSITY, 314
CURRY COLLEGE, 234
CUYAHOGA COMMUNITY COLLEGE, 414
DAEMEN COLLEGE, 356
DARTMOUTH COLLEGE, 325
DE ANZA COLLEGE, 33
DEAN JUNIOR COLLEGE, 234
UNIVERSITY OF DELAWARE, 79
DELTA COLLEGE, 251
DENISON UNIVERSITY, 416
UNIVERSITY OF DENVER, 64
DEPAUL UNIVERSITY, 129
DEPAUW UNIVERSITY, 154
FAIRLEIGH DICKINSON UNIVERSITY, 331
DIXIE COLLEGE, 554
DONNELLY COLLEGE, 185
DOUGLASS COLLEGE, 331
DRAKE UNIVERSITY, 169
DREW UNIVERSITY, 332
DUKE UNIVERSITY, 390
DUTCHESS COMMUNITY COLLEGE, 357
D'YOUVILLE COLLEGE, 358
EARLHAM COLLEGE, 155
EAST CAROLINA UNIVERSITY, 391
EAST STROUDSBURG STATE COLLEGE, 460
EAST TENNESSEE STATE UNIVERSITY, 500
EASTERN KENTUCKY UNIVERSITY, 200
EASTERN MICHIGAN UNIVERSITY, 252
EASTERN WASHINGTON STATE COLLEGE, 578
ECKERD COLLEGE, 88
EDGEWOOD COLLEGE, 595
ELMIRA COLLEGE, 358
ELON COLLEGE, 391
EMERSON COLLEGE, 235
FAIRMOUNT CENTER FOR CREATIVE & PERFORMING ARTS, 417
FAYETTEVILLE STATE UNIVERSITY, 392
FEDERAL CITY COLLEGE, 82
FISK UNIVERSITY, 501
FLORIDA JUNIOR COLLEGE, 90
FLORIDA SOUTHERN COLLEGE, 91
FLORIDA STATE UNIVERSITY, 92
UNIVERSITY OF FLORIDA, 93

FOOTHILL COLLEGE, 34
FORDHAM UNIVERSITY, LINCOLN CENTER, 359
FORT HAYS STATE UNIVERSITY, 185
FRANCONIA COLLEGE, 325
FRANKLIN AND MARSHALL COLLEGE, 461
FRESNO CITY COLLEGE, 34
FULLERTON COLLEGE, 35
FURMAN UNIVERSITY, 486
GADSDEN STATE JUNIOR COLLEGE, 1
GARDEN CITY COMMUNITY COLLEGE, 187
GEORGE PEABODY COLLEGE FOR TEACHERS, 501
GEORGE WASHINGTON UNIVERSITY, 83
GEORGIA STATE UNIVERSITY, 111
GLASSBORO STATE COLLEGE, 333
GONZAGA UNIVERSITY, 579
GREENBRIER COLLEGE, 588
GROSSMONT COLLEGE, 36
GROVE CITY COLLEGE, 462
GULF PARK COLLEGE, 282
HAMPTON INSTITUTE, 565
HANOVER COLLEGE, 157
HARLEM SCHOOL OF THE ARTS, INC, 360
THE HARTFORD CONSERVATORY, 73
HARTNELL COLLEGE, 37
HARTWICK COLLEGE, 360
HARVARD UNIVERSITY, 237
HASTING COLLEGE, 315
UNIVERSITY OF HAWAII, 118
HAWKEN SCHOOL, 417
HEBREW ARTS SCHOOL FOR MUSIC AND DANCE, 361
HENDERSON COUNTY JUNIOR COLLEGE, 520
HIGH SCHOOL FOR THE PERFORMING AND VISUAL ARTS, 521
HIGHLINE COMMUNITY COLLEGE, 580
HILLSDALE COLLEGE, 254
HOFSTRA UNIVERSITY, 362
HOLLINS COLLEGE, 566
HOPE COLLEGE, 254
UNIVERSITY OF HOUSTON, CENTRAL CAMPUS, 522
HUMBOLDT STATE UNIVERSITY, 37
HUNTER COLLEGE, CITY UNIVERSITY OF NEW YORK, 363
HUTCHINSON COMMUNITY COLLEGE, 187
UNIVERSITY OF IDAHO, 121
ILLINOIS CENTRAL COLLEGE, 132
ILLINOIS STATE UNIVERSITY, 134
ILLINOIS WESLEYAN UNIVERSITY, 133
IMPERIAL VALLEY COLLEGE, 38
INDIANA STATE UNIVERSITY, 157
INDIANA UNIVERSITY - PURDUE UNIVERSITY AT FORT WAYNE,
  158
INDIANA UNIVERSITY, BLOOMINGTON, 159
INDIANA UNIVERSITY NORTHWEST, 160
INDIANA UNIVERSITY OF PENNSYLVANIA, 463
INTERLOCHEN ARTS ACADEMY, 255
INTERNATIONAL COLLEGE, 38
IOWA LAKES COMMUNITY COLLEGE, 171
IOWA STATE UNIVERSITY, 171
ITHACA COLLEGE, 364
JACKSONVILLE UNIVERSITY, 94
JAMES MADISON UNIVERSITY, 566
JERSEY CITY STATE COLLEGE, 333
THE JOY OF MOVEMENT CENTER, 238
JUDSON COLLEGE, 2
THE JUILLIARD SCHOOL, 365
KALAMAZOO COLLEGE, 256
KANSAS STATE UNIVERSITY, 189
UNIVERSITY OF KANSAS, 190

UNIVERSITY OF TAMPA, 103
TARRANT COUNTY JUNIOR COLLEGE, SOUTH CAMPUS, 541
TEMPLE UNIVERSITY, 475
UNIVERSITY OF TENNESSEE, KNOXVILLE, 509
UNIVERSITY OF TENNESSEE, MARTIN, 510
TEXAS CHRISTIAN UNIVERSITY, 542
TEXAS SOUTHERN UNIVERSITY, 544
TEXAS SOUTHMOST COLLEGE, 544
TEXAS TECH UNIVERSITY, 545
TEXAS WOMEN'S UNIVERSITY, 546
UNIVERSITY OF TEXAS - AUSTIN, 546
UNIVERSITY OF TOLEDO, 427
TOWSON STATE UNIVERSITY, 225
TRANSYLVANIA UNIVERSITY, 204
TRINITY COLLEGE, 75
TRINITY COLLEGE, 85
TRINITY UNIVERSITY, 547
TULANE UNIVERSITY, 214
U S COAST GUARD ACADEMY, 76
UNION COLLEGE, 385
UNITED STATES INTERNATIONAL UNIVERSITY, 56
UNIVERSITY OF CALIFORNIA, RIVERSIDE, 56
UNIVERSITY OF DALLAS, 548
UNIVERSITY OF DETROIT, MARYGROVE COLLEGE, 266
UNIVERSITY OF ILLINOIS, 151
THE UNIVERSITY OF IOWA, 177
UNIVERSITY OF NORTH CAROLINA, 403
UNIVERSITY OF REDLANDS, 57
UNIVERSITY OF RICHMOND, 572
UNIVERSITY OF SOUTHERN CALIFORNIA, 57
UNIVERSITY OF SOUTHERN MISSISSIPPI, 288
UNIVERSITY OF TEXAS, AUSTIN, 549
UNIVERSITY OF TEXAS, EL PASO, 549
UNIVERSITY OF VERMONT, 562
UTAH STATE UNIVERSITY, 555
UNIVERSITY OF UTAH, 555
THE VICTORIA COLLEGE, 550
VILLA JULIE COLLEGE, 226
VINCENNES UNIVERSITY, 166
VIRGINIA INTERMONT COLLEGE, 574
UNIVERSITY OF VIRGINIA, 575
VITERBO COLLEGE, 600
WAGNER COLLEGE, 386
WAKE FOREST UNIVERSITY, 404
WALNUT HILL SCHOOL OF PERFORMING ARTS, 246
WARTBURG COLLEGE, 179
WASHBURN UNIVERSITY OF TOPEKA, 196
WASHINGTON COLLEGE, 226
WASHINGTON UNIVERSITY, 305
UNIVERSITY OF WASHINGTON, 583
WEBER STATE COLLEGE, 556
WEBSTER COLLEGE, 306
WELLS COLLEGE, 386
WESLEYAN UNIVERSITY, 76
WEST CHESTER STATE COLLEGE, 477
WEST HILLS COLLEGE, 58
WEST TEXAS STATE UNIVERSITY, 551
WEST VIRGINIA WESLEYAN COLLEGE, 591
WESTERN CONNECTICUT STATE COLLEGE, 77
WESTERN KENTUCKY UNIVERSITY, 205
WESTERN MICHIGAN UNIVERSITY, 267
WESTERN WASHINGTON STATE COLLEGE, 584
WESTFIELD STATE COLLEGE, 247
WESTMONT COLLEGE, 58
WILLIAM JEWELL COLLEGE, 307
WILLIAM WOODS - WESTMINISTER COLLEGE, 308

WILLIAMS COLLEGE, 247
WILLMAR COMMUNITY COLLEGE, 280
WILSON COLLEGE, 478
WINDHAM COLLEGE, 562
WINTHROP COLLEGE, 489
WISCONSIN COLLEGE CONSERVATORY, 601
UNIVERSITY OF WISCONSIN, EAU CLAIRE, 602
UNIVERSITY OF WISCONSIN, GREEN BAY, 602
UNIVERSITY OF WISCONSIN, LA CROSSE, 603
UNIVERSITY OF WISCONSIN, MADISON, 603
UNIVERSITY OF WISCONSIN, MARSHFIELD/WOOD CO CENTER, 604
THE UNIVERSITY OF WISCONSIN, MILWAUKEE SCHOOL OF FINE ARTS, 604
UNIVERSITY OF WISCONSIN, OSHKOSH, 605
UNIVERSITY OF WISCONSIN, SHEBOYGAN, 606
UNIVERSITY OF WISCONSIN, STEVENS POINT, 607
UNIVERSITY OF WISCONSIN, SUPERIOR, 608
UNIVERSITY OF WISCONSIN, WHITEWATER, 608
WRIGHT STATE UNIVERSITY, 430

Music

ABILENE CHRISTIAN UNIVERSITY, 512
ABRAHAM BALDWIN AGRICULTURAL COLLEGE, 105
ADAMS STATE COLLEGE, 60
ADELPHI UNIVERSITY, 346
ADIRONDACK COMMUNITY COLLEGE, 346
ADRIAN COLLEGE, 249
AGNES SCOTT COLLEGE, 105
UNIVERSITY OF AKRON COLLEGE OF FINE AND APPLIED ARTS, 408
UNIVERSITY OF ALABAMA, BIRMINGHAM, 1
UNIVERSITY OF ALASKA COLLEGE OF ARTS & LETTERS, 7
UNIVERSITY OF ALASKA, ANCHORAGE, 7
ALBANO BALLET AND PERFORMING ARTS ACADEMY, INC, 70
ALBANY STATE COLLEGE, 106
ALBERTUS MAGNUS COLLEGE, 70
ALBION COLLEGE, 249
ALBRIGHT COLLEGE, 452
ALCORN AGRICULTURAL & MECHANICAL COLLEGE, 281
ALDERSON - BROADDUS COLLEGE, 586
ALFRED UNIVERSITY, 347
ALICE LLOYD COLLEGE, 197
ALL NEWTON MUSIC SCHOOL, 228
ALLAN HANCOCK COLLEGE, 17
ALLEGHENY COLLEGE, 452
ALLEGHENY COUNTY COMMUNITY COLLEGE, 452
ALLEN COUNTY COMMUNITY JUNIOR COLLEGE, 180
ALLEN UNIVERSITY, 483
ALMA COLLEGE, 249
ALMA WHITE COLLEGE, 329
ALPENA COMMUNITY COLLEGE, 250
ALPHONSUS COLLEGE, 329
ALVERNO COLLEGE, 593
ALVIN JUNIOR COLLEGE, 512
AMARILLO COLLEGE, 512
AMBASSADOR COLLEGE, 17
AMERICAN CONSERVATORY OF MUSIC, 124
AMERICAN MUSICAL AND DRAMATIC ACADEMY, INC, 347
THE AMERICAN UNIVERSITY ACADEMY FOR THE PERFORMING ARTS, 81
AMHERST COLLEGE, 228
ANDERSON COLLEGE, 153
ANDERSON COLLEGE, 483
ANDREW COLLEGE, 106

ANDREWS UNIVERSITY, 250
ANGELO STATE UNIVERSITY, 512
ANNA MARIA COLLEGE, 228
ANNHURST COLLEGE, 70
ANTIOCH COLLEGE, 409
APPALACHIAN STATE UNIVERSITY, 387
AQUINAS COLLEGE, 250
ARAPAHOE COMMUNITY COLLEGE, 60
ARIZONA STATE UNIVERSITY, 8
UNIVERSITY OF ARIZONA, 8
ARKANSAS COLLEGE, 12
ARKANSAS STATE UNIVERSITY, 12
ARKANSAS TECH UNIVERSITY, 12
UNIVERSITY OF ARKANSAS, PINE BLUFF, 13
UNIVERSITY OF ARKANSAS, MONTICELLO, 13
UNIVERSITY OF ARKANSAS, LITTLE ROCK, 14
ARMSTRONG STATE COLLEGE, 106
ASBURY COLLEGE, 197
ASHLAND COLLEGE, 409
ASPEN MUSIC SCHOOL, 60
ATLANTIC CHRISTIAN COLLEGE, 387
ATLANTIC UNION COLLEGE THAYER CONSERVATORY OF MU-
    SIC, 229
AUGSBURG COLLEGE, 269
AUGUSTANA COLLEGE, 124
AUGUSTANA COLLEGE, 491
AURORA COLLEGE, 124
AUSTIN COLLEGE, 513
AUSTIN PEAY STATE UNIVERSITY, 497
AVILA COLLEGE, 290
BACONE COLLEGE, 432
BAKER UNIVERSITY, 180
BAKERSFIELD COLLEGE, 18
BALDWIN - WALLACE COLLEGE, 409
BALL STATE UNIVERSITY, 153
BAPTIST BIBLE COLLEGE, 453
BARAT COLLEGE, 125
BARD COLLEGE, 348
BARRINGTON COLLEGE, 480
BARRY COLLEGE, 86
BARTLESVILLE WESLEYAN COLLEGE, 432
BARTON COUNTY COMMUNITY COLLEGE, 180
BATES COLLEGE, 216
BAY PATH JUNIOR COLLEGE, 229
BAYLOR UNIVERSITY, 513
BEAVER COLLEGE, 453
BEE COUNTY COLLEGE, 514
BELHAVEN COLLEGE, 281
BELLARMINE COLLEGE, 197
BELMONT COLLEGE, 497
BELMONT MUSIC SCHOOL, 229
BELOIT COLLEGE, 593
BEMIDJI STATE COLLEGE, 269
BENEDICT COLLEGE, 483
BENEDICTINE COLLEGE, 181
BENNETT COLLEGE, 348
BENNETT COLLEGE, 387
BENNINGTON COLLEGE, 558
BEREA COLLEGE, 198
BERGEN COMMUNITY COLLEGE, 329
BERKLEE COLLEGE OF MUSIC, 230
BERKSHIRE CHRISTIAN COLLEGE, 230
BERKSHIRE MUSIC CENTER, TANGLEWOOD, 230
BERRY COLLEGE, 107
BETHANY BIBLE COLLEGE, 18
BETHANY COLLEGE, 181

BETHANY COLLEGE, 586
BETHANY LUTHERAN COLLEGE, 270
BETHANY NAZARENE COLLEGE, 432
BETHEL COLLEGE, 153
BETHEL COLLEGE, 182
BETHEL COLLEGE, 270
BETHEL COLLEGE, 497
BETHUNE - COOKMAN COLLEGE, 86
BISCAYNE COLLEGE, 86
BISHOP COLLEGE, 514
BISMARK JUNIOR COLLEGE, 406
BLACK HAWK COLLEGE, 125
BLACK HILLS STATE COLLEGE, 491
BLACKBURN COLLEGE, 126
BLINN COLLEGE, 514
BLOOMFIELD COLLEGE, 329
BLOOMSBURG STATE COLLEGE, 453
BLUE MOUNTAIN COLLEGE, 281
BLUE MOUNTAIN COMMUNITY COLLEGE, 442
BLUEFIELD COLLEGE, 563
BLUEFIELD COLLEGE, 586
BLUFFTON COLLEGE, 409
BOB JONES UNIVERSITY, 484
BOISE STATE UNIVERSITY, 120
BOSTON CONSERVATORY OF MUSIC, 231
BOSTON UNIVERSITY SCHOOL FOR THE ARTS, 231
BOWDOIN COLLEGE, 216
BOWIE STATE COLLEGE, 219
BOWLING GREEN STATE UNIVERSITY, 410
BRADFORD COLLEGE, 232
BRADLEY UNIVERSITY, 126
BRAINERD COMMUNITY COLLEGE, 270
BRANDEIS UNIVERSITY, 232
BRANDYWINE COLLEGE, 79
BRENAU COLLEGE, 107
BRESCIA COLLEGE, 198
BREVARD COLLEGE, 388
BRIARCLIFF COLLEGE, 349
UNIVERSITY OF BRIDGEPORT, 71
BRIDGEWATER COLLEGE, 563
BRIDGEWATER STATE COLLEGE, 232
BRIGHAM YOUNG UNIVERSITY, 553
BRIGHAM YOUNG UNIVERSITY - HAWAII CAMPUS, 118
BRONX COMMUNITY COLLEGE, 349
BROOKDALE COMMUNITY COLLEGE, 329
BROOKLYN COLLEGE SCHOOL OF PERFORMING ARTS, 349
BROWARD COMMUNITY COLLEGE, 86
BROWN UNIVERSITY, 480
BRYN MAWR COLLEGE, 453
BRYON COLLEGE, 498
BUCKNELL UNIVERSITY, 454
BUCKS COUNTY COMMUNITY COLLEGE, 454
BUENA VISTA COLLEGE, 167
BUNKER HILL COMMUNITY COLLEGE, 233
BUTLER COUNTY COMMUNITY JUNIOR COLLEGE, 182
BUTLER UNIVERSITY JORDAN COLLEGE OF MUSIC, 154
BUTTE COLLEGE, 18
CALDWELL COLLEGE, 330
SOUTHERN CALIFORNIA COLLEGE, 19
THE CALIFORNIA INSTITUTE OF THE ARTS, 19
CALIFORNIA INSTITUTE OF TECHNOLOGY, 20
CALIFORNIA LUTHERAN COLLEGE, 20
CALIFORNIA STATE COLLEGE, 455
CALIFORNIA STATE COLLEGE, BAKERSFIELD, 20
CALIFORNIA STATE COLLEGE, STANISLAUS, 21
CALIFORNIA STATE UNIVERSITY - DOMINGUEZ HILLS, 22

CALIFORNIA STATE UNIVERSITY, CHICO, 22
CALIFORNIA STATE UNIVERSITY, FRESNO, 23
CALIFORNIA STATE UNIVERSITY, FULLERTON, 23
CALIFORNIA STATE UNIVERSITY, LONG BEACH, 24
CALIFORNIA STATE UNIVERSITY, LOS ANGELES, 25
CALIFORNIA STATE UNIVERSITY, NORTHRIDGE, 25
CALIFORNIA STATE UNIVERSITY, SACRAMENTO, 26
UNIVERSITY OF CALIFORNIA, DAVIS, 26
UNIVERSITY OF CALIFORNIA, IRVINE, 27
UNIVERSITY OF CALIFORNIA, LOS ANGELES, 27
UNIVERSITY OF CALIFORNIA, SAN DIEGO, 28
UNIVERSITY OF CALIFORNIA, SANTA CRUZ, 28
CALVIN COLLEGE, 251
CAMDEN COUNTY COLLEGE, 330
CAMPBELL COLLEGE, 388
CAMPBELLSVILLE COLLEGE, 198
CANADA COLLEGE, 28
CANTOR'S INSTITUTE & SEMINARY COLLEGE OF JEWISH MU-
    SIC, 350
CAPE COD CONSERVATORY OF MUSIC AND ARTS, 233
CAPITAL UNIVERSITY, 410
CARDINAL STRITCH COLLEGE, 593
CARLETON COLLEGE, 271
CARLOW COLLEGE, 455
CARNEGIE - MELLON UNIVERSITY, 455
CARROLL COLLEGE, 309
CARROLL COLLEGE, 594
CARSON - NEWMAN COLLEGE, 498
CARTHAGE COLLEGE, 594
CASE WESTERN RESERVE UNIVERSITY, 411
CASPER COLLEGE, 610
CASTLETON STATE COLLEGE, 558
CATAWBA COLLEGE, 389
CATHERINE SPAULDING COLLEGE, 199
THE CATHOLIC UNIVERSITY OF AMERICA, 81
CAYUGA COUNTY COMMUNITY COLLEGE, 350
CECIL COMMUNITY COLLEGE, 219
CEDAR CREST COLLEGE, 456
CENTENARY COLLEGE FOR WOMEN, 331
CENTENARY COLLEGE OF LOUISANA, 206
CENTRAL ARIZONA COLLEGE, 9
UNIVERSITY OF CENTRAL ARKANSAS, 14
CENTRAL BIBLE COLLEGE, 290
CENTRAL COLLEGE, 167
CENTRAL COLLEGE, 182
CENTRAL CONNECTICUT STATE COLLEGE, 71
CENTRAL FLORIDA COMMUNITY COLLEGE, 87
CENTRAL METHODIST COLLEGE, 290
CENTRAL MICHIGAN UNIVERSITY, 251
CENTRAL MISSOURI STATE UNIVERSITY, 291
CENTRAL OREGON COMMUNITY COLLEGE, 442
CENTRAL STATE UNIVERSITY, 412
CENTRAL STATE UNIVERSITY, 432
CENTRAL TEXAS COLLEGE, 515
CENTRAL WASHINGTON UNIVERSITY, 577
CENTRAL WESLEYAN COLLEGE, 484
CENTRAL WYOMING COLLEGE, 610
CENTRALIA COLLEGE, 577
CENTRE COLLEGE OF KENTUCKY, 199
CERRO COSO COMMUNITY COLLEGE, 29
CHADRON STATE COLLEGE, 313
CHAMINADE UNIVERSITY OF HONOLULU, 118
CHATHAM COLLEGE, 456
CHESTNUT HILL COLLEGE, 457
CHEYNEY STATE COLLEGE, 457
CHICAGO CITY COLLEGE, OLIVE - HARVEY COLLEGE, 127

CHICAGO CONSERVATORY COLLEGE, 127
CHICAGO STATE UNIVERSITY, 127
CHIPOLA JUNIOR COLLEGE, 87
CHOWAN COLLEGE, 389
CHRISTIAN BROTHERS COLLEGE, 498
CHRISTOPHER NEWPORT COLLEGE, 563
THE CINCINNATI BIBLE SEMINARY, 412
UNIVERSITY OF CINCINNATI COLLEGE-CONSERVATORY OF MU-
    SIC, 412
CISCO JUNIOR COLLEGE, 515
THE CITY COLLEGE, CITY UNIVERSITY OF NEW YORK, 351
CITY UNIVERSITY OF NEW YORK HERBERT H LEHMAN COL-
    LEGE, 351
CITY UNIVERSITY OF NEW YORK, QUEENS COLLEGE, 352
CITY UNIVERSITY OF NEW YORK, YORK COLLEGE, 352
CLAFLIN COLLEGE, 484
CLAREMONT GRADUATE SCHOOL, 29
CLAREMORE JUNIOR COLLEGE, 433
CLARION STATE COLLEGE - CLARION CAMPUS, 457
CLARION STATE COLLEGE - VENANGO CAMPUS, 458
CLARK UNIVERSITY, 233
CLARKE COLLEGE, 167
CLARKE COLLEGE, 281
CLATSOP COMMUNITY COLLEGE, 442
CLEVELAND INSTITUTE OF MUSIC, 413
CLEVELAND MUSIC SCHOOL SETTLEMENT, 413
CLEVELAND STATE COMMUNITY COLLEGE, 499
CLEVELAND STATE UNIVERSITY, 414
CLINCH VALLEY COLLEGE OF THE UNIVERSITY OF VIRGINIA,
    563
CLOUD COUNTY COMMUNITY COLLEGE, 183
COASTAL CAROLINA COLLEGE OF THE UNIVERSITY OF SOUTH
    CAROLINA, 484
COE COLLEGE, 168
COFFEYVILLE COMMUNITY JUNIOR COLLEGE, 183
COKER COLLEGE, 485
COLBY COLLEGE, 217
COLBY COLLEGE, 325
COLBY COMMUNITY COLLEGE, 183
COLEGIO CESAR CHEVEZ, 442
COLGATE UNIVERSITY, 353
COLLEGE OF THE ALBEMARLE, 389
COLLEGE OF ARTESIA, 342
COLLEGE OF THE CANYONS, 29
COLLEGE OF DU PAGE, 128
COLLEGE OF EASTERN UTAH, 553
COLLEGE OF EMPORIA, 184
COLLEGE OF GREAT FALLS, 309
COLLEGE OF THE MAINLAND, 515
COLLEGE OF MARIN, 30
COLLEGE MISERICORDIA, 458
COLLEGE OF NOTRE DAME, 30
COLLEGE OF SAINT BENEDICT, 271
COLLEGE OF SAINT CATHERINE, 271
COLLEGE OF SAINT FRANCIS, 128
COLLEGE OF SAINT MARY, 313
COLLEGE OF SAINT ROSE, 353
COLLEGE OF SAINT TERESA, 272
COLLEGE OF SAINT THOMAS, 272
COLLEGE OF SAN MATEO, 30
COLLEGE OF SANTA FE, 342
COLLEGE OF THE SEQUOIAS, 31
COLLEGE OF THE SISKIYOUS, 31
THE COLLEGE OF WHITE PLAINS OF PACE UNIVERSITY, 354
COLLEGE OF WILLIAM AND MARY, 564
COLORADO COLLEGE, 61

EMORY AND HENRY COLLEGE, 564
EMORY UNIVERSITY, 109
EMPORIA STATE UNIVERSITY, 185
ENDICOTT COLLEGE, 236
ERSKINE COLLEGE, 486
ESSEX COMMUNITY COLLEGE, 220
EUREKA COLLEGE, 130
EVANGEL COLLEGE, 293
FAIRMONT STATE COLLEGE, 587
FAIRMOUNT CENTER FOR CREATIVE & PERFORMING ARTS, 417
FAITH BAPTIST BIBLE COLLEGE, 169
FAYETTEVILLE STATE UNIVERSITY, 392
FEDERAL CITY COLLEGE, 82
FELICIAN COLLEGE, 131
FELICIAN COLLEGE, 332
FERRIS STATE COLLEGE, 252
FERRUM COLLEGE, 565
FINCH COLLEGE, 359
FINDLAY COLLEGE, 417
FISK UNIVERSITY, 501
FLATHEAD VALLEY COMMUNITY COLLEGE, 310
FLORIDA AGRICULTURAL & MECHANICAL UNIVERSITY, 89
FLORIDA ATLANTIC UNIVERSITY, 89
FLORIDA COLLEGE, 90
FLORIDA INTERNATIONAL UNIVERSITY, 90
FLORIDA JUNIOR COLLEGE, 90
FLORIDA KEYS COMMUNITY COLLEGE, 91
FLORIDA MEMORIAL COLLEGE, 91
FLORIDA SOUTHERN COLLEGE, 91
FLORIDA STATE UNIVERSITY, 92
FLORIDA TECHNOLOGICAL UNIVERSITY, 92
UNIVERSITY OF FLORIDA, 93
FONTBONNE COLLEGE, 294
FOOTHILL COLLEGE, 34
FORDHAM UNIVERSITY, LINCOLN CENTER, 359
FORT HAYS STATE UNIVERSITY, 185
FORT LEWIS COLLEGE, 64
FORT SCOTT COMMUNITY JUNIOR COLLEGE, 186
FORT WAYNE BIBLE COLLEGE, 155
FORT WORTH CHRISTIAN COLLEGE, 519
FORT WRIGHT COLLEGE OF THE HOLY NAMES, 579
FRANCONIA COLLEGE, 325
FRANK PHILLIPS COLLEGE, 519
FRANKLIN AND MARSHALL COLLEGE, 461
FRANKLIN COLLEGE, 156
FREE WILL BAPTIST COLLEGE, 501
FRESNO CITY COLLEGE, 34
FRESNO PACIFIC COLLEGE, 35
FRIENDS UNIVERSITY, 186
FROSTBURG STATE COLLEGE, 220
FULLERTON COLLEGE, 35
FURMAN UNIVERSITY, 486
GADSDEN STATE JUNIOR COLLEGE, 1
GAINESVILLE JUNIOR COLLEGE, 109
GARDEN CITY COMMUNITY COLLEGE, 187
GARDNER - WEBB COLLEGE, 392
GAVILAN COLLEGE, 36
GENESEE COMMUNITY COLLEGE, 359
GENEVA COLLEGE, 461
GEORGE FOX COLLEGE, 443
GEORGE PEABODY COLLEGE FOR TEACHERS, 501
GEORGE WASHINGTON UNIVERSITY, 83
GEORGIA COLLEGE, 110
GEORGIA SOUTHERN COLLEGE, 110
GEORGIA SOUTHWESTERN COLLEGE, 111
GEORGIA STATE UNIVERSITY, 111

UNIVERSITY OF GEORGIA, 111
GEORGIAN COURT COLLEGE, 333
GETTYSBURG COLLEGE, 462
GLASSBORO STATE COLLEGE, 333
GLEN OAKS COMMUNITY COLLEGE, 253
GLENDALE COMMUNITY COLLEGE, 9
GLENVILLE STATE COLLEGE, 588
GODDARD COLLEGE, 559
GOLDEN VALLEY LUTHERAN COLLEGE, 273
GOLDOVSKY OPERA INSTITUTE, 236
GONZAGA UNIVERSITY, 579
GORDON COLLEGE, 236
GOSHEN COLLEGE, 156
GOUCHER COLLEGE, 221
GRACE COLLEGE, 156
GRACE COLLEGE OF THE BIBLE, 315
GRACELAND COLLEGE, 170
GRAMBLING COLLEGE OF LOUISIANA, 207
GRAND CANYON COLLEGE, 9
GRAND RAPIDS BAPTIST COLLEGE, 253
GRAND RAPIDS JUNIOR COLLEGE, 253
GRAYSON COUNTY COLLEGE, 520
GREEN MOUNTAIN COLLEGE, 559
GREENBRIER COLLEGE, 588
GREENSBORO COLLEGE, 392
GREENVILLE COLLEGE, 131
GRINNELL COLLEGE, 170
GROSSMONT COLLEGE, 36
GROVE CITY COLLEGE, 462
GULF COAST COMMUNITY COLLEGE, 93
GULF PARK COLLEGE, 282
GUSTAVUS ADOLPHUS COLLEGE, 274
HAMILTON COLLEGE, 360
HAMLINE UNIVERSITY, 274
HAMPTON INSTITUTE, 565
HANNIBAL LA GRANGE COLLEGE, 294
HANOVER COLLEGE, 157
HARDIN - SIMMONS UNIVERSITY, 520
HARDING COLLEGE, 15
HARLEM SCHOOL OF THE ARTS, INC, 360
HARRISBURG AREA COMMUNITY COLLEGE, 463
THE HARTFORD CONSERVATORY, 73
UNIVERSITY OF HARTFORD, 74
HARTNELL COLLEGE, 37
HARTWICK COLLEGE, 360
HARVARD UNIVERSITY, 237
HASTING COLLEGE, 315
HASTINGS TALENT EDUCATION CENTRE, INC, 361
HAVERFORD COLLEGE, 463
UNIVERSITY OF HAWAII, 118
UNIVERSITY OF HAWAII AT HILO - HILO COLLEGE, 119
HAWKEN SCHOOL, 417
HAZARD COMMUNITY COLLEGE, 200
HEBREW ARTS SCHOOL FOR MUSIC AND DANCE, 361
HEBREW UNION COLLEGE - JEWISH INSTITUTE OF RELIGION
   SCHOOL OF SACRED MUSIC, 361
HEIDELBURG COLLEGE, 418
HENDERSON COUNTY JUNIOR COLLEGE, 520
HENDRIX COLLEGE, 15
HENRY FORD COMMUNITY COLLEGE, 253
HESSTON COLLEGE, 187
HIGH POINT COLLEGE, 393
HIGH SCHOOL FOR THE PERFORMING AND VISUAL ARTS, 521
HIGHLINE COMMUNITY COLLEGE, 580
HILL JUNIOR COLLEGE, 521
HILLSBOROUGH COMMUNITY COLLEGE, YBOR CAMPUS, 93

HILLSDALE COLLEGE, 254
HINDS JUNIOR COLLEGE, 283
HIRAM COLLEGE, 418
HIRAM SCOTT COLLEGE, 316
HOBART & WILLIAM SMITH COLLEGES, 362
HOFSTRA UNIVERSITY, 362
HOLLINS COLLEGE, 566
HOLMES JUNIOR COLLEGE, 283
HOLY CROSS COLLEGE, 237
HOLY FAMILY COLLEGE, 595
HOLYOKE COMMUNITY COLLEGE, 237
HOOD COLLEGE, 221
HOPE COLLEGE, 254
HOUGHTON COLLEGE, 362
HOUSTON BAPTIST UNIVERSITY, 522
UNIVERSITY OF HOUSTON, CENTRAL CAMPUS, 522
UNIVERSITY OF HOUSTON, DOWNTOWN COLLEGE, 523
HOWARD COLLEGE, BIG SPRING, 523
HOWARD PAYNE COLLEGE, 523
HOWARD UNIVERSITY, 83
HUDSON VALLEY COMMUNITY COLLEGE, 363
HUMBOLDT STATE UNIVERSITY, 37
HUNTER COLLEGE, CITY UNIVERSITY OF NEW YORK, 363
HUNTINGTON COLLEGE, 157
HURON COLLEGE, 492
HUSTON - TILLOTSON COLLEGE, 523
HUTCHINSON COMMUNITY COLLEGE, 187
IDAHO STATE UNIVERSITY, 120
THE COLLEGE OF IDAHO, 121
UNIVERSITY OF IDAHO, 121
ILLINOIS BENEDICTINE COLLEGE, 132
ILLINOIS CENTRAL COLLEGE, 132
ILLINOIS COLLEGE, 132
ILLINOIS STATE UNIVERSITY, 134
ILLINOIS WESLEYAN UNIVERSITY, 133
UNIVERSITY OF ILLINOIS AT CHICAGO CIRCLE, 133
IMMACULATA COLLEGE, 463
IMMACULATA COLLEGE OF WASHINGTON, 84
IMPERIAL VALLEY COLLEGE, 38
INCARNATE WORD COLLEGE, 524
INDEPENDENCE COMMUNITY JUNIOR COLLEGE, 188
INDIAN RIVER JUNIOR COLLEGE, 94
INDIANA STATE UNIVERSITY, 157
INDIANA UNIVERSITY - PURDUE UNIVERSITY AT FORT WAYNE, 158
INDIANA UNIVERSITY - PURDUE UNIVERSITY, INDIANAPOLIS, 159
INDIANA UNIVERSITY, BLOOMINGTON, 159
INDIANA UNIVERSITY, EAST, 159
INDIANA UNIVERSITY NORTHWEST, 160
INDIANA UNIVERSITY OF PENNSYLVANIA, 463
INDIANA UNIVERSITY AT SOUTH BEND, 160
INDIANA UNIVERSITY, SOUTHEAST, 161
INTERLOCHEN ARTS ACADEMY, 255
INTERNATIONAL COLLEGE, 38
IOWA CENTRAL COMMUNITY COLLEGE, EAGLE GROVE, 170
IOWA CENTRAL COMMUNITY COLLEGE, FT DODGE, 170
IOWA LAKES COMMUNITY COLLEGE, 171
IOWA STATE UNIVERSITY, 171
IOWA WESLEYAN COLLEGE, 172
ITAWAMBA JUNIOR COLLEGE, 283
ITHACA COLLEGE, 364
JACKSON COMMUNITY COLLEGE, 255
JACKSON STATE COLLEGE, 283
JACKSON STATE COMMUNITY COLLEGE, 502
JACKSONVILLE COLLEGE, 524

JACKSONVILLE UNIVERSITY, 94
JAMES MADISON UNIVERSITY, 566
JEFFERSON STATE JUNIOR COLLEGE, 2
JERSEY CITY STATE COLLEGE, 333
JEWISH THEOLOGICAL SEMINARY OF AMERICA, 364
JOHN CARROLL UNIVERSITY, 418
JOHN F KENNEDY COLLEGE, 316
JOHNSON BIBLE COLLEGE, 502
JOHNSON C SMITH UNIVERSITY, 393
JOHNSON STATE COLLEGE, 559
JOLIET JUNIOR COLLEGE, 134
JONES COUNTY JUNIOR COLLEGE, 284
JUDSON BAPTIST COLLEGE, 444
JUDSON COLLEGE, 2
THE JUILLIARD SCHOOL, 365
JUNIATA COLLEGE, 464
KALAMAZOO COLLEGE, 256
KANSAS CITY KANSAS COMMUNITY COLLEGE, 188
KANSAS NEWMAN COLLEGE, 188
KANSAS STATE UNIVERSITY, 189
KANSAS WESLEYAN UNIVERSITY, 190
UNIVERSITY OF KANSAS, 190
KASKASKIA COLLEGE, 135
KEAN COLLEGE OF NEW JERSEY, 334
KEARNEY STATE COLLEGE, 316
KEENE STATE COLLEGE, 326
KELLOGG COMMUNITY COLLEGE, 256
KENNEDY - KING COLLEGE, 135
KENT STATE UNIVERSITY, 418
KENT STATE UNIVERSITY, TUSCARAWAS CAMPUS, 420
KENTUCKY STATE UNIVERSITY, 201
KENTUCKY WESLEYAN COLLEGE, 201
UNIVERSITY OF KENTUCKY, 201
UNIVERSITY OF KENTUCKY, HENDERSON COMMUNITY COL-
  LEGE, 202
KENYON COLLEGE, 420
KEUKA COLLEGE, 365
KILGORE COLLEGE, 524
THE KING'S COLLEGE, 365
KIRKLAND COLLEGE, 366
KIRKWOOD COMMUNITY COLLEGE, 172
KIRTLAND COMMUNITY COLLEGE, 257
KISHWAUKEE COLLEGE, 135
KNOX COLLEGE, 135
KNOXVILLE COLLEGE, 502
KODALY CENTER OF AMERICA, 238
KUTZTOWN STATE COLLEGE, 465
LA GRANGE COLLEGE, 112
LA SALLE COLLEGE, 465
LABETTE COMMUNITY JUNIOR COLLEGE, 191
LAKE CITY COMMUNITY COLLEGE, 94
LAKE ERIE COLLEGE, 420
LAKE FOREST COLLEGE, 136
LAKE LAND COLLEGE, 136
LAKE MICHIGAN COLLEGE, 257
LAKE SUMTER COMMUNITY COLLEGE, 95
LAKELAND COLLEGE, 595
LAKELAND COMMUNITY COLLEGE, 420
LAMAR COMMUNITY COLLEGE, 65
LAMAR UNIVERSITY, 524
LANDER COLLEGE, 487
LANE COLLEGE, 503
LANEY COLLEGE, 38
LANGSTON UNIVERSITY, 434
LANSING COMMUNITY COLLEGE, 257
LAREDO JUNIOR COLLEGE, 525

LAWRENCE UNIVERSITY, 596
LEBANON VALLEY COLLEGE, 465
LEE COLLEGE, 503
LEE COLLEGE, 525
LEES McRAE COLLEGE, 393
LEHIGH UNIVERSITY, 466
LEMOYNE - OWEN COLLEGE, 503
LENOIR - RHYNE COLLEGE, 394
LESLEY COLLEGE, 239
LEWIS & CLARK COMMUNITY COLLEGE, 137
LEWIS AND CLARK COLLEGE, 444
LEWIS UNIVERSITY, 137
LIMESTONE COLLEGE, 487
LINCOLN COLLEGE, 137
LINCOLN LAND COMMUNITY COLLEGE, 138
LINCOLN MEMORIAL UNIVERSITY, 504
LINCOLN TRAIL COLLEGE, 138
LINCOLN UNIVERSITY, 294
LINCOLN UNIVERSITY, 466
LINDENWOOD COLLEGE, 295
LIVINGSTONE COLLEGE, 394
LOCK HAVEN STATE COLLEGE, 466
LOMA LINDA UNIVERSITY, 39
LON MORRIS COLLEGE, 526
LONE MOUNTAIN COLLEGE, SAN FRANCISCO, 39
LONGVIEW COMMUNITY COLLEGE, 295
LONGWOOD COLLEGE, 567
LONGY SCHOOL OF MUSIC, 239
LOOP COLLEGE, 138
LORAS COLLEGE, 172
LORETTO HEIGHTS COLLEGE, 65
LOS ANGELES BAPTIST COLLEGE, 40
LOS ANGELES HARBOR COLLEGE, 40
LOS ANGELES SOUTHWEST COLLEGE, 40
LOS ANGELES VALLEY COLLEGE, 41
LOUISANA STATE UNIVERSITY, 207
LOUISIANA COLLEGE, 207
LOUISIANA POLYTECHNIC INSTITUTE, 208
LOUISIANA TECHNICAL UNIVERSITY, 208
UNIVERSITY OF LOUISVILLE, 202
UNIVERSITY OF LOWELL, 239
LOWER COLUMBIA COLLEGE, 580
LOYOLA UNIVERSITY, 208
LUBBOCK CHRISTIAN COLLEGE, 526
LUREEN B WALLACE STATE JUNIOR COLLEGE, 2
LUTHER COLLEGE, 173
LYCOMING COLLEGE, 467
LYNCHBURG COLLEGE, 568
LYNDON STATE COLLEGE, 560
MACALESTER COLLEGE, 275
MACMURRAY COLLEGE, 139
MACOMB COUNTY COMMUNITY COLLEGE - CENTER CAMPUS, 258
MACOMB COUNTY COMMUNITY COLLEGE - SOUTH CAMPUS, 258
MACON JUNIOR COLLEGE, 112
MADISON AREA TECHNICAL COLLEGE, 596
MADONNA COLLEGE, 259
UNIVERSITY OF MAINE AT PORTLAND - GORHAM, 217
UNIVERSITY OF MAINE, ORONO, 217
MALONE COLLEGE, 421
MANATEE JUNIOR COLLEGE, 95
MANCHESTER COLLEGE, 161
MANHATTAN SCHOOL OF MUSIC, 366
MANHATTANVILLE COLLEGE, 366
MANKATO STATE UNIVERSITY, 275

MANNES COLLEGE OF MUSIC, 367
MANOR JUNIOR COLLEGE, 467
MANSFIELD STATE COLLEGE, 467
MAPLE WOODS COMMUNITY COLLEGE, 295
MARIA REGINA COLLEGE, 367
MARIAN COLLEGE OF FOND DU LAC, 596
MARIAN COLLEGE, INDIANAPOLIS, 162
MARIETTA COLLEGE, 421
MARION COLLEGE, 162
MARJORIE WEBSTER JUNIOR COLLEGE, 84
MARLBORO COLLEGE, 560
MARS HILL COLLEGE, 394
MARSHALL UNIVERSITY, 588
MARTIN COLLEGE, 504
MARY BALDWIN COLLEGE, 568
MARY HARDIN - BAYLOR COLLEGE, 526
MARY HOLMES JUNIOR COLLEGE, 284
MARY MANSE COLLEGE, 421
MARY WASHINGTON COLLEGE, 569
MARYCREST COLLEGE, 174
UNIVERSITY OF MARYLAND, 221
UNIVERSITY OF MARYLAND, EASTERN SHORE, 222
MARYLHURST EDUCATION CENTER, 445
MARYMONT MANHATTAN COLLEGE, 368
MARYMOUNT COLLEGE, 191
MARYMOUNT COLLEGE, 368
MARYVILLE COLLEGE, 504
MARYWOOD COLLEGE, 468
UNIVERSITY OF MASSACHUSETTS, 239
UNIVERSITY OF MASSACHUSETTS, BOSTON, 240
MATTATUK COMMUNITY COLLEGE, 74
MAYLAND TECHNICAL INSTITUTE, 395
MAYVILLE STATE COLLEGE, 406
McCOOK COLLEGE, 316
McKENDREE COLLEGE, 139
McLENNAN COMMUNITY COLLEGE, 527
McMURRY COLLEGE, 527
McNEESE STATE UNIVERSITY, 209
McPHERSON COLLEGE, 191
MEMPHIS STATE UNIVERSITY, 504
MERCER UNIVERSITY, ATLANTA, 112
MERCY COLLEGE, 368
MERCY COLLEGE OF DETROIT, 259
MERCYHURST COLLEGE, 468
MEREDITH COLLEGE, 395
MERIDIAN JUNIOR COLLEGE, 284
MESA COLLEGE, 65
MESA COMMUNITY COLLEGE, 10
MESABI COMMUNITY COLLEGE, 275
MESSIAH COLLEGE, 469
METHODIST COLLEGE, 395
METROPOLITAN COMMUNITY COLLEGE, 276
METROPOLITAN STATE COLLEGE, 66
MIAMI - DADE COMMUNITY COLLEGE - NEW WORLD CENTER, 96
MIAMI - DADE COMMUNITY COLLEGE - NORTH CAMPUS, 96
MIAMI - DADE COMMUNITY COLLEGE, SOUTH CAMPUS, 96
MIAMI UNIVERSITY, 422
UNIVERSITY OF MIAMI, 96
MICHIGAN CHRISTIAN JUNIOR COLLEGE, 259
MICHIGAN STATE UNIVERSITY, 260
THE UNIVERSITY OF MICHIGAN, 261
UNIVERSITY OF MICHIGAN, FLINT, 261
MIDDLE GEORGIA COLLEGE, 113
MIDDLE TENNESSEE STATE UNIVERSITY, 505
MIDDLEBURY COLLEGE, 561

MIDLAND COLLEGE, 528
MIDLAND LUTHERAN COLLEGE, 317
MIDWESTERN STATE UNIVERSITY, 528
MILES COMMUNITY COLLEGE, 310
MILLERSVILLE STATE COLLEGE, 469
MILLIGAN COLLEGE, 505
MILLIKIN UNIVERSITY, 140
MILLSAPS COLLEGE, 284
MILTON COLLEGE, 597
MINERAL AREA JUNIOR COLLEGE, 296
UNIVERSITY OF MINNESOTA, MORRIS, 276
UNIVERSITY OF MINNESOTA, DULUTH - SCHOOL OF FINE ARTS, 277
MINOT STATE COLLEGE, 406
MIRA COSTA COMMUNITY COLLEGE, 41
MISSISSIPPI COLLEGE, 284
MISSISSIPPI GULF COAST JUNIOR COLLEGE, PERKINSTON CAMPUS, 285
MISSISSIPPI INDUSTRIAL COLLEGE, 285
MISSISSIPPI STATE UNIVERSITY, 285
MISSISSIPPI UNIVERSITY FOR WOMEN, 286
MISSISSIPPI VALLEY STATE COLLEGE, 286
UNIVERSITY OF MISSISSIPPI, 286
MISSOURI SOUTHERN STATE COLLEGE, 296
MISSOURI VALLEY COLLEGE, 296
MISSOURI WESTERN STATE COLLEGE, 297
UNIVERSITY OF MISSOURI, 297
UNIVERSITY OF MISSOURI - KANSAS CITY CONSERVATORY OF MUSIC, 298
UNIVERSITY OF MISSOURI, SAINT LOUIS, 298
MITCHELL COMMUNITY COLLEGE, 396
MODERN SCHOOL OF MUSIC, 84
MODESTO JUNIOR COLLEGE, 42
MOHAWK VALLEY COMMUNITY COLLEGE, 368
MONMOUTH COLLEGE, 140
MONROE COUNTY COMMUNITY COLLEGE, 261
MONTANA STATE UNIVERSITY, 310
UNIVERSITY OF MONTANA, SCHOOL OF FINE ARTS, 311
MONTCLAIR STATE COLLEGE, 335
MONTGOMERY COLLEGE, 222
MONTREAT ANDERSON COLLEGE, 396
MOODY BIBLE INSTITUTE, 141
MOORHEAD STATE UNIVERSITY, 343
MORAVIAN COLLEGE, 469
MOREHEAD STATE UNIVERSITY, 202
MOREHOUSE COLLEGE, 113
MORGAN STATE COLLEGE, 223
MORNINGSIDE COLLEGE, 174
MORRIS BROWN COLLEGE, 113
MORRIS HARVEY COLLEGE, 589
MORTON COLLEGE, 141
MOTLOW STATE COMMUNITY COLLEGE, 506
MOUNT ALOYSIUS JUNIOR COLLEGE, 470
MOUNT HOLYOKE COLLEGE, 241
MOUNT HOOD COMMUNITY COLLEGE, 434
MOUNT HOOD COMMUNITY COLLEGE, 445
MOUNT KISCO SCHOOL OF MUSIC, 369
MOUNT MARTY COLLEGE, 493
MOUNT MARY COLLEGE, 597
MOUNT OLIVE COLLEGE, 396
MOUNT SAINT CLARE COLLEGE, 174
MOUNT SAINT JOSEPH ON THE OHIO COLLEGE, 422
MOUNT SAINT MARY'S COLLEGE, 42
MOUNT SAN ANTONIO COLLEGE, 43
MOUNT SAN JACINTO COLLEGE, 43
MOUNT SCENARIO COLLEGE, 598

MOUNT UNION COLLEGE, 422
MOUNT VERNON COLLEGE, 84
MOUNT VERNON NAZERENE COLLEGE, 423
MOUNTAIN VIEW COLLEGE, 528
MUHLENBERG COLLEGE, 470
MUNDELEIN COLLEGE, 141
MURRAY STATE COLLEGE, 435
MURRAY STATE UNIVERSITY, 203
MUSIC & ARTS INSTITUTE OF SAN FRANCISCO, 44
THE MUSIC SCHOOL OF NORTH SHORE COMMUNITY COLLEGE, 241
MUSKEGON COMMUNITY COLLEGE, 262
MUSKINGUM COLLEGE, 423
NAPA COLLEGE, 44
NATIONAL COLLEGE OF EDUCATION, 142
NATIONAL MUSIC CAMP, 262
NAVARRO COLLEGE, 529
NAZARETH COLLEGE OF ROCHESTER, 369
NEBRASKA CHRISTIAN COLLEGE, 317
NEBRASKA WESLEYAN UNIVERSITY, 317
NEBRASKA WESTERN COLLEGE, 318
UNIVERSITY OF NEBRASKA, LINCOLN, 318
THE UNIVERSITY OF NEBRASKA, OMAHA, 319
UNIVERSITY OF NEVADA, LAS VEGAS, 323
UNIVERSITY OF NEVADA, RENO, 323
NEW COLLEGE OF THE UNIVERSITY OF SOUTH FLORIDA, 97
NEW ENGLAND COLLEGE, 326
NEW ENGLAND CONSERVATORY OF MUSIC, 241
UNIVERSITY OF NEW HAMPSHIRE, 327
UNIVERSITY OF NEW HAVEN, 75
NEW MEXICO HIGHLANDS UNIVERSITY, 343
NEW MEXICO JUNIOR COLLEGE, 344
NEW MEXICO MILITARY INSTITUTE, 344
NEW MEXICO STATE UNIVERSITY, 344
UNIVERSITY OF NEW MEXICO, 345
NEW ORLEANS BAPTIST THEOLOGICAL SEMINARY, 210
UNIVERSITY OF NEW ORLEANS, 210
THE NEW SCHOOL FOR MUSIC STUDY, 335
NEW SCHOOL OF MUSIC, 470
NEW YORK UNIVERSITY, 369
NEWBERRY COLLEGE, 488
NICHOLLS STATE UNIVERSITY, 210
NORFOLK STATE COLLEGE, 569
NORMANDALE COMMUNITY COLLEGE, 277
NORTH CAROLINA AGRICULTURE AND TECHNICAL STATE UNIVERSITY, 396
NORTH CAROLINA CENTRAL UNIVERSITY, 397
NORTH CAROLINA SCHOOL OF THE ARTS, 397
NORTH CAROLINA WESLEYAN COLLEGE, 398
UNIVERSITY OF NORTH CAROLINA, ASHEVILLE, 398
UNIVERSITY OF NORTH CAROLINA, CHARLOTTE, 399
UNIVERSITY OF NORTH CAROLINA, GREENSBORO, 399
UNIVERSITY OF NORTH CAROLINA, WILMINGTON, 400
NORTH CENTRAL BIBLE COLLEGE, 277
NORTH CENTRAL COLLEGE, 142
NORTH DAKOTA STATE UNIVERSITY, 406
NORTH DAKOTA STATE UNIVERSITY OF AGRICULTURE & APPLIED SCIENCE, 407
NORTH FLORIDA JUNIOR COLLEGE, 97
UNIVERSITY OF NORTH FLORIDA, 98
NORTH GEORGIA COLLEGE, 114
NORTH IDAHO COLLEGE, 122
NORTH IOWA AREA COMMUNITY COLLEGE, 175
NORTH PARK COLLEGE, 142
NORTH PLATTE COLLEGE, 319
NORTH TEXAS STATE UNIVERSITY, 529

NORTHAMPTON COUNTY AREA COMMUNITY COLLEGE, 471
NORTHEAST LOUISIANA UNIVERSITY, 211
NORTHEAST MISSISSIPPI JUNIOR COLLEGE, 287
NORTHEAST MISSOURI STATE UNIVERSITY, 299
NORTHEAST OKLAHOMA STATE UNIVERSITY, 435
NORTHEASTERN COLLEGIATE BIBLE INSTITUTE, 335
NORTHEASTERN ILLINOIS UNIVERSITY, 143
NORTHEASTERN JUNIOR COLLEGE, 67
NORTHEASTERN NEBRASKA COLLEGE, 319
NORTHEASTERN OKLAHOMA A & M COLLEGE, 435
NORTHEASTERN STATE COLLEGE, 435
NORTHEASTERN UNIVERSITY, 242
NORTHERN ARIZONA UNIVERSITY COLLEGE OF CREATIVE ARTS, 10
UNIVERSITY OF NORTHERN COLORADO, 67
NORTHERN ILLINOIS UNIVERSITY, 143
UNIVERSITY OF NORTHERN IOWA, 175
NORTHERN MICHIGAN UNIVERSITY, 263
NORTHERN MONTANA COLLEGE, 311
NORTHERN OKLAHOMA COLLEGE, 436
NORTHERN STATE COLLEGE, 493
NORTHLAND COLLEGE, 598
NORTHWEST CHRISTIAN COLLEGE, 446
NORTHWEST COLLEGE, 580
NORTHWEST COMMUNITY COLLEGE, 611
NORTHWEST MISSISSIPPI JUNIOR COLLEGE, 287
NORTHWEST MISSOURI STATE UNIVERSITY, 299
NORTHWEST NAZARENE COLLEGE, 122
NORTHWESTERN COLLEGE, 175
NORTHWESTERN MICHIGAN COLLEGE, 263
NORTHWESTERN OKLAHOMA STATE UNIVERSITY, 436
NORTHWESTERN STATE UNIVERSITY OF LOUISIANA, 211
NORTHWESTERN UNIVERSITY, 144
NORWICH UNIVERSITY, 561
NOTRE DAME COLLEGE, 327
NOTRE DAME COLLEGE OF OHIO, 423
COLLEGE OF NOTRE DAME OF MARYLAND, 223
NYACK COLLEGE, 370
OAKLAND CITY COLLEGE, 162
OAKLAND COMMUNITY COLLEGE, 264
OAKLAND UNIVERSITY, 264
OAKWOOD COLLEGE, 3
OBERLIN COLLEGE, 423
OCEAN COUNTY COLLEGE, 336
ODESSA COLLEGE, 530
OHIO NORTHERN UNIVERSITY, 424
OHIO UNIVERSITY, 425
OHIO WESLEYAN UNIVERSITY, 425
OHLONE COLLEGE, 44
OKALOOSA - WALTON JUNIOR COLLEGE, 98
OKLAHOMA BAPTIST UNIVERSITY, 437
OKLAHOMA CITY SOUTHWESTERN COLLEGE, 437
OKLAHOMA CITY UNIVERSITYSCHOOL OF MUSIC AND PERFORMING ARTS, 437
OKLAHOMA STATE UNIVERSITY, 438
UNIVERSITY OF OKLAHOMA, 438
UNIVERSITY OF SCIENCE AND ARTS OF OKLAHOMA, 439
OLD DOMINION UNIVERSITY, 569
OLIVET COLLEGE, 264
OLIVET NAZARENE COLLEGE, 144
ONONDAGA COMMUNITY COLLEGE, 370
ORAL ROBERTS UNIVERSITY, 439
ORANGE COAST COLLEGE, 45
OREGON COLLEGE OF EDUCATION, 446
OREGON STATE UNIVERSITY, 447
UNIVERSITY OF OREGON, 447

OSCAR ROSE JUNIOR COLLEGE, 440
OTERO JUNIOR COLLEGE, 67
OTTAWA UNIVERSITY, 192
OTTERBEIN COLLEGE, 426
OTTUMWA HEIGHTS COLLEGE, 176
OUR LADY OF THE LAKE COLLEGE, 530
PACIFIC LUTHERAN UNIVERSITY, 580
PACIFIC UNION COLLEGE, 45
PACIFIC UNIVERSITY, 448
UNIVERSITY OF THE PACIFIC, 46
PALM BEACH JUNIOR COLLEGE, 99
PALOMAR COLLEGE, 46
PAN AMERICAN UNIVERSITY, 530
PANHANDLE STATE UNIVERSITY, 440
PANOLA JUNIOR COLLEGE, 531
PARIS JUNIOR COLLEGE, 531
PARK COLLEGE, 300
PASADENA CITY COLLEGE, 47
PAUL QUINN COLLEGE, 531
PEABODY INSTITUTE OF THE JOHNS HOPKINS UNIVERSITY, 224
PEACE COLLEGE, 400
PEARL RIVER JUNIOR COLLEGE, 287
PEMBROKE STATE UNIVERSITY, 401
PENN HALL JUNIOR COLLEGE AND PREPARATORY SCHOOL, 471
PENN VALLEY COMMUNITY COLLEGE, 300
PENNSYLVANIA STATE UNIVERSITY, 471
PENSACOLA JUNIOR COLLEGE, 99
PEPPERDINE UNIVERSITY, SEAVER COLLEGE, 47
PERU STATE COLLEGE, 320
PFEIFFER COLLEGE, 401
PHILADELPHIA COLLEGE OF BIBLE, 472
PHILADELPHIA COLLEGE OF THE PERFORMING ARTS, 472
PHILLIPS COUNTY COMMUNITY COLLEGE, 15
PHILLIPS UNIVERSITY, 440
PIEDMONT COLLEGE, 114
PIKEVILLE COLLEGE, 203
PINE MANOR COLLEGE, 242
PITTSBURGH STATE UNIVERSITY, 192
UNIVERSITY OF PITTSBURGH, 472
PITTSFIELD COMMUNITY MUSIC SCHOOL, 242
PLATTE TECHNICAL COMMUNITY COLLEGE, 320
PLATTE VALLEY BIBLE COLLEGE, 320
PLYMOUTH STATE COLLEGE, 328
POINT LOMA COLLEGE, 48
PORTLAND STATE UNIVERSITY, 448
UNIVERSITY OF PORTLAND, 449
C W POST CENTER OF LONG ISLAND UNIVERSITY, 371
POTOMAC STATE COLLEGE, 589
PRATT COMMUNITY COLLEGE, 193
PRESBYTERIAN COLLEGE, 488
PRINCE GEORGES COMMUNITY COLLEGE, 224
PRINCETON UNIVERSITY, 337
PRINCIPIA COLLEGE, 145
UNIVERSITY OF PUGET SOUND, 581
PURDUE UNIVERSITY, 162
QUEENS COLLEGE, 402
QUEENSBOROUGH COMMUNITY COLLEGE, CITY UNIVERSITY OF NEW YORK, 372
QUINCY COLLEGE, 145
QUINNIPIAC COLLEGE, 75
RADCLIFFE COLLEGE, 243
RADFORD COLLEGE, 570
RAINY RIVER COMMUNITY COLLEGE, 278
RAMAPO COLLEGE, 337

SOUTHEASTERN BAPTIST COLLEGE, 288
SOUTHEASTERN BIBLE COLLEGE, 4
SOUTHEASTERN LOUISIANA UNIVERSITY, 212
SOUTHEASTERN MASSACHUSETTS UNIVERSITY, 245
SOUTHEASTERN OKLAHOMA STATE UNIVERSITY, 441
SOUTHERN ARKANSAS UNIVERSITY, 16
SOUTHERN BAPTIST THEOLOGICAL SEMINARY SCHOOL OF CHURCH MUSIC, 204
SOUTHERN BENEDICTINE COLLEGE, 4
UNIVERSITY OF SOUTHERN CALIFORNIA, 54
UNIVERSITY OF SOUTHERN COLORADO, 68
SOUTHERN CONNECTICUT STATE COLLEGE, 75
COLLEGE OF SOUTHERN IDAHO, 123
SOUTHERN ILLINOIS UNIVERSITY, 148
SOUTHERN ILLINOIS UNIVERSITY AT EDWARDSVILLE, 149
SOUTHERN METHODIST UNIVERSITY, 538
SOUTHERN MISSIONARY COLLEGE, 506
SOUTHERN OREGON COLLEGE, 450
SOUTHERN SEMINARY JUNIOR COLLEGE, 571
SOUTHERN STATE COLLEGE, 495
SOUTHERN UNIVERSITY, BATON ROUGE, 213
SOUTHERN UTAH STATE COLLEGE, 555
SOUTHWEST BAPTIST COLLEGE, 302
SOUTHWEST MISSISSIPPI JUNIOR COLLEGE, 288
SOUTHWEST MISSOURI STATE UNIVERSITY, 302
SOUTHWEST TEXAS JUNIOR COLLEGE, 538
SOUTHWEST TEXAS STATE UNIVERSITY, 538
SOUTHWESTERN ADVENTIST COLLEGE, 538
SOUTHWESTERN ASSEMBLY OF GOD COLLEGE, 538
SOUTHWESTERN BAPTIST THEOLOGICAL SEMINARY, 538
SOUTHWESTERN COLLEGE, 194
SOUTHWESTERN COLLEGE, 54
UNIVERSITY OF SOUTHWESTERN LOUISANA, 213
SOUTHWESTERN AT MEMPHIS, 507
SOUTHWESTERN OKLAHOMA STATE UNIVERSITY, 441
SOUTHWESTERN STATE COLLEGE, 450
SOUTHWESTERN UNIVERSITY AT GEORGETOWN, 539
THE UNIVERSITY OF THE SOUTH, 507
SPELMAN COLLEGE, 115
SPRING ARBOR COLLEGE, 266
SPRING HILL COLLEGE, 5
SPRINGFIELD COLLEGE, 245
SPRINGFIELD COLLEGE, ILLINOIS, 149
STANFORD UNIVERSITY, 55
STATE UNIVERSITY OF NEW YORK, ALBANY, 376
STATE UNIVERSITY OF NEW YORK, BINGHAMTON, 376
STATE UNIVERSITY OF NEW YORK, BUFFALO, 377
STATE UNIVERSITY OF NEW YORK COLLEGE, BROCKPORT, 377
STATE UNIVERSITY OF NEW YORK COLLEGE, CORTLAND, 378
STATE UNIVERSITY OF NEW YORK COLLEGE, FREDONIA, 378
STATE UNIVERSITY OF NEW YORK COLLEGE AT GENESEO, 378
STATE UNIVERSITY OF NEW YORK COLLEGE, NEW PALTZ, 379
STATE UNIVERSITY OF NEW YORK COLLEGE, ONEONTA, 379
STATE UNIVERSITY OF NEW YORK COLLEGE, OSWEGO, 380
STATE UNIVERSITY OF NEW YORK COLLEGE, PLATTSBURGH, 380
STATE UNIVERSITY OF NEW YORK COLLEGE, POTSDAM, 380
STATE UNIVERSITY OF NEW YORK COLLEGE, PURCHASE PROFESSIONAL SCHOOL OF ARTS, 381
STATE UNIVERSITY OF NEW YORK, OSWEGO, 381
STATE UNIVERSITY OF NEW YORK, STONY BROOK, 382
STATEN COLLEGE COMMUNITY COLLEGE, CITY UNIVERSITY OF NEW YORK, 382
STEPHEN F AUSTIN STATE UNIVERSITY, 539
STEPHENS COLLEGE, 304
STERLING COLLEGE, 195

STETSON UNIVERSITY, 102
STILLMAN COLLEGE, 5
STOCKTON STATE COLLEGE, 339
STUART OSTROW FOUNDATION, INC, 383
SUFFOLK COMMUNITY COLLEGE, 384
SUFFOLK COUNTY COMMUNITY COLLEGE, 384
SUL ROSS STATE UNIVERSITY, 540
SULLINS COLLEGE, 571
SUSQUEHANNA UNIVERSITY, 474
SWARTHMORE COLLEGE, 475
SWEET BRIAR COLLEGE, 572
SYMPHONY SCHOOL OF AMERICA, 600
SYRACUSE UNIVERSITY, 384
TABOR COLLEGE, 195
TALLADEGA COLLEGE, 5
UNIVERSITY OF TAMPA, 103
TARKIO COLLEGE, 304
TARLETON STATE UNIVERSITY, 540
TARRANT COUNTY JUNIOR COLLEGE, NORTHEAST CAMPUS, 541
TARRANT COUNTY JUNIOR COLLEGE, SOUTH CAMPUS, 541
TAYLOR UNIVERSITY, 164
TEMPLE JUNIOR COLLEGE, 541
TEMPLE UNIVERSITY, 475
TENNESSEE STATE UNIVERSITY, 508
TENNESSEE TECHNOLOGICAL UNIVERSITY, 508
TENNESSEE TEMPLE COLLEGE, 508
TENNESSEE WESLEYAN COLLEGE, 508
UNIVERSITY OF TENNESSEE AT CHATTANOOGA, 509
UNIVERSITY OF TENNESSEE, KNOXVILLE, 509
UNIVERSITY OF TENNESSEE, MARTIN, 510
TEXARKANA COLLEGE, 542
TEXAS AGRICULTURAL & INDUSTRIAL UNIVERSITY, KINGSVILLE, 542
TEXAS CHRISTIAN UNIVERSITY, 542
TEXAS COLLEGE, 543
TEXAS LUTHERAN COLLEGE, 543
TEXAS SOUTHERN UNIVERSITY, 544
TEXAS SOUTHMOST COLLEGE, 544
TEXAS TECH UNIVERSITY, 545
TEXAS WESLEYAN COLLEGE, 545
TEXAS WOMEN'S UNIVERSITY, 546
UNIVERSITY OF TEXAS - AUSTIN, 546
THIEL COLLEGE, 476
THORNTON COMMUNITY COLLEGE, 149
THREE RIVERS COMMUNITY COLLEGE, 305
TIDEWATER COMMUNITY COLLEGE, FREDERICK CAMPUS, 572
TIFT COLLEGE, 116
UNIVERSITY OF TOLEDO, 427
TOUGALOO COLLEGE, 288
TOWSON STATE UNIVERSITY, 225
TRANSYLVANIA UNIVERSITY, 204
TREASURE VALLEY COMMUNITY COLLEGE, 450
TRENTON STATE COLLEGE, 339
TREVECCA NAZARENE COLLEGE, 510
TRINIDAD STATE COLLEGE, 68
TRINITY CHRISTIAN COLLEGE, 150
TRINITY COLLEGE, 75
TRINITY COLLEGE, 85
TRINITY UNIVERSITY, 547
TRITON COLLEGE, 150
TROY STATE UNIVERSITY, 6
TULANE UNIVERSITY, 214
TUSCULUM COLLEGE, 510
TUSKEGEE INSTITUTE, 6
TYLER JUNIOR COLLEGE, 548

U S COAST GUARD ACADEMY, 76
UNION COLLEGE, 204
UNION COLLEGE, 321
UNION COLLEGE, 385
UNION UNIVERSITY, 511
UNITED STATES INTERNATIONAL UNIVERSITY, 56
UNITED WESLEYAN COLLEGE, 476
UNIVERSITY OF ALBUQUERQUE, 345
UNIVERSITY OF CALIFORNIA, RIVERSIDE, 56
UNIVERSITY OF DETROIT, MARYGROVE COLLEGE, 266
UNIVERSITY OF DUBUQUE, 177
UNIVERSITY OF EVANSVILLE, 165
UNIVERSITY OF ILLINOIS, 151
THE UNIVERSITY OF IOWA, 177
UNIVERSITY OF MINNESOTA, 279
UNIVERSITY OF MONTEVALLO, 6
UNIVERSITY OF NORTH CAROLINA, 403
UNIVERSITY OF NOTRE DAME, 165
UNIVERSITY OF PENNSYLVANIA, 476
UNIVERSITY OF REDLANDS, 57
UNIVERSITY OF RICHMOND, 572
UNIVERSITY OF SOUTHERN CALIFORNIA, 57
UNIVERSITY OF SOUTHERN MISSISSIPPI, 288
UNIVERSITY OF TEXAS, ARLINGTON, 548
UNIVERSITY OF TEXAS, AUSTIN, 549
UNIVERSITY OF TEXAS, EL PASO, 549
UNIVERSITY OF TULSA, 441
UNIVERSITY OF VERMONT, 562
UPPER IOWA UNIVERSITY, 178
UPSALA COLLEGE, 340
URSULINE COLLEGE, 428
UTAH STATE UNIVERSITY, 555
UNIVERSITY OF UTAH, 555
VALDOSTA STATE COLLEGE, 116
VALLEY CITY STATE COLLEGE, 407
VALPARAISO UNIVERSITY, 165
VASSAR COLLEGE, 385
VICTOR VALLEY COLLEGE, 57
THE VICTORIA COLLEGE, 550
VILLA JULIE COLLEGE, 226
VILLA MARIA COLLEGE OF BUFFALO, 385
VINCENNES UNIVERSITY, 166
VIRGINIA COMMONWEALTH UNIVERSITY, 573
VIRGINIA INTERMONT COLLEGE, 574
VIRGINIA POLYTECHNIC INSTITUTE AND STATE UNIVERSITY, 574
VIRGINIA STATE COLLEGE, 575
VIRGINIA UNION UNIVERSITY, 575
VIRGINIA WESLEYAN COLLEGE, 575
UNIVERSITY OF VIRGINIA, 575
VITERBO COLLEGE, 600
WABASH COLLEGE, 166
WAGNER COLLEGE, 386
WAKE FOREST UNIVERSITY, 404
WALDORF COLLEGE, 178
WALLA WALLA COLLEGE, 582
WALNUT HILL SCHOOL OF PERFORMING ARTS, 246
WARNER PACIFIC COLLEGE, 450
WARREN WILSON COLLEGE, 404
WARTBURG COLLEGE, 179
WASHBURN UNIVERSITY OF TOPEKA, 196
WASHINGTON AND JEFFERSON COLLEGE, 477
WASHINGTON AND LEE UNIVERSITY, 575
WASHINGTON COLLEGE, 226
WASHINGTON STATE UNIVERSITY, 583
WASHINGTON UNIVERSITY, 305

UNIVERSITY OF WASHINGTON, 583
WAUBONSEE COMMUNITY COLLEGE, 151
WAYLAND BAPTIST COLLEGE, 550
WAYNE STATE COLLEGE, 321
WAYNE STATE UNIVERSITY, 267
WEATHERFORD COLLEGE, 550
WEBER STATE COLLEGE, 556
WEBSTER COLLEGE, 306
WELLESLEY COLLEGE, 246
WELLS COLLEGE, 386
WESLEY COLLEGE, 80
WESLEYAN COLLEGE, 117
WESLEYAN UNIVERSITY, 76
WEST CHESTER STATE COLLEGE, 477
UNIVERSITY OF WEST FLORIDA, 103
WEST GEORGIA COLLEGE, 117
WEST HILLS COLLEGE, 58
WEST LIBERTY STATE COLLEGE, 590
WEST TEXAS STATE UNIVERSITY, 551
WEST VALLEY COLLEGE, 58
WEST VIRGINIA INSTITUTE OF TECHNOLOGY, 590
WEST VIRGINIA STATE COLLEGE, 591
WEST VIRGINIA UNIVERSITY - CREATIVE ARTS CENTER, 591
WEST VIRGINIA WESLEYAN COLLEGE, 591
WESTERN BAPTIST BIBLE COLLEGE, 451
WESTERN CAROLINA UNIVERSITY, 405
WESTERN COLLEGE OF MIAMI UNIVERSITY, 428
WESTERN CONNECTICUT STATE COLLEGE, 77
WESTERN ILLINOIS UNIVERSITY, 151
WESTERN KENTUCKY UNIVERSITY, 205
WESTERN MARYLAND COLLEGE, 227
WESTERN MICHIGAN UNIVERSITY, 267
WESTERN MONTANA COLLEGE, 312
WESTERN NEW MEXICO UNIVERSITY, 307
WESTERN STATE COLLEGE, 68
WESTERN WASHINGTON STATE COLLEGE, 584
WESTERN WYOMING COMMUNITY COLLEGE, 611
WESTFIELD STATE COLLEGE, 247
WESTMAR COLLEGE, 179
WESTMINISTER CHOIR COLLEGE, 340
WESTMINISTER COLLEGE, 307
WESTMINISTER COLLEGE, 556
WESTMINSTER COLLEGE, 478
WESTMONT COLLEGE, 58
WHARTON COUNTY JUNIOR COLLEGE, 551
WHEATON COLLEGE, 152
WHEATON COLLEGE, 247
WHITMAN COLLEGE, 584
WHITWORTH COLLEGE, 289
WHITWORTH COLLEGE, 585
WICHITA STATE UNIVERSITY, 196
WILBUR WRIGHT COLLEGE, CITY COLLEGE OF CHICAGO, 152
WILEY COLLEGE, 551
WILKES COLLEGE, 478
WILLAMETTE UNIVERSITY, 451
WILLIAM CAREY COLLEGE, 289
WILLIAM JEWELL COLLEGE, 307
WILLIAM PATERSON COLLEGE, 341
WILLIAM RAINEY HARPER COLLEGE, 152
WILLIAM WOODS - WESTMINISTER COLLEGE, 308
WILLIAMS COLLEGE, 247
WILLMAR COMMUNITY COLLEGE, 280
WILMINGTON COLLEGE, 428
WILMINGTON MUSIC SCHOOL, 80
WILSON COLLEGE, 478
WINONA STATE UNIVERSITY, 280

WINSTON - SALEM STATE UNIVERSITY, 405
WINTHROP COLLEGE, 489
UNIVERSITY OF WISCONSIN CENTER, MANITOWOC COUNTY, 600
WISCONSIN COLLEGE CONSERVATORY, 601
UNIVERSITY OF WISCONSIN, RIVER FALLS, 601
UNIVERSITY OF WISCONSIN, EAU CLAIRE, 602
UNIVERSITY OF WISCONSIN, GREEN BAY, 602
UNIVERSITY OF WISCONSIN, LA CROSSE, 603
UNIVERSITY OF WISCONSIN, MADISON, 603
UNIVERSITY OF WISCONSIN, MARSHFIELD/WOOD CO CENTER, 604
THE UNIVERSITY OF WISCONSIN, MILWAUKEE SCHOOL OF FINE ARTS, 604
UNIVERSITY OF WISCONSIN, OSHKOSH, 605
UNIVERSITY OF WISCONSIN, PARKSIDE, 606
THE UNIVERSITY OF WISCONSIN, PLATTEVILLE, 606
UNIVERSITY OF WISCONSIN, SHEBOYGAN, 606
UNIVERSITY OF WISCONSIN, STEVENS POINT, 607
UNIVERSITY OF WISCONSIN, SUPERIOR, 608
UNIVERSITY OF WISCONSIN, WHITEWATER, 608
WITTENBERG UNIVERSITY, 429
WOOD JUNIOR COLLEGE, 289
THE COLLEGE OF WOOSTER, 429
WRIGHT STATE UNIVERSITY, 430
UNIVERSITY OF WYOMING, 611
XAVIER UNIVERSITY OF LOUISANA, 214
YALE UNIVERSITY, 77
YANKTON COLLEGE, 496
YESHIVA UNIVERSITY, 386
YORK COLLEGE, 322
YORK COLLEGE OF PENNSYLVANIA, 479
YOUNG HARRIS COLLEGE, 117
YOUNGSTOWN STATE UNIVERSITY, 430

Theatre

ABILENE CHRISTIAN UNIVERSITY, 512
ABRAHAM BALDWIN AGRICULTURAL COLLEGE, 105
ACADEMY THEATRE SCHOOL OF PERFORMING ARTS, 105
ADAMS STATE COLLEGE, 60
ADELPHI UNIVERSITY, 346
ADIRONDACK COMMUNITY COLLEGE, 346
ADRIAN COLLEGE, 249
AGNES SCOTT COLLEGE, 105
UNIVERSITY OF AKRON COLLEGE OF FINE AND APPLIED ARTS, 408
UNIVERSITY OF ALABAMA, BIRMINGHAM, 1
UNIVERSITY OF ALASKA COLLEGE OF ARTS & LETTERS, 7
UNIVERSITY OF ALASKA, ANCHORAGE, 7
ALBANO BALLET AND PERFORMING ARTS ACADEMY, INC, 70
ALBANY STATE COLLEGE, 106
ALBERTUS MAGNUS COLLEGE, 70
ALBION COLLEGE, 249
ALBRIGHT COLLEGE, 452
ALDERSON - BROADDUS COLLEGE, 586
ALFRED UNIVERSITY, 347
ALICE LLOYD COLLEGE, 197
ALLAN HANCOCK COLLEGE, 17
ALLEGHENY COLLEGE, 452
ALLEGHENY COUNTY COMMUNITY COLLEGE, 452
ALLEN UNIVERSITY, 483
ALLENTOWN COLLEGE OF SAINT FRANCIS DE SALES, 453
ALMA COLLEGE, 249
ALPENA COMMUNITY COLLEGE, 250
ALPHONSUS COLLEGE, 329

ALVERNO COLLEGE, 593
ALVIN JUNIOR COLLEGE, 512
AMARILLO COLLEGE, 512
AMBASSADOR COLLEGE, 17
AMERICAN ACADEMY OF DRAMATIC ARTS, 347
AMERICAN CENTER FOR THE PERFORMING ARTS, 228
AMERICAN MUSICAL AND DRAMATIC ACADEMY, INC, 347
THE AMERICAN UNIVERSITY ACADEMY FOR THE PERFORMING ARTS, 81
AMHERST COLLEGE, 228
ANDERSON COLLEGE, 153
ANDERSON COLLEGE, 483
ANGELO STATE UNIVERSITY, 512
ANNE ARUNDEL COMMUNITY COLLEGE, 219
ANTIOCH COLLEGE, 409
APPALACHIAN STATE UNIVERSITY, 387
ARAPAHOE COMMUNITY COLLEGE, 60
ARIZONA STATE UNIVERSITY, 8
UNIVERSITY OF ARIZONA, 8
ARKANSAS COLLEGE, 12
ARKANSAS STATE UNIVERSITY, 12
ARKANSAS TECH UNIVERSITY, 12
UNIVERSITY OF ARKANSAS, PINE BLUFF, 13
UNIVERSITY OF ARKANSAS, LITTLE ROCK, 14
ARMSTRONG STATE COLLEGE, 106
ASHLAND COLLEGE, 409
ATLANTIC CHRISTIAN COLLEGE, 387
AUGSBURG COLLEGE, 269
AUGUSTANA COLLEGE, 124
AUGUSTANA COLLEGE, 491
AURORA COLLEGE, 124
AUSTIN COLLEGE, 513
AUSTIN PEAY STATE UNIVERSITY, 497
AVILA COLLEGE, 290
BAKERSFIELD COLLEGE, 18
BALDWIN - WALLACE COLLEGE, 409
BALL STATE UNIVERSITY, 153
BAPTIST BIBLE COLLEGE, 453
BARAT COLLEGE, 125
BARD COLLEGE, 348
BARRINGTON COLLEGE, 480
BARRY COLLEGE, 86
BARTON COUNTY COMMUNITY COLLEGE, 180
BATES COLLEGE, 216
BAY DE NOC COMMUNITY COLLEGE, 251
BAY PATH JUNIOR COLLEGE, 229
BAYLOR UNIVERSITY, 513
BEAVER COLLEGE, 453
BEE COUNTY COLLEGE, 514
BELMONT COLLEGE, 497
BELOIT COLLEGE, 593
BEMIDJI STATE COLLEGE, 269
BENEDICTINE COLLEGE, 181
BENNETT COLLEGE, 348
BENNETT COLLEGE, 387
BENNINGTON COLLEGE, 558
BEREA COLLEGE, 198
BERKSHIRE COMMUNITY COLLEGE, 230
BERRY COLLEGE, 107
BETHANY COLLEGE, 586
BETHANY LUTHERAN COLLEGE, 270
BETHEL COLLEGE, 153
BETHEL COLLEGE, 182
BETHEL COLLEGE, 270
BETHEL COLLEGE, 497
BISCAYNE COLLEGE, 86

BISHOP COLLEGE, 514
BLACK HAWK COLLEGE, 125
BLACK HILLS STATE COLLEGE, 491
BLACKBURN COLLEGE, 126
BLOOMFIELD COLLEGE, 329
BLOOMSBURG STATE COLLEGE, 453
BLUE MOUNTAIN COLLEGE, 281
BLUE MOUNTAIN COMMUNITY COLLEGE, 442
BLUEFIELD COLLEGE, 563
BLUEFIELD COLLEGE, 586
BLUFFTON COLLEGE, 409
BOB JONES UNIVERSITY, 484
BOISE STATE UNIVERSITY, 120
BOSTON COLLEGE, 231
BOSTON CONSERVATORY OF MUSIC, 231
BOSTON UNIVERSITY SCHOOL FOR THE ARTS, 231
BOWDOIN COLLEGE, 216
BOWIE STATE COLLEGE, 219
BOWLING GREEN STATE UNIVERSITY, 410
BOWLING GREEN STATE UNIVERSITY - FIRELANDS CAMPUS, 410
BRADFORD COLLEGE, 232
BRADLEY UNIVERSITY, 126
BRAINERD COMMUNITY COLLEGE, 270
BRANDEIS UNIVERSITY, 232
BRANDYWINE COLLEGE, 79
BRAZOSPORT COLLEGE, 5150
BRENAU COLLEGE, 107
BRESCIA COLLEGE, 198
BREVARD COLLEGE, 388
BRIARCLIFF COLLEGE, 349
UNIVERSITY OF BRIDGEPORT, 71
BRIDGEWATER STATE COLLEGE, 232
BRIGHAM YOUNG UNIVERSITY, 553
BRIGHAM YOUNG UNIVERSITY - HAWAII CAMPUS, 118
BRONX COMMUNITY COLLEGE, 349
BROOKDALE COMMUNITY COLLEGE, 329
BROOKLYN COLLEGE SCHOOL OF PERFORMING ARTS, 349
BROWARD COMMUNITY COLLEGE, 86
BROWN UNIVERSITY, 480
BRYN MAWR COLLEGE, 453
BUCKNELL UNIVERSITY, 454
BUCKS COUNTY COMMUNITY COLLEGE, 454
BUENA VISTA COLLEGE, 167
BUNKER HILL COMMUNITY COLLEGE, 233
BUTLER COUNTY COMMUNITY JUNIOR COLLEGE, 182
BUTLER UNIVERSITY JORDAN COLLEGE OF MUSIC, 154
BUTTE COLLEGE, 18
CALDWELL COLLEGE, 330
SOUTHERN CALIFORNIA COLLEGE, 19
THE CALIFORNIA INSTITUTE OF THE ARTS, 19
CALIFORNIA INSTITUTE OF TECHNOLOGY, 20
CALIFORNIA LUTHERAN COLLEGE, 20
CALIFORNIA STATE COLLEGE, 455
CALIFORNIA STATE COLLEGE, STANISLAUS, 21
CALIFORNIA STATE UNIVERSITY - DOMINGUEZ HILLS, 22
CALIFORNIA STATE UNIVERSITY, CHICO, 22
CALIFORNIA STATE UNIVERSITY, FRESNO, 23
CALIFORNIA STATE UNIVERSITY, FULLERTON, 23
CALIFORNIA STATE UNIVERSITY, LONG BEACH, 24
CALIFORNIA STATE UNIVERSITY, LOS ANGELES, 25
CALIFORNIA STATE UNIVERSITY, NORTHRIDGE, 25
CALIFORNIA STATE UNIVERSITY, SACRAMENTO, 26
UNIVERSITY OF CALIFORNIA, DAVIS, 26
UNIVERSITY OF CALIFORNIA, IRVINE, 27
UNIVERSITY OF CALIFORNIA, SAN DIEGO, 28

UNIVERSITY OF CALIFORNIA, SANTA CRUZ, 28
CALVIN COLLEGE, 251
CAMDEN COUNTY COLLEGE, 330
CAMPBELL COLLEGE, 388
CAMPBELLSVILLE COLLEGE, 198
CANADA COLLEGE, 28
CARLETON COLLEGE, 271
CARLOW COLLEGE, 455
CARNEGIE - MELLON UNIVERSITY, 455
CARROLL COLLEGE, 309
CARROLL COLLEGE, 594
CARSON - NEWMAN COLLEGE, 498
CARTHAGE COLLEGE, 594
CASE WESTERN RESERVE UNIVERSITY, 411
CASPER COLLEGE, 610
CASTLETON STATE COLLEGE, 558
CATAWBA COLLEGE, 389
CATHERINE SPAULDING COLLEGE, 199
THE CATHOLIC UNIVERSITY OF AMERICA, 81
CAYUGA COUNTY COMMUNITY COLLEGE, 350
CECIL COMMUNITY COLLEGE, 219
CEDAR CREST COLLEGE, 456
CENTENARY COLLEGE FOR WOMEN, 331
CENTENARY COLLEGE OF LOUISANA, 206
UNIVERSITY OF CENTRAL ARKANSAS, 14
CENTRAL COLLEGE, 167
CENTRAL CONNECTICUT STATE COLLEGE, 71
CENTRAL FLORIDA COMMUNITY COLLEGE, 87
CENTRAL METHODIST COLLEGE, 290
CENTRAL MICHIGAN UNIVERSITY, 251
CENTRAL MISSOURI STATE UNIVERSITY, 291
CENTRAL STATE UNIVERSITY, 432
CENTRAL TEXAS COLLEGE, 515
CENTRAL WASHINGTON UNIVERSITY, 577
CENTRAL WYOMING COLLEGE, 610
CENTRALIA COLLEGE, 577
CENTRE COLLEGE OF KENTUCKY, 199
CERRO COSO COMMUNITY COLLEGE, 29
CHADRON STATE COLLEGE, 313
CHAMINADE UNIVERSITY OF HONOLULU, 118
CHATHAM COLLEGE, 456
CHEYNEY STATE COLLEGE, 457
CHICAGO CITY COLLEGE, AMUNDSEN - MAYFAIR COLLEGE, 126
CHICAGO CITY COLLEGE, MALCOLM X COLLEGE, 126
CHICAGO CITY COLLEGE, OLIVE - HARVEY COLLEGE, 127
CHICAGO CITY COLLEGE, SOUTHWEST COLLEGE, 127
UNIVERSITY OF CHICAGO, 127
CHIPOLA JUNIOR COLLEGE, 87
CHRISTIAN BROTHERS COLLEGE, 498
CHRISTOPHER NEWPORT COLLEGE, 563
UNIVERSITY OF CINCINNATI COLLEGE-CONSERVATORY OF MUSIC, 412
CISCO JUNIOR COLLEGE, 515
THE CITY COLLEGE, CITY UNIVERSITY OF NEW YORK, 351
CITY UNIVERSITY OF NEW YORK HERBERT H LEHMAN COLLEGE, 351
CITY UNIVERSITY OF NEW YORK, QUEENS COLLEGE, 352
CLAREMORE JUNIOR COLLEGE, 433
CLARION STATE COLLEGE - CLARION CAMPUS, 457
CLARK UNIVERSITY, 233
CLARKE COLLEGE, 167
CLATSOP COMMUNITY COLLEGE, 442
CLEVELAND STATE UNIVERSITY, 414
CLINCH VALLEY COLLEGE OF THE UNIVERSITY OF VIRGINIA, 563

CATEGORICAL — Theatre

CLOUD COUNTY COMMUNITY COLLEGE, 183
COASTAL CAROLINA COLLEGE OF THE UNIVERSITY OF SOUTH
   CAROLINA, 484
COE COLLEGE, 168
COFFEYVILLE COMMUNITY JUNIOR COLLEGE, 183
COKER COLLEGE, 485
COLBY COLLEGE, 217
COLBY COLLEGE, 325
COLBY COMMUNITY COLLEGE, 183
COLEGIO CESAR CHEVEZ, 442
COLGATE UNIVERSITY, 353
COLLEGE OF THE ALBEMARLE, 389
COLLEGE OF ARTESIA, 342
COLLEGE OF THE CANYONS, 29
COLLEGE OF DU PAGE, 128
COLLEGE OF EASTERN UTAH, 553
COLLEGE OF EMPORIA, 184
COLLEGE OF GREAT FALLS, 309
COLLEGE OF THE MAINLAND, 515
COLLEGE OF MARIN, 30
COLLEGE MISERICORDIA, 458
COLLEGE OF NOTRE DAME, 30
COLLEGE OF SAINT BENEDICT, 271
COLLEGE OF SAINT CATHERINE, 271
COLLEGE OF SAINT FRANCIS, 128
COLLEGE OF SAINT ROSE, 353
COLLEGE OF SAINT TERESA, 272
COLLEGE OF SAINT THOMAS, 272
COLLEGE OF SAN MATEO, 30
COLLEGE OF SANTA FE, 342
COLLEGE OF THE SEQUOIAS, 31
COLLEGE OF THE SISKIYOUS, 31
THE COLLEGE OF STEUBENVILLE, 414
THE COLLEGE OF WHITE PLAINS OF PACE UNIVERSITY, 354
COLLEGE OF WILLIAM AND MARY, 564
COLORADO COLLEGE, 61
COLORADO MOUNTAIN COLLEGE, EAST CAMPUS, 61
COLORADO MOUNTAIN COLLEGE WEST CAMPUS, 61
COLORADO STATE UNIVERSITY, 62
COLORADO WOMEN'S COLLEGE, 63
UNIVERSITY OF COLORADO, BOULDER, 63
COLUMBIA COLLEGE, 291
COLUMBIA COLLEGE, 485
COLUMBIA STATE COMMUNITY COLLEGE, 499
COLUMBIA UNIVERSITY, 354
COLUMBIA UNIVERSITY, BARNARD COLLEGE, 354
COLUMBUS COLLEGE, 108
COMMUNITY COLLEGE OF BALTIMORE, 220
COMPTON COMMUNITY COLLEGE, 32
CONCORD COLLEGE, 587
CONCORDIA COLLEGE, 273
CONCORDIA COLLEGE, 443
CONCORDIA TEACHERS COLLEGE, 129
CONCORDIA TEACHERS COLLEGE, 313
CONNECTICUT COLLEGE, 72
UNIVERSITY OF CONNECTICUT, 72
COOKE COUNTY JUNIOR COLLEGE, 516
CORNELL UNIVERSITY, 355
CORNING COMMUNITY COLLEGE, 356
CORNISH INSTITUTE OF ALLIED ARTS, 578
CORPUS CHRISTI STATE UNIVERSITY, 516
COTTEY COLLEGE, 292
COWLEY COUNTY COMMUNITY COLLEGE, 184
CREIGHTON UNIVERSITY, 314
CROWDER COLLEGE, 292
CULVER-STOCKTON COLLEGE, 292

CUMBERLAND COLLEGE, 200
CUMBERLAND COUNTY COLLEGE, 331
CURRY COLLEGE, 234
CUYAHOGA COMMUNITY COLLEGE, 414
CYPRESS COLLEGE, 33
DAEMEN COLLEGE, 356
DAKOTA STATE COLLEGE, 492
DAKOTA WESLEYAN UNIVERSITY, 492
DALLAS BAPTIST COLLEGE, 517
DALLAS THEATER CENTER, 517
DANA COLLEGE, 314
DARTMOUTH COLLEGE, 325
DAVID LIPSCOMB COLLEGE, 499
DAVIDSON COLLEGE, 390
DAVIS & ELKINS COLLEGE, 587
DAWSON COMMUNITY COLLEGE, 309
DAYTONA BEACH JUNIOR COLLEGE, 88
UNIVERSITY OF DAYTON, 415
DE ANZA COLLEGE, 33
DEAN JUNIOR COLLEGE, 234
DEKALB COMMUNITY COLLEGE, 109
DEL MAR COLLEGE, 517
DELAWARE STATE COLLEGE, 79
UNIVERSITY OF DELAWARE, 79
DELTA STATE UNIVERSITY, 282
DENISON UNIVERSITY, 416
COMMUNITY COLLEGE OF DENVER, NORTH CAMPUS, 63
UNIVERSITY OF DENVER, 64
DEPAUW UNIVERSITY, 154
DICKINSON COLLEGE, 459
FAIRLEIGH DICKINSON UNIVERSITY, 331
DILLARD UNIVERSITY, 206
DISTRICT OF COLUMBIA TEACHERS COLLEGE, 82
DIXIE COLLEGE, 554
DOANE COLLEGE, 315
DONNELLY COLLEGE, 185
DORDT COLLEGE, 168
DOUGLASS COLLEGE, 331
DRAKE UNIVERSITY, 169
DREW UNIVERSITY, 332
DREXEL UNIVERSITY, 459
DRURY COLLEGE, 293
DUKE UNIVERSITY, 390
DUQUESNE UNIVERSITY, 459
DUTCHESS COMMUNITY COLLEGE, 357
DYERSBURG STATE COMMUNITY COLLEGE, 500
D'YOUVILLE COLLEGE, 358
EARLHAM COLLEGE, 155
EAST CAROLINA UNIVERSITY, 391
EAST CENTRAL JUNIOR COLLEGE, 282
EAST CENTRAL OKLAHOMA STATE UNIVERSITY, 433
EAST MISSISSIPPI JUNIOR COLLEGE, 282
EAST STROUDSBURG STATE COLLEGE, 460
EAST TENNESSEE STATE UNIVERSITY, 500
EAST TEXAS BAPTIST COLLEGE, 518
EASTERN BAPTIST COLLEGE, 460
EASTERN ILLINOIS UNIVERSITY, 129
EASTERN KENTUCKY UNIVERSITY, 200
EASTERN MENNONITE COLLEGE, 564
EASTERN MICHIGAN UNIVERSITY, 252
EASTERN MONTANA COLLEGE, 309
EASTERN NEW MEXICO UNIVERSITY, PORTALES, 342
EASTERN OKLAHOMA STATE COLLEGE, 434
EASTERN OREGON STATE COLLEGE, 443
EASTERN WASHINGTON STATE COLLEGE, 578
EASTERN WYOMING COLLEGE, 611

EASTFIELD COLLEGE, 519
ECKERD COLLEGE, 88
EDGECLIFF COLLEGE, 416
EDGEWOOD COLLEGE, 595
EDINBORO STATE COLLEGE, 460
EDISON COMMUNITY COLLEGE, 88
EL CENTRO COLLEGE, 519
EL PASO COMMUNITY COLLEGE, 64
ELIZABETH SETON COLLEGE, 358
ELIZABETHTOWN COLLEGE, 461
ELMHURST COLLEGE, 130
ELMIRA COLLEGE, 358
ELON COLLEGE, 391
EMERSON COLLEGE, 235
EMORY UNIVERSITY, 109
EMPORIA STATE UNIVERSITY, 185
ERSKINE COLLEGE, 486
ESSEX COMMUNITY COLLEGE, 220
EUREKA COLLEGE, 130
EVANGEL COLLEGE, 293
FAIRMONT STATE COLLEGE, 587
FAIRMOUNT CENTER FOR CREATIVE & PERFORMING ARTS, 417
FAYETTEVILLE STATE UNIVERSITY, 392
FEDERAL CITY COLLEGE, 82
FELICIAN COLLEGE, 332
FERRIS STATE COLLEGE, 252
FERRUM COLLEGE, 565
FINCH COLLEGE, 359
FINDLAY COLLEGE, 417
FISK UNIVERSITY, 501
FLATHEAD VALLEY COMMUNITY COLLEGE, 310
FLORIDA AGRICULTURAL & MECHANICAL UNIVERSITY, 89
FLORIDA ATLANTIC UNIVERSITY, 89
FLORIDA COLLEGE, 90
FLORIDA INTERNATIONAL UNIVERSITY, 90
FLORIDA JUNIOR COLLEGE, 90
FLORIDA SOUTHERN COLLEGE, 91
FLORIDA STATE UNIVERSITY, 92
FLORIDA TECHNOLOGICAL UNIVERSITY, 92
UNIVERSITY OF FLORIDA, 93
FONTBONNE COLLEGE, 294
FOOTHILL COLLEGE, 34
FORDHAM UNIVERSITY, LINCOLN CENTER, 359
FORT HAYS STATE UNIVERSITY, 185
FORT LEWIS COLLEGE, 64
FORT WORTH CHRISTIAN COLLEGE, 519
FORT WRIGHT COLLEGE OF THE HOLY NAMES, 579
FRANCONIA COLLEGE, 325
FRANK PHILLIPS COLLEGE, 519
FRANKLIN AND MARSHALL COLLEGE, 461
FREE WILL BAPTIST COLLEGE, 501
FRESNO CITY COLLEGE, 34
FRESNO PACIFIC COLLEGE, 35
FRIENDS UNIVERSITY, 186
FROSTBURG STATE COLLEGE, 220
FULLERTON COLLEGE, 35
FURMAN UNIVERSITY, 486
GADSDEN STATE JUNIOR COLLEGE, 1
GAINESVILLE JUNIOR COLLEGE, 109
GALLAUDET COLLEGE, 83
GARDEN CITY COMMUNITY COLLEGE, 187
GAVILAN COLLEGE, 36
GENESEE COMMUNITY COLLEGE, 359
GEORGE FOX COLLEGE, 443
GEORGE PEABODY COLLEGE FOR TEACHERS, 501
GEORGE WASHINGTON UNIVERSITY, 83

GEORGETOWN UNIVERSITY, 83
GEORGIA COLLEGE, 110
GEORGIA SOUTHERN COLLEGE, 110
GEORGIA SOUTHWESTERN COLLEGE, 111
GEORGIA STATE UNIVERSITY, 111
UNIVERSITY OF GEORGIA, 111
GETTYSBURG COLLEGE, 462
GLASSBORO STATE COLLEGE, 333
GLENDALE COMMUNITY COLLEGE, 9
GLENVILLE STATE COLLEGE, 588
GODDARD COLLEGE, 559
GOLDEN VALLEY LUTHERAN COLLEGE, 273
GOLDOVSKY OPERA INSTITUTE, 236
GONZAGA UNIVERSITY, 579
GOODMAN SCHOOL OF DRAMA
GOSHEN COLLEGE, 156
GOUCHER COLLEGE, 221
GRACE COLLEGE, 156
GRACELAND COLLEGE, 170
GRAHM JUNIOR COLLEGE, 237
GRAMBLING COLLEGE OF LOUISIANA, 207
GRAND CANYON COLLEGE, 9
GRAND RAPIDS BAPTIST COLLEGE, 253
GRAYSON COUNTY COLLEGE, 520
GREEN MOUNTAIN COLLEGE, 559
GREENBRIER COLLEGE, 588
GREENSBORO COLLEGE, 392
GRINNELL COLLEGE, 170
GROSSMONT COLLEGE, 36
GROVE CITY COLLEGE, 462
GULF COAST COMMUNITY COLLEGE, 93
GULF PARK COLLEGE, 282
HAMILTON COLLEGE, 360
HAMLINE UNIVERSITY, 274
HAMPTON INSTITUTE, 565
HANOVER COLLEGE, 157
HARCUM JUNIOR COLLEGE, 462
HARDIN - SIMMONS UNIVERSITY, 520
HARDING COLLEGE, 15
HARLEM SCHOOL OF THE ARTS, INC, 360
HARRISBURG AREA COMMUNITY COLLEGE, 463
HARTFORD COLLEGE FOR WOMEN, 73
UNIVERSITY OF HARTFORD, 74
HARTNELL COLLEGE, 37
HARTWICK COLLEGE, 360
HARVARD UNIVERSITY, 237
HASTING COLLEGE, 315
HAWAII LOA COLLEGE, 118
UNIVERSITY OF HAWAII, 118
UNIVERSITY OF HAWAII AT HILO - HILO COLLEGE, 119
HAWKEN SCHOOL, 417
HAZARD COMMUNITY COLLEGE, 200
HEDGEROW THEATRE SCHOOL, 463
HEIDELBURG COLLEGE, 418
HENDERSON COUNTY JUNIOR COLLEGE, 520
HENDRIX COLLEGE, 15
HENRY FORD COMMUNITY COLLEGE, 253
HERKIMER COUNTY COMMUNITY COLLEGE, 361
HESSTON COLLEGE, 187
HIGH POINT COLLEGE, 393
HIGH SCHOOL FOR THE PERFORMING AND VISUAL ARTS, 521
HIGHLINE COMMUNITY COLLEGE, 580
HILL JUNIOR COLLEGE, 521
HILLSBOROUGH COMMUNITY COLLEGE, YBOR CAMPUS, 93
HINDS JUNIOR COLLEGE, 283

LONGWOOD COLLEGE, 567
LOOP COLLEGE, 138
LORAS COLLEGE, 172
LORETTO HEIGHTS COLLEGE, 65
LOS ANGELES HARBOR COLLEGE, 40
LOS ANGELES SOUTHWEST COLLEGE, 40
LOS ANGELES VALLEY COLLEGE, 41
LOUISANA STATE UNIVERSITY, 207
LOUISIANA COLLEGE, 207
LOUISIANA POLYTECHNIC INSTITUTE, 208
LOUISIANA TECHNICAL UNIVERSITY, 208
UNIVERSITY OF LOUISVILLE, 202
LOWER COLUMBIA COLLEGE, 580
LOYOLA UNIVERSITY, 208
LOYOLA UNIVERSITY OF CHICAGO, 139
LUBBOCK CHRISTIAN COLLEGE, 526
LUREEN B WALLACE STATE JUNIOR COLLEGE, 2
LUTHER COLLEGE, 173
LYCOMING COLLEGE, 467
LYNCHBURG COLLEGE, 568
LYNDON STATE COLLEGE, 560
MACALESTER COLLEGE, 275
MACMURRAY COLLEGE, 139
MACOMB COUNTY COMMUNITY COLLEGE - CENTER CAMPUS, 258
MACOMB COUNTY COMMUNITY COLLEGE - SOUTH CAMPUS, 258
MACON JUNIOR COLLEGE, 112
MADISON AREA TECHNICAL COLLEGE, 596
UNIVERSITY OF MAINE AT PORTLAND - GORHAM, 217
UNIVERSITY OF MAINE, ORONO, 217
MALONE COLLEGE, 421
MANATEE JUNIOR COLLEGE, 95
MANCHESTER COLLEGE, 161
MANHATTANVILLE COLLEGE, 366
MANKATO STATE UNIVERSITY, 275
MANSFIELD STATE COLLEGE, 467
MAPLE WOODS COMMUNITY COLLEGE, 295
MARIAN COLLEGE, INDIANAPOLIS, 162
MARIETTA COLLEGE, 421
MARJORIE WEBSTER JUNIOR COLLEGE, 84
MARLBORO COLLEGE, 560
MARQUETTE UNIVERSITY, 597
MARS HILL COLLEGE, 394
MARY BALDWIN COLLEGE, 568
MARY HARDIN - BAYLOR COLLEGE, 526
MARY MANSE COLLEGE, 421
MARY WASHINGTON COLLEGE, 569
MARYCREST COLLEGE, 174
UNIVERSITY OF MARYLAND, 221
UNIVERSITY OF MARYLAND, EASTERN SHORE, 222
MARYMOUNT MANHATTAN COLLEGE, 368
MARYMOUNT COLLEGE, 191
MARYMOUNT COLLEGE, 368
MARYVILLE COLLEGE, 504
MARYWOOD COLLEGE, 468
UNIVERSITY OF MASSACHUSETTS, 239
MASSASOIT COMMUNITY COLLEGE, 240
MASSON COLLEGE, 218
MATTATUK COMMUNITY COLLEGE, 74
MAYVILLE STATE COLLEGE, 406
MCKENDREE COLLEGE, 139
McLENNAN COMMUNITY COLLEGE, 527
McMURRY COLLEGE, 527
McNEESE STATE UNIVERSITY, 209

McPHERSON COLLEGE, 191
MEMPHIS STATE UNIVERSITY, 504
MERCER UNIVERSITY, ATLANTA, 112
MERCY COLLEGE, 368
MERCY COLLEGE OF DETROIT, 259
MERCYHURST COLLEGE, 468
MEREDITH COLLEGE, 395
MERIDIAN JUNIOR COLLEGE, 284
MESA COLLEGE, 65
MESA COMMUNITY COLLEGE, 10
MESABI COMMUNITY COLLEGE, 275
MESSIAH COLLEGE, 469
METHODIST COLLEGE, 395
METROPOLITAN COMMUNITY COLLEGE, 276
METROPOLITAN STATE COLLEGE, 66
MIAMI - DADE COMMUNITY COLLEGE - NEW WORLD CENTER, 96
MIAMI - DADE COMMUNITY COLLEGE - NORTH CAMPUS, 96
MIAMI - DADE COMMUNITY COLLEGE, SOUTH CAMPUS, 96
MIAMI UNIVERSITY, 422
UNIVERSITY OF MIAMI, 96
MICHIGAN STATE UNIVERSITY, 260
THE UNIVERSITY OF MICHIGAN, 261
UNIVERSITY OF MICHIGAN, FLINT, 261
MIDDLE GEORGIA COLLEGE, 113
MIDDLE TENNESSEE STATE UNIVERSITY, 505
MIDDLEBURY COLLEGE, 561
MIDLAND COLLEGE, 528
MIDLAND LUTHERAN COLLEGE, 317
MIDWESTERN STATE UNIVERSITY, 528
MILES COMMUNITY COLLEGE, 310
MILLERSVILLE STATE COLLEGE, 469
MILLIGAN COLLEGE, 505
MILLIKIN UNIVERSITY, 140
MILLSAPS COLLEGE, 284
UNIVERSITY OF MINNESOTA, MORRIS, 276
UNIVERSITY OF MINNESOTA, DULUTH - SCHOOL OF FINE ARTS, 277
MINOT STATE COLLEGE, 406
MIRA COSTA COMMUNITY COLLEGE, 41
MISSISSIPPI COLLEGE, 284
MISSISSIPPI STATE UNIVERSITY, 285
MISSISSIPPI UNIVERSITY FOR WOMEN, 286
UNIVERSITY OF MISSISSIPPI, 286
MISSOURI SOUTHERN STATE COLLEGE, 296
MISSOURI VALLEY COLLEGE, 296
MISSOURI WESTERN STATE COLLEGE, 297
UNIVERSITY OF MISSOURI, 297
UNIVERSITY OF MISSOURI, KANSAS CITY, 298
MITCHELL COLLEGE, 74
MITCHELL COMMUNITY COLLEGE, 396
MODESTO JUNIOR COLLEGE, 42
MONMOUTH COLLEGE, 140
MONROE COUNTY COMMUNITY COLLEGE, 261
MONTANA STATE UNIVERSITY, 310
UNIVERSITY OF MONTANA, SCHOOL OF FINE ARTS, 311
MONTCLAIR STATE COLLEGE, 335
MONTGOMERY COLLEGE, 222
MOORHEAD STATE UNIVERSITY, 343
MORAVIAN COLLEGE, 469
MOREHEAD STATE UNIVERSITY, 202
MOREHOUSE COLLEGE, 113
MORGAN STATE COLLEGE, 223
MORNINGSIDE COLLEGE, 174
MORRIS HARVEY COLLEGE, 589
MORTON COLLEGE, 141

TRANSYLVANIA UNIVERSITY, 204
TRENTON STATE COLLEGE, 339
TREVECCA NAZARENE COLLEGE, 510
TRINIDAD STATE COLLEGE, 68
TRINITY COLLEGE, 75
TRINITY COLLEGE, 85
TRINITY UNIVERSITY, 547
TRITON COLLEGE, 150
TROY STATE UNIVERSITY, 6
TULANE UNIVERSITY, 214
TUSCULUM COLLEGE, 510
TUSKEGEE INSTITUTE, 6
TYLER JUNIOR COLLEGE, 548
U S COAST GUARD ACADEMY, 76
UNION COLLEGE, 204
UNION COLLEGE, 340
UNION COLLEGE, 385
UNION UNIVERSITY, 511
UNITED STATES INTERNATIONAL UNIVERSITY, 56
UNIVERSITY OF ALBUQUERQUE, 345
UNIVERSITY OF CALIFORNIA, RIVERSIDE, 56
UNIVERSITY OF DALLAS, 548
UNIVERSITY OF DETROIT, MARYGROVE COLLEGE, 266
UNIVERSITY OF DUBUQUE, 177
UNIVERSITY OF ILLINOIS, 151
THE UNIVERSITY OF IOWA, 177
UNIVERSITY OF MINNESOTA, 279
UNIVERSITY OF MONTEVALLO, 6
UNIVERSITY OF NORTH CAROLINA, 403
UNIVERSITY OF NOTRE DAME, 165
UNIVERSITY OF PENNSYLVANIA, 476
UNIVERSITY OF REDLANDS, 57
UNIVERSITY OF RICHMOND, 572
UNIVERSITY OF SOUTHERN CALIFORNIA, 57
UNIVERSITY OF SOUTHERN MISSISSIPPI, 288
UNIVERSITY OF TEXAS, ARLINGTON, 548
UNIVERSITY OF TEXAS, AUSTIN, 549
UNIVERSITY OF TEXAS, EL PASO, 549
UNIVERSITY OF TULSA, 441
UNIVERSITY OF VERMONT, 562
UPPER IOWA UNIVERSITY, 178
UPSALA COLLEGE, 340
URSULINE COLLEGE, 428
UTAH STATE UNIVERSITY, 555
UNIVERSITY OF UTAH, 555
VALDOSTA STATE COLLEGE, 116
VALPARAISO UNIVERSITY, 165
VANDERBILT UNIVERSITY, 511
VASSAR COLLEGE, 385
VICTOR VALLEY COLLEGE, 57
VILLA JULIE COLLEGE, 226
VILLANOVA UNIVERSITY, 477
VINCENNES UNIVERSITY, 166
VIRGINIA COMMONWEALTH UNIVERSITY, 573
VIRGINIA INTERMONT COLLEGE, 574
VIRGINIA POLYTECHNIC INSTITUTE AND STATE UNIVERSITY, 574
VIRGINIA WESLEYAN COLLEGE, 575
UNIVERSITY OF VIRGINIA, 575
VITERBO COLLEGE, 600
WAGNER COLLEGE, 386
WAKE FOREST UNIVERSITY, 404
WALDORF COLLEGE, 178
WALNUT HILL SCHOOL OF PERFORMING ARTS, 246
WARNER PACIFIC COLLEGE, 450
WARREN WILSON COLLEGE, 404

WARTBURG COLLEGE, 179
WASHBURN UNIVERSITY OF TOPEKA, 196
WASHINGTON AND JEFFERSON COLLEGE, 477
WASHINGTON AND LEE UNIVERSITY, 575
WASHINGTON COLLEGE, 226
WASHINGTON STATE UNIVERSITY, 583
WASHINGTON UNIVERSITY, 305
UNIVERSITY OF WASHINGTON, 583
WAUBONSEE COMMUNITY COLLEGE, 151
WAYLAND BAPTIST COLLEGE, 550
WAYNE STATE COLLEGE, 321
WAYNE STATE UNIVERSITY, 267
WEATHERFORD COLLEGE, 550
WEBER STATE COLLEGE, 556
WEBSTER COLLEGE, 306
WELLESLEY COLLEGE, 246
WELLS COLLEGE, 386
WESLEYAN COLLEGE, 117
WESLEYAN UNIVERSITY, 76
WEST CHESTER STATE COLLEGE, 477
UNIVERSITY OF WEST FLORIDA, 103
WEST GEORGIA COLLEGE, 117
WEST HILLS COLLEGE, 58
WEST LIBERTY STATE COLLEGE, 590
WEST TEXAS STATE UNIVERSITY, 551
WEST VALLEY COLLEGE, 58
WEST VIRGINIA STATE COLLEGE, 591
WEST VIRGINIA UNIVERSITY - CREATIVE ARTS CENTER, 591
WEST VIRGINIA WESLEYAN COLLEGE, 591
WESTERN CAROLINA UNIVERSITY, 405
WESTERN COLLEGE OF MIAMI UNIVERSITY, 428
WESTERN CONNECTICUT STATE COLLEGE, 77
WESTERN ILLINOIS UNIVERSITY, 151
WESTERN KENTUCKY UNIVERSITY, 205
WESTERN MARYLAND COLLEGE, 227
WESTERN MICHIGAN UNIVERSITY, 267
WESTERN NEW MEXICO UNIVERSITY, 307
WESTERN STATE COLLEGE, 68
WESTERN WASHINGTON STATE COLLEGE, 584
WESTFIELD STATE COLLEGE, 247
WESTMAR COLLEGE, 179
WESTMINISTER COLLEGE, 307
WESTMINISTER COLLEGE, 556
WESTMINSTER COLLEGE, 478
WESTMONT COLLEGE, 58
WHARTON COUNTY JUNIOR COLLEGE, 551
WHITMAN COLLEGE, 584
WHITWORTH COLLEGE, 585
WILBUR WRIGHT COLLEGE, CITY COLLEGE OF CHICAGO, 152
WILLAMETTE UNIVERSITY, 451
WILLIAM CAREY COLLEGE, 289
WILLIAM JEWELL COLLEGE, 307
WILLIAM PATERSON COLLEGE, 341
WILLIAM WOODS - WESTMINISTER COLLEGE, 308
WILLIAMS COLLEGE, 247
WILLMAR COMMUNITY COLLEGE, 280
WILMINGTON COLLEGE, 428
WILMINGTON COLLEGE, 80
WINDHAM COLLEGE, 562
WINONA STATE UNIVERSITY, 280
WINTHROP COLLEGE, 489
UNIVERSITY OF WISCONSIN CENTER, MANITOWOC COUNTY, 600
UNIVERSITY OF WISCONSIN, RIVER FALLS, 601
UNIVERSITY OF WISCONSIN, EAU CLAIRE, 602
UNIVERSITY OF WISCONSIN, GREEN BAY, 602

UNIVERSITY OF WISCONSIN, LA CROSSE, 603
UNIVERSITY OF WISCONSIN, MADISON, 603
UNIVERSITY OF WISCONSIN, MARSHFIELD/WOOD CO CENTER, 604
THE UNIVERSITY OF WISCONSIN, MILWAUKEE SCHOOL OF FINE ARTS, 604
UNIVERSITY OF WISCONSIN, OSHKOSH, 605
UNIVERSITY OF WISCONSIN, PARKSIDE, 606
THE UNIVERSITY OF WISCONSIN, PLATTEVILLE, 606
UNIVERSITY OF WISCONSIN, SHEBOYGAN, 606
UNIVERSITY OF WISCONSIN, STEVENS POINT, 607
UNIVERSITY OF WISCONSIN, SUPERIOR, 608
UNIVERSITY OF WISCONSIN, WHITEWATER, 608
WITTENBERG UNIVERSITY, 429
WOOD JUNIOR COLLEGE, 289
THE COLLEGE OF WOOSTER, 429
WRIGHT STATE UNIVERSITY, 430
XAVIER UNIVERSITY, 430
XAVIER UNIVERSITY OF LOUISANA, 214
YALE UNIVERSITY, 77
YANKTON COLLEGE, 496
YESHIVA UNIVERSITY, 386
YORK COLLEGE, 322
YORK COLLEGE OF PENNSYLVANIA, 479
YOUNG HARRIS COLLEGE, 117
YOUNGSTOWN STATE UNIVERSITY, 430

TV, Radio and Film

ABILENE CHRISTIAN UNIVERSITY, 512
ADELPHI UNIVERSITY, 346
UNIVERSITY OF AKRON COLLEGE OF FINE AND APPLIED ARTS, 408
UNIVERSITY OF ALABAMA, BIRMINGHAM, 1
UNIVERSITY OF ALASKA COLLEGE OF ARTS & LETTERS, 7
ALBRIGHT COLLEGE, 452
ALFRED UNIVERSITY, 347
ALLAN HANCOCK COLLEGE, 17
THE AMERICAN UNIVERSITY ACADEMY FOR THE PERFORMING ARTS, 81
ANDERSON COLLEGE, 153
ANDREWS UNIVERSITY, 250
ANTIOCH COLLEGE, 409
APPALACHIAN STATE UNIVERSITY, 387
ARAPAHOE COMMUNITY COLLEGE, 60
ARIZONA STATE UNIVERSITY, 8
UNIVERSITY OF ARIZONA, 8
ARKANSAS COLLEGE, 12
UNIVERSITY OF ARKANSAS, MONTICELLO, 13
ASHLAND COLLEGE, 409
AUGUSTANA COLLEGE, 124
AUGUSTANA COLLEGE, 491
AUSTIN COLLEGE, 513
AVILA COLLEGE, 290
BAKERSFIELD COLLEGE, 18
BARD COLLEGE, 348
BARTON COUNTY COMMUNITY COLLEGE, 180
BAYLOR UNIVERSITY, 513
BEMIDJI STATE COLLEGE, 269
BENEDICTINE COLLEGE, 181
BENNETT COLLEGE, 387
BEREA COLLEGE, 198
BERRY COLLEGE, 107
BETHANY COLLEGE, 586
BISHOP COLLEGE, 514
BLACK HAWK COLLEGE, 125

BLOOMSBURG STATE COLLEGE, 453
BLUE MOUNTAIN COMMUNITY COLLEGE, 442
BOB JONES UNIVERSITY, 484
BOISE STATE UNIVERSITY, 120
BOWDOIN COLLEGE, 216
BOWIE STATE COLLEGE, 219
BOWLING GREEN STATE UNIVERSITY, 410
BRAINERD COMMUNITY COLLEGE, 270
UNIVERSITY OF BRIDGEPORT, 71
BRIGHAM YOUNG UNIVERSITY, 553
BRONX COMMUNITY COLLEGE, 349
BROOKDALE COMMUNITY COLLEGE, 329
BROWARD COMMUNITY COLLEGE, 86
BUCKS COUNTY COMMUNITY COLLEGE, 454
BUENA VISTA COLLEGE, 167
BUNKER HILL COMMUNITY COLLEGE, 233
BUTTE COLLEGE, 18
THE CALIFORNIA INSTITUTE OF THE ARTS, 19
CALIFORNIA LUTHERAN COLLEGE, 20
CALIFORNIA STATE COLLEGE, 455
CALIFORNIA STATE UNIVERSITY - DOMINGUEZ HILLS, 22
CALIFORNIA STATE UNIVERSITY, CHICO, 22
CALIFORNIA STATE UNIVERSITY, FRESNO, 23
CALIFORNIA STATE UNIVERSITY, FULLERTON, 23
CALIFORNIA STATE UNIVERSITY, LOS ANGELES, 25
UNIVERSITY OF CALIFORNIA, IRVINE, 27
UNIVERSITY OF CALIFORNIA, SAN DIEGO, 28
UNIVERSITY OF CALIFORNIA, SANTA CRUZ, 28
CALVIN COLLEGE, 251
CAMDEN COUNTY COLLEGE, 330
CARROLL COLLEGE, 594
CASPER COLLEGE, 610
CATAWBA COLLEGE, 389
THE CATHOLIC UNIVERSITY OF AMERICA, 81
CAYUGA COUNTY COMMUNITY COLLEGE, 350
CECIL COMMUNITY COLLEGE, 219
CENTRAL MICHIGAN UNIVERSITY, 251
CENTRAL MISSOURI STATE UNIVERSITY, 291
CENTRAL STATE UNIVERSITY, 412
CENTRAL TEXAS COLLEGE, 515
CENTRAL WASHINGTON UNIVERSITY, 577
CENTRALIA COLLEGE, 577
CHATHAM COLLEGE, 456
CHRISTIAN BROTHERS COLLEGE, 498
CHRISTOPHER NEWPORT COLLEGE, 563
UNIVERSITY OF CINCINNATI COLLEGE - CONSERVATORY OF MUSIC, 412
THE CITY COLLEGE, CITY UNIVERSITY OF NEW YORK, 351
CLARION STATE COLLEGE - CLARION CAMPUS, 457
CLARK UNIVERSITY, 233
CLATSOP COMMUNITY COLLEGE, 442
COFFEYVILLE COMMUNITY JUNIOR COLLEGE, 183
COKER COLLEGE, 485
COLBY COLLEGE, 325
COLBY COMMUNITY COLLEGE, 183
COLGATE UNIVERSITY, 353
COLLEGE OF DU PAGE, 128
COLLEGE OF MARIN, 30
COLLEGE OF SAINT CATHERINE, 271
COLLEGE OF SAINT ROSE, 353
COLLEGE OF SAINT TERESA, 272
COLLEGE OF SAN MATEO, 30
COLLEGE OF THE SEQUOIAS, 31
THE COLLEGE OF STEUBENVILLE, 414
COLORADO COLLEGE, 61
COLORADO MOUNTAIN COLLEGE WEST CAMPUS, 61

COLORADO STATE UNIVERSITY, 62
UNIVERSITY OF COLORADO, BOULDER, 63
COLUMBIA STATE COMMUNITY COLLEGE, 499
COMMUNITY COLLEGE OF BALTIMORE, 220
COMPTON COMMUNITY COLLEGE, 32
CONCORDIA COLLEGE, 273
CONNECTICUT COLLEGE, 72
UNIVERSITY OF CONNECTICUT, 72
CORNELL UNIVERSITY, 355
CORPUS CHRISTI STATE UNIVERSITY, 516
CULVER-STOCKTON COLLEGE, 292
DALLAS BAPTIST COLLEGE, 517
DARTMOUTH COLLEGE, 325
DAVIDSON COLLEGE, 390
DE ANZA COLLEGE, 33
DENISON UNIVERSITY, 416
UNIVERSITY OF DENVER, 64
FAIRLEIGH DICKINSON UNIVERSITY, 331
DIXIE COLLEGE, 554
DONNELLY COLLEGE, 185
DRAKE UNIVERSITY, 169
DREW UNIVERSITY, 332
DREXEL UNIVERSITY, 459
DUQUESNE UNIVERSITY, 459
DUTCHESS COMMUNITY COLLEGE, 357
EAST CAROLINA UNIVERSITY, 391
EAST STROUDSBURG STATE COLLEGE, 460
EAST TENNESSEE STATE UNIVERSITY, 500
EASTERN CONNECTICUT STATE COLLEGE, 73
EASTERN KENTUCKY UNIVERSITY, 200
EASTERN MICHIGAN UNIVERSITY, 252
EASTERN WASHINGTON STATE COLLEGE, 578
EDINBORO STATE COLLEGE, 460
EL PASO COMMUNITY COLLEGE, 64
ELIZABETHTOWN COLLEGE, 461
EMERSON COLLEGE, 235
ENDICOTT COLLEGE, 236
EUREKA COLLEGE, 130
FAIRMONT STATE COLLEGE, 587
FAYETTEVILLE STATE UNIVERSITY, 392
FEDERAL CITY COLLEGE, 82
FELICIAN COLLEGE, 332
FERRIS STATE COLLEGE, 252
FERRUM COLLEGE, 565
FINDLAY COLLEGE, 417
FISK UNIVERSITY, 501
FLORIDA SOUTHERN COLLEGE, 91
FLORIDA STATE UNIVERSITY, 92
FLORIDA TECHNOLOGICAL UNIVERSITY, 92
FOOTHILL COLLEGE, 34
FORT HAYS STATE UNIVERSITY, 185
FRANCONIA COLLEGE, 325
FRANKLIN AND MARSHALL COLLEGE, 461
FRESNO CITY COLLEGE, 34
GADSDEN STATE JUNIOR COLLEGE, 1
GAVILAN COLLEGE, 36
GENESEE COMMUNITY COLLEGE, 359
GEORGE PEABODY COLLEGE FOR TEACHERS, 501
GEORGIA SOUTHERN COLLEGE, 110
GEORGIA STATE UNIVERSITY, 111
GLENDALE COMMUNITY COLLEGE, 9
GODDARD COLLEGE, 559
GONZAGA UNIVERSITY, 579
GRACELAND COLLEGE, 170
GRAND RAPIDS JUNIOR COLLEGE, 253
GRAYSON COUNTY COLLEGE, 520

GREENBRIER COLLEGE, 588
GROSSMONT COLLEGE, 36
GROVE CITY COLLEGE, 462
GULF PARK COLLEGE, 282
HAMPTON INSTITUTE, 565
HARDING COLLEGE, 15
HARTNELL COLLEGE, 37
HARVARD UNIVERSITY, 237
HENRY FORD COMMUNITY COLLEGE, 253
HERKIMER COUNTY COMMUNITY COLLEGE, 361
HIGH POINT COLLEGE, 393
HIGH SCHOOL FOR THE PERFORMING AND VISUAL ARTS, 521
HOFSTRA UNIVERSITY, 362
HOPE COLLEGE, 254
UNIVERSITY OF HOUSTON, CENTRAL CAMPUS, 522
HOWARD COLLEGE, BIG SPRING, 523
HUMBOLDT STATE UNIVERSITY, 37
HUNTER COLLEGE, CITY UNIVERSITY OF NEW YORK, 363
HUNTINGTON COLLEGE, 157
HUTCHINSON COMMUNITY COLLEGE, 187
IDAHO STATE UNIVERSITY, 120
UNIVERSITY OF IDAHO, 121
ILLINOIS CENTRAL COLLEGE, 132
ILLINOIS STATE UNIVERSITY, 134
IMPERIAL VALLEY COLLEGE, 38
INDIANA STATE UNIVERSITY, 157
INDIANA UNIVERSITY - PURDUE UNIVERSITY AT FORT WAYNE, 158
INDIANA UNIVERSITY, BLOOMINGTON, 159
INDIANA UNIVERSITY OF PENNSYLVANIA, 463
INTERNATIONAL COLLEGE, 38
ITHACA COLLEGE, 364
JACKSON STATE COMMUNITY COLLEGE, 502
JAMES MADISON UNIVERSITY, 566
JEFFERSON STATE JUNIOR COLLEGE, 2
JERSEY CITY STATE COLLEGE, 333
JOHN CARROLL UNIVERSITY, 418
JUNIATA COLLEGE, 464
KALAMAZOO COLLEGE, 256
KANSAS STATE UNIVERSITY, 189
UNIVERSITY OF KANSAS, 190
KEAN COLLEGE OF NEW JERSEY, 334
KEARNEY STATE COLLEGE, 316
KELLOGG COMMUNITY COLLEGE, 256
KENNEDY - KING COLLEGE, 135
KENT STATE UNIVERSITY, 418
KENTUCKY STATE UNIVERSITY, 201
KENTUCKY WESLEYAN COLLEGE, 201
UNIVERSITY OF KENTUCKY, HENDERSON COMMUNITY COLLEGE, 202
KING'S COLLEGE, 464
KUTZTOWN STATE COLLEGE, 465
LA SALLE COLLEGE, 465
LABETTE COMMUNITY JUNIOR COLLEGE, 191
LAKE ERIE COLLEGE, 420
LAKE FOREST COLLEGE, 136
LAKE LAND COLLEGE, 136
LAKELAND COMMUNITY COLLEGE, 420
LANE COMMUNITY COLLEGE, 444
LANEY COLLEGE, 38
LEE COLLEGE, 525
LEMOYNE COLLEGE, 366
LINCOLN COLLEGE, 137
LINCOLN LAND COMMUNITY COLLEGE, 138
LINDENWOOD COLLEGE, 295
LINFIELD COLLEGE, 445

CATEGORICAL — TV, Radio and Film

WILBUR WRIGHT COLLEGE, CITY COLLEGE OF CHICAGO, 152
WILLIAM JEWELL COLLEGE, 307
WILLIAM PATERSON COLLEGE, 341
WILLIAM WOODS - WESTMINISTER COLLEGE, 308
WINONA STATE UNIVERSITY, 280
UNIVERSITY OF WISCONSIN, RIVER FALLS, 601
UNIVERSITY OF WISCONSIN, EAU CLAIRE, 602
UNIVERSITY OF WISCONSIN, LA CROSSE, 603
UNIVERSITY OF WISCONSIN, MADISON, 603
THE UNIVERSITY OF WISCONSIN, MILWAUKEE SCHOOL OF FINE ARTS, 604
UNIVERSITY OF WISCONSIN, OSHKOSH, 605
UNIVERSITY OF WISCONSIN, PARKSIDE, 606
THE UNIVERSITY OF WISCONSIN, PLATTEVILLE, 606
UNIVERSITY OF WISCONSIN, SHEBOYGAN, 606
UNIVERSITY OF WISCONSIN, STEVENS POINT, 607
UNIVERSITY OF WISCONSIN, SUPERIOR, 608
UNIVERSITY OF WISCONSIN, WHITEWATER, 608
THE COLLEGE OF WOOSTER, 429
WRIGHT STATE UNIVERSITY, 430
UNIVERSITY OF WYOMING, 611
XAVIER UNIVERSITY, 430
XAVIER UNIVERSITY OF LOUISANA, 214
YALE UNIVERSITY, 77
YORK COLLEGE OF PENNSYLVANIA, 479
YOUNGSTOWN STATE UNIVERSITY, 430

Visual Arts

ABILENE CHRISTIAN UNIVERSITY, 512
ABRAHAM BALDWIN AGRICULTURAL COLLEGE, 105
ADAMS STATE COLLEGE, 60
ADELPHI UNIVERSITY, 346
ADIRONDACK COMMUNITY COLLEGE, 346
ADRIAN COLLEGE, 249
AGNES SCOTT COLLEGE, 105
UNIVERSITY OF AKRON COLLEGE OF FINE AND APPLIED ARTS, 408
UNIVERSITY OF ALABAMA, BIRMINGHAM, 1
UNIVERSITY OF ALASKA COLLEGE OF ARTS & LETTERS, 7
UNIVERSITY OF ALASKA, ANCHORAGE, 7
ALBANY STATE COLLEGE, 106
ALBERTUS MAGNUS COLLEGE, 70
ALBION COLLEGE, 249
ALBRIGHT COLLEGE, 452
ALCORN AGRICULTURAL & MECHANICAL COLLEGE, 281
ALDERSON - BROADDUS COLLEGE, 586
ALFRED UNIVERSITY, 347
ALICE LLOYD COLLEGE, 197
ALLAN HANCOCK COLLEGE, 17
ALLEGHENY COUNTY COMMUNITY COLLEGE, 452
ALLEN COUNTY COMMUNITY JUNIOR COLLEGE, 180
ALLEN UNIVERSITY, 483
ALMA COLLEGE, 249
ALPENA COMMUNITY COLLEGE, 250
ALPHONSUS COLLEGE, 329
ALVERNO COLLEGE, 593
THE AMERICAN UNIVERSITY ACADEMY FOR THE PERFORMING ARTS, 81
AMHERST COLLEGE, 228
ANDERSON COLLEGE, 153
ANDERSON COLLEGE, 483
ANDREWS UNIVERSITY, 250
ANGELO STATE UNIVERSITY, 512
ANNA MARIA COLLEGE, 228
ANTIOCH COLLEGE, 409

APPALACHIAN STATE UNIVERSITY, 387
ARAPAHOE COMMUNITY COLLEGE, 60
ARIZONA STATE UNIVERSITY, 8
UNIVERSITY OF ARIZONA, 8
ARKANSAS TECH UNIVERSITY, 12
UNIVERSITY OF ARKANSAS, PINE BLUFF, 13
UNIVERSITY OF ARKANSAS, MONTICELLO, 13
UNIVERSITY OF ARKANSAS, LITTLE ROCK, 14
ARMSTRONG STATE COLLEGE, 106
ASHLAND COLLEGE, 409
ATLANTIC CHRISTIAN COLLEGE, 387
ATLANTIC UNION COLLEGE THAYER CONSERVATORY OF MUSIC, 229
AUGSBURG COLLEGE, 269
AUGUSTANA COLLEGE, 491
AUSTIN COLLEGE, 513
AUSTIN PEAY STATE UNIVERSITY, 497
AVILA COLLEGE, 290
BAKER UNIVERSITY, 180
BALL STATE UNIVERSITY, 153
BARAT COLLEGE, 125
BARD COLLEGE, 348
BARRINGTON COLLEGE, 480
BARRY COLLEGE, 86
BARTON COUNTY COMMUNITY COLLEGE, 180
BATES COLLEGE, 216
BAY DE NOC COMMUNITY COLLEGE, 251
BAY PATH JUNIOR COLLEGE, 229
BAYLOR UNIVERSITY, 513
BEAVER COLLEGE, 453
BEE COUNTY COLLEGE, 514
BELHAVEN COLLEGE, 281
BELOIT COLLEGE, 593
BEMIDJI STATE COLLEGE, 269
BENEDICT COLLEGE, 483
BENEDICTINE COLLEGE, 181
BENNETT COLLEGE, 387
BENNINGTON COLLEGE, 558
BEREA COLLEGE, 198
BERGEN COMMUNITY COLLEGE, 329
BERKSHIRE COMMUNITY COLLEGE, 230
BERRY COLLEGE, 107
BETHANY COLLEGE, 181
BETHANY COLLEGE, 586
BETHANY LUTHERAN COLLEGE, 270
BETHEL COLLEGE, 182
BETHEL COLLEGE, 270
BETHEL COLLEGE, 497
BISHOP COLLEGE, 514
BLACK HAWK COLLEGE, 125
BLACK HILLS STATE COLLEGE, 491
BLINN COLLEGE, 514
BLOOMFIELD COLLEGE, 329
BLOOMSBURG STATE COLLEGE, 453
BLUE MOUNTAIN COMMUNITY COLLEGE, 442
BLUEFIELD COLLEGE, 586
BLUFFTON COLLEGE, 409
BOB JONES UNIVERSITY, 484
BOISE STATE UNIVERSITY, 120
BOSTON UNIVERSITY SCHOOL FOR THE ARTS, 231
BOWDOIN COLLEGE, 216
BOWIE STATE COLLEGE, 219
BOWLING GREEN STATE UNIVERSITY, 410
BRADFORD COLLEGE, 232
BRADLEY UNIVERSITY, 126
BRAINERD COMMUNITY COLLEGE, 270

BRANDEIS UNIVERSITY, 232
BRANDYWINE COLLEGE, 79
BRENAU COLLEGE, 107
BRESCIA COLLEGE, 198
UNIVERSITY OF BRIDGEPORT, 71
BRIDGEWATER COLLEGE, 563
BRIDGEWATER STATE COLLEGE, 232
BRIGHAM YOUNG UNIVERSITY, 553
BRIGHAM YOUNG UNIVERSITY - HAWAII CAMPUS, 118
BRONX COMMUNITY COLLEGE, 349
BROOKDALE COMMUNITY COLLEGE, 329
BROWARD COMMUNITY COLLEGE, 86
BUCKNELL UNIVERSITY, 454
BUCKS COUNTY COMMUNITY COLLEGE, 454
BUENA VISTA COLLEGE, 167
BUNKER HILL COMMUNITY COLLEGE, 233
BUTLER COUNTY COMMUNITY JUNIOR COLLEGE, 182
BUTLER UNIVERSITY JORDAN COLLEGE OF MUSIC, 154
BUTTE COLLEGE, 18
THE CALIFORNIA INSTITUTE OF THE ARTS, 19
CALIFORNIA STATE COLLEGE, 455
CALIFORNIA STATE COLLEGE, BAKERSFIELD, 20
CALIFORNIA STATE COLLEGE, STANISLAUS, 21
CALIFORNIA STATE UNIVERSITY - DOMINGUEZ HILLS, 22
CALIFORNIA STATE UNIVERSITY, CHICO, 22
CALIFORNIA STATE UNIVERSITY, FULLERTON, 23
CALIFORNIA STATE UNIVERSITY, LONG BEACH, 24
CALIFORNIA STATE UNIVERSITY, LOS ANGELES, 25
CALIFORNIA STATE UNIVERSITY, NORTHRIDGE, 25
UNIVERSITY OF CALIFORNIA, SAN DIEGO, 28
UNIVERSITY OF CALIFORNIA, SANTA CRUZ, 28
CALVIN COLLEGE, 251
CAMDEN COUNTY COLLEGE, 330
CAMPBELLSVILLE COLLEGE, 198
CANADA COLLEGE, 28
CAPITAL UNIVERSITY, 410
CARDINAL STRITCH COLLEGE, 593
CARLETON COLLEGE, 271
CARROLL COLLEGE, 309
CARROLL COLLEGE, 594
CARSON - NEWMAN COLLEGE, 498
CASE WESTERN RESERVE UNIVERSITY, 411
CASPER COLLEGE, 610
CASTLETON STATE COLLEGE, 558
CATAWBA COLLEGE, 389
CATHERINE SPAULDING COLLEGE, 199
CAYUGA COUNTY COMMUNITY COLLEGE, 350
CECIL COMMUNITY COLLEGE, 219
CEDAR CREST COLLEGE, 456
CENTRAL ARIZONA COLLEGE, 9
CENTRAL COLLEGE, 167
CENTRAL COLLEGE, 182
CENTRAL FLORIDA COMMUNITY COLLEGE, 87
CENTRAL METHODIST COLLEGE, 290
CENTRAL MICHIGAN UNIVERSITY, 251
CENTRAL MISSOURI STATE UNIVERSITY, 291
CENTRAL OREGON COMMUNITY COLLEGE, 442
CENTRAL STATE UNIVERSITY, 412
CENTRAL STATE UNIVERSITY, 432
CENTRAL TEXAS COLLEGE, 515
CENTRAL WASHINGTON UNIVERSITY, 577
CENTRE COLLEGE OF KENTUCKY, 199
CHADRON STATE COLLEGE, 313
CHAMINADE UNIVERSITY OF HONOLULU, 118
CHATHAM COLLEGE, 456
CHESTNUT HILL COLLEGE, 457

CHEYNEY STATE COLLEGE, 457
CHICAGO CITY COLLEGE, AMUNDSEN - MAYFAIR COLLEGE, 126
CHICAGO CITY COLLEGE, MALCOLM X COLLEGE, 126
CHIPOLA JUNIOR COLLEGE, 87
CHRISTIAN BROTHERS COLLEGE, 498
CHRISTOPHER NEWPORT COLLEGE, 563
UNIVERSITY OF CINCINNATI COLLEGE - CONSERVATORY OF MU-
   SIC, 412
THE CITY COLLEGE, CITY UNIVERSITY OF NEW YORK, 351
CITY UNIVERSITY OF NEW YORK HERBERT H LEHMAN COL-
   LEGE, 351
CITY UNIVERSITY OF NEW YORK, QUEENS COLLEGE, 352
CITY UNIVERSITY OF NEW YORK, YORK COLLEGE, 352
CLAFLIN COLLEGE, 484
CLAREMORE JUNIOR COLLEGE, 433
CLARION STATE COLLEGE - CLARION CAMPUS, 457
CLARK UNIVERSITY, 233
CLARKE COLLEGE, 167
CLARKE COLLEGE, 281
CLATSOP COMMUNITY COLLEGE, 442
CLEVELAND STATE UNIVERSITY, 414
COASTAL CAROLINA COLLEGE OF THE UNIVERSITY OF SOUTH
   CAROLINA, 484
COFFEYVILLE COMMUNITY JUNIOR COLLEGE, 183
COKER COLLEGE, 485
COLBY COLLEGE, 325
COLBY COMMUNITY COLLEGE, 183
COLEGIO CESAR CHEVEZ, 442
COLGATE UNIVERSITY, 353
COLLEGE OF THE ALBEMARLE, 389
COLLEGE OF ARTESIA, 342
COLLEGE OF THE CANYONS, 29
COLLEGE OF DU PAGE, 128
COLLEGE OF EASTERN UTAH, 553
COLLEGE OF EMPORIA, 184
COLLEGE OF GREAT FALLS, 309
COLLEGE OF THE MAINLAND, 515
COLLEGE OF MARIN, 30
COLLEGE MISERICORDIA, 458
COLLEGE OF SAINT BENEDICT, 271
COLLEGE OF SAINT CATHERINE, 271
COLLEGE OF SAINT FRANCIS, 128
COLLEGE OF SAINT MARY, 313
COLLEGE OF SAINT ROSE, 353
COLLEGE OF SAINT THOMAS, 272
COLLEGE OF SAN MATEO, 30
COLLEGE OF SANTA FE, 342
COLLEGE OF THE SEQUOIAS, 31
COLLEGE OF WILLIAM AND MARY, 564
COLORADO COLLEGE, 61
COLORADO MOUNTAIN COLLEGE, EAST CAMPUS, 61
COLORADO MOUNTAIN COLLEGE WEST CAMPUS, 61
COLORADO STATE UNIVERSITY, 62
COLORADO WOMEN'S COLLEGE, 63
UNIVERSITY OF COLORADO, BOULDER, 63
COLUMBIA COLLEGE, 485
COLUMBIA UNION COLLEGE, 219
COLUMBIA UNIVERSITY, BARNARD COLLEGE, 354
COMMUNITY COLLEGE OF BALTIMORE, 220
COMPTON COMMUNITY COLLEGE, 32
CONCORD COLLEGE, 587
CONCORDIA COLLEGE, 273
CONCORDIA TEACHERS COLLEGE, 129
CONCORDIA TEACHERS COLLEGE, 313
CONNECTICUT COLLEGE, 72
UNIVERSITY OF CONNECTICUT, 72

CATEGORICAL — Visual Arts

CONNORS STATE COLLEGE, 414
CONVERSE COLLEGE, 486
CORNELL UNIVERSITY, 355
CORNISH INSTITUTE OF ALLIED ARTS, 578
CORPUS CHRISTI STATE UNIVERSITY, 516
COWLEY COUNTY COMMUNITY COLLEGE, 184
CREIGHTON UNIVERSITY, 314
CULVER-STOCKTON COLLEGE, 292
CUMBERLAND COLLEGE, 200
CUMBERLAND COLLEGE, 499
CUMBERLAND COUNTY COLLEGE, 331
CURRY COLLEGE, 234
CUYAHOGA COMMUNITY COLLEGE, 414
CYPRESS COLLEGE, 33
DAKOTA STATE COLLEGE, 492
DALLAS BAPTIST COLLEGE, 517
DANA COLLEGE, 314
DARTMOUTH COLLEGE, 325
DAVID LIPSCOMB COLLEGE, 499
DAVIDSON COLLEGE, 390
DAVIS & ELKINS COLLEGE, 587
UNIVERSITY OF DAYTON, 415
DE ANZA COLLEGE, 33
DEAN JUNIOR COLLEGE, 234
DEFIANCE COLLEGE, 415
DEKALB COMMUNITY COLLEGE, 109
DEL MAR COLLEGE, 517
DELAWARE STATE COLLEGE, 79
DENISON UNIVERSITY, 416
UNIVERSITY OF DENVER, 64
DEPAUL UNIVERSITY, 129
DEPAUW UNIVERSITY, 154
DICKINSON COLLEGE, 459
FAIRLEIGH DICKINSON UNIVERSITY, 331
DISTRICT OF COLUMBIA TEACHERS COLLEGE, 82
DIXIE COLLEGE, 554
DOANE COLLEGE, 315
DOMINICAN COLLEGE, 518
DOUGLASS COLLEGE, 331
DOWLING COLLEGE, 325
DRAKE UNIVERSITY, 169
DREW UNIVERSITY, 332
DREXEL UNIVERSITY, 459
DRURY COLLEGE, 293
DUTCHESS COMMUNITY COLLEGE, 357
EARLHAM COLLEGE, 155
EAST CAROLINA UNIVERSITY, 391
EAST CENTRAL JUNIOR COLLEGE, 282
EAST CENTRAL MISSOURI DISTRICT JUNIOR COLLEGE, 293
EAST MISSISSIPPI JUNIOR COLLEGE, 282
EAST STROUDSBURG STATE COLLEGE, 460
EAST TENNESSEE STATE UNIVERSITY, 500
EAST TEXAS BAPTIST COLLEGE, 518
EASTERN BAPTIST COLLEGE, 460
EASTERN CONNECTICUT STATE COLLEGE, 73
EASTERN ILLINOIS UNIVERSITY, 129
EASTERN KENTUCKY UNIVERSITY, 200
EASTERN MENNONITE COLLEGE, 564
EASTERN MICHIGAN UNIVERSITY, 252
EASTERN MONTANA COLLEGE, 309
EASTERN NEW MEXICO UNIVERSITY, PORTALES, 342
EASTERN OREGON STATE COLLEGE, 443
EASTERN WASHINGTON STATE COLLEGE, 578
EASTERN WYOMING COLLEGE, 611
EASTFIELD COLLEGE, 519
ECKERD COLLEGE, 88

EDGECLIFF COLLEGE, 416
EDGEWOOD COLLEGE, 595
EDINBORO STATE COLLEGE, 460
EDISON COMMUNITY COLLEGE, 88
EL CENTRO COLLEGE, 519
ELIZABETHTOWN COLLEGE, 461
ELMHURST COLLEGE, 130
ELMIRA COLLEGE, 358
ELON COLLEGE, 391
EMERSON COLLEGE, 235
EMMANUEL COLLEGE, 236
EMORY UNIVERSITY, 109
EMPORIA STATE UNIVERSITY, 185
ENDICOTT COLLEGE, 236
EUREKA COLLEGE, 130
EVANGEL COLLEGE, 293
FAIRMONT STATE COLLEGE, 587
FAIRMOUNT CENTER FOR CREATIVE & PERFORMING ARTS, 417
FEDERAL CITY COLLEGE, 82
FELICIAN COLLEGE, 131
FELICIAN COLLEGE, 332
FERRIS STATE COLLEGE, 252
FERRUM COLLEGE, 565
FINCH COLLEGE, 359
FINDLAY COLLEGE, 417
FISK UNIVERSITY, 501
FLATHEAD VALLEY COMMUNITY COLLEGE, 310
FLORIDA AGRICULTURAL & MECHANICAL UNIVERSITY, 89
FLORIDA INTERNATIONAL UNIVERSITY, 90
FLORIDA JUNIOR COLLEGE, 90
FLORIDA KEYS COMMUNITY COLLEGE, 91
FLORIDA STATE UNIVERSITY, 92
FLORIDA TECHNOLOGICAL UNIVERSITY, 92
UNIVERSITY OF FLORIDA, 93
FONTBONNE COLLEGE, 294
FOOTHILL COLLEGE, 34
FORDHAM UNIVERSITY, LINCOLN CENTER, 359
FORT HAYS STATE UNIVERSITY, 185
FORT SCOTT COMMUNITY JUNIOR COLLEGE, 186
FORT WORTH CHRISTIAN COLLEGE, 519
FORT WRIGHT COLLEGE OF THE HOLY NAMES, 579
FRANCONIA COLLEGE, 325
FRANKLIN AND MARSHALL COLLEGE, 461
FRESNO CITY COLLEGE, 34
FRESNO PACIFIC COLLEGE, 35
FRIENDS UNIVERSITY, 186
FROSTBURG STATE COLLEGE, 220
FULLERTON COLLEGE, 35
FURMAN UNIVERSITY, 486
GADSDEN STATE JUNIOR COLLEGE, 1
GARDEN CITY COMMUNITY COLLEGE, 187
GAVILAN COLLEGE, 36
GENESEE COMMUNITY COLLEGE, 359
GENEVA COLLEGE, 461
GEORGE PEABODY COLLEGE FOR TEACHERS, 501
GEORGETOWN UNIVERSITY, 83
GEORGIA COLLEGE, 110
GEORGIA SOUTHWESTERN COLLEGE, 111
GEORGIA STATE UNIVERSITY, 111
GEORGIAN COURT COLLEGE, 333
GETTYSBURG COLLEGE, 462
GLASSBORO STATE COLLEGE, 333
GODDARD COLLEGE, 559
GOLDEN VALLEY LUTHERAN COLLEGE, 273
GOSHEN COLLEGE, 156
GOUCHER COLLEGE, 221

POTOMAC STATE COLLEGE, 589
PRATT COMMUNITY COLLEGE, 193
PRATT INSTITUTE, 371
PRESBYTERIAN COLLEGE, 488
PRINCETON UNIVERSITY, 337
PRINCIPIA COLLEGE, 145
PURDUE UNIVERSITY, 162
QUEENS COLLEGE, 402
QUEENSBOROUGH COMMUNITY COLLEGE, CITY UNIVERSITY OF NEW YORK, 372
RADCLIFFE COLLEGE, 243
RADFORD COLLEGE, 570
RAINY RIVER COMMUNITY COLLEGE, 278
RANDOLPH - MACON COLLEGE, 570
RANGER JUNIOR COLLEGE, 532
REED COLLEGE, 449
REGIS COLLEGE, 243
REND LAKE COLLEGE, 146
RHODE ISLAND COLLEGE, 481
UNIVERSITY OF RHODE ISLAND, 481
RICE UNIVERSITY, 532
RICKS COLLEGE, 122
RIDER COLLEGE, 337
RIO HONDO COLLEGE, 48
RIPON COLLEGE, 599
RIVERSIDE CITY COLLEGE, 49
RIVIER COLLEGE, 328
ROANOKE COLLEGE, 571
ROBERTS WESLEYAN COLLEGE, 372
ROCKY MOUNTAIN COLLEGE, 312
ROSARY COLLEGE, 147
RUST COLLEGE, 287
RUTGERS UNIVERSITY, CAMDEN COLLEGE OF ARTS & SCIENCES, 338
RUTGERS UNIVERSITY, DOUGLASS COLLEGE, 338
RUTGERS UNIVERSITY, NEWARK, 339
SAGINAW VALLEY COLLEGE, 265
SAINT AMBROSE COLLEGE, 176
SAINT ANDREWS PRESBYTERIAN COLLEGE, 402
SAINT AUGUSTINE'S COLLEGE, 403
SAINT CLOUD STATE UNIVERSITY, 278
SAINT EDWARDS UNIVERSITY, 533
SAINT FRANCIS COLLEGE, 162
SAINT JOHNS RIVER JUNIOR COLLEGE FLORIDA SCHOOL OF THE ARTS, 100
SAINT JOSEPH'S COLLEGE, 163
SAINT LAWRENCE UNIVERSITY, 374
SAINT LEO COLLEGE, 101
SAINT LOUIS COMMUNITY COLLEGE AT MERAMEC, 300
SAINT LOUIS UNIVERSITY, 301
SAINT MARTIN'S COLLEGE, 581
SAINT MARY COLLEGE, 193
SAINT MARY OF THE PLAINS COLLEGE, 194
SAINT MARY-OF-THE-WOODS COLLEGE, 163
SAINT MARY'S COLLEGE, 164
SAINT MARY'S COLLEGE OF MARYLAND, 224
SAINT MARY'S DOMINICAN COLLEGE, 212
SAINT MARY'S UNIVERSITY, 533
SAINT MICHAEL'S COLLEGE, 561
SAINT NORBERT COLLEGE, 599
SAINT OLAF COLLEGE, 278
SAINT PETERSBURG COLLEGE, 101
SAINT VINCENT COLLEGE, 473
SALEM COLLEGE, 403
SALESIAN COLLEGE, 339
SALISBURY STATE COLLEGE, 225

SAM HOUSTON STATE UNIVERSITY, 534
SAMFORD UNIVERSITY, 3
SAN ANTONIO COLLEGE, 535
SAN DIEGO CITY COLLEGE, 49
SAN FRANCISCO STATE UNIVERSITY, 50
UNIVERSITY OF SAN FRANCISCO, 50
SAN JOAQUIN DELTA COLLEGE, 51
SANGAMON STATE UNIVERSITY, 148
SANTA BARBARA CITY COLLEGE CONTINUING EDUCATION DIVISION, 51
SANTA MONICA COLLEGE, 51
SANTA ROSA JUNIOR COLLEGE, 52
SARAH LAWRENCE COLLEGE, 374
SCHOOL OF CONTEMPORARY MUSIC, 243
SCHOOL OF FINE ARTS, 426
SCHOOL OF THE OZARKS, 301
SCHOOLCRAFT COLLEGE, 265
SCHREINER COLLEGE, 536
SCRIPPS COLLEGE, 52
SEATTLE PACIFIC UNIVERSITY, 582
SEATTLE UNIVERSITY, 582
SETON HILL COLLEGE, 473
SEWARD COUNTY COMMUNITY COLLEGE, 194
SHAW UNIVERSITY, 403
SHEPHERD COLLEGE, 590
SIENA HEIGHTS COLLEGE, 266
SIERRA COLLEGE, 52
SILVER LAKE COLLEGE, 599
SIMON'S ROCK EARLY COLLEGE, 243
SINCLAIR COMMUNITY COLLEGE, 427
SIOUX FALLS COLLEGE, 493
SKIDMORE COLLEGE, 375
SKYLINE COLLEGE, 53
SMITH COLLEGE, 244
UNIVERSITY OF SOUTH ALABAMA, 4
SOUTH CAROLINA STATE COLLEGE, 488
THE UNIVERSITY OF SOUTH DAKOTA, 494
SOUTH DAKOTA STATE UNIVERSITY, 494
UNIVERSITY OF SOUTH DAKOTA AT SPRINGFIELD, 495
UNIVERSITY OF SOUTH FLORIDA, 102
SOUTH GEORGIA COLLEGE, 115
THE SOUTH SHORE CONSERVATORY OF MUSIC, INC, 244
SOUTHAMPTON COLLEGE OF LONG ISLAND UNIVERSITY, 375
SOUTHEASTERN LOUISIANA UNIVERSITY, 212
SOUTHEASTERN MASSACHUSETTS UNIVERSITY, 245
SOUTHERN ARKANSAS UNIVERSITY, 16
UNIVERSITY OF SOUTHERN CALIFORNIA, 54
UNIVERSITY OF SOUTHERN COLORADO, 68
SOUTHERN CONNECTICUT STATE COLLEGE, 75
COLLEGE OF SOUTHERN IDAHO, 123
SOUTHERN ILLINOIS UNIVERSITY, 148
SOUTHERN ILLINOIS UNIVERSITY AT EDWARDSVILLE, 149
SOUTHERN METHODIST UNIVERSITY, 538
SOUTHERN MISSIONARY COLLEGE, 506
SOUTHERN OREGON COLLEGE, 450
SOUTHERN STATE COLLEGE, 495
SOUTHERN UNIVERSITY, BATON ROUGE, 213
SOUTHERN UTAH STATE COLLEGE, 555
SOUTHWEST MISSOURI STATE UNIVERSITY, 302
SOUTHWEST TEXAS STATE UNIVERSITY, 538
SOUTHWESTERN COLLEGE, 194
UNIVERSITY OF SOUTHWESTERN LOUISIANA, 213
SOUTHWESTERN AT MEMPHIS, 507
SOUTHWESTERN STATE COLLEGE, 450
SOUTHWESTERN UNIVERSITY AT GEORGETOWN, 539
THE UNIVERSITY OF THE SOUTH, 507

SPRING HILL COLLEGE, 5
STATE UNIVERSITY OF NEW YORK, ALBANY, 376
STATE UNIVERSITY OF NEW YORK, BINGHAMTON, 376
STATE UNIVERSITY OF NEW YORK, BUFFALO, 377
STATE UNIVERSITY OF NEW YORK COLLEGE, CORTLAND, 378
STATE UNIVERSITY OF NEW YORK COLLEGE, FREDONIA, 378
STATE UNIVERSITY OF NEW YORK COLLEGE AT GENESEO, 378
STATE UNIVERSITY OF NEW YORK COLLEGE, NEW PALTZ, 379
STATE UNIVERSITY OF NEW YORK COLLEGE, ONEONTA, 379
STATE UNIVERSITY OF NEW YORK COLLEGE, OSWEGO, 380
STATE UNIVERSITY OF NEW YORK COLLEGE, PLATTSBURGH, 380
STATE UNIVERSITY OF NEW YORK COLLEGE, POTSDAM, 380
STATE UNIVERSITY OF NEW YORK COLLEGE, PURCHASE PRO-
   FESSIONAL SCHOOL OF ARTS, 381
STATE UNIVERSITY OF NEW YORK, OSWEGO, 381
STATEN COLLEGE COMMUNITY COLLEGE, CITY UNIVERSITY OF
   NEW YORK, 382
STEPHENS COLLEGE, 304
STERLING COLLEGE, 195
STILLMAN COLLEGE, 5
STOCKTON STATE COLLEGE, 339
STUART OSTROW FOUNDATION, INC, 383
SUFFOLK COUNTY COMMUNITY COLLEGE, 384
SUFFOLK UNIVERSITY, 245
SUL ROSS STATE UNIVERSITY, 540
SULLINS COLLEGE, 571
SUSQUEHANNA UNIVERSITY, 474
SWARTHMORE COLLEGE, 475
SWEET BRIAR COLLEGE, 572
SYRACUSE UNIVERSITY, 384
TABOR COLLEGE, 195
UNIVERSITY OF TAMPA, 103
TARLETON STATE UNIVERSITY, 540
TARRANT COUNTY JUNIOR COLLEGE, NORTHEAST CAMPUS, 541
TARRANT COUNTY JUNIOR COLLEGE, SOUTH CAMPUS, 541
TAYLOR UNIVERSITY, 164
TEMPLE JUNIOR COLLEGE, 541
TEMPLE UNIVERSITY, 475
TENNESSEE STATE UNIVERSITY, 508
TENNESSEE TECHNOLOGICAL UNIVERSITY, 508
TENNESSEE WESLEYAN COLLEGE, 508
UNIVERSITY OF TENNESSEE AT CHATTANOOGA, 509
UNIVERSITY OF TENNESSEE, MARTIN, 510
TEXARKANA COLLEGE, 542
TEXAS AGRICULTURAL & INDUSTRIAL UNIVERSITY, KINGS-
   VILLE, 542
TEXAS CHRISTIAN UNIVERSITY, 542
TEXAS COLLEGE, 543
TEXAS LUTHERAN COLLEGE, 543
TEXAS SOUTHERN UNIVERSITY, 544
TEXAS SOUTHMOST COLLEGE, 544
TEXAS TECH UNIVERSITY, 545
TEXAS WESLEYAN COLLEGE, 545
TEXAS WOMEN'S UNIVERSITY, 546
UNIVERSITY OF TEXAS - AUSTIN, 546
THIEL COLLEGE, 476
THOMAS MORE COLLEGE, 204
THREE RIVERS COMMUNITY COLLEGE, 305
UNIVERSITY OF TOLEDO, 427
TOUGALOO COLLEGE, 288
TOWSON STATE UNIVERSITY, 225
TREASURE VALLEY COMMUNITY COLLEGE, 450
TRENTON STATE COLLEGE, 339
TREVECCA NAZARENE COLLEGE, 510

TRINITY CHRISTIAN COLLEGE, 150
TRINITY COLLEGE, 75
TRINITY COLLEGE, 85
TRINITY UNIVERSITY, 547
TRITON COLLEGE, 150
TROY STATE UNIVERSITY, 6
TULANE UNIVERSITY, 214
TUSCULUM COLLEGE, 510
TUSKEGEE INSTITUTE, 6
TYLER JUNIOR COLLEGE, 548
UNION COLLEGE, 321
UNION COLLEGE, 340
UNION COLLEGE, 385
UNION UNIVERSITY, 511
UNITED STATES INTERNATIONAL UNIVERSITY, 56
UNIVERSITY OF ALBUQUERQUE, 345
UNIVERSITY OF DALLAS, 548
UNIVERSITY OF DETROIT, MARYGROVE COLLEGE, 266
UNIVERSITY OF ILLINOIS, 151
THE UNIVERSITY OF IOWA, 177
UNIVERSITY OF MONTEVALLO, 6
UNIVERSITY OF NOTRE DAME, 165
UNIVERSITY OF PENNSYLVANIA, 476
UNIVERSITY OF REDLANDS, 57
UNIVERSITY OF RICHMOND, 572
UNIVERSITY OF SOUTHERN MISSISSIPPI, 288
UNIVERSITY OF TEXAS, AUSTIN, 549
UNIVERSITY OF TEXAS, EL PASO, 549
UNIVERSITY OF TULSA, 441
UNIVERSITY OF VERMONT, 562
UPPER IOWA UNIVERSITY, 178
URSULINE COLLEGE, 428
UNIVERSITY OF UTAH, 555
VALDOSTA STATE COLLEGE, 116
VALLEY CITY STATE COLLEGE, 407
VALPARAISO UNIVERSITY, 165
VASSAR COLLEGE, 385
VICTOR VALLEY COLLEGE, 57
VILLA JULIE COLLEGE, 226
VILLA MARIA COLLEGE OF BUFFALO, 385
VINCENNES UNIVERSITY, 166
VIRGINIA COMMONWEALTH UNIVERSITY, 573
VIRGINIA INTERMONT COLLEGE, 574
VIRGINIA STATE COLLEGE, 575
VIRGINIA WESLEYAN COLLEGE, 575
VITERBO COLLEGE, 600
WABASH COLLEGE, 166
WAGNER COLLEGE, 386
WAKE FOREST UNIVERSITY, 404
WALNUT HILL SCHOOL OF PERFORMING ARTS, 246
WARNER PACIFIC COLLEGE, 450
WARREN WILSON COLLEGE, 404
WARTBURG COLLEGE, 179
WASHBURN UNIVERSITY OF TOPEKA, 196
WASHINGTON COLLEGE, 226
WASHINGTON STATE UNIVERSITY, 583
WASHINGTON UNIVERSITY, 305
WAUBONSEE COMMUNITY COLLEGE, 151
WAYNE STATE COLLEGE, 321
WAYNE STATE UNIVERSITY, 267
WEATHERFORD COLLEGE, 550
WEBER STATE COLLEGE, 556
WEBSTER COLLEGE, 306
WESLEY COLLEGE, 80
WESLEYAN COLLEGE, 117
WESLEYAN UNIVERSITY, 76

WEST CHESTER STATE COLLEGE, 477
UNIVERSITY OF WEST FLORIDA, 103
WEST GEORGIA COLLEGE, 117
WEST HILLS COLLEGE, 58
WEST LIBERTY STATE COLLEGE, 590
WEST TEXAS STATE UNIVERSITY, 551
WEST VALLEY COLLEGE, 58
WEST VIRGINIA STATE COLLEGE, 591
WEST VIRGINIA UNIVERSITY - CREATIVE ARTS CENTER, 591
WESTERN CAROLINA UNIVERSITY, 405
WESTERN COLLEGE OF MIAMI UNIVERSITY, 428
WESTERN CONNECTICUT STATE COLLEGE, 77
WESTERN ILLINOIS UNIVERSITY, 151
WESTERN MARYLAND COLLEGE, 227
WESTERN MONTANA COLLEGE, 312
WESTERN STATE COLLEGE, 68
WESTFIELD STATE COLLEGE, 247
WESTMAR COLLEGE, 179
WESTMINISTER COLLEGE, 307
WESTMINISTER COLLEGE, 556
WESTMINSTER COLLEGE, 478
WHARTON COUNTY JUNIOR COLLEGE, 551
WHEATON COLLEGE, 247
WHITMAN COLLEGE, 584
WHITWORTH COLLEGE, 289
WHITWORTH COLLEGE, 585
WICHITA STATE UNIVERSITY, 196
WILKES COLLEGE, 478
WILLAMETTE UNIVERSITY, 451
WILLIAM JEWELL COLLEGE, 307
WILLIAM RAINEY HARPER COLLEGE, 152
WILLIAMS COLLEGE, 247
WILLMAR COMMUNITY COLLEGE, 280
WILMINGTON COLLEGE, 428
WILMINGTON COLLEGE, 80
WILSON COLLEGE, 478
WINDHAM COLLEGE, 562
WINONA STATE UNIVERSITY, 280
WINTHROP COLLEGE, 489
UNIVERSITY OF WISCONSIN CENTER, MANITOWOC COUNTY, 600
UNIVERSITY OF WISCONSIN, RIVER FALLS, 601
UNIVERSITY OF WISCONSIN, EAU CLAIRE, 602
UNIVERSITY OF WISCONSIN, GREEN BAY, 602
UNIVERSITY OF WISCONSIN, LA CROSSE, 603
UNIVERSITY OF WISCONSIN, MADISON, 603
THE UNIVERSITY OF WISCONSIN, MILWAUKEE SCHOOL OF FINE ARTS, 604
UNIVERSITY OF WISCONSIN, OSHKOSH, 605
UNIVERSITY OF WISCONSIN, PARKSIDE, 606
UNIVERSITY OF WISCONSIN, SHEBOYGAN, 606
UNIVERSITY OF WISCONSIN, STEVENS POINT, 607
UNIVERSITY OF WISCONSIN, SUPERIOR, 608
UNIVERSITY OF WISCONSIN, WHITEWATER, 608
THE COLLEGE OF WOOSTER, 429
WRIGHT STATE UNIVERSITY, 430
UNIVERSITY OF WYOMING, 611
YALE UNIVERSITY, 77
YANKTON COLLEGE, 496
YESHIVA UNIVERSITY, 386
YORK COLLEGE OF PENNSYLVANIA, 479
YOUNG HARRIS COLLEGE, 117

YOUNGSTOWN STATE UNIVERSITY, 430

Other Specialties

UNIVERSITY OF ALASKA COLLEGE OF ARTS & LETTERS, 7
THE AMERICAN UNIVERSITY ACADEMY FOR THE PERFORMING ARTS, 81
UNIVERSITY OF ARIZONA, 8
ARKANSAS STATE UNIVERSITY, 12
ASPEN MUSIC SCHOOL, 60
AUGUSTANA COLLEGE, 491
AURORA COLLEGE, 124
BALL STATE UNIVERSITY, 153
BAPTIST COLLEGE AT CHARLESTON, 483
BARAT COLLEGE, 125
BENNINGTON COLLEGE, 558
BETHEL COLLEGE, 153
BOSTON UNIVERSITY SCHOOL FOR THE ARTS, 231
BRIGHAM YOUNG UNIVERSITY, 553
BROOKDALE COMMUNITY COLLEGE, 329
BUCKS COUNTY COMMUNITY COLLEGE, 454
BUTTE COLLEGE, 18
CALIFORNIA STATE COLLEGE, 455
CALIFORNIA STATE COLLEGE, SAN BERNARDINO, 21
UNIVERSITY OF CALIFORNIA, SANTA CRUZ, 28
CEDARVILLE COLLEGE, 411
CENTRAL ARIZONA COLLEGE, 9
CENTRAL WASHINGTON UNIVERSITY, 577
CHRISTOPHER NEWPORT COLLEGE, 563
THE CINCINNATI BIBLE SEMINARY, 412
COLGATE UNIVERSITY, 353
COMPTON COMMUNITY COLLEGE, 32
DICKINSON COLLEGE, 459
DIXIE COLLEGE, 554
DUQUESNE UNIVERSITY, 459
EAST STROUDSBURG STATE COLLEGE, 460
EASTERN KENTUCKY UNIVERSITY, 200
EASTERN WYOMING COLLEGE, 611
ELIZABETHTOWN COLLEGE, 461
EMPORIA STATE UNIVERSITY, 185
FLORIDA STATE UNIVERSITY, 92
FREED-HARDEMAN COLLEGE, 501
GEORGIA SOUTHERN COLLEGE, 110
GETTYSBURG COLLEGE, 462
HANNIBAL LA GRANGE COLLEGE, 294
HOLYOKE COMMUNITY COLLEGE, 237
INTERLOCHEN ARTS ACADEMY, 255
ITHACA COLLEGE, 364
JOHNSON C SMITH UNIVERSITY, 393
KENNEDY - KING COLLEGE, 135
LAKE FOREST COLLEGE, 136
LAKE MICHIGAN COLLEGE, 257
LELAND POWERS SCHOOL, 238
LINCOLN COLLEGE, 137
LINCOLN UNIVERSITY, 294
LINDENWOOD COLLEGE, 295
LINFIELD COLLEGE, 445
LONE MOUNTAIN COLLEGE, SAN FRANCISCO, 39
LONGY SCHOOL OF MUSIC, 239
LOUISANA STATE UNIVERSITY, 207
LOUISIANA TECHNICAL UNIVERSITY, 208
LOYOLA UNIVERSITY, 208
MACOMB COUNTY COMMUNITY COLLEGE - SOUTH CAMPUS, 258
MERCER COUNTY COMMUNITY COLLEGE, 334
MERCER UNIVERSITY, ATLANTA, 112

METROPOLITAN STATE COLLEGE, 66
MIAMI UNIVERSITY, 422
MICHIGAN STATE UNIVERSITY, 260
MISSOURI VALLEY COLLEGE, 296
MITCHELL COLLEGE, 74
MORNINGSIDE COLLEGE, 174
MOUNT HOOD COMMUNITY COLLEGE, 434
NEW COLLEGE OF THE UNIVERSITY OF SOUTH FLORIDA, 97
UNIVERSITY OF NEW HAVEN, 75
NEW YORK INSTITUTE OF TECHNOLOGY, 369
NORTH CAROLINA SCHOOL OF THE ARTS, 397
UNIVERSITY OF NORTH CAROLINA, ASHEVILLE, 398
UNIVERSITY OF NORTH CAROLINA, CHARLOTTE, 399
NORTH GEORGIA COLLEGE, 114
NORTHEAST MISSOURI STATE UNIVERSITY, 299
NORTHERN OKLAHOMA COLLEGE, 436
UNIVERSITY OF OKLAHOMA, 438
UNIVERSITY OF SCIENCE AND ARTS OF OKLAHOMA, 439
OLIVET NAZARENE COLLEGE, 144
UNIVERSITY OF OREGON, 447
PARK COLLEGE, 300
PASADENA CITY COLLEGE, 47
PEPPERDINE UNIVERSITY, SEAVER COLLEGE, 47
QUINNIPIAC COLLEGE, 75
SAINT CLOUD STATE UNIVERSITY, 278
SAINT LAWRENCE UNIVERSITY, 374
SALEM COLLEGE, 589
SAN DIEGO CITY COLLEGE, 49
SAN FRANCISCO STATE UNIVERSITY, 50
SAN JOAQUIN DELTA COLLEGE, 51
SHEPHERD COLLEGE, 590
SIMON'S ROCK EARLY COLLEGE, 243
SOUTH PLAINS COLLEGE, 536
SOUTHERN MISSIONARY COLLEGE, 506
SOUTHWESTERN BAPTIST THEOLOGICAL SEMINARY, 538
STATE UNIVERSITY OF NEW YORK, ALBANY, 376
STEPHEN F AUSTIN STATE UNIVERSITY, 539
UNIVERSITY OF TAMPA, 103
TEMPLE UNIVERSITY, 475
TOWSON STATE UNIVERSITY, 225
TRINITY COLLEGE, 150
UNITED STATES INTERNATIONAL UNIVERSITY, 56
UNIVERSITY OF EVANSVILLE, 165
UNIVERSITY OF ILLINOIS, 151
WAKE FOREST UNIVERSITY, 404
WARREN WILSON COLLEGE, 404
WAYLAND BAPTIST COLLEGE, 550
WAYNE STATE COLLEGE, 321
WAYNE STATE UNIVERSITY, 267
WEATHERFORD COLLEGE, 550
UNIVERSITY OF WISCONSIN, MADISON, 603
UNIVERSITY OF WYOMING, 611

ALPHABETICAL INDEX

ALPHABETICAL INDEX

FRANKLIN COLLEGE, 156
FREE WILL BAPTIST COLLEGE, 501
FREED-HARDEMAN COLLEGE, 501
FRESNO CITY COLLEGE, 34
FRESNO PACIFIC COLLEGE, 35
FRIENDS UNIVERSITY, 186
FROSTBURG STATE COLLEGE, 220
FULLERTON COLLEGE, 35
FURMAN UNIVERSITY, 486
GADSDEN STATE JUNIOR COLLEGE, 1
GAINESVILLE JUNIOR COLLEGE, 109
GALLAUDET COLLEGE, 83
GARDEN CITY COMMUNITY COLLEGE, 187
GARDNER - WEBB COLLEGE, 392
GAVILAN COLLEGE, 36
GENESEE COMMUNITY COLLEGE, 359
GENEVA COLLEGE, 461
GEORGE FOX COLLEGE, 443
GEORGE PEABODY COLLEGE FOR TEACHERS, 501
GEORGE WASHINGTON UNIVERSITY, 83
GEORGETOWN UNIVERSITY, 83
GEORGIA COLLEGE, 110
GEORGIA SOUTHERN COLLEGE, 110
GEORGIA SOUTHWESTERN COLLEGE, 111
GEORGIA STATE UNIVERSITY, 111
UNIVERSITY OF GEORGIA, 111
GEORGIAN COURT COLLEGE, 333
GETTYSBURG COLLEGE, 462
GLASSBORO STATE COLLEGE, 333
GLEN OAKS COMMUNITY COLLEGE, 253
GLENDALE COMMUNITY COLLEGE, 9
GLENVILLE STATE COLLEGE, 588
GODDARD COLLEGE, 559
GOLDEN VALLEY LUTHERAN COLLEGE, 273
GOLDOVSKY OPERA INSTITUTE, 236
GONZAGA UNIVERSITY, 579
GOODMAN SCHOOL OF DRAMA., 131
GORDON COLLEGE, 236
GOSHEN COLLEGE, 156
GOUCHER COLLEGE, 221
GRACE COLLEGE, 156
GRACE COLLEGE OF THE BIBLE, 315
GRACELAND COLLEGE, 170
GRAHM JUNIOR COLLEGE, 237
GRAMBLING COLLEGE OF LOUISIANA, 207
GRAND CANYON COLLEGE, 9
GRAND RAPIDS BAPTIST COLLEGE, 253
GRAND RAPIDS JUNIOR COLLEGE, 253
GRAYSON COUNTY COLLEGE, 520
GREEN MOUNTAIN COLLEGE, 559
GREENBRIER COLLEGE, 588
GREENSBORO COLLEGE, 392
GREENVILLE COLLEGE, 131
GRINNELL COLLEGE, 170
GROSSMONT COLLEGE, 36
GROVE CITY COLLEGE, 462
GULF COAST COMMUNITY COLLEGE, 93
GULF PARK COLLEGE, 282
GUSTAVUS ADOLPHUS COLLEGE, 274
HAMILTON COLLEGE, 360
HAMLINE UNIVERSITY, 274
HAMPTON INSTITUTE, 565
HANNIBAL LA GRANGE COLLEGE, 294
HANOVER COLLEGE, 157
HARCUM JUNIOR COLLEGE, 462
HARDIN - SIMMONS UNIVERSITY, 520

HARDING COLLEGE, 15
HARLEM SCHOOL OF THE ARTS, INC, 360
HARRISBURG AREA COMMUNITY COLLEGE, 463
HARTFORD COLLEGE FOR WOMEN, 73
THE HARTFORD CONSERVATORY, 73
UNIVERSITY OF HARTFORD, 74
HARTNELL COLLEGE, 37
HARTWICK COLLEGE, 360
HARVARD UNIVERSITY, 237
HASTING COLLEGE, 315
HASTINGS TALENT EDUCATION CENTRE, INC, 361
HAVERFORD COLLEGE, 463
HAWAII LOA COLLEGE, 118
UNIVERSITY OF HAWAII, 118
UNIVERSITY OF HAWAII AT HILO - HILO COLLEGE, 119
HAWKEN SCHOOL, 417
HAZARD COMMUNITY COLLEGE, 200
HEBREW ARTS SCHOOL FOR MUSIC AND DANCE, 361
HEBREW UNION COLLEGE - JEWISH INSTITUTE OF RELIGION
    SCHOOL OF SACRED MUSIC, 361
HEDGEROW THEATRE SCHOOL, 463
HEIDELBURG COLLEGE, 418
HENDERSON COUNTY JUNIOR COLLEGE, 520
HENDRIX COLLEGE, 15
HENRY FORD COMMUNITY COLLEGE, 253
HERKIMER COUNTY COMMUNITY COLLEGE, 361
HESSTON COLLEGE, 187
HIGH POINT COLLEGE, 393
HIGH SCHOOL FOR THE PERFORMING AND VISUAL ARTS,
    521
HIGHLINE COMMUNITY COLLEGE, 580
HILL JUNIOR COLLEGE, 521
HILLSBOROUGH COMMUNITY COLLEGE, YBOR CAMPUS, 93
HILLSDALE COLLEGE, 254
HINDS JUNIOR COLLEGE, 283
HIRAM COLLEGE, 418
HIRAM SCOTT COLLEGE, 316
HOBART & WILLIAM SMITH COLLEGES, 362
HOFSTRA UNIVERSITY, 362
HOLLINS COLLEGE, 566
HOLMES JUNIOR COLLEGE, 283
HOLY CROSS COLLEGE, 237
HOLY FAMILY COLLEGE, 595
HOLYOKE COMMUNITY COLLEGE, 237
HOOD COLLEGE, 221
HOPE COLLEGE, 254
HOUGHTON COLLEGE, 362
HOUSTON BAPTIST UNIVERSITY, 522
UNIVERSITY OF HOUSTON, CENTRAL CAMPUS, 522
UNIVERSITY OF HOUSTON, DOWNTOWN COLLEGE, 523
HOWARD COLLEGE, BIG SPRING, 523
HOWARD PAYNE COLLEGE, 523
HOWARD UNIVERSITY, 83
HUDSON VALLEY COMMUNITY COLLEGE, 363
HUMBOLDT STATE UNIVERSITY, 37
HUNTER COLLEGE, CITY UNIVERSITY OF NEW YORK, 363
HUNTINGTON COLLEGE, 157
HURON COLLEGE, 492
HUSTON - TILLOTSON COLLEGE, 523
HUTCHINSON COMMUNITY COLLEGE, 187
IDAHO STATE UNIVERSITY, 120
THE COLLEGE OF IDAHO, 121
UNIVERSITY OF IDAHO, 121
ILLINOIS BENEDICTINE COLLEGE, 132
ILLINOIS CENTRAL COLLEGE, 132
ILLINOIS COLLEGE, 132

Alphabetical Index